THE MEDICAL DEPARTMENT: HOSPITALIZATION AND EVACUATION, ZONE OF INTERIOR

UNITED STATES ARMY IN WORLD WAR II

The Technical Services

THE MEDICAL DEPARTMENT: HOSPITALIZATION AND EVACUATION, ZONE OF INTERIOR

by

Clarence McKittrick Smith

CENTER OF MILITARY HISTORY

UNITED STATES ARMY

WASHINGTON, D.C., 1989

Library of Congress Catalog Card Number: 54-60005

First Printed 1956—CMH Pub 10-7

For sale by the Superintendent of Documents, U.S. Government Printing Office
Washington, DC 20402

UNITED STATES ARMY IN WORLD WAR II

Kent Roberts Greenfield, General Editor*

*General Editor of the Technical Service volumes, Lt. Col. Leo J. Meyer, Deputy Chief Historian.

. . . to Those Who Served

Foreword

Few Army activities are subject to closer scrutiny than those of protecting the health of the troops and binding up the wounds of those who have borne the battle. As in the matter of feeding and clothing, the general public has well-established civilian standards against which it can measure the efficiency of those responsible for the Army's medical service. When conducted with speed and professional competence this service is a source of comfort to both the man in uniform and his family and friends; when it fails to equal or excel the system of medical care to which American society is accustomed it is subject to immediate and strong protest from a people able and willing to criticize. The successful conduct of a military medical service therefore requires not only a knowledge of contemporary civilian medical practice but also administrative talent capable of adjusting the demands of the public and the medical profession to the Army's needs in time of war with the minimum of friction.

This is the first volume of a series which relates the hospitalization and evacuation experience of the Army in World War II. It should prove enlightening both to military men directly or indirectly concerned with the Army's medical service and to that large group of doctors and hospital administrators who daily face policy and management problems similar to those recounted here.

A. C. SMITH
Major General, USA
Chief, Military History

Washington, D. C.
25 June 1954

Introductory Note

The medical histories of the Civil War and the First World War which were published under the auspices of earlier Surgeons General contain lengthy descriptions of hospitalization and evacuation in rear areas. The present volume therefore continues the Army Medical Service's tradition of presenting a detailed account of these operations during a great war.

The contrasts between World War II and earlier wars in matters of hospitalization and evacuation are of course striking. The Army provided—at a maximum—more than twice as many hospital beds in the United States in World War II as it did in World War I, although curiously enough the number of beds in the zone of interior hospitals of World War I was very little larger than that in the Federal rear-area ("general") hospitals of the Civil War. The process of transporting and regulating the flow of patients to these hospitals in World War II differed in important respects from the methods used earlier. Yet despite these—and many other—changes, real elements of continuity existed. The convalescent hospitals and specialty centers, which became outstanding features of the World War II hospital system, existed on a smaller scale in World War I. The horse-drawn ambulance of the Civil War gave way to the motor ambulance of the two world wars, but hospital trains carried large numbers of patients in 1864 as in 1918 and 1945. Even the use of airplanes for transporting Army patients in the United States, an important factor in evacuation during World War II, had its small beginnings in World War I.

These observations are not meant to imply that the recent changes in hospitalization and evacuation outside the combat areas were less numerous or important than the features which remained essentially the same. They are merely a reminder that the full meaning of this volume can only be grasped if it is read with some knowledge of earlier events. Even without this background, however, readers who now or in the future are engaged in the work of hospitalization and evacuation should find much in the account to help them build on the achievements and avoid the pitfalls of the past. If the book serves that purpose, the work of the author and his assistants will be amply justified, as will the interest of the many officers and civilians who responded so freely when called upon for their personal knowledge of the events described.

The author of *Hospitalization and Evacuation, Zone of Interior,* Clarence McK. Smith, is a graduate of Newberry College, South Carolina, has an M.A. degree from Harvard, and except for a dissertation, has completed the requirements for a Ph.D. degree at Duke University. He taught history at Newberry College from 1940 until he entered the Army in World War II. During the war he served as an officer in the Medical Administrative Corps of the Army. From 1946 to 1954, he was a member of the Historical Division of the Office of The Surgeon General.

GEORGE E. ARMSTRONG
Major General, U.S. Army
The Surgeon General

Washington, D. C.
11 January 1955

Preface

This volume is one of several planned for a series on the history of the Medical Department of the United States Army during World War II. It deals primarily with the logistics of hospitalization and evacuation. As used here, therefore, the term "hospitalization" means all of the instrumentalities—buildings, equipment, supplies, and personnel—which directly served sick and wounded soldiers[1] in the attempt to restore them to physical fitness; and the term "evacuation" includes all of the means necessary to move patients from one place to another, whether from the battlefield to a hospital in the rear of combat zones, or from one hospital to another in the United States. The professional care of patients is not discussed in this volume; this subject will be treated fully in other studies being prepared by specialists in the various fields of medicine and surgery. Nor are details of the internal administration and operation of hospitals and evacuation units described here except to the extent necessary to explain the evolution of general policies and practices affecting the system of hospitalization and evacuation as a whole. Also, this volume confines itself almost entirely to events in the zone of interior (that is, the United States). This approach excludes any account of overseas hospitalization and evacuation operations, but not a discussion of the plans and preparations for them in the United States. Hospitalization and evacuation in theaters of operations will be covered elsewhere in this series. Treatment in this volume of the evacuation of patients from theaters to the United States might seem illogical unless the reader understands that the Army considered this operation a function of the zone of interior.

While hospitalization and evacuation are closely related, each is a complicated operation within itself. For simplicity and clarity they are treated in this volume as separate subjects, the first three parts dealing with hospitalization and the fourth with evacuation. Any account of hospitalization and evacuation involves some consideration of such elements as supplies and personnel. This volume therefore necessarily overlaps to some extent the subject matter of other volumes planned for this series. An effort has been made to keep such duplication to a minimum, with the result that some subjects may seem to have been slighted and others—such as the services of the Red Cross in hospitals—overlooked. Fuller information on these topics will be found in other volumes being written by the Army and by other agencies.

[1] A system of hospitalization and evacuation for army animals was also maintained by the Medical Department, but was of small dimensions and is not dealt with in this volume.

Though many agencies of the War Department were involved in the actions required to provide the Army with hospitalization and evacuation services—the War Department General Staff, especially its G–4 Division; the offices of The Surgeon General, the Air Surgeon, and the Ground Surgeon in Washington, and of surgeons of local commands elsewhere; the headquarters of the Army Ground, Air, and Service Forces; and the offices of chiefs of various technical services—emphasis has been placed in this volume on the work of The Surgeon General and his Office. While the history is not written with any conscious partiality for the viewpoint of The Surgeon General, it is written from his vantage point. There are several reasons for this approach. Most important is that The Surgeon General by tradition and directive is the chief health officer of the Army, and it is to him that the public looks when matters of health and medical care are concerned. A more practical reason is that the records of the Surgeon General's Office were more readily available than those of the offices of other surgeons. Finally, concentrating upon activities of the Surgeon General's Office is a very useful means of limiting the scope of this work and of giving it focus, without excluding consideration of actions affecting hospitalization and evacuation by agencies on higher, parallel, and lower levels of authority.

This volume is based almost entirely on records filed in various collections under the jurisdiction of the Department of the Army. With minor exceptions the author had free and unlimited access to them. Because of The Surgeon General's decision not to request "top secret" clearance for historians, the writer was not permitted to use the few files retaining that classification. This limitation is believed to have been of little consequence, because most of the once top-secret documents either had been given lower classifications or had been declassified altogether by the time they were needed. The author was also denied access to files of The Inspector General containing confidential complaints made to his representative during inspections of individual installations, but reports of more general inspections and investigations of hospitalization and evacuation by the chief medical officer on the staff of The Inspector General were made available. Compared with the records actually used, those to which access was denied are probably insignificant in quality as well as quantity. Publicity already given to the "tons of documents" through which one must search in the preparation of a volume of this kind makes it unnecessary to comment further on that subject.

Because of the nature of the source material for this volume, the form of its footnotes may appear unconventional to some readers. The following general observations will help in understanding them. Normally, a document is first identified by its type, file number (in some instances), sender, addressee, date, and subject. Its location is then given by indicating the collection of files and the specific folder in that collection in which it is found. The security classification of documents is not given.

Numerous technical terms have been used in this work, despite an earnest effort to avoid employing words and phrases in a manner understood by members of the military establishment but not by general readers. As a rule, technical terms and general terms given a special meaning by the Army are explained when they are first introduced in the text. Abbreviations have been used freely, especially in the footnotes. In most instances they are those authorized by the Army. Reference to a list of abbreviations at the end of the volume will help the reader interpret many of them.

The problem of how to designate Army officers whose ranks changed from time to time has been settled by giving the rank an officer held at the time of the action discussed. An effort also has been made to mention at some point in the work the highest rank an officer held during (but not after) the war.

A word of caution is in order about the statistical data in this volume. They were compiled from documents used in wartime operations, and further investigation by statisticians may eventually result in figures that are somewhat different. Nevertheless, it is believed that any variations will be inconsequential and will not diminish the historical significance of the data used here.

It is impossible to acknowledge in detail all of the help which the author received in the preparation of this work. Many acknowledgements will be found in footnotes throughout the volume. As for others, the author is especially indebted to Miss Zelma E. McIlvain and Mr. Hubert E. Potter for their assistance. Miss McIlvain did the major portion of research for Part Four and prepared preliminary drafts for much of Chapters XXII, XXIII and XXIV. Mr. Potter assisted in research for parts of Chapters XXII, XXIII, XXIV and XXV, and prepared preliminary drafts for certain portions of them. In addition, he assisted the writer immeasurably in obtaining important, hard-to-find documents.

The author is also indebted to the entire staff of the Historical Unit. Mrs. Josephine P. Kyle, Chief of its Archives and Research Branch, and her staff were indefatigable in searching for and locating not only large blocks of files but also individual documents requested by the writer. Typists of the Administrative Branch spent many weary hours making extracts from documents and typing drafts and final copies of chapters. Editorial clerks of this Branch prepared the tables in this volume and carefully checked and rechecked the manuscript before it was finally submitted for publication. My colleagues in the Historians Branch, and especially its chief, Dr. Donald O. Wagner, who supervised the preparation of this study, reviewed the manuscript and made many helpful suggestions for its improvement. The Armed Forces Institute of Pathology prepared the organization charts, under the supervision of Miss Sylvia Gottwerth, formerly of the Historical Unit. Finally, Col. Joseph H. McNinch, MC, Col. Roger G. Prentiss, Jr., MC, and Col. Calvin H. Goddard, MC—successive chiefs of the Historical Unit—gave the author and his assistants unflinching support, especially by their scholarly attitude toward the preparation of this volume.

A word of appreciation is also due to many persons outside the present Surgeon General's Office. Many officers who participated in events discussed in this volume—now retired or serving in other assignments—gave the author valuable help. Those interviewed usually spoke freely and frankly of their experiences. Others made excellent critical comments on drafts of chapters submitted to them for review. The information which they thus furnished was especially helpful in filling in the background of important documents and events. The names of many appear in footnotes throughout the volume, but two deserve special mention here—the wartime Surgeons General, Maj. Gen. James C. Magee and Maj. Gen. Norman T. Kirk. The author is also grateful for criticisms and editorial assistance from Col. Leo J. Meyer, Deputy Chief Historian, Office of the Chief of Military History, and from members of the Editorial Branch of the same Office.

Washington, D. C.
10 March 1953

CLARENCE McK. SMITH

Contents

PART ONE

Hospitalization during the Emergency Period, 8 September 1939—7 December 1941

PART TWO

Hospitalization in the Early War Years, 7 December 1941—Mid-1943

PART THREE

Hospitalization in the Later War Years, Mid–1943—1946

PART FOUR

Evacuation to and in the Zone of Interior

Tables

Charts

Illustrations

All illustrations are from the files of the Department of Defense except those on pp. 386, 387 which were obtained from American Car and Foundry Co.

PART ONE

HOSPITALIZATION DURING THE EMERGENCY PERIOD 8 SEPTEMBER 1939—7 DECEMBER 1941

Introduction

The State of Army Hospitalization, 1939

When President Roosevelt proclaimed a "limited national emergency" on 8 September 1939, just one week after Germany invaded Poland, the Medical Department of the United States Army was operating 7 general hospitals and 119 station hospitals. Five of the general hospitals were located in the United States—Walter Reed at Washington, D. C.; Army and Navy at Hot Springs, Ark.; Fitzsimons at Denver, Colo.; Letterman at San Francisco, Calif.; and William Beaumont at El Paso, Tex. The other two were in overseas possessions—Tripler in the Hawaiian Islands and Sternberg in the Philippines. Of the station hospitals 104 were on Army posts in the United States and Alaska, while the remainder were divided among the Philippine Islands, the Hawaiian Islands, and the Panama Canal Zone. Each station hospital was designated by the name of the post on which it was located and each general hospital, except one, was named for a deceased medical officer. Hence, station and general hospitals in the United States in both peace and war, as well as those in overseas possessions in peacetime, were called "named hospitals."

Station hospitals and general hospitals had different functions. The former served local and ordinary needs, usually receiving patients from stations where located and treating those with minor ills and injuries only. General hospitals, on the other hand, were designed to serve general and special needs. By transfer from station hospitals they received patients who suffered from severe or obscure diseases as well as those who needed complicated surgery.

Capacities of named hospitals depended largely upon troop populations served. Other factors also influenced their capacities, such as climate, prevalence of disease, general physical condition of troops, and types of activities in which the latter were engaged. Hospital capacities and hospital requirements were expressed in terms of beds, which in the Army meant not only beds themselves but also shelter, equipment, utilities, and personnel that went with them. For an Army strength of 135,749 in the United States and Alaska in June 1939 there were 4,136 general hospital beds and 8,234 station hospital beds. This represented a bed ratio to strength of approximately 3 percent for general hospitals and 6 percent for station hospitals. For a strength of 10,993 in the Philippines there were 317 general hospital beds and 360 station hospital beds. In the Hawaiian Islands, the most healthful of overseas possessions, there were 350 general hospital beds and 360 station hospital beds for a strength of 20,601. The Panama Canal Zone, with next to the highest sick rate in the Army, had only 269 station hospital beds for a strength of 13,533, a ratio of 1.98 percent. This unusual situation resulted from the fact that civilian Canal Zone hospitals—Gorgas, Colon, and Corozal—staffed with Army Medical Corps officers but under the control of the Governor of the Canal Zone, cared for a considerable portion of the Army's patients in that area.[1]

The Surgeon General believed that the Army's hospitals were inadequate, even for peacetime needs. He had begun a long-range program in 1934 to improve and expand them but funds appropriated by Congress for Medical Department construction had been sufficient for little more than essential maintenance of existing buildings. As a result, the Army's hospitals in 1939 were poorly suited to any increase in its strength. In Panama only fifty beds were located in a hospital building. The remainder were crowded into buildings erected for other purposes. Hospital plants in the Hawaiian and Philippine Islands needed repairs and alterations. In the United States hospital buildings were small and widely scattered among a number of permanent Army posts. Erected twenty-five to thirty years before, many lacked facilities for the separation of patients according to grade, sex, and disease, and for such modern diagnostic and treatment procedures as basal metabolism, X-ray, and oxygen and physical therapy. Of the entire number, The Surgeon General considered only twenty-five as modern, fire-resistant buildings and only fifty of the remainder as worth modernization. The others, he believed, should be replaced with new buildings.[2]

For the care of patients in theaters of operations in wartime the Medical Department had a doctrine of hospitalization and evacuation that dated from the Civil War and had been successfully applied during both the Spanish-American War and World War I. Casualties were given emergency treatment at a series of medical stations established in the forward areas of combat zones. To provide such treatment as well as the transportation of patients, when necessary, from one station to another farther to the rear, every regiment and separate battalion of all arms and services, except medical, had a medical detachment, and every division had a medical regiment, medical battalion, or medical squadron. To furnish as near the front as possible a higher type of treatment than first aid or emergency medical care, hospitals designed for easy movement and hence called "mobile hospitals" were assigned to field armies. They were of three types: surgical hospitals, evacuation hospitals, and convalescent hospitals. Surgical hospitals were planned for use in either division or army areas of combat zones. In division areas they were to carry out emergency procedures, such as treatment of shock, control of stubborn hemorrhage, reconstitution of blood following hemorrhage, and fixation of complex fractures, in order to prepare men with serious injuries for further removal to the rear. In army areas they performed much the same function as evacuation hospitals. Evacuation hospitals normally served only in the rear areas of combat zones. They provided definitive treatment for evacuees from forward areas and for the sick and

[1] *Annual Report of The Surgeon General, U.S. Army, 1939* (Washington, 1940), pp. 170, 250; *1940* (Washington, 1941), p. 1 (cited hereafter as *Annual Report . . . Surgeon General*). Only Puerto Rico, with a mean annual strength of 1,312, had a slightly higher admission rate than Panama. Puerto Rico had no Army hospital in the middle of 1939.

[2] (1) *Annual Report . . . Surgeon General, 1937* (1937), pp. 167–68; *1939* (1940), p. 253; *1940* (1941), p. 265. (2) *Hearings before the Subcommittee of the Committee on Appropriations, House of Representatives, 76th Cong, 1st session* [H. R. 6791] *Supplemental Military Appropriation Bill for 1940* (Washington, 1939), pp. 157–58. (3) Statement of MD Activities by Maj Gen James C. Magee, SG, USA, for the Subcmtee of the House Cmtee on Mil Approps (1939). HD: 321.6–1. (4) Preliminary Estimates, QMC, FY 1941 (25 May 39). Off file, Hosp Cons Div, SGO. (5) An Rpts, CA Surgs. SG: 319.1–2. (6) C. M. Walson, "Observations at Army Hospitals," *Army Medical Bulletin,* No. 42 (1937), pp. 65–72.

injured of surrounding areas. They returned some patients to duty after short periods of treatment, transferred others with prospect of early recovery to convalescent hospitals, and prepared still others for transportation to general hospitals for continuation of treatment. Convalescent hospitals were not staffed and equipped to perform major surgery. Their chief function was to restore to physical fitness patients received from evacuation hospitals, to treat cases of venereal disease, and to care for patients from units located near by.

For service in communications zones there were station and general hospitals. The latter received patients not only from station hospitals but mainly from evacuation and surgical hospitals. They returned some to duty in theaters of operations and transferred others for further treatment to general hospitals in the zone of interior. Since it was expected that hospitals in communications zones would rarely need to be moved, station and general hospitals were called "fixed hospitals." When several were grouped in one location they might be combined into a hospital center with a 1,000-bed convalescent camp. All hospitals in theaters of operations, whether fixed or mobile, were designated by numbers rather than by names and locations, and hence were called "numbered hospitals." [3]

Unlike named hospitals in the United States, numbered hospitals had standard capacities, staffs, and equipment that were established by tables of organization, tables of basic allowances, and equipment lists. Tables of organization for hospitals showed the capacities of installations which different units were designed to operate. While tables of basic allowances listed equipment authorized for units and their members, they did not itemize such articles as drugs and biologicals, surgical gauzes, surgical instruments, dental supplies and equipment, laboratory supplies and equipment, X-ray supplies and equipment, and operating-room equipment. These were included under one heading as an "assemblage." Items for hospital assemblages were listed individually and by amounts in Medical Department equipment lists.

For use in theaters of operations in June 1939 the Medical Department had little more than doctrine. Only five Medical Department field units were in existence—four medical regiments (two of which were overseas) and one medical squadron. According to The Surgeon General, failure to have other units in training resulted from a shortage of Medical Department enlisted men. Congress limited their number to 5 percent of the strength of the Army, and use of more than 4 percent in named hospitals and other peacetime installations left few for field units. Early in 1939 The Surgeon General had sought an increase in the Medical Department's allowance of enlisted men, but without success.[4]

To provide officers for wartime hospitals—physicians, dentists, and nurses—The Surgeon General had proposed in March 1939 the revival of "affiliated units." These were reserve units sponsored by civilian hospitals and medical schools. Such units had been organized by the American Red Cross during World War I and had contributed substantially to Army hospital service in France. "I am convinced," wrote Surgeon General Charles R. Reynolds, "that the Medical Department can have reserve hospital

[3] AR 40-580, MD, Hosps—Gen Provisions, 29 Jun 29.

[4] (1) Cmtee to Study the MD, 1942, Testimony of Col Albert G. Love, p. 2. HD. (2) *Annual Report . . . Surgeon General, 1939* (1940), pp. 179-82.

units ready to function as required . . . only by civil institutions sponsoring these units, especially those needed within the early periods of mobilization. . . ."[5] In August 1939 the Secretary of War approved in principle The Surgeon General's plan to organize affiliated units to staff 32 general, 17 evacuation, and 13 surgical hospitals. Full approval was given several months later.[6]

The only reserve equipment which the Medical Department had on hand was that stored after World War I. It was "of 1918 vintage, incomplete in modern operating-room equipment, wholly deficient in essential laboratory equipment, totally lacking in X-ray, physical therapy and hydrotherapy equipment, and stocked with scientific items now obsolete and rapidly becoming obsolescent."[7] Moreover, with few exceptions, tables of organization and tables of basic allowances for field medical units, including hospitals, had not been changed since 1929, and the preparation of new equipment lists for them had just been begun in January 1939.[8] To prepare for war the Medical Department had to start almost from scratch.

Effect of the War in Europe

The period of the emergency in the United States was for the Medical Department a time of partial preparation for war through the provision of the hospitalization actually required for an expanding Army. Its steps in this direction were sometimes painful and often halting. Several factors accounted for this. Formal mobilization planning of the Medical Department, like that of the rest of the Army, was based upon a belief that the anticipated force of 1,000,000 to 1,200,000 men would be called up only if the United States or its possessions were attacked. It was therefore essentially defensive in nature. Moreover, there was uncertainty about the nature of increases of the Army—whether rises in the authorized strength of the Regular Army were temporary or permanent and whether or not the mobilization that finally occurred was for a year of training only, as it purported to be. Furthermore, funds which the General Staff could secure for the entire Army, let alone the Medical Department, were limited by the caution of the President and the sentiment of Congress. Finally, The Surgeon General and his associates, like many others in the Army and the Government at large, found it difficult to break peacetime habits of thought and action in order to plan imaginatively for a second World War.[9]

---

[5] (1) Ltr, SG to TAG, 17 Mar 39, sub: Affiliation of MD Units with Civ Insts. HD: 326.01-1 (Affiliated Units). (2) *The Medical Department of the United States Army in the World War* (Washington, 1923), vol. I, p. 102 (cited hereafter as *The Medical Department . . . in the World War*).

[6] (1) Cmtee to Study the MD, 1942, Testimony, pp. 8–10. HD. (2) *Annual Report . . . Surgeon General, 1940* (1941). pp. 177–78. (3) For a full discussion of the revival of affiliated units see John H. McMinn and Max Levin, Personnel (manuscript for a companion volume in this series). HD.

[7] Ltr, SG to TAG, 6 Apr 40, sub: Status of MD for War. AG: 381 (4–6–40) (1).

[8] (1) Tables of organization and tables of basic allowances that were available in June 1939 are on file in HD. (2) Incl 2, Ltr, Brig Gen Harry D. Offutt to Col H. W. Doan, 10 Jun 48. HD: 322. (3) Interv, MD Historians with Gen Offutt, 10 Nov 49. HD: 000.71.

[9] Mark S. Watson, *Chief of Staff: Prewar Plans and Preparations* (Washington, 1950), pp. 15–56, 126–71, in UNITED STATES ARMY IN WORLD WAR II, discusses plans and preparations of the General Staff, along with limiting factors and influences, in considerable detail. Robert E. Sherwood, *Roosevelt and Hopkins: An Intimate History* (New York, 1950), pp. 157–62, discusses the difficulty Government Departments displayed in adjusting to planning for a global war.

The war in Europe had almost immediate effects upon the Army and the Medical Department. In September 1939 the authorized enlisted strength of the Regular Army was increased from 210,000 to 227,000. The next spring, as the Nazi war machine rolled toward the English Channel, it was again raised—to 280,000 in May and to 375,000 in June. Then, in the latter part of 1940, after the fall of France, Congress approved a peacetime mobilization. From September of that year until December 1941, the Army's strength grew from 438,254 officers and enlisted men to 1,686,403. The Medical Department had to expand its operations accordingly. This involved mainly building up facilities in the United States, where 85 to 90 percent of the troops were stationed, but hospitals in overseas possessions also had to be expanded and additional ones provided for new Atlantic defense bases. While a regular system of field hospitalization and evacuation was as yet unnecessary, medical units had to be organized and prepared for such service.[10]

The expansion of hospital facilities in the United States involved many considerations. Decisions had to be made as to the types of housing to be used and the number of beds that would be needed. Means had to be found for providing suitable hospital plants in as short a time as possible. New hospitals had to be manned and the staffs of old ones augmented. "Green" officers had to organize hospitals and establish procedures for their administration. Supplies and equipment had to be placed in hospital plants at appropriate times. Finally, it was necessary to develop procedures for the operation of the greatly expanded hospital system.

The preparation of hospital units for field service sometimes conflicted with these activities, for such units also demanded personnel and equipment. The amount they should be given while in training was a moot question. The number of such units to be activated had to be determined. After they were organized they needed to be trained. Before most of these steps could be taken, tables and lists governing their organization, manning, and equipment had to be revised and modernized.

The challenge of an expanding Regular Army and a peacetime mobilization affected only slightly the organizational structure of the Army for hospitalization. Yet this structure and its changes must be understood before the actions of various agencies in providing hospitalization are discussed.

[10] *Biennial Report of the Chief of Staff of the United States Army, July 1, 1939 to June 30, 1941, to the Secretary of War* (Washington, 1941) (cited hereafter as *Biennial Report . . . Chief of Staff, 1939-41*). Figures on strength of the Army were supplied by the Strength Accounting Branch, AGO.

CHAPTER I

Organization and Responsibilities for Hospitalization

Hospitalization, like other activities of the Medical Department, was planned and supervised by medical officers called surgeons. The commander of every non-medical military organization, from headquarters of the Army in Washington (War Department) to battalions in the field, had on his staff a surgeon whose duties were both advisory and administrative. As a staff officer he advised on matters affecting the health of all members of a command and exercised technical control (that is, professional and medical as opposed to administrative and military) over all medical activities under the jurisdiction of his commander. As an administrative officer he also exercised command control over his own office and in some instances over certain medical units and organizations such as hospitals.[1]

The Surgeon General's Position in the War Department

The chief medical officer of the Army was The Surgeon General.[2] He served as medical adviser to the Chief of Staff and was directly responsible to him for the planning and technical supervision of all Army hospitals. In his capacity as head of a service he commanded, beside the personnel in his own Office, medical "field installations" of the War Department. Like the chiefs of other arms and services, such as the Chief of Infantry, the Chief of the Air Corps, and The Quartermaster General, The Surgeon General was subject to supervision by the War Department General Staff.

The General Staff, while it had no authority to command, in actual practice did so, issuing directives and orders and approving or disapproving recommendations of The Surgeon General. In such instances it acted in the name of the Chief of Staff or the Secretary of War. The Staff had five divisions, each of which repre-

[1] (1) AR 40–10, MD, The MC—Gen Provisions, 6 Jun 24. (2) Blanche B. Armfield, Organization and Administration (manuscript for a companion volume in this series), has a full discussion of the organization of the Medical Department.

[2] The War Department capitalized the definite article in the formal designations of certain general officers, presumably to distinguish them from others with similar titles.

sented a functional grouping of duties of the Chief of Staff. They were the Personnel (G–1), Military Intelligence (G–2), Organization and Training (G–3), Supply (G–4), and War Plans (WPD) Divisions. The Supply Division was charged by Army regulations with the preparation of plans and policies for hospitalization and evacuation and the supervision of such activities. In peacetime it limited itself in this field primarily to matters of construction and supply. The Personnel Division handled matters pertaining to personnel that were Army-wide in scope; the Organization and Training Division, those relating to the organization, training, and use of field units. Direct communication between divisions of the General Staff and any chief of service (such as The Surgeon General) was authorized by Army regulations, but formal requests and decisions were normally channeled through the Office of The Adjutant General, the War Department's office of record.[3]

In the latter part of 1940, after mobilization began, medical officers were assigned to several War Department agencies having a direct interest in hospitalization and evacuation. In October 1940 Brig. Gen. (later Maj. Gen.) Howard McC. Snyder was assigned to the Office of The Inspector General and remained in that position until the end of the war. Shortly afterward a medical officer was transferred from the Surgeon General's Office to General Headquarters (GHQ), an organization established in July 1940 to supervise the training of field forces, including medical units. About the same time Lt. Col. (later Brig. Gen.) Frederick A. Blesse was placed in the G–4 division of the General Staff. During 1941 he was transferred to GHQ and was succeeded in G–4 by Maj. (later Col.) William L. Wilson.[4]

The Surgeon General's Office

When President Roosevelt proclaimed the emergency, The Surgeon General was Maj. Gen. James C. Magee. He had succeeded Maj. Gen. Charles R. Reynolds the preceding June. Most divisions of his Office had something to do with hospitalization and evacuation. Particularly concerned was the Planning and Training Division, headed by Col. (later Brig. Gen.) Albert G. Love. It had three subdivisions: Planning, Training, and Hospital Construction and Repair. The last of these operated almost independently, its chief, Lt. Col. (later Col.) John R. Hall, having direct access to General Magee.[5] This subdivision handled all of The Surgeon General's construction problems, estimating bed requirements and planning hospitals. In this work it collaborated with the War Department's constructing agencies—the Quartermaster Corps and the Corps of Engineers. This subdivision grew from 2 officers, 3 civilian architects, and 4 clerks in September 1940 to 4 officers, 4 architects, and 7 clerks by the end of 1941.[6] The remainder of the Planning and Training Division dealt with medical field units. It

[3] (1) Mark S. Watson, *Chief of Staff: Prewar Plans and Preparations* (Washington, 1950), pp. 57–84, in UNITED STATES ARMY IN WORLD WAR II, has an excellent discussion of the origin and powers of the General Staff. (2) AR 10–15, Gen Staff, Orgn and Gen Duties, 18 Aug 36. (3) FM 101–5, Staff Officers' Field Manual, 19 Aug 40.

[4] (1) Armfield, *op. cit.* (2) Kent R. Greenfield, Robert R. Palmer and Bell I. Wiley, *The Organization of Ground Combat Troops* (Washington, 1947), pp. 1–32, in UNITED STATES ARMY IN WORLD WAR II, have a discussion of the development of GHQ.

[5] Interv, MD Historian with Col Love, 27 Aug 47. HD: 000.71.

[6] Achilles L. Tynes, Data for Preparation of Historical Record of Construction Branch of The Surgeon General's Office during the Expansion Period of the Army and World War II (1945) (cited hereafter as Tynes, Construction Branch). HD.

estimated the number that would be required and prepared or revised their tables of organization and equipment. Until GHQ was established in July 1940, this Division also supervised the training and use in the United States of hospital and other medical units. The Finance and Supply Division furnished hospitals with supplies and equipment and allotted them funds for the employment of civilians. The Military Personnel, Dental, Veterinary, and Nursing Divisions handled military personnel and certain professional matters. The Professional Service Division established policies for medical care and treatment and issued technical directives to maintain professional standards.[7]

In recognition of the growing importance of problems of hospitalization during mobilization, a Hospitalization Subdivision was set up in the Professional Service Division in February 1941. Two months later it was separated and became the Hospitalization Division. Lt. Col. (later Col.) Harry D. Offutt was made its chief and continued in that capacity throughout General Magee's administration. Established with one officer and one clerk, this division expanded to three officers and three clerks by the end of June 1941. Although it was charged with the development of plans and policies for hospitalization and evacuation through liaison with other divisions of the Surgeon General's Office, it had neither the authority nor the staff to make comprehensive plans and coordinate the actions of others in making such plans effective.[8]

The Surgeon General's Control Over Hospitals and Hospital Units

While all hospitals were under the technical supervision of The Surgeon General, not all were subject to the same control by his Office. The degree varied according to the command structure of the War Department. For administrative purposes the United States was divided into nine corps areas, each in charge of a corps area commander under the jurisdiction of the Chief of Staff. Overseas possessions were organized into three departments that corresponded administratively to corps areas in the United States. All stations in departments and most in corps areas were under the command-control of department and corps area commanders respectively. Located within corps areas but beyond the jurisdiction of their commanders were field installations of the War Department. They operated directly under the chiefs of various arms and services in Washington and were therefore called "exempted stations."

Hospitals classified as War Department field installations were subject to the greatest amount of control by The Surgeon General because they were under his command. All general hospitals in the United States were in this category. In only one instance was an intermediate commander between The Surgeon General and a general hospital commander. Walter Reed General Hospital was under the jurisdiction of the commandant of the Army Medical Center (Washington, D. C.), who was in turn under the command of The Sur-

[7] Armfield, *op. cit.*

[8] SG OOs 32, 13 Feb 41; 87, 18 Apr 41. In an interview on 15 November 1949 Brig Gen H. D. Offutt stated that he never felt handicapped by a lack of personnel in his division. HD: 000.71. In an interview on 10 November 1950 Maj Gen James C. Magee (Ret) stated that no one division could have exercised authority over all factors involved in hospitalization and that vesting such authority in one division would have subordinated other divisions of the Surgeon General's Office to a sort of overlordship. HD: 314 (Correspondence on MS) III.

geon General. Despite this intermediate step, Walter Reed actually received closer supervision from the Surgeon General's Office than did other general hospitals, largely because of its proximity. Next in line in degree of control were hospitals of exempted stations of all other services and of all arms except the Air Corps. For example Fort Benning (Georgia), including its station hospital, was under the Chief of Infantry and Fort Belvoir (Virginia) was under the Chief of Engineers. The chiefs of arms and services normally had no surgeons on their staffs and were therefore prone to refer problems connected with hospitalization to The Surgeon General. He employed corps area surgeons as his own field representatives to supervise hospitals of exempted stations. Corps area hospitals, under the command-control of corps area commanders, were supervised by corps area surgeons in their dual capacities as local staff officers and technical representatives of The Surgeon General. Hospitals furthest removed from the latter's influence were those in overseas departments, not only because of their distance from Washington but also because department surgeons did not serve as field representatives of The Surgeon General.[9]

Although hospitals of the Air Corps were theoretically in the same class as those of exempted stations of other arms and services, they were actually in a somewhat different category. The Chief of the Air Corps had in his Office a Medical Division, whose head was analogous to a staff surgeon and therefore assumed considerable authority over Air Corps station hospitals. During 1940 and 1941, as the Air Corps expanded, the number of such hospitals increased. Soon after a reorganization of the air forces in June 1941, which established the Army Air Forces and gave it control over the Air Corps, the Secretary of War directed a blanket exemption of all Air Corps stations—new as well as old—from corps area control. The following October the head of the Air Corps Medical Division, Col. (later Maj. Gen.) David N. W. Grant, was assigned to AAF headquarters and designated "Air Surgeon." This series of events tended to separate Air Corps hospitals from other Army hospitals and to place them more under control of AAF headquarters at the expense of the Surgeon General's Office.[10]

A shift of responsibility which affected The Surgeon General's control over medical units, including those for numbered hospitals, had meanwhile occurred. Until late 1940 certain corps area commanders and surgeons acted also as commanders and surgeons of the four field armies in the United States. Corps area surgeons were therefore responsible, under their commanders and The Surgeon General, for supervising the training of field medical units. In October 1940, the command of field armies was taken away from corps area commanders and placed in the hands of separate army commanders responsible to GHQ in Washington. GHQ and army headquarters were charged with the training and use on maneuvers of all field units. Actually, this transfer of training functions was not so complete as anticipated,[11] even though in November 1940 all table-of-

[9] (1) AR 170–10, CAs and Depts, Admin, 10 Oct 39. (2) AR 350–105, Mil Educ, Gen and Spec Serv Schs—Desig, Loc, and Orgn, 1 Oct 38. (3) Armfield, *op. cit.*

[10] (1) Rad MX–F, TAG to CGs of CAs, 27 Jun 41. (2) Ltr, TAG to CofAAF and ACofS G–4 WDGS, 12 Sep 41, sub: Trf of Gen Staff Functions . . . to AAF. Both in AG: 322.2 (6–18–41)(1) Sec 2. (3) Hubert A. Coleman, Organization and Administration, AAF Medical Services in the Zone of Interior (1948), pp. 45–76. HD.

[11] See below, pp. 43–48.

organization units in the United States, including those of the Medical Department, were either assigned or attached to armies or corps.[12]

In the changes just enumerated were seeds that were eventually to grow into bitter weeds for The Surgeon General. Among them were the trend of the Army Air Forces toward separatism and its development of a separate set of hospitals, the establishment of medical officers in headquarters on a higher level of authority than The Surgeon General, and the latter's partial loss of authority over medical field units. Understanding something of these changes and of responsibilities and relationships of various War Department agencies, one may now turn to a consideration of the manner in which the Army provided hospitalization during the emergency period.

[12] (1) Greenfield *et al.*, *op. cit.*, pp. 3-4, 6-9. (2) Armfield, *op. cit.* (3) Ltr, TAG to CGs all Armies, Army Corps, CAs, CofS GHQ, etc., 4 Nov 40, sub: Units Asgd and Atchd to GHQ, Armies, and Corps. . . . AG: 320.2 (8-2-40)(4) Sec 3.

CHAPTER II

Planning for and Expanding Hospitals in the United States

Hospital Construction

Early Basic Decisions

Any large-scale expansion of "hospital facilities"—that is, wards, offices, and clinics normally found in civilian hospitals, plus housing for commissioned and enlisted personnel, storage for medical and military supplies and equipment, and administrative space for nonmedical military activities—demanded a simple method of estimating requirements and authorizing beds. Such expansion also demanded that additional housing be provided as rapidly and inexpensively as possible.

The method prescribed by mobilization regulations for estimating bed requirements was one that Colonel Love had devised from World War I experience. It involved computation of the number of beds needed for successive 15-day periods of mobilization on the basis of average daily admission rates, the rate of accumulation of patients in hospitals by 15-day periods, and increases and decreases in troop strengths during these periods. When hospitals were expanded for the September 1939 increase in the Army, this method proved too complicated for general use and The Surgeon General included in his Protective Mobilization Plan of December 1939 a simpler one, also devised by Colonel Love—the multiplication of troop strength by a predetermined percentage of beds. In August 1940 G–4 adopted the latter, and its simplicity made its ready acceptance by all agencies of the War Department a foregone conclusion.[1]

Opinion differed on the proper percentage to use in estimating and authorizing station hospital beds. The Surgeon General used 4 percent in calculating requirements in the fall of 1939, and G–4 began to use this figure in planning for mobilization in August 1940. Experience of the previous winter made some surgeons believe it provided insufficient beds for "green troops,"[2] and on 6 September 1940 General Magee asked the General Staff to consider 5 percent as the probable

[1] (1) Albert G. Love, "War Casualties," *Army Medical Bulletin*, No. 24 (1931), pp. 18, 37, 38, 68. (2) MR 4–3, 2 Apr 34; MR 4–2, 13 Feb 40; and SG PMP, 1939, Annex No 29. (3) Ltr AG 600.12 (8–6–40)M–D–M, TAG to C of Arms and Servs, CGs of CAs, and COs of Exempted Stas, 7 Aug 40, sub: Supp No 2 to WD Cons Policy. SG: 600.12–1.

[2] (1) Synopsis Ltr, Surg 4th CA to Surg Ft McClellan, 13 Aug 40, sub: Expansion of Hosp Fac, and 8 inds. SG: 632.–1 (Ft McClellan)N. (2) Ltr, Surg 7th CA to SG, 10 Sep 40, sub: Hosp . . . NG. SG: 632.–1 (7th CA)AA.

requirement for station hospital beds.[3] G-4's Construction Branch verbally approved this ratio, but the Assistant Chief of Staff, G-4, Brig. Gen. Richard C. Moore, later reversed this action, authorizing station hospital beds for only 4 percent of the strength served but permitting provisions for expansion to 5 percent if necessary.[4] This meant in the case of new hospitals that wards would be constructed with space for beds for 4 percent of a command but that utilities, administrative buildings, and clinical facilities would be constructed to serve a hospital with beds for 5 percent. Thus additional wards could be erected later without overloading the "chassis" of a hospital. The ratio of beds in general hospitals to the total strength of the Army—1 percent—received official sanction at the same time. General Magee did not protest the decision as to station hospitals but observed a policy during the following year of supporting local requests or initiating action for increases in bed ratios in specific instances.[5]

The manner of providing additional housing was a subject on which The Surgeon General and the General Staff eventually came to marked disagreement. Based on a belief that unnecessary construction should be avoided and a fear that sudden attack would require mobilization before requisite construction could be completed, War Department policy in 1939 was to use existing housing to the maximum extent possible.[6] Mobilization regulations therefore called for the use of existing Army hospitals, with emergency expansions, for the initial beds required. To house additional beds other buildings would be used in the following order: (1) Federal hospitals, (2) civilian hospitals, (3) vacated Army posts, and (4) public and private buildings such as schools and hotels. Finally, as a last resort, new station and general hospitals would be constructed.[7]

For all new buildings the War Department planned to use one-story frame construction, called "cantonment-type." It required The Quartermaster General to keep on file standard plans for such buildings.[8] Those for hospitals had been prepared in 1935 in collaboration with The Surgeon General's Hospital Construction and Repair Subdivision. They consisted of forty-nine drawings: forty-five for administrative offices, clinics, wards, messes, quarters for personnel, and service buildings, and four for twenty different combinations of these buildings to make hospitals ranging in size from 25 to 2,000 beds. Most of the buildings were of a standard size. To reduce the danger of fire, all were separated by a minimum of fifty feet. For each group of not more than five, this space was increased to 100 feet. Each hospital therefore covered a large area, a 500-bed installation spreading over twenty acres. Advantages of this hospital were its relatively low cost, the rapidity with which it could be erected, and the small number

[3] Ltr, SG (Magee) to TAG, 6 Sep 40, sub: MD in Mob. AG: 381 (1-1-40) Sec 3.

[4] (1) Memo, SG for ACofS G-4 WDGS, 10 Sep 40. (2) D/S, ACofS G-4 WDGS to SG, 13 Sep 40, sub: Hosp . . . Mob. . . . (3) Memo, Cons Br G-4 WDGS for Maj Gen [Eugene] Reybold, 7 Mar 41, sub: Four Percent Hosp. All in HRS: G-4/29135-12.

[5] (1) Synopsis Ltr, CG Ft Jackson to TAG, 11 Dec 40, sub: Cons Sta Hosp, and 4 inds. SG: 632.-1 (Ft Jackson)N. (2) 5th ind, Surg Ft Sill to CG 8th CA, 12 Mar 41, on cy Ltr, CG Ft Sill to TAG, 10 Dec 40, sub: Add Hosp, Ft Sill. SG: 632.-1 (Ft Sill)N. (3) Ltr SG to TAG, 27 May 41, sub: Add Hosp Fac. . . . SG: 632.-1. (4) Ltr, CG 4th CA to TAG, 1 May 41, sub: Add Hosp Bed Reqmts, and 11 inds. SG: 632.-1 (4th CA)AA.

[6] The War Department Mobilization Plan, speech by Lt Col Harry L. Twaddle, GSC, Chief Mob Br G-3 Div WDGS, 30 Sep 39. G-3 Course No 13 and 13A, AWC, 1939-40.

[7] MR 4-3, 2 Apr 34; MR 4-3, C-1, 31 Dec 34; and MR 4-2, 13 Feb 40.

[8] MR 4-1, Sup; Cons; Trans, 5 Jan 40.

of highly skilled workmen needed to construct it. Its most obvious disadvantages were the danger of fire and the administrative difficulties caused by the wide area covered.[9]

The hospital construction policy enunciated in mobilization regulations was not made the official guide for the provision of hospitals for Regular Army expansions in 1939 and 1940, but certain aspects of it were followed. Thus, although apparently no attempt was made to use non-Army buildings, existing Army hospitals were expanded and new construction was authorized only at stations not served by such. For example, essential units of a 350-bed cantonment-type hospital—a mess hall, a clinical building, and several wards—were constructed at Camp Jackson (South Carolina), a National Guard encampment. Regular Army posts which already possessed hospitals, such as Fort McClellan (Alabama) and Fort Benning (Georgia), expanded them by converting hospital porches, barracks, and other available buildings into hospital wards.[10] In such instances results were unsatisfactory. At Fort Benning, for example, the surgeon had to enlarge a 230-bed hospital, built for a garrison of 4,000, to serve a strength of 19,000 in January 1940. He did this by adding 334 beds in porches, barracks, and a portable wooden building. The operating rooms, clinics, laboratory, and mess halls of the permanent hospital were then too small for the greater bed capacity. Thus there was created, he explained, "a relative giant with inadequate heart and internal viscera."[11]

Despite this experience, in the spring of 1940 G–4 planned to establish the practice of expanding existing hospitals as official policy for subsequent increases in the Regular Army. Both The Surgeon General and The Quartermaster General opposed this move. Among the many objections they raised, probably the most important from the medical viewpoint was the one just noted—limits upon expansion of bed capacity imposed by the size of operating rooms and clinical facilities. Of equal importance, from the construction viewpoint, was the unsuitability of many barracks for hospital use because of their location or structural characteristics. Moreover, it was improbable that their conversion and eventual reconversion would be cheaper in the long run than the erection of cantonment-type hospitals. On 24 May 1940, therefore, Colonel Love, Acting The Surgeon General, recommended that all additional beds should be housed in new cantonment-type hospitals. G–4 disapproved this recommendation, perhaps because of shortages of funds and uncertainty about the nature of increases in the Regular Army, and on 7 June 1940 issued an official "Policy for Hospitalization during the Emergency." It authorized cantonment-type hospitals for new stations but required the expansion of existing hospitals on all Regular Army posts.[12]

---

[9] (1) Floyd Kramer, "Mobilization Type Hospitals," *Army Medical Bulletin,* No. 31 (1935), pp. 1–19. (2) Tynes, Construction Branch, HD.

[10] See correspondence in SG: 632.–1 (Cp Jackson)D. 632.–1 (Ft McClellan)N, and 632.–1 (Ft Benning)N.

[11] Ltr, Surg Ft Benning to SG, 19 Jan 40, sub: An Rpt of Sta Hosp. SG: 632.–1 (Ft Benning)N.

[12] (1) Memo, Exec Off G–4 for Cons Br G–4 WDGS, 22 May 40, sub: Hosp. (2) Memo QM 600.1 C–C, QMG for ACofS G–4 WDGS, 28 May 40, sub: Util of Bks for Temp Hosp Accommodations. (3) Memo, Act SG for ACofS G–4 WDGS, 24 May 40, sub: Hosp for Increase in the Army above 227,000. (4) Memo, Chief Cons Br G–4 for ACofS G–4 WDGS, 3 Jun 40, sub: Util of Bks for Temp Hosp Accommodations. (5) Memo, Chief Cons Br G–4 for ACofS G–4 WDGS, 5 Jun 40, sub: Hosp for Increases of Army. (6) Ltr AG 705 (6–5–40)M–DM, TAG to CGs of all CAs, COs of Exempted Stas, and CofArms and Servs, 7 Jun 40, sub: Policy for Hosp during Emergency. All in HRS: G–4/31757.

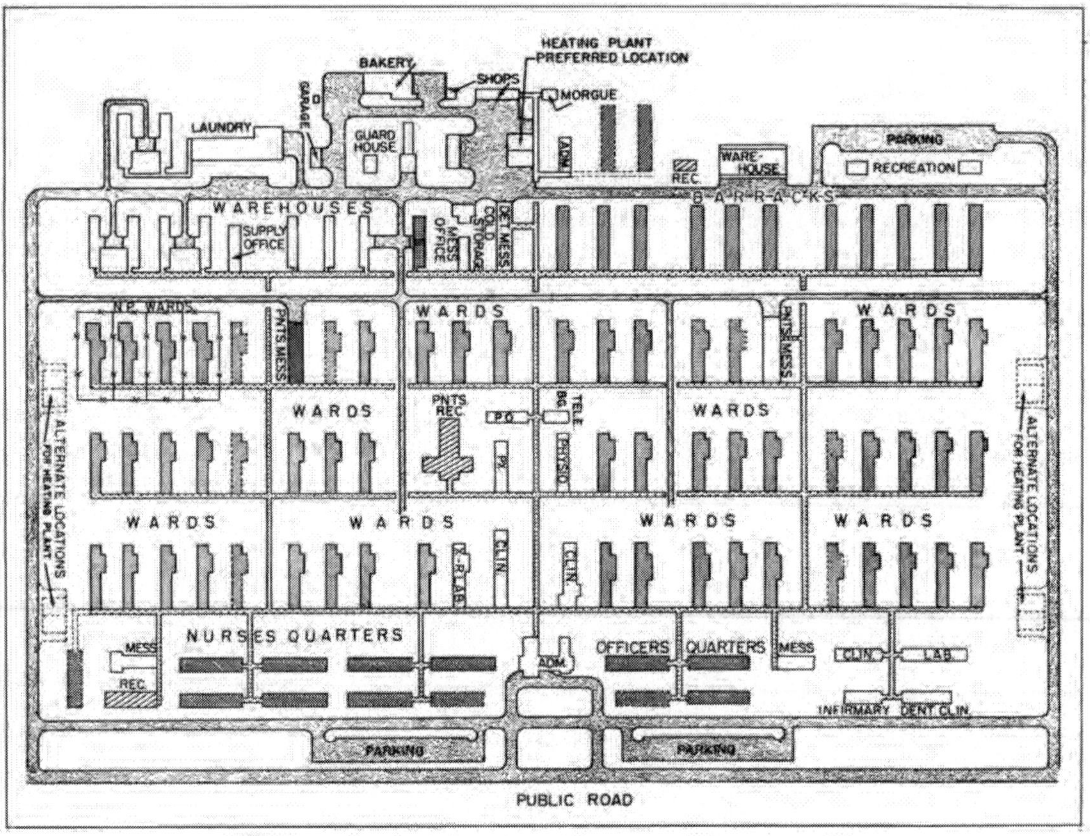

PLAN FOR CANTONMENT-TYPE HOSPITAL

The inapplicability of this policy soon became apparent. For example, despite a recommendation by The Surgeon General that a 550-bed cantonment-type hospital be constructed for Camp Ord, G-4 directed on 6 June 1940 that the camp continue to use an expanded hospital at the Presidio of Monterey. The Surgeon, the Quartermaster, and G-4 of the Ninth Corps Area opposed this decision. They pointed out that the hospital and barracks at Monterey did not have enough total space to accommodate all the beds needed and that some cantonment-type construction would be necessary. In addition, both the barracks and the hospital were old and in need of repairs, were potential firetraps, were separated by a public road, and were located six miles from the troops at Ord. In view of these arguments, the General Staff reversed its decision and authorized the construction of a cantonment-type hospital at Camp Ord.[13]

As plans were made to receive draftees in the fall of 1940, dissatisfaction with the existing policy increased and The Surgeon General attempted to get it changed. His

[13] (1) Ltr, SG to Surg 9th CA, 6 Jun 40, sub: Hosp for Cantonment Garrison, Cp Ord, with 3 inds. SG: 632.-1 (Cp Ord)C. (2) Rad 265 WVY V 50 WD, CG 9th CA to TAG, 15 Jul 40. Same file. (3) Correspondence in SG: 632.-1 (Ft Sill)N.

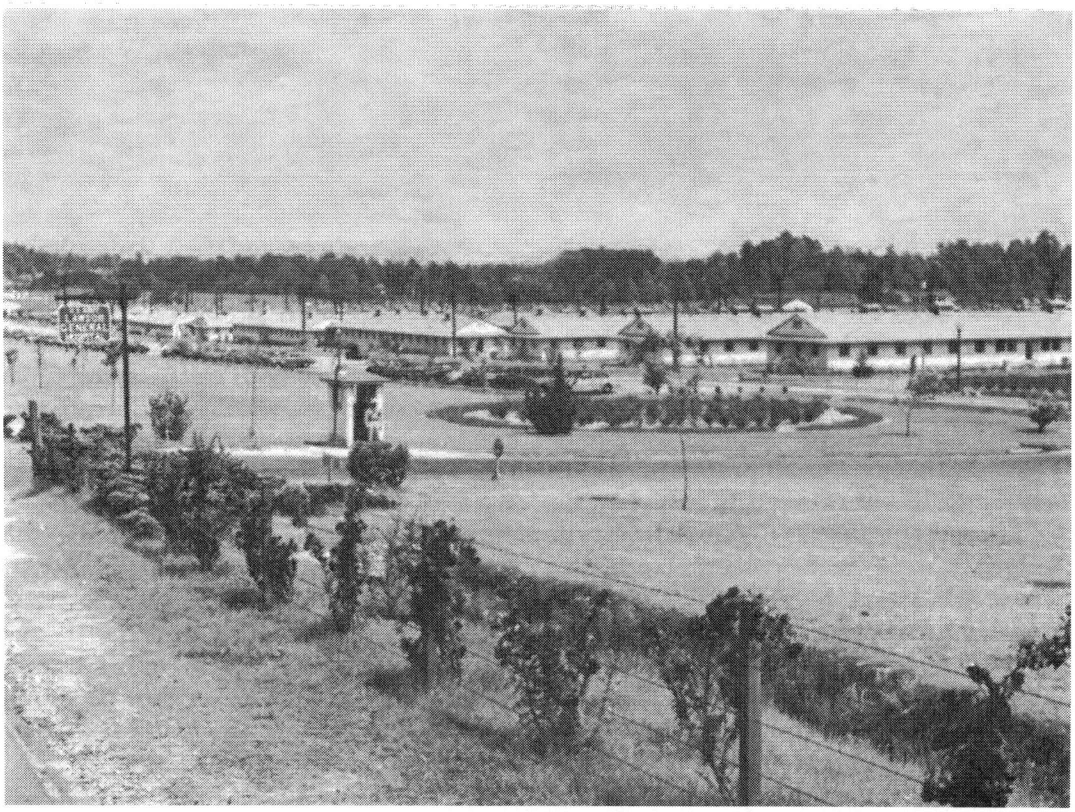

LAWSON GENERAL, A CANTONMENT-TYPE HOSPITAL

Office supported requests of local surgeons for exemption from its provisions.[11] On 5 September 1940 General Magee conferred with General Moore and the next day sent him a personal note. Referring to the impossibility of providing an adequate hospital at Fort Benning under the established policy, he stated: "There is so much dynamite in this that I think you should know about it." [15] Nevertheless, the War Department did not immediately revise the policy, and G–4 permitted few exceptions to it.[16] As a result the situation became so serious by mid-September that the Chief of Staff asked The Inspector General to investigate the rights and wrongs of interchanges between G–4 and The Surgeon General as well as delays in deciding the type of construction to be used.[17] Apparently The Inspector Gen-

[11] For example, see: Memo, SG for ACofS G–4 WDGS, 11 Sep 40, sub: Hosp, Ft McClellan. SG: 632.–1 (Ft McClellan)N.

[15] Memo, Maj Gen J[ames] C. Magee for Brig Gen R[ichard] C. Moore. 6 Sep 40. SG: 632.–1 (Ft Benning)N.

[16] (1) Rad AG 600.12 (9–5–40), TAG to CG 9th CA, 10 Sep 40. SG 632.–1 (Ft Lewis)N. (2) Ltr, Surg Ft Benning to SG, 21 Aug 40, sub: Cons of Med Fac, and 3 inds. SG: 632.–1 (Ft Benning)N. (3) Synopsis Ltr, CG Ft Bragg to CG 4th CA, 6 Sep 40, and 5 inds. SG: 632.–1 (Ft Bragg)N.

[17] Memo, CofSA for IG, 14 Sep 40. HRS: OCS 17749-225. The reply to this memorandum has not been located in War Department files.

eral's report favored The Surgeon General's position, for soon afterward the Chief of Staff personally approved General Magee's recommendation "that the erection of cantonment hospitals be announced as the normal procedure" for all large posts, whether Regular Army or not.[18]

The revised policy on hospital construction, issued by the War Department on 26 September 1940, discarded the long-established plan to construct additional buildings for hospitals as a last resort only. Thereafter peacetime hospitals were to be expanded only on small posts where clinical facilities were generally sufficient for additional patients. Cantonment-type hospitals were to be constructed elsewhere.[19] Without this change hospitals on Regular Army posts would have consisted of a hodgepodge of small permanent hospitals, permanent barracks, and temporary buildings required to supplement them. Delay in making the revision was responsible for much confusion and some delay in the erection of suitable hospital buildings on Regular Army posts,[20] but it had no effect on hospitals for new posts because cantonment-type construction had been authorized for them since June 1940.

Planning for Construction and Selecting Sites of Hospitals

Planning for station hospitals was done on a day-to-day rather than a long-term basis, because their size, number, and location depended almost entirely upon a constantly changing troop distribution. In the fall of 1940 the Surgeon General's Office prepared two studies showing the additional beds that would be required by June 1941 at each post in the United States,[21] but lack of information about ultimate troop distribution and changes in station strengths limited their value. In some instances three or more increases in authorized strengths required the same number of revisions of hospital construction plans for a single post.[22] As information about stations and their strengths became available, the Construction and Repair Subdivision prepared plans for hospital construction for each. Consisting of the number of beds needed, the types and numbers of buildings required, and the layout or arrangement of buildings, these plans amounted only to recommendations. Final decisions on hospital construction were made by G-4 for ground force stations and by the Chief of the Air Corps for air stations. Because of the day-to-day type of planning and the lack of information about action on his recommendations, The Surgeon General found it difficult to keep track of station hospitals authorized for construction.[23]

Planning for general hospitals was on a more comprehensive basis. Although it

---

[18] (1) Memo, SG for ACofS G-4 WDGS, 20 Sep 40, and note thereon signed G. C. M[arshall]. (2) D/S, ACofS G-4 WDGS to TAG, sub: Revised Policy for Hosp during Emergency. Both in HRS: G-4/31757.

[19] Ltr AG 600.12 (9-25-40) MD, TAG to CofArms and Servs, CGs of CAs, and COs of exempted Stas, 26 Sep 40, sub: Revised Policy for Hosp during Emergency. HRS: G-4/31757.

[20] SG: 632.-1 (Ft McClellan)N; 632.-1 (Ft Benning)N; 632.-1 (Ft Bragg)N.

[21] SG Ltrs, 1 Oct and 7 Nov 40, sub: Bed Reqmt Study. SG: 632.-2.

[22] SG: 632.-1 (Ft Jackson)N, 1940; SG: 632.-1 (Ft Ord)C, 1940; SG: 632.-1 (Ft Bragg)N, 1940.

[23] (1) Ltr, CofAC to SG, 17 Apr 41, sub: Increases in Str for Pilot Tng Sch, and 9 inds. AAF: 632B Hosp and Infirmaries. (2) Ltr AG 600.12 (9-28-40)M-D, TAG to QMG, 3 Oct 40, sub: Temp Cons . . . 5th CA. SG: 632.-1 (5th CA)AA. (3) Memo, SG for QMG, 7 Oct 40, sub: Ft Knox. SG: 632.-1 (Ft Knox)N. (4) Ltr, SG to Fed Bd of Hosp, 5 May 41. SG: 632.-1.

depended to some extent upon troop distribution, the fact that general hospitals would serve more than one post and would operate directly under The Surgeon General gave him considerable latitude in determining their size, number, and location. On 10 August 1940 G–4 sought information on increases in general hospitals that passage of the Selective Service Act would require.[24] In response The Surgeon General proposed the construction of ten new general hospitals with a total capacity of 9,500 beds—one each in the First, Second, Fifth, Sixth, and Seventh Corps Areas; three in the Fourth, where the troop concentration would be heaviest; and two in the Ninth, where troops would be spread from Canada to Mexico. In the Eighth Corps Area, he proposed redesignation of the 1,700-bed Fort Sam Houston (Texas) Station Hospital as a general hospital, since it was already performing the functions of both types.[25] Plans had already been made to increase the capacity of Walter Reed General Hospital, in the Third Corps Area, by relieving it of station-hospital cases which it had previously received from near-by posts.[26] With the general hospitals already in operation, this plan would have provided a total of over 15,000 general hospital beds in the United States for an expected Army strength of 1,400,000.

The expansion of general hospitals during 1941 followed basically The Surgeon General's plan. On 25 September 1940 G–4 approved the construction of ten general hospitals, with a total capacity of 10,000 beds, in locations substantially the same as those recommended by The Surgeon General.[27] Objections of the commander of the Eighth Corps Area to redesignation of the Fort Sam Houston Station Hospital caused The Surgeon General to withdraw that proposal.[28] During 1941, therefore, the following general hospitals were added to the five the Army already had: Lovell at Fort Devens, Mass.; Tilton at Fort Dix, N. J.; Stark at Charleston, S. C.; Lawson at Atlanta, Ga.; LaGarde at New Orleans, La.; Billings at Fort Benjamin Harrison, Ind.; O'Reilly at Springfield, Mo.; Hoff at Santa Barbara, Calif.; and Barnes at Vancouver Barracks, Wash.[29] No additional ones were required until September 1941, when an increase in the size of the Army was anticipated. At that time The Surgeon General submitted a proposal for a proportionate increase in the number of general hospital beds,[30] but it was later merged with a larger plan to meet the needs of a wartime Army.

Selection of proper sites was an essential factor in planning for hospital construction. It was important, for instance, for both station and general hospitals to have sufficient space for future expansion; to be free from objectionable neighbors such as factories, railroad yards, warehouses, utilities areas, and training grounds; and

[24] Memo, ACofS G–4 WDGS for SG, 10 Aug 40, sub: Increase in Number of Gen Hosps. HRS: G–4/29135–11.

[25] 1st ind, SG to TAG, 23 Aug 40, on Memo G–4/29135–11, ACofS G–4 WDGS for SG, 10 Aug 40, sub: Increase in Number of Gen Hosps. AG: 322.3 Gen Hosp (8–10–40)(1).

[26] 4th ind SGO 701.–1, SG to TAG, 5 Aug 40, and 7th ind, TAG to SG, 30 Sep 40, on Ltr, SG to TAG, 15 Jul 40, sub: Gen Hosp Beds for Enlarged Army. AG: 322.3 Gen Hosp (7–15–40)(1) Sec 1.

[27] D/S, ACofS G–4 WDGS to TAG, 25 Sep 40, sub: Increase in Number of Gen Hosps. HRS: G–4/29135–11.

[28] Ltr, SG to TAG, 9 Oct 40, sub: New Gen Hosp (Ft Sam Houston, Tex), with 2d ind, CG 8th CA to TAG, 7 Nov 40, and 4th ind, SG to QMG, 9 Dec 40. AG: 322.3 Gen Hosp (8–10–40)(1).

[29] SG: 632.–1, 1941, for each hospital named.

[30] Memo, SG for ACofS G–4 WDGS, 19 Sep 41, sub: DF G–4/20052–103, Augmented PMP, 1942. SG: 632.–1.

to be located on terrain that was moderately level and properly drained. The accessibility of good highway and railroad nets was especially important for general hospitals, whose function was to receive patients from other hospitals. The availability of good water supplies and of adequate utilities connections had also to be considered. The Quartermaster General's chief interest in hospital sites lay in their suitability from an engineering and construction standpoint.

During the emergency period The Quartermaster General selected construction sites in collaboration with other interested War Department agencies. For hospitals, this meant both The Surgeon General and corps area commanders.[31] In the early phases of mobilization the selection of sites for station hospitals was left in many instances to local authorities, for The Surgeon General's Hospital Construction and Repair Subdivision had little personnel to spare for such activities. Sites so selected were generally satisfactory but sometimes had undesirable features, such as promixity to training areas, poor drainage, or inadequate space for expansion. As the press of work abated during 1941, The Surgeon General began to exercise more direct supervision over site selection through visits of his representatives to stations where hospital construction was anticipated.[32] The selection of sites for general hospitals was more complicated and time consuming, even though the general areas in which they were to be located were first approved by the General Staff. As a rule, the War Department directed corps area commanders to appoint boards, with medical representatives, to make investigations and recommendations. Their surveys required considerable time and their recommendations in some instances were deemed unsatisfactory. In such cases, the Secretary of War appointed other boards representing The Surgeon General, The Quartermaster General, the General Staff, and corps area surgeons to make further surveys and recommendations.[33]

Difficulties in Providing Satisfactory Hospital Plants

The Surgeon General and The Quartermaster General disagreed about the manner in which the Medical Department as the using agency should exercise advisory supervision over hospital construction. The Surgeon General insisted that his office should review each building schedule which was sent out and each change in plans proposed by the field. He believed that this procedure was necessary to maintain the proper division of space among various hospital services, an appropriate relationship among different buildings of a hospital plant, and the possibility of future expansion. In his opinion experience justified this position. For example, hospital construction at Fort Francis E. Warren (Wyoming) was delayed from early November 1940 until

[31] Memo QM 322.2 C-OT (Gen Hosps), QMG for ACofS G-4 WDGS, 11 Jan 41, sub: Gen Hosps, and D/S G-4/32445, ACofS G-4 WDGS to TAG, 15 Jan 41, sub: Control of Cons Projects. AG: 322.2 Gen Hosp (7-15-40)(1) Sec 1.

[32] (1) Tynes, Construction Branch, p. 32. (2) Memos from offs of Hosp Cons and Repair Subdiv dated 18 Jan, 11 Apr, 28 Jul, 20 Aug, 22 Aug, 2 Sep, and 16 Sep 41. HD: 333(Hosp).

[33] (1) Memo, ACofS G-4 WDGS for DepCofSA, 14 Nov 40, sub: Gen Hosps. HRS: G-4/29135-11. (2) Ltr, TAG to CG 4th CA, 29 Sep 40, sub: Cons of Cantonment Hosps 4th CA (Atlanta, Charleston, New Orleans). AG: 322.3 Gen Hosp (9-27-40) M-D. (3) Rad, TAG to CG 7th CA, 19 Dec 40, and D/S G-4/29135-14, ACofS G-4 WDGS to TAG, 14 Jan 41, sub: Convening a WD Board . . . . AG: 322.3 Gen Hosps (7-15-40) (1) Sec 4.

January 1941 because The Quartermaster General sent out plans which The Surgeon General had not approved and against which local authorities protested. At Fort Rosecrans (California) local quartermaster and medical officers erected a two-story wooden hospital which The Surgeon General considered unsafe. In other places, such as Camp Wallace (Texas), Camp Custer (Michigan), Camp Roberts (California), and Camp Leonard Wood (Missouri), local changes in approved plans produced hospitals considered unsatisfactory by The Surgeon General.[34]

Hoping to speed construction, The Quartermaster General proposed standardization and decentralization—the use of standard building schedules (that is, lists of buildings for hospitals ranging in size from 25 to 2,000 beds) approved initially by the Surgeon General's Office and subject to no further changes by it, and the delegation of authority to make changes in hospital layouts and building plans to medical and quartermaster officers in the field.[35] Nevertheless, because of The Surgeon General's insistence, both the Quartermaster Corps and the Corps of Engineers followed the practice of referring hospital building schedules and layouts to his Office for approval and twice during 1941 The Quartermaster General instructed his field agents not to change hospital construction plans without prior approval of the Surgeon General's Office.[36]

Centralization of the Medical Department's advisory supervision over hospital construction did not necessarily assure erection of satisfactory hospital buildings. That depended considerably upon the plans used. Drawn in 1935, they were simply pulled "off the shelf" when needed. The medical officer (Col. Floyd Kramer) who had helped prepare them warned the Surgeon General's Office that they would not be entirely satisfactory, and in October 1940 Colonel Hall, of the Hospital Construction and Repair Subdivision, indicated that he was "by no means certain" that they would "suit our 1940 ideas."[37] It soon appeared that they did not. Hospitals built on such plans had insufficient space for some activities and none at all for others. X-ray clinics and laboratories were too small for use in modern medicine. Administration buildings had insufficient space for extensive records required for patients and civilian employees and were cut up into too many small rooms for efficient use. Post dental work required more room than originally expected. General hospitals needed more space for quartermaster activities. Inadequate kitchens and mess storerooms became the source of frequent complaints. Offices for the medical supply officer and the medical detachment commander, recreation buildings for patients and for nurses, post exchange

[34] (1) Ltr, SG to QMG, 5 Jan 41, sub: Unauth Changes in Cantonment Hosps. . . , with 2d ind, SG to QMG, 14 Feb 41. SG: 632.-1. (2) 1st ind, SG to QMG, 17 Jul 41, on Synopsis Ltr, QMG to SG, 17 Jul 41. Same file. (3) SG: 632.-1 (Ft F. E. Warren)N, 1940-41 and (Ft Rosecrans)N, 1940-41.

[35] (1) 1st ind QM 632 C-ED, QMG to SG, 8 Feb 41, on Ltr, SG to QMG, 5 Jan 41, sub: Unauth Changes in Cantonment Hosps. . . . (2) Synopsis Ltr, QMG to SG, 17 Jul 41. Both in SG: 632.-1.

[36] (1) Ltr QM 632 C-EP Hosp Fac, QMG to SG, 9 Aug 41, sub: Add Hosp Fac. SG: 632.-1. (2) 2d ind, CofAC to CofEngrs, 11 Aug 41, on Ltr, SG to CofEngrs, 31 Jul 41, sub: Hosp Insp, AC Sta, 8th CA. Same file. (3) Ltr, QMG to Cons QMs, 8 Feb 41, sub: Hosp Layouts. Same file. (4) Ltr QM 632 C-EP (Zone VII), QMG to Zone Cons QM, Zone VII, 12 Sep 41, sub: Revisions in Hosp Plans and Layouts. Off file, Hosp Cons Div SGO, "Policy File."

[37] (1) Lessons Learned from Planning and Constructing Army Hospitals, Speech by Col John R. Hall, 16 Sep 43. HD: 632.-1. (2) Ltr, Col J. R. Hall to Col H. C. Coburn, Jr, MC, Sta Hosp Ft Bragg, 16 Oct 40. SG: 632.-1 (Ft Bragg)N.

buildings, ambulance garages, and strong rooms for safeguarding narcotics as required by Federal law were not included in existing plans. Of equal importance, neuropsychiatric wards for which plans were provided lacked sufficient strength and safety features to prevent patients from attempting escape or suicide.[38]

The question of whether to revise existing plans completely or to make piecemeal changes arose in the fall of 1940. General Love, Chief of the Planning and Training Division, advocated their complete revision, but Colonel Hall demurred on the ground that he would encounter delays and difficulties in securing approval of G–4 and co-operation of The Quartermaster General.[39] That his position had some basis in fact is indicated by a controversy from August through October over proposed changes for separate buildings. After The Quartermaster General complained that requests of The Surgeon General for piecemeal changes were delaying construction, their offices hurled charges and countercharges against each other until G–4 forbade further changes in standard designs without Staff approval, and the chief of the G–4 Construction Branch, concluding that further argument was useless, closed the controversy by recommending on 18 October 1940 that all papers pertaining to it be filed.[40] Two months later The Quartermaster General proposed a complete revision of cantonment-type hospital plans, but Colonel Hall maintained his former position, this time for a different reason. "It is the opinion of this office," he wrote, "that sufficient experience with the plants to be erected according to the present plans has not yet been had to make a complete and satisfactory revision possible at this time."[41]

As soon as hospitals built on the 1935 plans were received from contractors, steps had to be taken to correct their defects and overcome their deficiencies. Several methods were adopted. One was to rearrange the use of space. For example, local commanders converted wards into X-ray clinics and laboratories and used the space vacated in clinical buildings to increase surgical facilities. To replace the bed ca pacity thus lost, The Surgeon General obtained additional wards.[42] Another method was to modify the buildings erected. Changes in neuropsychiatric wards, such as the removal of exposed pipes, were made to increase the safety of mentally disturbed patients; and kitchens and mess halls were enlarged by adjacent construction.[43] A third method was to construct additional buildings, such as storehouses,

[38] (1) An Rpts, 1941, Sta Hosps at Fts Knox and Bragg, Cps Lee, Roberts, Claiborne, and Bowie, and O'Reilly Gen Hosp. HD. (2) Memo, IG for ACofS G–4 WDGS 22 Apr 41, sub: Cons Defects. HRS: G–4/32900. (3) Tynes, Construction Branch, pp. 16–18. (4) Rpt, Conf of SG with CA Surgs, 10–12 Mar 41. HD: 337.

[39] Interv, MD Historian with Col Albert G. Love, 27 Aug 47. HD: 000.71.

[40] (1) Ltr AG 600.12(8–15–40), TAG to SG, 17 Aug 40, sub: Changes in Standard Design, with 3d ind, QMG to TAG, 7 Sep 40, 4th ind, TAG to SG, 20 Sep 40, and 5th ind, SG to TAG, 8 Oct 40. SG: 632.–1. (2) Memo, Lt Col Stephen J. Chamberlin for ACofS G–4 WDGS, 18 Oct 40, same sub. HRS: G–4/31741.

[41] Memo, SG (Hall) for QMG, 17 Dec 40. SG: 632.–1.

[42] (1) An Rpts, 1941, Sta Hosps at Ft Bragg and Cp Roberts and O'Reilly Gen Hosp. HD. (2) Ltr, SG to TAG, 7 May 41, sub: Request for Urgent Emergency Cons, and 2d ind AG 600.12 (5–7–41), TAG to QMG, 5 Jul 41. SG: 632.–1. (3) Ltr, SG to QMG, 14 Jul 41, same sub. Same file.

[43] (1) Memo, Col John R. Hall for SG, 28 Jul 41, sub: Rpt of Insp, 8th CA. HD: 333. (2) 2d ind, SG to Hq AAF, 9 May 42, on Ltr, Surg Southeast AC Tng Ctr to SG, 5 May 42, sub: Hosp Messes. SG: 632.–1. (3) Ltr QM 300.5 C–ED(Gen), QMG to all Cons QMs, 21 May 41, sub: Piping—Detention Wards. SG: 632.–1.

ambulance garages, post exchanges, and strong rooms.[44] Finally, existing plans for a few buildings, such as neuropsychiatric wards, kitchens, and messes, were revised during 1941 for subsequent use, in order to prevent perpetuation of the process of building and changing.[45]

Development of a New Type of Hospital Plant

In the spring of 1941 complaints were made in both military and civilian circles that the hospitals constructed not only lacked space for certain activities but also were unsatisfactory from an administrative and safety viewpoint.[46] Wide dispersal of buildings intensified administrative problems without assuring adequate fire protection. As early as January 1941 the offices of The Quartermaster General and The Surgeon General had agreed upon a program of installing draft-stops in closed corridors that connected different buildings of hospital plants, as a fire-protection measure.[47] In May the Chief of the Air Corps secured appropriations for the installation of automatic fire-sprinkler systems in fifty-eight Air Corps hospitals and The Quartermaster General made plans for their installation in all other hospitals with 400 or more beds. By December 1941 the installation of such systems in all the wards, except detention wards, and in the patients' kitchens of cantonment-type hospitals became War Department policy.[48]

Meanwhile work had begun on the development of a new type of hospital. When complaints about existing plants were first made, Colonel Hall expressed The Surgeon General's preference for more compact hospitals built of fire-resistant materials.[49] Soon afterward his Office began to collaborate with the Quartermaster General's in designing such a plant. It consisted of buildings that were generally two stories high with exterior walls of masonry and interiors of slow-burning materials. Such construction permitted a more compact arrangement of structures than had previously been possible. Ward buildings were placed opposite each other on a central connecting corridor permitting one diet kitchen and one ward office and examining room to serve two wards. Two-story corridors connected the buildings of a hospital group, and ramps were placed at suitable intervals to give access from one story to the other. To allow more

[44] (1) Ltr, SG to Off of Budget Off, 26 Dec 40, sub: Supp Est, FY 1941. SG: 632.-1. (2) D/S G-4/29135-17, ACofS G-4 WDGS to TAG for transmittal to SG, 13 Jan 41, sub: Med Fac. . . . AG: 322.3 Gen Hosp (7-15-40)(1) Sec 1. (3) Ltr, SG to ACofS G-4 WDGS, 15 Mar 41, sub: PXs for Hosps. SG: 632.-1. (4) Ltr AG 600.12 (8-4-41)MO-D-M, TAG to CGs of all Depts *et al.*, 19 Aug 41, sub: WD Cons Policy. HD: 600.12-1.

[45] (1) Ltr, SG to Cons Div OQMG, 4 Jun 41, sub: Plans for Ward 8—NP Bldgs. (2) Ltr, SG to QMG, 7 Aug 41, sub: Modification of M-16 Mess, with 1st ind QM 633 C-ED(Danville GH), QMG to SG, 4 Sep 41. Both in SG: 632.-1.

[46] (1) Ltr, Nathaniel O. Gould, Architect and Engr, Detroit, to SecWar, 27 Mar 41. AG: 600.12 (3-27-41)(1). (2) Ltr, F. A. Arnold to SG USPHS, 4 Apr 41. SG: 632.-1. (3) Ltr, CofEngrs to SG, 9 May 41, sub: Type of Hosp Cons. Same file. (4) Memo, Exec Asst OCE for Engr Div OCE, 3 May 41, and Memo, Head Engr for Exec Asst OCE, 6 May 41, sub: Hosp Layouts. CE: 632 Pt I.

[47] Memo, SG (Hall) for QMG, 29 Jan 41. SG: 632.-1.

[48] (1) Synopsis Ltr, CofAC to CofEngrs, 9 May 41, sub: Fire Prevention in Hosps, with 1st ind, CofEngrs to CofAC, 17 May 41, and three subsequent inds. SG: 671.2. (2) Memo QM 632 C-ED (Gen), Design Sec OQMG for Chief Design Sec OQMG, 13 May 41, sub: Sprinkler and Alarm Systs—Hosps. CE: 671.3 Pt 1. (3) 3d ind AG 671.7 (10-21-41)MO-D, TAG to CofEngrs, 26 Dec 41, on Ltr QM 671 C-RU (Gen), QMG to TAG, 21 Oct 41, sub: Fire Protection. Same file.

[49] 2d ind SGO 600.12-1, SG (Hall) for TAG, 16 Apr 41, on Ltr, Nathaniel O. Gould to SecWar, 27 Mar 41. AG: 600.12 (3-27-41)(1).

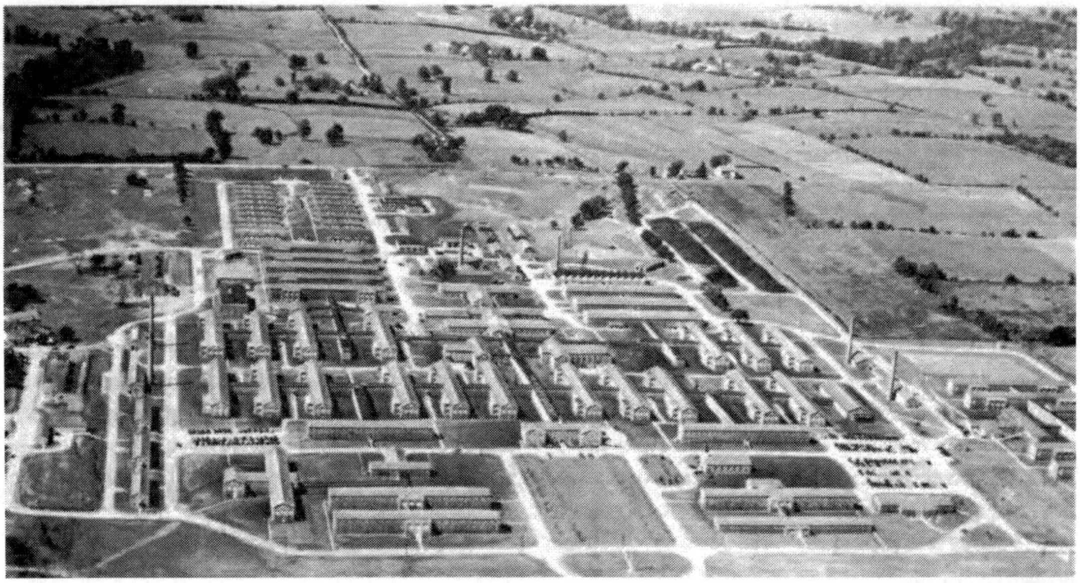

VALLEY FORGE GENERAL, A SEMIPERMANENT-TYPE HOSPITAL

space for medical care, the width of all wards, clinics, and other key buildings was increased from twenty-five to thirty-two feet, and facilities that were either lacking or inadequate in cantonment-type hospitals were introduced or redesigned in plans for the new type.[50] On 6 August 1941 the Staff authorized the construction of two-story, semipermanent, fire-resistant plants for all future hospitals.[51] Final drawings were not completed for several months, and before they could be put into general use the United States was at war.

Evaluation of Hospital Construction Program

Although hospitals constructed during the period of peacetime mobilization did not "even approach the ideal," in Colonel Hall's opinion the wonder was "not that so many mistakes were made but rather that we have been able in a somewhat satisfactory manner to meet our obligation to the sick and wounded."[52] Hospital beds had to be provided on a scale unknown in ordinary times. Between September 1940 and December 1941 the number of normal beds (that is, those for which 100 square feet of space each was provided in ward buildings) in station hospitals increased from 7,391 to 58,736 and in general hospitals, from 4,925 to 15,533. *(Chart 1)* Only in the fall and winter of 1940–41 was there a shortage of normal beds. At that time the Medical Department used emergency and expansion beds (that is, those set up on the basis of seventy-two square feet each not only in

[50] (1) Tynes, Construction Branch, pp. 39–40. (2) Ltr, SG to CofEngrs, 7 Feb 42, sub: Fire-Resistant Type of Hosp. SG: 632.–1.

[51] 2d ind AG 632 (7–7–41)MO–D, TAG to QMG and SG in turn, 6 Aug 41, on Ltr, SG to TAG, 7 Jul 41, sub: Fire-Resistant Type of Cons for Hosp. SG: 632.–1.

[52] Lessons Learned from Planning and Constructing Army Hospitals, speech by Col Hall, 16 Sep 43. HD: 632.–1.

Chart 1—Status of Station and General Hospital Beds in Continental United States: August 1940–December 1941

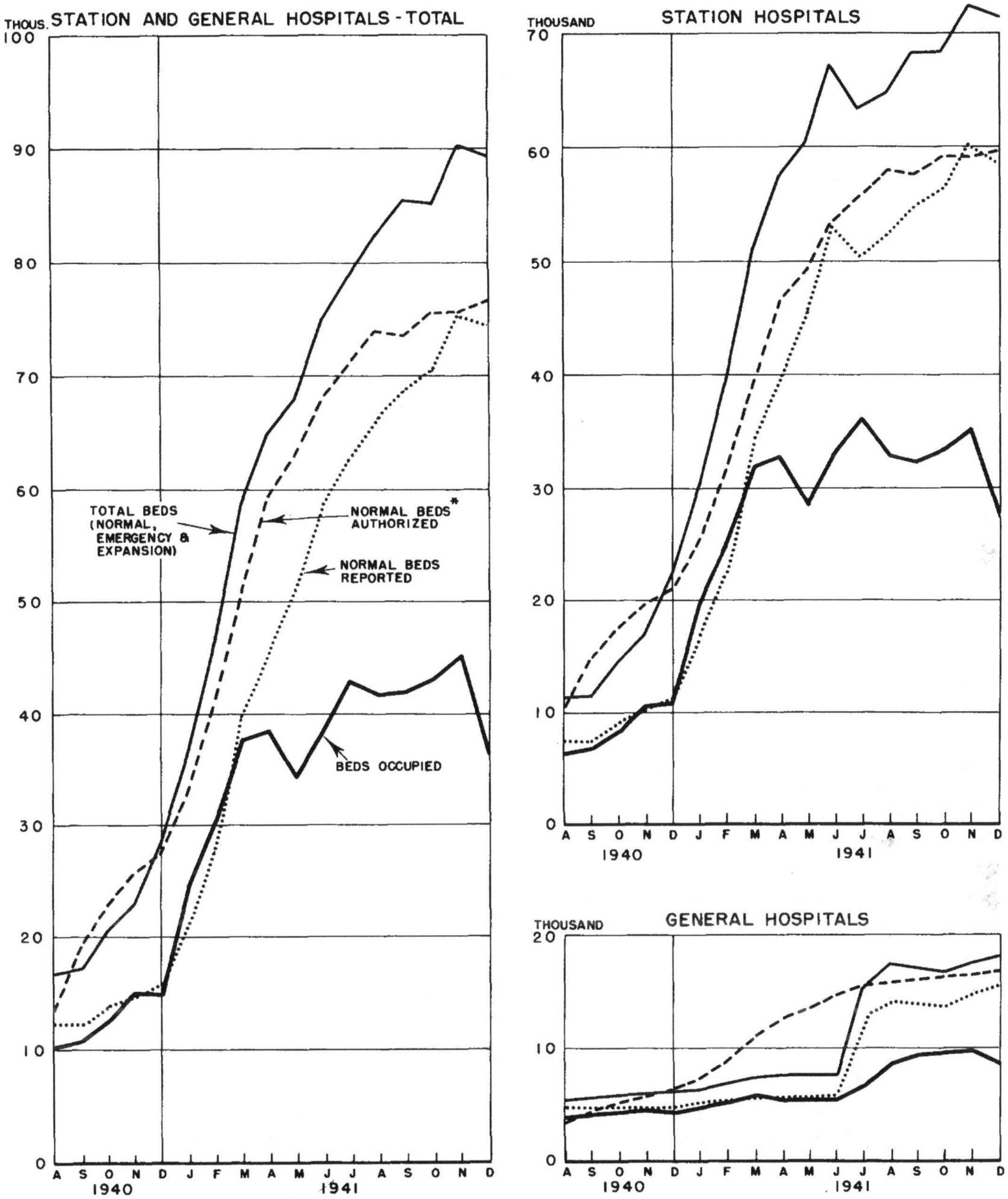

* Based on War Department determined percentage of troop strength.

Source: Figures for total beds, normal beds reported, and beds occupied, as of the last full week of each month, shown in Bed Status Reports, Health Reports Br, Med Statistics Div, SGO.

wards but also in porches, halls, barracks, and tents) and sent some patients to nearby civilian and Veterans Administration hospitals.[53] It also continued a policy, begun early in 1940, of reducing the number of Civilian Conservation Corps and Veterans Administration patients in Army hospitals and in December secured War Department approval of a policy of limiting sharply the hospitalization of dependents of military personnel.[54] In the spring of 1941 construction began to catch up with needs and after March the number of patients in hospitals at no time exceeded the total number of normal beds. *(See Chart 1.)*

Hospital Administration

Internal Organization and Administrative Procedures

When mobilization began, the only guide to the organization and administration of Army hospitals was an Army regulation published in the mid-1930's. It gave hospital commanders much discretion in both fields and lacked detailed instructions for inexperienced officers to follow.[55] A more specific guide was therefore necessary. In October 1940 the Medical Department devoted an entire issue of the *Army Medical Bulletin* to an article prepared by Col. Charles M. Walson, then surgeon of the Second Corps Area, entitled "Station Hospital Organization Chart, Regulations, and Medical Department Questionnaire." During the first half of 1941 the Training Subdivision of the Surgeon General's Office revised this article and the War Department issued it in July as a technical manual.[56]

The manual described hospital organization in considerable detail, advocating the separation of activities into two major categories, administrative and professional, and the grouping of professional activities into services composed of subunits called sections. For example, the surgical service of a station hospital might contain sections devoted to general surgery, orthopedics, obstetrics and gynecology, urology, eye-ear-nose-and-throat disorders, anesthesia, roentgenology, and physiotherapy; the medical service, sections for general medicine, contagious diseases, dermatology, neuropsychiatry, and detention. The manual also provided for a headquarters, or commanding officer's staff, separate from other administrative units of general hospitals. In addition, it described the duties and responsibilities of staff officers, as well as important administrative procedures, and contained checklists for chiefs of services to use in measuring the efficiency of operations. While it was somewhat more specific than the Army regulation governing hospital administration, this manual also gave local commanders considerable autonomy. *(Chart 2)*

[53] (1) An Rpts, 1941, Sta Hosps at Cps Beauregard, Shelby, Blanding, Custer, and Roberts, and Fts Leonard Wood, Sill, and Bragg. HD. (2) AR 40–1080, par 2 *n* (1), (2), and (3), 31 Dec 34, and C 2, AR 40–1080, par 2 *n* (1), (2), and (3), 16 Mar 40. (3) Ltr, CO Sta Hosp Ft Snelling to Surg 7th CA, 9 Sep 40, sub: Auth to Reduce Floor Space. . . , and 3 inds. SG: 632.-1(Ft Snelling)N.

[54] (1) Rpt, Conf of SG with CA Surgs, 14–16 Oct 40, and 10–12 Mar 41. HD: 337. (2) Memo, ACofS G-4 WDGS for CofSA, 5 Dec 40, sub: Reply of SecWar to VA. HRS: G-4/28901-17. (3) Ltr, SG to TAG, 28 Nov 40, sub: Med Care for Dependents . . . and cy Ltr AG 702 (11-28-40) M-A-M, TAG to CGs of CAs and Depts and COs of Exempted Stas, 18 Dec 40, same sub. HD: 701.-1.

[55] AR 40–590, 21 Nov 35, The Admin of Hosps, Gen Provisions.

[56] (1) *Army Medical Bulletin*, No. 54, (1940). (2) TM 8–260, Fixed Hosps of the MD (Gen and Sta Hosps), Jul 41. (3) Memo for Record on D/S G-3/44468, ACofS G-3 WDGS to TAG, 17 Apr 41, sub: TM 8-260. AG: 300.7 TM 8-260 (4-15-41)(1).

Chart 2—Hospital Organization as Suggested by TM 8-260, July 1941

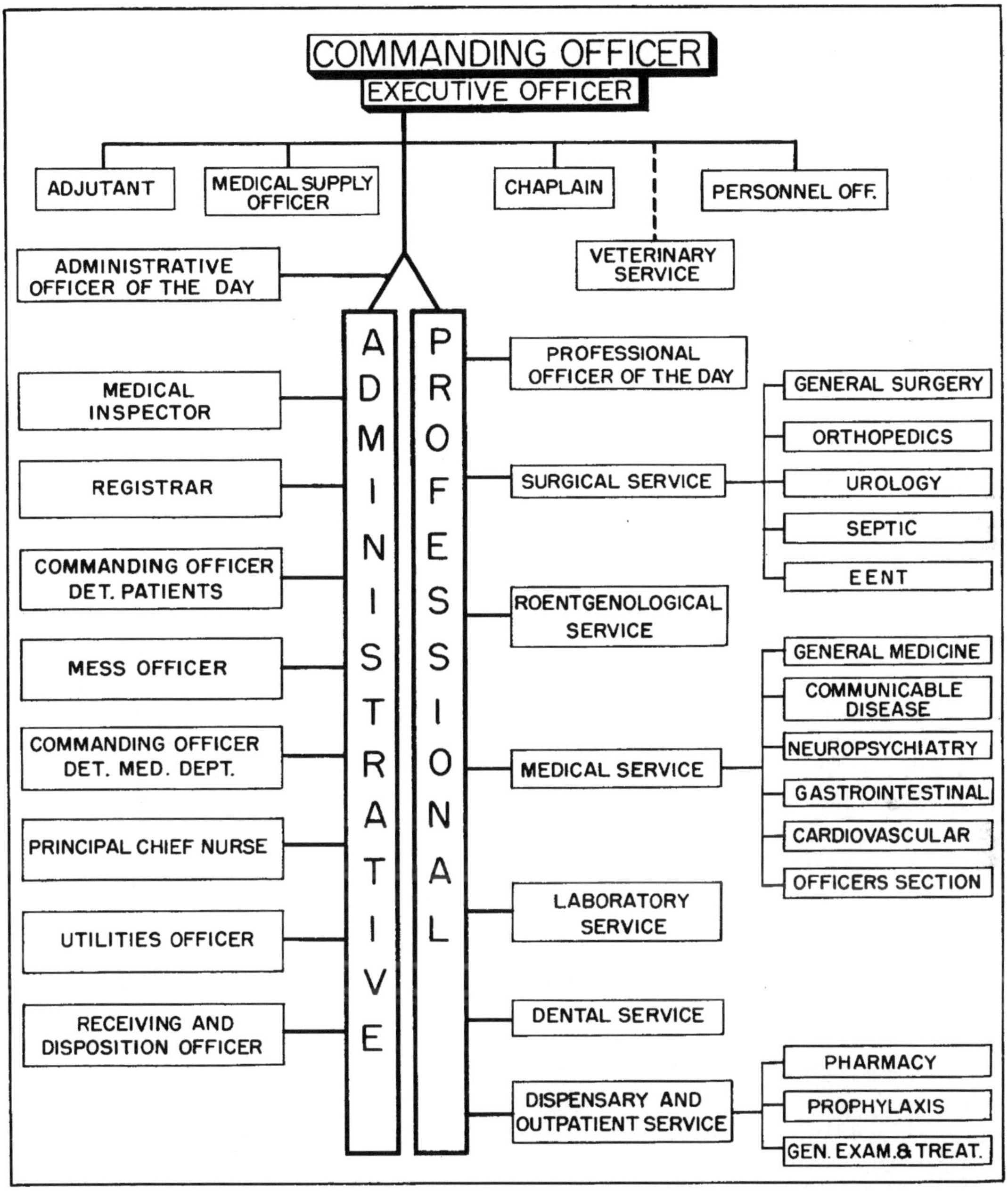

Lack of a specific directive requiring standard hospital organization resulted in many local variations.[57] The one general point of similarity was the separation of administrative from professional activities. In most hospitals the latter were organized as sections that were grouped in services: medical, surgical, dental, and laboratory. Some hospitals looked upon nursing as a separate professional service, although the manual recommended that the nursing unit be considered an administrative one. Others gave activities that might have been included as sections of either the medical or surgical service a higher status. For example, the station hospitals at Fort Lewis (Washington) and Fort Knox (Kentucky) possessed orthopedic services; that at Fort Ord (California) had separate genitourinary and eye-ear-nose-and-throat services; and that at Fort Bragg (North Carolina), a separate neuropsychiatric service. On the other hand there were but three professional services at the 1,200-bed station hospital at Camp Bowie (Texas): medical, surgical, and nursing.

Administrative units were usually not grouped in services, and their number varied from one hospital to another. For example at Stark General Hospital there were 29, including staff offices; at LaGarde, 14; while the number proposed in the manual was 12. Station hospitals likewise varied. On some posts they were under the supervision of station surgeons, who supplied certain administrative services. In one such instance the station surgeon handled all hospital personnel and supply activities. On other posts, a single officer served both as station surgeon and as hospital commander. The Fort Bragg Station Hospital, which was divided into three sections located from one quarter of a mile to a mile apart, had separate commanders for each unit, but possessed a central registrar's office, medical supply section, nursing section, mess and hospital fund, military and civilian personnel divisions, and medical detachment. General hospitals not located on Army posts usually had administrative sections not found in station hospitals, such as the finance and provost marshal's offices.

Neither Army regulations nor the manual on organization limited the number of officers a hospital commander could supervise directly. Thus the number of individuals reporting to him varied as did the organization of administrative and professional activities. As a rule, only chiefs of professional services, not of sections under them, reported to the commanding officer, but in most hospitals the chief of each administrative section reported directly to the commander or his executive officer. Thus the officers supervised directly by a hospital commander sometimes reached large numbers. For example, at Stark General Hospital the chiefs of four professional services and twenty-nine different administrative sections reported directly to the commander. In some instances the number of officers actually reporting was smaller than it seemed, because one officer frequently held several positions. *(Chart 3)*

Administrative procedures likewise varied from hospital to hospital. Since there was no manual covering hospital operations in detail, hospital commanders were free to supplement general procedures outlined in Army regulations as they saw

[57] (1) The following three paragraphs are based on: An Rpts, 1941, Sta Hosps at Fts Knox, Leonard Wood, Lewis, Bragg, Sill, Ord, and G. G. Meade, and Cp Bowie, and Stark, Billings, Hoff, LaGarde, and Lawson Gen Hosps. HD. (2) See also: Edward J. Morgan and Donald O. Wagner, The Organization of the Medical Department in the Zone of the Interior (1946), pp. 102–06. HD.

Chart 3—Organization of Lawson General Hospital, 1941

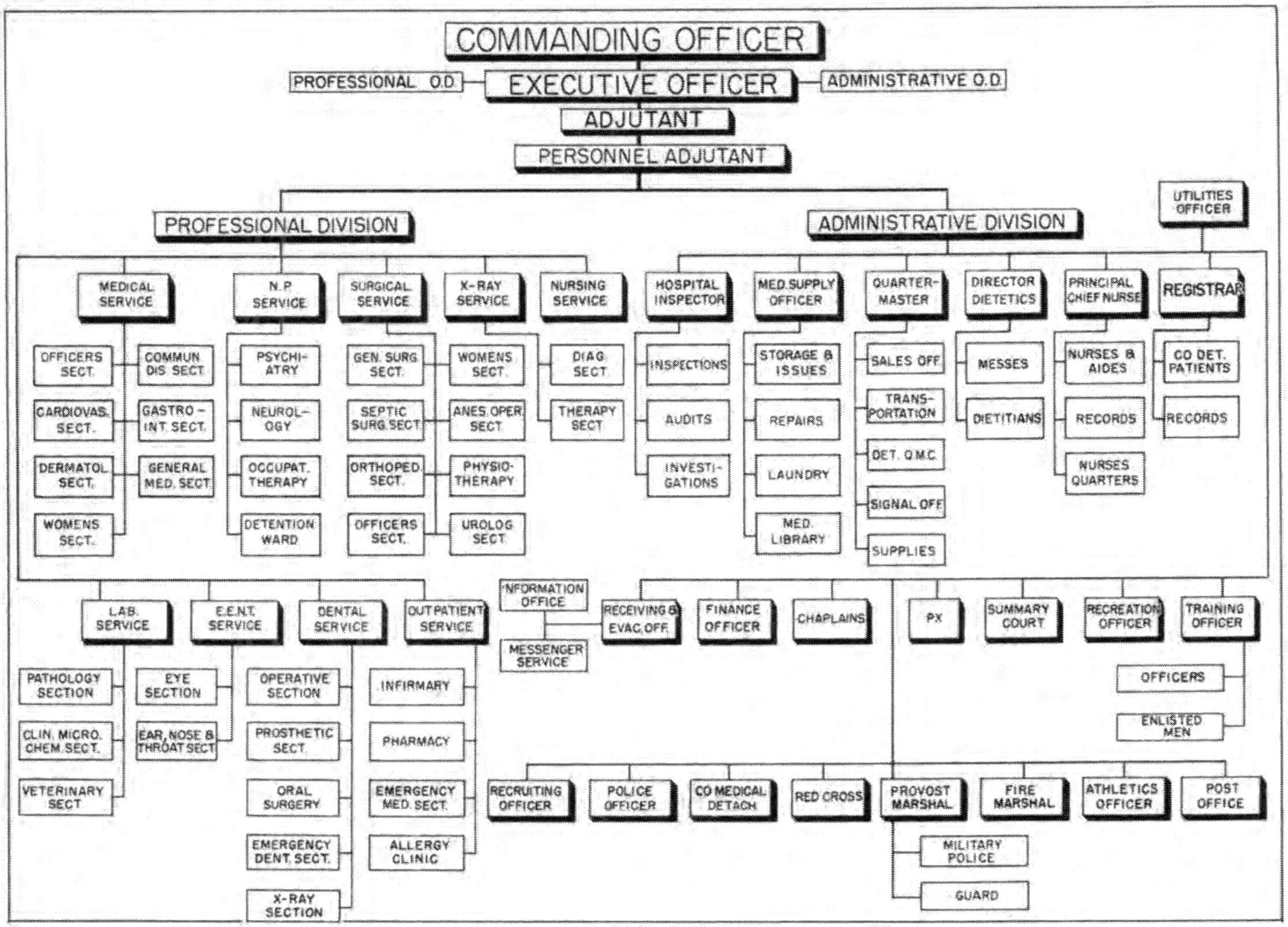

fit. Hospital regulations published in the *Army Medical Bulletin* in October 1940 and in Technical Manual 8–260 in July 1941 were probably of value to some, but officers opening new hospitals often borrowed copies of regulations and administrative forms of other hospitals to use as guides in establishing their own administrative procedures.[58]

The Surgeon General supervised and directed the professional work of hospitals through inspections by members of his Office and the issuance of technical instructions, but he exercised little direct control during this period over their administrative activities. Rather he depended on The Inspector General and corps area authorities to keep hospitals in line with Army procedures and to report administrative problems that arose.[59]

The question of whether the autonomy given hospital commanders resulted in less efficient operations than might have otherwise been the case was not discussed during the period under consideration. Arguments might have been raised in favor of flexibility which permitted accommodation to local situations. Later on, lack of uniformity in organization and administration became a subject of much discussion and efforts were made to develop standardized organizations and simplified administrative procedures.[60]

Manning of Hospitals: Manning Guides and Personnel Problems

In September 1940 there was no up-to-date guide for manning named hospitals. Since they were then small, few in number, and widely different in construction none was needed, for personnel requirements of each installation could be determined best on an individual basis. With the opening of large hospitals built on standard plans, corps area surgeons began to need a guide to use in computing requirements and distributing personnel. The only available one was a 1929 table of organization for wartime station hospitals in the zone of interior.[61] Although named hospitals were not being organized under it the General Staff early in 1940 had given the Third Corps Area permission to use this table as a guide, pending the publication of a "table for converting bed requirements into personnel requirements." Preparation of the latter in the Surgeon General's Office was delayed until December 1940, because the revision of tables of organization for field force units had priority.[62]

As submitted to the General Staff, the new guide called for more personnel, especially officers and enlisted men, than did the old one. For example, a 500-bed station hospital under the old table was to have 25 officers, 60 nurses, and 200 enlisted men; under the new guide, 37 officers, 60 nurses, and 275 enlisted men. The Surgeon General thought that the old table did not provide sufficient personnel for "a present day hospital." Although G–1 agreed that the amount called for by

[58] (1) Interv, MD Historian with Maj Gen Howard McC. Snyder, 25 May 48. HD: 000.71. (2) See also: An Rpt, 1941, Lovell Gen Hosp. HD.

[59] (1) Interv, MD Historian with Col Albert G. Love, 27 Aug 47. HD: 000.71. (2) Interv, MD Historian with Gen Snyder, 25 May 48. HD: 000.71.

[60] See below, pp. 121–24, 268–78.

[61] T/O 786 W, Sta Hosp, ZI, 1 Jul 29.

[62] (1) 2d ind, TAG to CG 3d CA, 28 Mar 40, on Ltr, Surg 3d CA to SG, 22 Jan 40, sub: Civ Employees in Sta Hosps. AG: 381 (1–1–40) Sec 1. (2) 1st ind SGO 370.01–1, SG to TAG, 9 Apr 40, on Ltr, TAG to CGs of CAs, COs of Exempted Stas, C of Arms and Servs, 28 Mar 40, same sub. Same file. (3) Ltr SGO 370.01–1, SG to TAG, 19 Dec 40, sub: Guide for Determining Pers Reqmts, Sta Hosps, ZI. AG: 381 (11–3–37) Sec 1–12.

the new guide was reasonable,[63] the Staff delayed its publication because it expressed requirements in terms of military personnel only and called for more enlisted men than the number already allotted to hospitals. The first objection was apparently removed in January 1941 when Maj. (later Col.) Arthur B. Welsh, of The Surgeon General's Planning and Training Division, stated that civilians could be substituted for enlisted men on an approximate man-for-man basis.[64] Two months later, incidentally, his superior officer, General Love, informed corps area surgeons that civilians should replace enlisted men on a three-for-two basis.[65] In view of continued disagreement among members of the General Staff over the total number of enlisted men involved, the question of publication was submitted in March 1941 to the Chief of Staff. As a result a "Guide for Determination of Medical Department Personnel" was published on 9 April 1941 with the understanding that it represented requirements, not availabilities.[66]

Publication of the guide did not mean that hospitals were to have the strength prescribed. The Surgeon General apparently had no trouble in getting the General Staff to authorize the number of physicians, dentists, and nurses whom he desired, but he encountered difficulty in procuring the number authorized.[67] During the fall and winter of 1940–41 hospitals considered the shortage of physicians and nurses acute. To alleviate it they employed civilian nurses on a temporary basis and used Medical Corps officers from field force units located near by. Medical Administrative Corps officers filled a few administrative positions, but the Army had few such officers and their substitution for Medical Corps officers in administrative work gained little headway prior to the war years. By the spring of 1941 the procurement situation had apparently improved and many hospital commanders reported that the number of officers and nurses assigned to them was adequate.[68]

The question of the number of enlisted men to be assigned to named hospitals was bound up with the use of civilian employees and the training of medical personnel. The Surgeon General contended that the Medical Department needed proportionately as many enlisted men in named hospitals during mobilization as in peacetime in order to train enlisted men in technical duties for use later as cadres and fillers for new units and installations. He insisted, therefore, that hospital staffs should have no higher proportion of civilians than 20 percent of the total enlisted

[63] (1) Memo, Act SG for ACofS G-1 WDGS, 1 Apr 41, sub: Approval of T/O for Sta Hosps in the ZI. HD: 322.052-1. (2) Memo G-1/13308-291, ACofS G-1 WDGS for ACofS G-4 WDGS, 14 Feb 41, sub: Guide for Determining Pers Reqmts, Sta Hosp, ZI. AG: 381(11-3-37) Sec 1-12.

[64] D/S G-4/31697, ACofS G-4 WDGS to TAG, 30 Dec 40, sub: Guide for Determining Pers Reqmts, Sta Hosp, ZI, and Memo G-1/13308-291, ACofS G-1 WDGS for ACofS G-4 WDGS, 8 Jan 41, same sub. AG: 381(11-7-37) Sec 1-12.

[65] Rpt, Conf of SG with CA Surgs, 10-12 Mar 41. HD: 337.

[66] (1) Memo G-1/13308-291, ACofS G-1 WDGS for ACofS G-4 WDGS, 14 Feb 41, sub: Guide for Determining Pers Reqmts, Sta Hosp, ZI. (2) Memo G-3/42107, ACofS G-3 WDGS for ACofS G-4 WDGS, 28 Feb 41, same sub. (3) Memo G-4/31697, ACofS G-4 WDGS for ACofS G-1 WDGS, 11 Mar 41, same sub. (4) Memo G-4/31697, ACofS G-4 WDGS for CofSA, 22 Mar 41, same sub. All in AG: 381(11-3-37) Sec 1-12. The Chief of Staff's stamp of approval for publication was dated 28 March 1941. (5) MR 4-2, Hospitalization, C-1, 9 Apr 41.

[67] John H. McMinn and Max Levin, Personnel (MS for companion vol. in Medical Dept. series), HD.

[68] An Apts, 1941, Hoff, O'Reilly, and Billings Gen Hosps and Sta Hosps at Cps Livingston and Forrest, Fts Knox and Jackson, and Indiantown Gap Mil Res. HD.

and civilian staff.[69] On the other hand, faced with the problem of dividing a given number of enlisted men among field force units (including numbered hospital units) and zone of interior installations of the various arms and services, the General Staff believed that civilians should constitute as much as 50 percent of the staffs of named hospitals. In this connection G–3 suggested that the Medical Department might affiliate (not explaining what it meant by this term) numbered hospital units with named hospitals to provide additional enlisted men for service in the named hospitals and at the same time to give the numbered hospital units the best possible training.[70] The Surgeon General planned to train numbered units in named hospitals, but he apparently expected the members of such units to be used not as regular operating personnel but as understudies of their opposite numbers. Repeatedly, therefore, he asked for greater allotments of enlisted men for fixed installations of the Medical Department, but without success.[71] Hence, the enlisted men authorized for assignment to general and station hospitals were fewer than The Surgeon General desired, and those received by hospitals were fewer than the number authorized. To supplement them hospitals used civilians and men from near-by field medical units, the former sometimes constituting more than half of the total enlisted and civilian staffs.[72]

In addition to having less military personnel than they considered desirable, hospitals received officers and enlisted men who needed further training. Nurses and Medical Corps Reserve officers were of course qualified by training and experience to care for the sick and injured, but most who entered the Army after September 1940 knew little about the administration of Army hospitals. In some instances this resulted in devotion of more time and energy to paper work than was ordinarily thought proper. Recognizing the need for training Reserve officers in administrative procedures before assigning them to hospitals, The Surgeon General authorized a program in November 1940 to train fifty Reserve and National Guard officers each month for such positions as registrar, detachment commander, receiving and disposition officer, adjutant, executive officer, medical supply officer, and mess officer. In general, though, the burden of training officers and nurses in administrative work fell upon the commanding officers of the hospitals to which they were assigned.[73]

A majority of enlisted men available for service in hospitals during 1941 lacked a knowledge of both military and technical matters. The number of Medical Department men in the enlisted Reserves was

[69] (1) Ltr, SG to TAG, 3 Sep 40, sub: Employment of Civs. AG: 381(1–1–40) Sec 3. (2) Ltr, SG (init J. C. M[agee]) to TAG, 6 Sep 40, sub: MD in Mob. Same file. (3) Memo, Act SG (Brig Gen A[lbert] G. Love) to ACofS G–1 WDGS, 1 Apr 41, sub: Increase in Auth for MD EM for . . . Overhead. HD: 322.052–1.

[70] Memo G–1/15081 Med, ACofS G–1 WDGS for ACofS G–3 WDGS, 13 Sep 40, sub: Allocation of MD Pers, and Memo G–3/6541 Med 68, ACofS G–3 WDGS for ACofS G–1 WDGS, same sub. AG: 381 (1–1–40) Sec 3.

[71] (1) For example, see: Memo, Act SG for ACofS G–1 WDGS, 1 Apr 41, sub: Increase in Auth for MD EM for CA, SvC, and WD Overhead. HD: 322.052–1. (2) Also see McMinn and Levin, *op. cit.*

[72] For example, see: An Rpts, 1941, Sta Hosps at Cps Blanding, Bowie, and Forrest, Fts Bragg and Knox, Indiantown Gap Mil Res, and Hoff Gen Hosp. HD.

[73] (1) Interv, MD Historian with Gen Snyder, 25 May 48. HD: 000.71. (2) An Rpts, 1940, Sta Hosps at Cps Livingston, Blanding, Edwards, Shelby, Forrest, J. T. Robinson, and Claiborne, Fts Jackson, Bragg, and Knox, and O'Reilly, Lawson, Hoff, Billings, and Tilton Gen Hosps. HD. (3) SG Ltrs 79, 7 Nov 40; 14, 26 Feb 41; and 32, 5 Apr 41.

negligible, and the Medical Department's replacement training centers and enlisted technicians' schools did not begin to turn out trained men in large numbers until the summer of 1941.[74] Regular Army enlisted men from hospitals already in operation formed the cadres of enlisted detachments of new hospitals. The remainder were usually men assigned direct from reception centers. The necessity of giving them basic military training interfered with their performance of technical duties, and hospital commanders generally preferred men from replacement training centers after they became available. To make up for the lack of technical training, hospitals instituted on-the-job training programs which varied in content and value from one installation to another.[75]

Civilians in Army hospitals were normally used in jobs traditionally held by such enlisted men as medical technicians, ward orderlies, clerks, cooks and cooks' helpers, repair and maintenance men, and janitors. In some instances civilian nurses were employed, and until the end of the first year of the war all female dietitians and physical therapy aides were in civilian status. The chief problem in the use of civilians was procurement. To reduce difficulties in that connection The Surgeon General in September 1940 decentralized to corps areas the employment of civilians for station hospitals, including those on exempted stations. He retained in his Office for a time the employment of civilians for named general hospitals.[76] Among local conditions that continued to hamper the procurement of sufficient numbers of qualified civilians, the most important were lack of housing near hospitals in isolated areas, inadequate transportation to such hospitals, absence of labor markets in some places, and competition of other government agencies for available civilians.[77]

Shortages of Supplies and Equipment

Another difficulty encountered in opening new hospitals was a shortage of suitable supplies and equipment, and complaints of hospital commanders on this score were frequent.[78] Depots met earliest needs by issuing reserves stored after World War I. As a result, much that hospitals received, such as surgical instruments, plaster of paris bandages, and ward furniture, was of 1918 vintage. When reserves proved insufficient, depots supplemented them with local emergency

[74] (1) *Annual Report of The Secretary of War, 1941* (Washington, 1941), pp. 95, 134. (2) McMinn and Levin, *op. cit.* (3) [Samuel M. Goodman], A Summary of the Training of Army Service Forces Medical Department Personnel, 1 July 1939–31 December 1944 ([1946]), pp. 38, 46–48.

[75] (1) An Rpts, 1941, Sta Hosps at Cps Livingston, Blanding, Edwards, Shelby, Forrest, J. T. Robinson, Bowie, and Claiborne, Fts Jackson, Bragg, and Knox, and O'Reilly, Lawson, Hoff, Billings, and Tilton Gen Hosps. HD.

[76] Ltr, SG (Fin and Sup Div) to Surgs CAs and Depts, 12 Sep 40, sub: Use of Civ Pers in Army Hosps, and Ltr, TAG to C of Arms and Servs, CGs of Exempted Stas, 31 Oct 40, sub: Provision for Civ Employees in Hosps of Exempted Stas. AG 381 (1-1-40) Sec 3.

[77] An Rpts, 1941, Sta Hosps at Cps Livingston, Blanding, Edwards, Shelby, Forrest, J. T. Robinson, Bowie, and Claiborne, Fts Jackson, Bragg, and Knox, and O'Reilly, Lawson, Hoff, Billings, and Tilton Gen Hosps. HD.

[78] Unless otherwise indicated, the following paragraphs are based upon annual reports of Barnes, Hoff, Lawson, and O'Reilly General Hospitals, and Camps Beauregard, Blanding, Claiborne, Croft, Forrest, Shelby, and Forts Bragg, Jackson, Lewis, and Leonard Wood Station Hospitals. In a conference on 10 November 1950, General Magee disagreed with the interpretation given here, stating that he personally found a high state of satisfaction with supplies when he inspected hospitals. (Notes filed in HD: 314 [Correspondence on MS] I.) For a statement about the general shortage of Army supplies in 1940, see Mark S. Watson, *Chief of Staff: Prewar Plans and Preparations* (Washington, 1950), p. 209, in UNITED STATES ARMY IN WORLD WAR II.

purchases but even so had to ship many assemblages 50- to 60-percent complete.[79] Hospitals thus failed initially to receive many critical items. Most frequently lacking were sterilizers, X-ray equipment, orthopedic equipment, dental operating units, cystoscopic instruments, and catheters.

To make up for shortages hospitals resorted to a variety of expedients. In some instances medical and dental officers sent home for their own instruments. At Camp Claiborne (Louisiana) they personally purchased medical supplies which they considered requisite. The station hospital at Camp Blanding (Florida) made up for its lack of laboratory supplies and equipment by borrowing from the University of Florida and the Florida State Board of Health, while the Camp Claiborne Station Hospital borrowed an X-ray developing tank from a dealer in Shreveport, Louisiana. In other instances Army authorities arranged locally to use the facilities of neighboring hospitals. For example, the Camp Beauregard (Louisiana) Station Hospital sent cases requiring X-ray and electrocardiographic work to the Veterans Administration Facility at Pineville, La.; used the diagnostic and clinical facilities of the Central Louisiana State Mental Hospital for neuropsychiatric patients; and sent fractures requiring reductions or large casts to the Baptist Hospital in Alexandria, La. Where office and ward furniture was lacking, hospitals improvised desks, chairs, and tables from boxes and lumber salvaged from the hospital's construction. Thus the improvisation and ingenuity of local personnel compensated to a great extent for shortages of supplies and equipment.

The above situation resulted initially from the inadequacy and obsolescence of the war reserve. It continued because considerable time was required both for industry to convert to the production of goods on the scale demanded and for the Medical Department to modify its peacetime methods of requirements-computation, purchasing, stock-control, storage, and distribution. Although the quantity of supplies became more adequate by the fall of 1941, the situation was by no means satisfactory at the end of the year and many items were still on "back order."[80]

Development of Procedures Affecting Operation of the Hospital System

As new station and general hospitals opened, broad policies and procedures to govern the hospital system in general became necessary and The Surgeon General's Hospitalization Division concentrated its efforts in those fields.[81] The need for a new policy to govern the selection of patients for transfer to general hospitals developed in the spring of 1941. Until that time hospital commanders and corps area surgeons decided which cases were sufficiently "serious, complicated, or obscure" to require treatment in the five general hospitals then in operation. Few restrictions were placed upon them: cases of resection and amputation requiring the fitting of prostheses were to be transferred to Walter Reed, Letterman, or Army and Navy General Hospitals; patients with tuberculosis, to Fitzsimons; and "cases of such diseases as the waters of the hot springs of Arkansas have an established reputation for benefiting," to Army and

[79] (1) Memo, Lt Col R. L. Black, Dir Storage and Maintenance Div SGO for HD SGO, 16 Nov 44, sub: Sup [Depot] Hist Highlights. HD: 400.24 (Storage and Distr). (2) Hist and Procedure Manual of the Toledo Med Depot, 1941–45. HD.

[80] Richard E. Yates, The Procurement and Distribution of Medical Supplies in the Zone of the Interior during World War II (1946), pp. 22–46. HD.

[81] Cmtee to Study the MD, 1942, Testimony of Col Harry D. Offutt, pp. 196–98. HD.

Navy.[82] To provide a more exact guide the Hospitalization Division developed a policy that was published on 26 March 1941.[83] While it did not relieve local surgeons of responsibility for selecting patients to be transferred, it provided generally that all requiring more than sixty days of hospitalization as well as those needing specialized treatment not available at station hospitals should be sent to general hospitals. Major elective[84] operations were to be performed at general hospitals only. Station hospitals were to dispose of enlisted neuropsychiatric or psychotic patients locally, but were to send officers, nurses, and warrant officers who were similarly affected or who had other disabilities which made them unfit for further military service to general hospitals for observation and disposition. Hospitals previously designated for the care and treatment of special cases were to continue to receive them as in the past.

Soon after this policy was established the Hospitalization Division developed a procedure to implement it. Under current Army regulations hospital commanders needed corps area approval for each transfer of a patient from a station to a general hospital.[85] As new hospitals opened, this requirement resulted in much paper work for corps area surgeons and in delayed treatment for patients. On 19 May 1941, therefore, The Surgeon General requested authority to set aside specific numbers of general hospital beds to which station hospitals might transfer patients without reference to corps area headquarters. The General Staff approved this request and on 21 June 1941 authorized the establishment of a system of bed credits. This permitted the Hospitalization Division to allot a certain number of beds in general hospitals to each large station hospital and, through corps area surgeons, to small ones. Thereafter post commanders normally transferred patients to general hospitals without reference to higher authority. When stations needed changes in allotments, they ordinarily requested them through corps area surgeons. In emergencies, they were authorized to communicate directly with The Surgeon General.[86]

The procedure for transferring patients from station to general hospitals was further simplified in the late summer of 1941. Until then Army regulations required each hospital to make extracts or copies of the clinical records, including case histories, of patients being transferred, to be sent along with them. As the number of patients increased, this time-consuming process began to delay their transfer and hence their treatment. The Surgeon General then secured approval of a change which permitted station hospital authorities to transfer to general hospitals, along with patients, the original clinical records of their cases. The transferring hospital kept only clinical-record briefs and cross references indicating the disposition of original records.[87]

Another problem for the Hospitalization Division was the disposition of patients. It concerned the Hospital Construction and Repair Subdivision also, for prompt disposition of patients reduces total bed requirements by making available for patient care more of the beds al-

[82] (1) AR 40–600, Gen Hosp, Gen Provisions, 31 Dec 34. (2) Mins, SGO Conf with CA Surgs, 10–12 Mar 41. SG: 337.–1.

[83] (1) SG Ltr 24, 26 Mar 41. (2) *Annual Report . . . Surgeon General, 1941* (1941), p. 253.

[84] Advantageous to the patient but not necessary to save life.

[85] AR 40–600, par 4 *a* (1), 31 Dec 34.

[86] (1) Ltr, SG to TAG, 19 May 41, sub: Trf of Pnts to Gen Hosps. SG: 705.–1. (2) WD Cir 120, 21 Jun 41.

[87] (1) Ltr, Brig Gen H. D. Offutt to Col H. W. Doan, 10 Jun 48, annex 1. HD: 322. (2) WD Cir 184, 26 Aug 41. (3) SG Ltr 94, 16 Sep 41.

ready set up. During 1941 there was considerable local dissatisfaction with difficulties and delays encountered in granting patients disability discharges from the Army. Believing that lack of experience on the part of many medical officers was responsible, one corps area surgeon issued a directive in 1940 to clarify procedures for handling such cases.[88] In general, the centralization in corps area headquarters of authority to discharge men on certificates of disability, rather than inefficient hospital procedures, seems to have been considered the most important reason for delays.[89] Apparently sharing this view, The Surgeon General secured authority in September 1941 for the commanders of general hospitals to grant disability discharges. At the same time, it should be noted, the War Department was further decentralizing such authority to other local commanders, including those of divisions, reception centers, replacement training centers, and exempted stations. The Surgeon General also secured authority for general hospital commanders to issue travel orders for men returning to duty or being discharged from the Army.[90]

In the fall of 1941 the Chief of Staff became concerned about delays in the retirement of disabled officer-patients. When General Marshall called a case of this kind to his attention, The Surgeon General replied that such delays were "chronic" but that they occurred in large part in Army administrative channels after general hospitals had completed their work and made their recommendations. Soon afterward he directed general hospital commanders to "personally assure themselves that the disposition of officer patients is expedited insofar as this can be done without prejudice to the interest of the individual or of the Government."[91] Further steps to speed the disposition of officer-patients were not taken at this time.

Partial simplification of the procedure for granting disability discharges went some distance, though not as far as possible, toward relieving Army hospitals of patients who were unnecessarily occupying beds. Action was also taken to relieve hospitals of certain other patients—that is, some of those suffering from tuberculosis, psychosis, and other chronic diseases. At the beginning of mobilization the President approved a recommendation of the Federal Board of Hospitalization that members of the armed forces who were injured or incurred disabilities "in line of duty" and whose physical rehabilitation by the Army or Navy was not feasible should be cared for by the Veterans Administration. Accordingly the Surgeon General's Office secured approval in March 1941 for the transfer to the Veterans Administration of most enlisted men who were permanently disabled by the development of pulmonary tuberculosis. Two months later this provision was extended to all classes of chronic disability cases. Three classes of tuberculous patients—those nearing retirement after thirty years of service, those in the first three noncommissioned grades whose recovery was probable within a year, and those whose cases were considered not to have been incurred in line of duty—were to be kept in the Army and transferred to Fitzsimons General Hospital. As soon as

[88] An Rpt, 1940, Surg 2d CA. HD.

[89] Rpt, Conf of SG with CA Surgs, 10–12 Mar 41. HD: 337.

[90] (1) Cmtee to Study the MD, 1942, Testimony of Col Offutt, pp. 196–98. HD. (2) WD Cirs 194, 17 Sep 41; 196, 19 Sep 41; and 187, 4 Sep 41.

[91] (1) Memo, CofSA for SG, 23 Sep 41. (2) Memo, CG WRGH for SG, 26 Sep 41. (3) Ltr, SG to COs Gen Hosps, n d, sub: Disposition of Off Pnts. (4) Memo, Act SG to CofSA, 6 Oct 41, same sub. All in SG: 705.-1. (5) WD Cir 217, 15 Oct 41.

patients in the last group were able, they were to be discharged to their own care or that of relatives.[92]

The removal of psychotic patients from Army hospitals was more complicated. Many could not be transferred to the Veterans Administration because their disabilities had existed before induction. State institutions were often reluctant to accept those who required care in locked wards. As a result psychotic patients began to accumulate in Army hospitals. Early in the mobilization period a large three-story section of Walter Reed General Hospital was converted into closed wards and the Medical Department arranged to use, as an annex to that section, 100 beds in St. Elizabeth's Hospital in Washington. One or two closed wards more than had been planned were constructed at each new general hospital erected during 1941. In the summer of that year, after Walter Reed General Hospital had demonstrated the rather elementary fact that transfer of psychotic patients to state institutions was expedited by addressing requests to proper state agencies or authorities, The Surgeon General issued a circular letter naming those in each state. About the same time his Office arranged to establish a special neuropsychiatric center in the just-completed and unused State Hospital at Danville, Ky. Called Darnall General Hospital, it was ready to receive patients a few months after the Japanese attacked Pearl Harbor.[93]

Starting almost from scratch in September 1939, the Medical Department reached a state of partial preparation for war by December 1941. To provide hospitals for a rapidly expanding Army in the United States, a simple method of computing requirements was adopted and ratios of beds to troop strength—smaller than The Surgeon General considered desirable—were officially established. Experience in expanding hospital facilities showed that it was impracticable to rely upon the use of existing Army hospitals and available non-Army buildings. It also revealed imperfections and shortcomings in cantonment-type hospitals planned in the thirties, with the result that a new type of hospital more compact and fire resistant was developed. As new hospitals opened, the Surgeon General's Office evolved general guides for their organization and administration but left hospital commanders with much autonomy in this field. Attention was focused not upon internal hospital administration but upon simplifying procedures affecting the hospital system in general. In this connection attempts were made to reduce unnecessary occupancy of beds by patients no longer needing treatment or of no further use to the Army. There were shortages of personnel, though authorized allotments for hospitals were generous, and it was necessary in many instances to substitute civilians for enlisted men. Shortages of supplies and equipment were alleviated by the ingenuity of hospital commanders and their staffs. Meanwhile, the Surgeon General's Office was also concerned with plans and preparations for overseas hospitalization, the subject to which the discussion now turns.

[92] (1) *Annual Report . . . Surgeon General, 1941* (1941), p. 253. (2) Ltr SGO 300.3-1, SG to TAG, 7 Apr 41, sub: Proposed Change in AR 615-360. AG: 220.8 (8-1-34) Case 1. (3) WD Cirs 100, 19 May 41; 44, 17 Mar 41; 226, 27 Oct 41; and 252, 11 Dec 41.

[93] (1) Ltr, Brig Gen H. D. Offutt to Col H. W. Doan, 10 Jun 48, incl. 1. HD: 322. (2) Ltr, SG to QMG, 17 Dec 40, sub: Add Fac for the Care of Insane, and 1st ind QM 632 C-EP (Gen Hosp), QMG to SG, 31 Jan 41. SG: 632.-1. (3) SG Ltr 64, 24 Jun 41, sub: Disposition of NP Pnts. (4) *Annual Report . . . Surgeon General, 1941* (1941), p. 165.

CHAPTER III

Plans and Preparations for Hospitalization in Overseas Areas

Mobilization Planning

Planning for field hospitalization in the event of mobilization involved determination of the numbers and types of medical units that would be needed for the force anticipated, provision of up-to-date guides for their organization and equipment, and arrangements for furnishing them with personnel and supplies. Until the fall of 1940 the defensive nature of all War Department mobilization planning combined with limitations upon available funds to hold Medical Department activities in this sphere largely within the realm of paper work.

Determining the Number of Medical Units Needed

Determination of the number of mobile medical units that would be needed was governed primarily by the number of combat units authorized. Each combat organization such as a regiment or division had a standard structure consisting of a specific number of units of the several arms and services, including medical, that were "organic" parts of the larger unit. Thus units designed to provide emergency medical care and transportation for patients in divisional areas of combat zones were automatically required along with the regiments and divisions of which they were a part. The organization of corps and armies, though not strictly governed by tables of organization, was also standardized. On recommendation of The Surgeon General in the winter of 1939 a "type army" (that is, a standard army) was authorized 3 medical regiments, 10 evacuation hospitals, 8 surgical hospitals, 1 convalescent hospital, 1 medical laboratory, and 1 medical supply depot. A corps was authorized either a medical regiment or a medical battalion. Other medical units varying in kind and number might be authorized as a General Headquarters (GHQ) reserve force. In July 1940 the War Department Protective Mobilization Plan listed as mobile medical units, for an anticipated force of approximately 1,150,000 men, 8 medical regiments, 5 "reinforcing" medical battalions, 1 horse-drawn ambulance company, 1 medical troop, 17 evacuation hospitals, 13 surgical hospitals, 1 convalescent hospital, 2 medical laboratories, 2 medical supply depots, and certain other miscellaneous units.[1]

There was no standard number of fixed medical units such as station and general hospitals for given combat forces. To estimate the number needed the Surgeon General's Office again turned to Colonel Love's analysis of World War I battle casualty experience. From this study some members of the Planning and Training Division believed that beds in fixed hospitals should equal 15 percent of a theater's strength. Others believed a lower ratio would suffice.[2] The Surgeon General indicated in his Protective Mobilization Plan of 1939 that 126,000 fixed beds would be needed by the end of the first year of mobilization.[3] The War Department Plan provided for only 35,000—in 32 general hospitals, 4 station hospitals, and 2 hospital centers. The Surgeon General considered this provision "alarmingly inadequate" and attempted during 1940 to secure an increase both in the number of beds authorized and in their scheduled rate of availability. In February he submitted a study showing that a minimum of 115,000 fixed beds would be required, but because G–3 believed that the majority of troops to be mobilized should be allotted to combat arms, The Surgeon General's recommendations received only partial approval. On 6 August 1940 the General Staff authorized an increase in the number of 1,000-bed general hospitals from 32 to 102. The number of station hospitals and hospital centers remained as originally planned.[4] *(Table 1)*

Revision of Tables of Organization and Equipment Lists

As a part of its mobilization planning the Surgeon General's Office undertook a general revision of tables of organization of all medical units and the preparation of up-to-date equipment lists for them. Although these projects had been started earlier, only the equipment list for medical regiments and the tables of organization for medical regiments and squadrons had been completed by the fall of 1939. After the President declared an emergency this work was pushed to completion by the end of 1940.

Changes in the tables of organization of medical units that supplied emergency medical care and transportation for patients in combat zones reflected changes in combat units to increase their mobility and flexibility. When the infantry division was "streamlined" and converted from a "square" to a "triangular" organization, its organic medical unit was reduced from a regiment to a battalion and appropriate tables for the latter were prepared. Likewise, the medical battalion eventually be-

[1] (1) Kent R. Greenfield, Robert R. Palmer, and Bell I. Wiley, *The Organization of Ground Combat Troops* (Washington, 1947), pp. 263–68, 275–80, in UNITED STATES ARMY IN WORLD WAR II. (2) 1st ind, SG to TAG, 11 Oct 39, on Ltr, TAG to C of Arms and Servs, 3 Oct 39, sub: Orgn of Army Troops. AG: 320.2(9-27-39)(1). (3) Ltr 320.3-1, SG to ACofS G-3 WDGS, 13 Jul 40, sub: Corps Med Units and Atchd Med, and Army Med Regts. HD: McKinney files. (4) War Department Protective Mobilization Plan, 1940, Annex No. 7, Pt. I. AG: Budget Div, WDGS files, A-45-7.

[2] Memo, GLM [Col Garfield L. McKinney] for Col [Albert G.] Love, 6 Feb 40. HD: McKinney files.

[3] SG PMP, 1939, Annex No. 29, Chart No 2.

[4] (1) Ltr, SG to TAG, 15 Feb 40, sub: Hosp under WD PMP 1939. AG: 381 (5-10-40) G-4/20052-134. (2) Ltr, SG to TAG, 8 Jul 40, sub: Hosp under WD PMP. 1939, with 1st ind AG 381 (7-8-40)M-C, TAG to SG, 6 Aug 40. HD: 370.01-1. (3) Memo G-3/6541-Med-64, ACofS G-3 WDGS for Sec Gen Staff, 14 Apr 40, sub: Status of MD for War. AG: 381 (4-6-40) (1). (4) The War Department Mobilization Plan, speech by Lt Col Harry L. Twaddle, GSC, Chief Mob Br G-3 Div WDGS, 30 Sep 39. G-3 Course No 13 and 13A, AWC, 1939-40.

TABLE 1—COMPARISON OF THE WAR DEPARTMENT'S PLAN AND THE SURGEON GENERAL'S RECOMMENDATION FOR FIXED BEDS FOR THEATERS OF OPERATIONS

Days of Mobilization	War Department Plan			The Surgeon General's Recommendation		
	Gen Hosp	Sta Hosp	Hosp Ctr	Gen Hosp	Sta Hosp	Hosp Ctr
M-Day	....	....	....	....	....	....
M+10/11	....	....	....	1,000	....	....
M+30/31	....	....	....	8,000	....	....
M+60/61	3,000	....	....	32,000	1,000	2,000
M+90/91	3,000	....	....	36,000	2,000	2,000
M+120/121	22,000	1,000	2,000	43,000	3,000	4,000
M+150/151	32,000	1,000	2,000	52,000	3,000	5,000
M+180/181	32,000	1,000	2,000	72,000	3,000	5,000
M+210/211	32,000	1,000	2,000	84,000	3,000	7,000
M+240/241	32,000	1,000	2,000	92,000	3,000	9,000
M+270/271	32,000	1,000	2,000	96,000	3,000	10,000
M+300	32,000	1,000	2,000	99,000	3,000	10,000
M+330	32,000	1,000	2,000	101,000	3,000	10,000
M+360	32,000	1,000	2,000	102,000	3,000	10,000

Source: Study accompanying ltr, SG to TAG, 14 Feb 40, sub: Hosp under WD PMP 1939. AG: 381 (5-10-40) G-4/20052-134.

came the organic unit of a corps. Plans for the organization of armored divisions required the preparation of tables of organization for medical units of that type of combat organization. In 1940 the tables of medical regiments and squadrons were again revised. Generally there was a tendency to increase the personnel in medical units of all sizes and to replace animal-drawn with motor vehicles. Basically, none of the changes made altered the Medical Department's long-established doctrine of hospitalization and evacuation in combat zones.[5]

Changes in tables of organization of hospital units reflected a growth in specialized medicine. New tables published during 1940 listed for the first time the specialists required as ward officers and chiefs of sections of professional services. They also allotted to hospitals more enlisted men having specialists' ratings and correspondingly fewer having only basic military training. For the first time, they provided for civilian dietitians, physical-therapy aides, and dental hygienists. In many cases the total number of officers and enlisted men was increased. For example, in a 1,000-bed general hospital the number of officers rose from 42, of whom 30 were physicians, to 73, of whom 55 were physicians, and of enlisted men from 400 to 500. These changes, the Surgeon General's Office believed, would enable military hospital units "to perform the necessary additional specialized medical

[5] (1) Documents on the revisions are in SG: 320.3-1, 1939 and 1940. (2) History of Organization and Equipment Allowance Branch [SGO], 1939-44. HD. (3) Ltr, Surg 4th CA to Corps and Div Surgs, 26 Mar 40, sub: Third Army Maneuvers. HD: McKinney files. (4) Memo, Capt Thomas N. Page for [Brig.] Gen [Albert G.] Love, 28 Dec 40, sub: Activities of the Planning Subdiv [SGO]. HD: McKinney files.

and surgical work required, in order to approach the standards of medicine and surgery as practiced in first class civilian hospitals. . . ."[6]

Although no new hospital unit was developed during the emergency period, a change in the surgical hospital indicated the Medical Department's awareness of the problem of developing a highly mobile unit to care for seriously wounded casualties near the front lines. The single-unit 250-bed surgical hospital developed after World War I was replaced by a new 400-bed surgical hospital to be organized under a table of organization issued on 1 December 1940.[7] Similar in some respects to the "mobile hospital" adapted from the French *auto-chir* during World War I,[8] the new hospital comprised a headquarters and three subordinate elements: a mobile surgical unit and two 200-bed hospitalization units. Each of the latter had its own headquarters. Since each subordinate unit was capable of independent operation, the surgical unit would be free to move forward, as soon as one hospitalization unit was immobilized with patients, to operate for the other hospitalization unit or to supplement the facilities of other medical stations. Some of the surgical units, the Surgeon General's Office anticipated, would have complete operating, sterilizing, X-ray, and medical supply rooms permanently installed on bus-type or van-type motor vehicles.[9]

Along with revised tables of organization, new equipment lists were prepared. At the beginning of 1939 the only ones available were shipping lists used during World War I. Like the medical supply catalog, they contained many articles that were obsolete and lacked others that had been developed in intervening years. To enable medical units to give modern medical and surgical treatmet, it was necessary to find out from manufacturers what articles were available and to analyze the functions and activities of each unit, from reveille to taps, to determine which were needed. Another factor, the transportation of units to theaters of operations, had to be considered. To conserve shipping tonnage an attempt was made to include only indispensable articles in equipment lists. This work was done by Colonel Offutt, assigned to the Army Medical Center in January 1939 and later transferred to the Surgeon General's Office. He collaborated with the Medical Field Service School (Carlisle Barracks, Pennsylvania), Walter Reed General Hospital, and The Surgeon General's Supply Division and Planning and Training Division. The first list completed (in June 1939) was for the medical regiment. Others—including those for hospitals—followed during the remainder of 1939 and the first ten months of 1940. As rapidly as they were approved by the Surgeon General's Office they were mimeographed and sent to the various medical supply depots. Concurrently, the table of basic allowances for the Medical Department was revised by The Surgeon

[6] (1) The above paragraph is based largely on a comparison of the following T/Os: Gen Hosps, T/O 683W (6 Jun 32) with T/O 8-507 (25 Jul 40); Sta Hosp, T/O 684W (1 Jul 29) with T/O 8-508 (25 Jul 40) and Evac Hosp, T/O 283W (1 Jul 29) with T/O 8-232 (1 Oct 40). (2) See also Ltr, SG to TAG, 11 Jul 40, sub: Publication of T/O 8-508 and T/O 8-507. AG: 320.6 (Med) (4-18-40) (1).

[7] T/O 8-231 (1 Dec 40) superseded T/O 284W (1 Jul 29).

[8] *The Medical Department . . . in the World War* (1925), vol. VIII, pp. 184-91.

[9] (1) Ltr, Maj Frank B. Wakeman, SGO to Lt Col Guy B. Denit, MC, C&GS Sch, Ft Leavenworth, 11 Feb 41. SG: 322.3-1. (2) For documents on the experimental development of these vehicles see SG: 322.15-17.

General's Planning and Training Division and was published on 1 November 1940.[10]

Efforts to Assure Availability of Equipment and Personnel for Units Planned

Revision of equipment lists emphasized the importance of modernizing World War I unit assemblages in storage. After the war in Europe began, Surgeon General Magee requested funds for this purpose. In April and again in May 1940 he informed the General Staff of the Medical Department's unpreparedness for war, stating: "I have not at the War Department's disposal for any emergency one complete, modern 1,000-bed general hospital for instant dispatch." [11] Funds which the General Staff could secure were limited.[12] Moreover, believing that The Surgeon General failed to recognize that increases in industrial capacity since World War I would make procurement easier and faster, G-4 opposed "piecemeal action" which favored the Medical Department alone. Hence the Staff only promised "consideration" of Medical Department requirements along with those of other services, and it was not until the month before the passage of the Selective Service Act that substantial funds for Medical Department equipment were included in the War Department's budget requests.[13]

To provide professional staffs for hospitals included in the Protective Mobilization Plan, The Surgeon General early in 1940 began to arrange with civilian medical institutions for the organization of authorized affiliated units. By June 1940 he requested an increase in their number, stating that the response of sponsoring institutions was more enthusiastic than he had expected. The next month the General Staff raised the numbers authorized to 68 general, 30 evacuation, and 23 surgical hospital units. About a year later the Surgeon General's Office reported success in the organization of affiliated units for 41 general, 11 evacuation, and 4 surgical hospitals—approximately the number originally authorized in 1939.[14]

Attempts to secure enlisted men for training in hospital units were only partially successful. Although draftees could be used to fill units scheduled for activation during mobilization, trained cadres would be required for each one and some units would have to be ready for action on M Day. Therefore some men needed to be trained in units before mobilization. Increases in the authorized enlisted strength of the Army during 1939 and 1940 and in the authorized strength of the Medical Department in May 1940 from 5 to 7 percent of Army's strength afforded some additional men. Since most of them were needed for organic medical units of divisions or for expanding named hospitals,

[10] (1) Hist of Basic Equip Lists for Med T/O Orgns, incl 2, to Ltr, Brig Gen Harry D. Offutt to Col H. W. Doan, 10 Jun 48. HD: 322. (2) Memo, Capt Thomas N. Page for Gen Love, 28 Dec 40, sub: Activities of the Planning Subdiv [SGO]. HD: McKinney files.

[11] Ltrs, SG to TAG, 6 Apr and 10 May 40, sub: Status of the MD for War. AG: 381 (4-6-40) (1).

[12] Mark S. Watson, *Chief of Staff: Prewar Plans and Preparations* (Washington, 1950), pp. 156-66, in UNITED STATES ARMY IN WORLD WAR II.

[13] (1) Memo G-4/20052-134, ACofS G-4 WDGS for CofSA, 20 Apr 40, sub: Status of MD for War. AG: 381(4-6-40) (1). (2) Ltr, TAG to SG, 23 May 40, same sub. Same file. (3) Memo G-4/20052-134, Act ACofS G-4 WDGS for CofSA, 19 Aug 40, same sub. (Marked "not used.") AG: 381(5-10-40).

[14] (1) Ltr, SG to Each Affiliating Inst, 16 May 40, sub: Affiliated Units, MD, USA. HD: 326.01-1. (2) Ltr, SG to TAG, 26 Jun 40, same sub, with 1st ind AG 381(6-26-40)M-A, TAG to SG, 22 Jul 40. Same file. (3) *Annual Report . . . Surgeon General, 1941* (1941), p. 145. (4) John H. McMinn and Max Levin, Personnel (MS for companion vol. in Medical Dept. series), HD.

the General Staff at first allotted none at all to nonorganic medical units and numbered hospitals. Insisting upon the necessity of training men in such units, The Surgeon General secured authority in June 1940 for the organization, along with one medical laboratory and one medical supply depot, of two evacuation and two surgical hospital units at half their table-of-organization enlisted strength, but it was not until 1 August 1940 that the first of these was activated.[15]

Preparing Hospitalization for Overseas Areas During a Peacetime Mobilization

Mobilization of the Army for a year of peacetime training reversed the situation which had been anticipated in mobilization plans. Instead of field medical units such as regimental medical detachments, medical battalions, medical regiments, and numbered hospitals to support combat forces engaged in defensive operations, the greatest need was for named hospitals in the United States. Hence, they had first call upon medical personnel and equipment. Moreover, since the United States was not at war, additional hospitalization required in bases and possessions outside its continental limits was provided on a peacetime basis—that is, in named hospitals. Nevertheless, medical units had to be organized and trained along with the combat forces they were designed to support.

Activation of Field Medical Units

When mobilization began in September 1940 the Army had, aside from the medical units that were organic parts of existing divisions, only the following field medical units: 2 surgical hospitals, 2 evacuation hospitals, 2 medical regiments, 1 medical supply depot, and 1 medical laboratory.[16] Additional organic medical units would be activated and trained along with their parent units, such as infantry divisions. Their number depended upon the number of parent units that would be called into being by the General Staff. The number of nonorganic units—those serving with armies, corps, and General Headquarters—that would be activated for training might differ from the number needed for combat operations. In anticipation of the passage of the Selective Service Act, The Surgeon General had recommended in July 1940 the activation at half strength of all such units in the Protective Mobilization Plan except hospital centers, hospital trains, the auxiliary surgical group, and the general dispensary.[17] The General Staff partially adopted this recommendation in preparing the 1941 troop basis. In December 1940, it authorized the following corps, army, and GHQ medical units: 8 medical battalions, 8 medical regiments, 1 medical supply depot, 1 medical laboratory, 1 general dispensary, 15 evacuation hospitals, 6 surgical hospitals, 22 general hospitals, and 22 station hospitals.[18] Approximately half of these

[15] (1) Memo, ACofS G-1 WDGS for TAG, 6 Nov 39, sub: Enl Pers, MD. G-1: 15081-Med. (2) Ltr AG 320.2 (5-13-40)M-D, TAG to SG, 14 May 40, sub: Adequacy of Serv Units as Contained in Proposed Trp Basis, with 1st ind, SG to TAG, 20 May 40. SG: 320.2-1. (3) Memo, SG for ACofS G-3 WDGS, 26 Jun 40, sub: Sta Lists. HD: McKinney files. (4) McMinn and Levin, *op. cit.*

[16] (1) *Annual Report . . . Surgeon General, 1940* (1941), p. 175, and *1941* (1941), p. 153. (2) Unit cards of the 1st and 3d Evac Hosps, 6th and 7th Surg Hosps, 2d Med Lab, and 4th Med Sup Depot. HD.

[17] Ltr SGO 370.01-1, SG to TAG, 17 Jul 40, sub: Mob of MD Units in President's Tng Mob, PMP. AG: 381(1-1-40) Sec 3.

[18] Ltr AG 320.2 (11-15-40)M(Ret) M-C, to CGs of all Armies *et al.*, 16 Dec 40, sub: Constitution and Activation of Units. AG: 320.2(11-15-40)(1) Sec 1.

units were to be activated in February 1941 and the rest in June. Early in 1941 the Staff revised the troop basis, and authorized an additional medical battalion and two additional medical regiments. By the end of June 1941 all of the units authorized had been activated. The next month two additional station hospital units were provided when two provisional hospitals, organized but not needed for a task force, were redesignated as numbered hospitals. Although plans were made later in the year for additional units, no more were authorized until after war came.[19]

Role of Hospital Units; Their Personnel and Equipment

Confusion existed about the purpose of the hospital units activated during this period. The character of the mobilization and the nature of the international situation were perhaps responsible for this. Under the Selective Service Act, Reservists and draftees could not legally be made to serve outside the United States except in its territories and possessions. Nevertheless, the Army being mobilized had to be prepared for action anywhere in the event of a threat to the security of the country.

The Surgeon General seems to have regarded authorized hospital units as primarily if not exclusively schools for tactical training that would furnish cadres for other similar units or would provide trained enlisted men as fillers for the hospitals that would be called up in case of war—that is, the affiliated units. Along with shortages of personnel and equipment and demands of named hospitals for both, this view undoubtedly influenced his recommendations and plans for supplying hospital units with these elements. As tactical training units, numbered hospitals would need—in The Surgeon General's opinion—officers and equipment for unit administration and field training only. Their enlisted members would be given technical training in named hospitals or in enlisted technicians' schools. Moreover, full assemblages of equipment and complete officer staffs were not available for numbered hospitals. Therefore, The Surgeon General planned to issue only field training equipment to numbered hospital units and he recommended that few officers, from two to five, should be assigned to each.[20]

The General Staff considered the 1941 hospital units not as training schools but as true hospitals which could operate in the United States (presumably on maneuvers) or in theaters of operations "in the event of an emergency." On 3 January 1941 it issued a letter to that effect.[21] Despite this view, the Staff adopted The Surgeon General's recommendation that hospital units be given only part of their personnel—perhaps because of the shortage of men and officers to meet various needs and demands.[22] Those formed dur-

[19] (1) *Annual Report . . . Surgeon General, 1941* (1941), pp. 153–54. (2) An Rpt, 1941, Surg GHQ. HD. (3) Ltr AG 320.2(5-14-41)MC-C-M, TAG to CofS GHQ; CGs of all Armies, CAs, and Depts; C of Arms and Servs, etc, 22 Nov 41, sub: Revision of Trp Unit Basis, FY 1942. SG: 320.2-1. (4) An Rpts, 1941, 267th and 168th Sta Hosps. HD.

[20] (1) Ltr cited n. 17. (2) *Annual Report . . . Surgeon General, 1941* (1941), p. 154. (3) 1st ind SGO 322.15–17. (Ft Knox)N, SG to Surg Ft Knox, 10 Sep 40, on Ltr, CO 6th Surg Hosp to SG, 5 Sep 40, sub: T/O&E. HD: McKinney files. (4) Ltr, SG to TAG, 25 Feb 41, sub: Unit Assemblages, with 3 inds. SG: 475.5–1.

[21] Ltr AG 322.2(12-6-40)M–C–M, TAG to CofS GHQ, CGs of Armies, *et al.*, 3 Jan 41, sub: Purpose and Tng of Certain MC Units to be Activated with Sel Serv Men. SG: 322.3–1.

[22] Ltr AG 111 (12–23–40)M–C–M, TAG to CofS GHQ; CGs Armies, CAs, and Depts, 31 Dec 40, sub: Trp Basis, PMP, 1941. AWC: 160–93.

ing 1941 received initially, in addition to cadres of Regular Army enlisted men, from two to five officers each and only enough selectees—either from reception centers or from replacement training centers—to provide them with about half of their table-of-organization enlisted strength.[23]

The position of the Staff on equipment differed from The Surgeon General's. In December 1940 it announced a supply policy for all Army units—they would obtain complete issues of authorized equipment, except controlled items (that is, those in short supply and issued only on special instructions by the War Department), by submitting requisitions to corps area headquarters. Two weeks later it issued another directive making this policy applicable specifically to Medical Department units,[24] but a shortage of supplies and equipment made compliance with this directive impossible when hospital units were first activated in 1941.[25]

Toward the middle of 1941 the views of The Surgeon General on the purpose of hospital units began to coincide with those of the General Staff. By that time he had been required to provide medical complements for hospitals being established in new overseas commands and to prepare medical support for task forces being formed to occupy the French West Indies when it was feared that area might fall into German hands.[26] For these purposes he drew personnel from named hospitals in the United States. In May 1941 he informed G–3 that he was having considerable difficulty in providing hospitals for "task forces destined for early dispatch." Explaining that he had to collect medical personnel from many scattered sources for this purpose, he pointed out that this was not only a disorderly process but also a threat to the medical service of the hospitals from which personnel was drawn. He therefore asked G–3 to authorize full complements of officers, nurses, and enlisted men for seventeen of the hospitals activated earlier in 1941. This would simplify the problem, he thought, of converting training units into functional units. At the same time he requested authority to withhold from such units all supplies and equipment, except training equipment, individual equipment, motor transportation, and controlled items, until their assignment to missions involving medical care.[27] Early in July the Staff approved sufficient increases in the personnel of eleven—but not seventeen—units to bring their number of enlisted men up to almost full table-of-organization strength and of officers and nurses up to 50 and 75 percent respectively. The Staff also approved The Surgeon General's proposal to withold the issuance of full hospital equipment to these

[23] An Rpts, 1941, 4th, 6th, 10th, 11th, 15th, 19th, 23d, and 27th Evac Hosps; 28th, 33d, 48th, 61st, 62d, and 74th Surg Hosps; 1st, 5th, 7th, 10th, 11th, 12th, 22d, 47th, and 109th Sta Hosps; and 53d, 56th, 63d, 66th, 148th, 208th, 209th, 210th, 212th, 213th, and 214th Gen Hosps. HD.

[24] (1) Ltr, TAG to CofS GHQ; CGs Armies, CAs, *et al.*, 30 Dec 40, sub: Current Sup Policies and Procedure. AG: 475 (8–12–40) (1) Sec 1. (2) Ltr AG 320.2(11–16–40)M–D–M, TAG to same, 14 Jan 41, sub: Orgn, Tng, and Admin of Med Units. SG: 322.3–1.

[25] (1) Equipment for only three hospital units was available in medical supply depots in June 1941. Memo for Record on Memo, Act ACofS G–4 WDGS for TAG, 13 Oct 41, sub: Equip forMed Units. . . . HRS: G–4/33344. (2) See An Rpts of numbered hosps cited above. HD.

[26] (1) See below, pp. 48 and 49. (2) An Rpts, 1943, 167th and 168th Sta Hosps. HD. These hospitals were originally organized as provisional hospitals, Station Hospitals A and B, for service with a task force being organized for the occupation of the French West Indies.

[27] Memo, SG for ACofS G–3 WDGS, 27 May 41, sub: Med Units, Task Forces. . . . AG: 320.2(5–27–41)(6).

eleven units, thus sanctioning, at least for this group, the practice already followed. The next month, G–4 refused to grant The Surgeon General's request to approve this practice as policy for all other numbered hospital units. Accordingly, when a "War Department Pool of Task Force Units" was formed in August 1941, raising the total number of hospital units earmarked for actual operations from eleven to thirty-one, different supply procedures prevailed for the two groups.[28]

In the fall of 1941 the difference of opinion about issuing hospital assemblages reached a crucial point when G–4 noted that only four assemblages had been completed by October, that demands of the Philippine Army and lend-lease aid might seriously interfere with the completion of others, and that, according to its observers, hospital units participating in maneuvers needed full issues of equipment. Accordingly G–4 asked The Surgeon General for recommendations on speeding up the equipment of units in the task force pool.[29] In reply The Surgeon General pointed to progress, stating on 5 November 1941 that five hospital assemblages had been issued, that twenty others were ready for issuance, and that still others were being packed. He attributed delays to slow deliveries by manufacturers and again requested permission to hold assemblages in depots until hospital units were assigned to missions involving the actual care of patients. In support of this request he argued that units in training did not need full equipment, storage for it in the field was inadequate, careless handling by unit members would cause breakage and deterioration, and units would be unable to repack assemblages for shipment.[30] Maintaining its position but recognizing the possibility of warehousing shortages, G–4 began a survey of corps area storage facilities on 6 December 1941 and directed The Surgeon General to earmark and hold all available equipment for specific units until further notified.[31]

Training and Use of Hospital Units

In accord with The Surgeon General's plan—that members of hospital units would receive tactical training in units but technical training in named hospitals—numbered hospital units were generally stationed near named hospitals, but confusion existed about the command that was responsible for their training and use. With the separation of field forces from

[28] (1) Ltr, TAG to CGs 2d, 3d, 4th, 7th, 8th, and 9th CAs, and SG, 7 Jul 41, sub: Orgn of Med Units. AG: 320.2 (5–27–41) (6). (2) Ltr, SG to TAG, 17 Jul 41, sub: Sup of Med Units, and 1st ind, TAG to SG, 6 Aug 41. SG: 475.5–1. (3) Ltr, AG 381 (7–28–41) MC–E–M, TAG to CofS GHQ, CGs of Armies *et al.*, 20 Aug 41, sub: Units for Emergency Expeditionary Forces. SG: 322.3–1.

[29] (1) Memo, Act ACofS G–4 WDGS for TAG, 13 Oct 41, sub: Equip of Med Units for WD Pool of Task Forces, with Memo for Record. HRS: G–4/33344. (2) 1st ind, SG to TAG, 16 Oct 41, and 2d ind, TAG to SG, 27 Oct 41, on Ltr, TAG to SG, 14 Oct 41, sub: Equip of Med Units for WD Pool of Task Forces. AG: 320.2(5–27–41)(6). (3) Memo G–4/33344, Lt Col Clarence P. Townsley, GSC, Chief Planning Sec [G–4] (init WLW[ilson]) for Col [Albert W] Waldron, [25 Nov 41], sub: Equip for Med Units for WD Pool of Task Forces. HD: Wilson files, "Vol. I, 15 May 41–20 Jan 42." (4) D/S, Act ACofS G–4 WDGS for TAG, 25 Oct 41, sub: Equip for Med Units for WD Pool of Task Forces, with Memo for Record. HRS: G–4/33344.

[30] (1) Ltr, SG to TAG, 5 Nov 41, sub: Equip for Med Units in WD Pool of Task Forces. SG: 475.5–1. (2) Memo, SG for ACofS G–4 WDGS, 19 Nov 41, sub: Comments on Draft of Ltr "Current policies and Procedures for Classification, Storage, and Issue of Sup." Same file.

[31] (1) Memo, Act ACofS G–4 WDGS for TAG, 27 Nov 41, sub: Equip forMed Units for WD Pool of Task Forces, with Memo for Record. HRS: G–4/33344. (2) 1st ind, TAG to SG, 6 Dec 41, on Ltr, SG to TAG, 5 Nov 41, same sub. AG: 320.2 (5–27–41) (6). (3) Ltr, TAG to CGs of CAs, 6 Dec 41, same sub. Same file.

corps areas late in 1940, the General Staff, it will be recalled, either assigned or attached to the four field armies all numbered medical units, including station and general hospitals that did not normally serve under the jurisdiction of field armies. At the same time, the Staff directed corps area commanders to make their medical facilities available for the training of hospital units, and it forbade army commanders to assume control over such units without the approval of corps area commanders. Furthermore, while one directive stated that the personnel and units of field forces on duty with corps areas would be controlled entirely by corps area commanders, another forbade the same commanders to assume jurisdiction over field force units undergoing training in corps area installations.[32] As a result, neither GHQ nor the Surgeon General's Office exercised any very direct control over numbered hospital units, and the units themselves were sometimes confused as to whether they were subject to army or corps area command.[33]

Without close supervision from higher authorities the training which hospital units received depended primarily upon the attitudes of local surgeons and unit commanders. In some instances, well-planned on-the-job training programs were established in named hospitals and were co-ordinated with unit field training. In others, the commanders of named hospitals assigned men from numbered units to vacant jobs regardless of their training value. In such cases technical training suffered because many men did only menial work, and controversies developed between hospital commanders responsible for post medical care and unit commanders responsible for the technical as well as the field training of their men.[34]

Confusion about the control of hospital units also affected their use on maneuvers. Explaining his lack of authority over hospital units, The Surgeon General suggested that the personnel of some should be used to augment the staffs of named hospitals and to assist medical detachments, battalions, and regiments engaged in maneuvers. He proposed that other units should be employed in giving medical care as they would in theaters of operations.[35] Their use in this manner was limited by incomplete staffs and lack of equipment. In some instances evacuation hospitals borrowed enough personnel and equipment from other medical units and from corps areas to enable them to provide limited hospitalization for troops in the field. After they were set up, such hospitals tended to become stationary. Army commanders then had to improvise mobile hospitals by using personnel and equipment of medical regiments. Generally armies had to rely upon corps areas for

[32] (1) Ltr AG 320.2(9-27-40)M-C, TAG to C of Arms and Servs, CGs of Armies, Army Corps, Divs, CAs and Depts, etc., 3 Oct 40, sub: Orgn, Tng, and Admin of Army. SG: 320.3-1. (2) Ltr, TAG to same, 4 Nov 40, sub: Units Asgd and Atchd to GHQ, Armies, Corps. . . . AG: 320.2(8-2-40) (4) Sec 3. (3) Ltr AG 320.2(11-16-40)M-D-M, TAG to same, 14 Jan 41, sub: Orgn, Tng, and Admin of Med Units. SG: 322.3-1. (4) Ltr, TAG to same, 8 Apr 41, sub: Asgmt and Atchmt of Fld Force Units to GHQ, Armies, Army Corps. . . . AG: 320.2(8-2-40)(4) Sec 3A, Pt 1.

[33] (1) Memo 2, incl to Ltr, Col Daniel J. Sheehan, MC, to Col Roger G. Prentiss, Jr, MC, 10 May 51. HD: 314 (Correspondence on MS) III. (2) An Rpts, 1940 and 41, 222d, 213th, 215th, and 183d Gen Hosps. HD.

[34] (1) Memo, Lt Col T. E. Huber for Historian, Tng Div SGO, 4 Jun 45, sub: Unit Tng, ASF, World War II. HD: 353. (2) Memo 2, incl to Ltr, Col Daniel J. Sheehan, MC, to Col Roger G. Prentiss, Jr, MC, 10 May 51. HD: 314 (Correspondence on MS) III.

[35] Rpt, Conf of SG with CA Surgs, 10-12 Mar 41. HD: 337.

hospitalization of troops on maneuvers. To assist corps area hospitals and at the same time to give members of numbered units some experience in the actual operation of hospitals, station, general, evacuation, and surgical hospital units were attached to named hospitals in maneuver areas. Because their members were usually integrated with the staffs of corps area hospitals, such units not only tended to lose their identities but also failed to acquire experience as functioning organizations.[36]

Furnishing Hospitalization for Overseas Areas

Even before war actually began, additional hospitalization had to be supplied for troops in garrisons in territorial possessions of the United States and on island bases leased from the British in September 1940. In the Hawaiian and Philippine Islands, the Panama Canal Zone, Puerto Rico, and Alaska, hospitals were expanded as in the United States and additional increments of supplies and personnel were sent to care for the expansion.[37] According to War Department plans, the Atlantic bases were to be garrisoned and operated on a peacetime basis. The Surgeon General's Office therefore planned hospitalization for them in the same way as for posts in the United States. After computing bed requirements on a 5 percent ratio, the Hospital Construction and Repair Subdivision collaborated with the Chief of Engineers (who was charged with the construction of those bases) in drawing plans for permanent or semipermanent hospital buildings of appropriate sizes. Meanwhile, other groups in the Office planned shipments of supplies and equipment and earmarked personnel to be drawn from existing installations for new hospitals.[38]

Implementation of the plans to garrison the Atlantic bases got under way early in 1941 before construction was completed. In January a few medical officers and a small detachment of enlisted men sailed with troops being sent to St. John's, Newfoundland. They operated a 40-bed hospital aboard the transport *Edmund B. Alexander* until it was ready to return to the United States about the middle of June. Then they moved into a rented estate at Northbank.[39] In April, a second group of medical personnel, consisting of 21 medical officers and 164 enlisted men, accompanied the garrisons bound for Trinidad and Bermuda. The detachment which accompanied the Trinidad base force established a hospital in a temporary, single-building structure. The one which went to Bermuda set itself up, along with base headquarters and other activities, in a hotel building. In other bases medical officers with small staffs operated dispensaries and arranged for the hospitalization of patients needing further treatment either

[36] An Rpts, 1941, Surg GHQ, First Army, Second Army, Third Army, Fourth Army, and 1st, 4th, 6th, 10th, 11th, and 23d Evac Hosps, 166th Sta Hosp, and Ft Bragg Sta Hosp. HD.

[37] (1) An Rpts, 1941, Surg Hawaiian, Puerto Rican, and Panama Canal Depts. HD. (2) HD: 322, Welsh file.

[38] (1) Memo, Lt Col H. D. Offutt for Maj Welsh, 8 Feb 41. HD: Atlantic Bases file folder. (2) Ltr, SG to CofEngrs, 25 Feb 41, sub: Floor Plans for MD Fac at Antigua, Bahama, British Guiana, and Saint Lucia. SG: 632.-1. (3) Memo, SG for Maj [Henry I.] Hodes, G-3, 28 Nov 40, sub: MD Pers for Atlantic Bases. HD: Atlantic Bases file folder. (4) Ltr, SG to CofEngrs, 10 Mar 41, sub: Med Sups and Equip . . . , and 1st ind, CofEngrs to SG, 31 Mar 41. Same file.

[39] An Rpt, 1941, Sta Hosp. Newfoundland Base Comd. HD.

in hospitals established by the Engineers for civilians working on Army construction or in hospitals operated by the British.[40]

In the fall of 1941 the first numbered hospital units were sent overseas. Under an agreement with the Icelandic Government, the United States established a force in Iceland as an outpost of defense. On 5 September 1941 the second echelon of this force, "the first United States expedition to depart with a complete plan and all means necessary to implement it,"[41] sailed from New York. The 11th, 167th, and 168th Station Hospitals accompanied it. The last two were composed of Regular Army men drawn from named hospitals in the United States and organized in mid-1941 as provisional Station Hospitals A and B for service with an expedition (later canceled) to the French West Indies. The other was made up primarily of drafted men who converted themselves into Regular Army soldiers by volunteering for three-year enlistments before sailing. Upon arriving in Iceland only one of these units actually operated a hospital in 1941. On 24 September the 168th opened in a permanent three-story frame building at Camp Laugarnes. The 11th and 167th were attached to the 168th and served as maintenance and construction forces on roads, utilities, and buildings.[42]

Plans and preparations for hospitalization in overseas areas were limited during the emergency period by meager funds and the uncertain nature of the peacetime mobilization. For this reason the Medical Department encountered difficulty—as it would later for other causes—in securing authority from the War Department General Staff to plan for and activate as many hospital units as it considered desirable. For estimating requirements the Surgeon General's Office had only World War I experience to rely upon, and there were differences of opinion as to how many fixed beds would be really needed. In order to enable units to give modern medical care, the tables governing their organization and equipment were revised. Although personnel authorized by such revisions was often increased, the General Staff began a practice—to be carried to greater lengths later—of requiring reductions in both personnel and equipment for table-of-organization units. Affiliated units were organized and some regular units were activated. The role of the latter was uncertain, but The Surgeon General gradually tended to agree with the General Staff that some of them at least would be used to give actual medical care. The rest would continue to train fillers for affiliated units. While The Surgeon General and the General Staff agreed upon the policy of providing hospital units with less than full quotas of officers and enlisted men, they disagreed upon the question of whether or not units in training should receive full issues of supplies and equipment. This dispute was to continue unabated during the first half of the war.

[40] (1) Memo, Maj A. B. Welsh for Brig Gen A. G. Love, 7 Apr 41, and Ltr AG 320.2(4-8-41)M-D-M, TAG to C of Arms and Servs, 8 Apr 41, sub: Immed garrison for Bermuda and Trinidad. . . . HD: Atlantic Base file folder. (2) A History of Medical Department Activities in the Caribbean Defense Command in World War II, vol I, pp. 245-46, 281-82, 311, 314, and 320. HD. (3) An Rpt, 1941, Surg Bermuda Base Comd. HD.

[41] Greenfield *et al.*, *op. cit.*, pp. 22-23. For a full discussion of the agreement with Iceland and the force sent for its defense, see Stetson Conn and Byron Fairchild, Defense of the Americas, Vol. II, a forthcoming volume in the series UNITED STATES ARMY IN WORLD WAR II.

[42] An Rpts, 1941, 1943, 168th Sta Hosp; 1941, 1942, 167th Sta Hosp; 1941, 11th Sta Hosp; 1942, Surg Iceland Base Comd. HD.

PART TWO

HOSPITALIZATION
IN THE EARLY WAR YEARS
7 DECEMBER 1941—MID-1943

Introduction

Despite its year of peacetime mobilization the United States was not prepared for the offensive when war came on 7 December 1941. An immediate necessity was the deployment of troops to protect the country and its overseas bases. At the same time the Nation's power had to be mobilized and co-ordinated with that of its Allies. The Army's total strength increased from 1,686,403 in December 1941 to 6,993,102 in June 1943. Although most troops were of necessity in training in the United States, enough were overseas by the latter part of 1942 to permit a transition from the defensive to the offensive with assaults upon the Japanese in the Solomons and the invasion of North Africa. By June 1943 the peak of the preparation phase was reached. The next month saw the beginning of a steady decline in the strength of the Army at home as more and more troops moved overseas. In the latter half of 1943 the invasion of Sicily and Italy occurred and the Pacific island-hopping, which was to culminate in the defeat of Japan, began.

The Medical Department, like the rest of the country, was unprepared to support offensive operations at the outbreak of the war. This lack of preparation is most evident in the field of hospitalization. Few hospital units were in training and equipment in the war reserve was inadequate and in part obsolete. Although hospitals in the United States were sufficient for the Army that had thus far been mobilized, additional beds had to be provided rapidly as the Army's numerical strength shot upward. The first year and a half of the war was therefore a period of "growing pains" for the Medical Department, during which it adjusted itself to the demands of global warfare and with some difficulty discarded or modified peacetime practices and procedures in favor of those required by far-flung offensives. It was a time of finding out what was wrong with prewar planning and of correcting errors; of meeting immediate needs in the quickest possible fashion and of preparing at the same time for future operations. Under General Magee's leadership, the Department exhibited certain conservative tendencies in hospital expansion and administration which sometimes irked those in higher positions of authority. Nevertheless many developments considered progressive in the later war years had their origins during this period.

At this time also a reorganization of the War Department shifted The Surgeon General to a new position in the official hierarchy. Affecting his responsibility and authority for hospitalization, it required major adjustments in the relationships of his Office with other War Department agencies. The main features of that reorganization and its effects, along with changes in units in the Surgeon General's Office concerned with hospitalization, need to be discussed before details of the expansion and administration of hospitals are considered.

CHAPTER IV

Changes in Organization and Responsibilities for Hospitalization

Since most changes occurring early in the war in the responsibilities of various agencies for hospitalization resulted from the reorganization of the War Department in March 1942, major outlines of the new organization must be described briefly here.[1] In this connection one should understand that difficulties in hospitalization and evacuation resulting from the reorganization were aspects of a larger problem involving activities of the Medical Department in general and that similar problems were often encountered by other technical and supply services.

Reorganization of the War Department

Under the new setup the General Staff was relieved of some of its administrative and operative functions in the zone of interior by the creation of three major commands—Army Air Forces, Army Ground Forces, and Services of Supply (called Army Service Forces after March 1943). The divisions of the General Staff were to devote themselves to planning, to the general supervision of matters for which they were traditionally responsible, and to the strategic direction of forces in theaters of operations. The three major commands were all subject to the supervision and control of the General Staff, under the Chief of Staff, General George C. Marshall. War Department charts placed them all on the same level, but differences of opinion subsequently developed over whether or not they were actually coequal in authority.

The Army Air Forces, which had been established in June 1941 and had attained a great deal of practical autonomy, had taken the lead and supplied the drive for the reorganization as a means of protecting and regularizing its current position. Colonel Grant continued as the Air Surgeon. The Army Ground Forces comprised the arms (such as Infantry, Cavalry, and Artillery) and was responsible for

[1] Fuller discussions may be found in other volumes: (1) John D. Millett, *The Organization and Role of the Army Service Forces* (Washington, 1954), pp. 23–42, 93–97, 132–37, 148, 298–309, Ray S. Cline, *Washington Command Post: The Operations Division* (Washington, 1951), pp. 61–74, 90–95, 111–19, and Kent R. Greenfield, Robert R. Palmer, and Bell I. Wiley, *The Organization of Ground Combat Troops* (Washington, 1947), pp. 142–45, 268–71, all in UNITED STATES ARMY IN WORLD WAR II. (2) Wesley Frank Craven and James Lea Cate, eds., *The Army Air Forces in World War II* (Chicago, 1948), Vol. I, pp. 257–67. (3) Blanche B. Armfield, Organization and Administration (MS for companion vol. in Medical Dept. series). HD.

preparing the ground army for combat. General Headquarters was now liquidated and much of its personnel was transferred to AGF headquarters. Colonel Blesse then became Chief Surgeon of the Army Ground Forces (or the Ground Surgeon). He remained in that position until December 1942, when he was succeeded by Col. William E. Shambora, and returned to it again in May 1944 for the rest of the war.

To the Services of Supply were assigned the corps areas, the technical and supply services such as the Medical Department and the Quartermaster Corps, certain War Department administrative services, and some of the functions and personnel of G–4. Lt. Gen. (later General) Brehon B. Somervell, Assistant Chief of Staff, G–4, of the War Department General Staff since 25 November 1941, became Commanding General, Services of Supply. Under his jurisdiction was The Surgeon General, the head of the Medical Department.

The Surgeon General's New Position

Uncertainty developed about the effect the reorganization had or should have on responsibilities and authority for hospitalization and other medical activities. While General Magee recognized that there were "changes in the flow of control from the Secretary of War to the Medical Department," he did not believe that the reorganization had altered the responsibility of The Surgeon General for the health and medical care of the entire Army.[2] Apparently he did not comprehend at the outset the full impact on his office of the interposition of an intermediate headquarters between himself and the General Staff. According to SOS doctrine General Somervell was responsible for all activities, including hospitalization, within the Services of Supply and was at the same time staff adviser to—and in some instances spokesman for—the Chief of Staff on supplies and services, including medical, for the entire Army.[3] In his new position, The Surgeon General was an adviser to General Somervell. In this capacity the extent to which General Magee could discharge what he considered to be his responsibilities depended primarily upon the degree to which General Somervell accepted his recommendations (1) regarding SOS medical matters as the basis of command decisions and (2) regarding Army-wide medical matters as a basis for action or advice to the Chief of Staff. So far as hospitalization and evacuation in particular were concerned, it depended—partially, at least—upon the role of a medical section in SOS headquarters.

When SOS headquarters was established in March 1942 a medical officer, Lt. Col. William L. Wilson,[4] was transferred from G–4 along with General Somervell, Brig. Gen. (later Lt. Gen.) LeRoy Lutes, and others. For several months he served in the Miscellaneous Branch of the SOS Operations Division under General Lutes. In July 1942, when SOS headquarters was reorganized, a

[2] (1) Ltr, SG to CG SOS, 25 Mar 42, sub: Med Serv of Army. HD: 321.6–1. (2) Cmtee to Study the MD, 1942, Testimony, p. 2055. HD.

[3] (1) Ltr, Gen Brehon B. Somervell to Col R[oger] G. Prentiss, Jr, ed, Hist of the MD in World War II, 13 Nov 50. HD: 314 (Correspondence on MS) III. (2) Ltr, Lt Gen LeRoy Lutes to same, 8 Nov 50. Same file. (3) The SOS viewpoint is explained in Millett, *op. cit.*, pp. 143–47.

[4] Colonel Wilson received his promotion from major to lieutenant colonel on 18 April 1942 but it was retroactive to 1 February 1942. This accounts for the fact that documents signed by him and cited in the footnotes show him as a major until the middle of April.

Hospitalization and Evacuation Branch was established in General Lutes' office and Colonel Wilson was made its chief. This Branch gained additional medical officers and by October 1942 it had, in addition to its chief, one Medical Administrative Corps and three Medical Corps officers. Lt. Col. William C. Keller, a physician formerly with the Pennsylvania Railroad, was in charge of a railway evacuation section. Maj. (later Col.) John C. Fitzpatrick, who had had experience as a transport surgeon, was in charge of a sea evacuation section. Maj. (later Lt. Col.) Henry McC. Greenleaf devoted his attention to hospitalization. The administrative officer, Maj. (later Col.) Harry J. Nelson, was in charge of office administration.[5]

The SOS statement of the functions of this Branch—to review plans for, co-ordinate activities related to, and insure the means for hospitalization and evacuation—was subject to different interpretations. General Magee believed that his Office was best equipped to decide upon medical matters and that his advice should be given preponderant weight. Accordingly, in his opinion any medical officer in a staff position of a higher headquarters should be a representative of The Surgeon General and should receive his instructions and advice from the Surgeon General's Office. He interpreted establishment of the Hospitalization and Evacuation Branch as representing a desire in SOS headquarters for a section to co-ordinate activities of various Army agencies in the transportation (or evacuation) of patients.[6]

The SOS viewpoint was different. In July 1942 General Lutes informed corps area commanders that the "Hospitalization and Evacuation Branch lays down the policies to the Surgeon General on Hospitalization and Evacuation," and that it then visited their areas to see if "policies and plans as laid down to the Surgeon General" were satisfactory and were being followed.[7] Colonel Wilson took the position that hospitalization and evacuation required supervision by a higher headquarters than the Surgeon General's Office. In explaining his position as chief of the SOS Hospitalization and Evacuation Branch, he emphasized that he had no authority as a staff officer to make decisions or to issue orders concerning hospitalization and evacuation (that could be done only by General Somervell or General Lutes) but that it was his responsibility to gather and evaluate information on such matters and to present it, along with recommendations for action, to Generals Lutes and Somervell. If his advice differed from The Surgeon General's, he stated, he gave the latter's opinion as well as his own.[8] In view of different conceptions of their respective responsibilities, it was perhaps inevitable that conflicts would develop between the SOS Hospitalization and Evacuation Branch and the Surgeon General's Office.[9]

[5] (1) WD Cir 59, Orgn Chart, SOS Orgn, 2 Mar 42. (2) Cmtee to Study the MD, 1942, Testimony, pp. 1274–76. HD. (3) History of Planning Division, ASF, Vol. 1, p. 77. HRS.

[6] (1) Cmtee to Study the MD, 1942, Testimony, pp. 1973–2022. HD. (2) Verbatim transcription of notes employed by Maj Gen James C. Magee in conf in HD AML, 10 Nov 50. HD: 314 (Correspondence on MS) III.

[7] Rpt, Conf of CGs, SOS, 2d sess, 30 Jul 42, pp. 52–53. HD: 337.

[8] (1) Memo, Maj W. L. Wilson for Gen Lutes, 18 Apr 42, sub: Hosp and Evac Oprs, SOS. HD: Wilson files, "No 472, Hosp and Evac, 1941–42." (2) Cmtee to Study the MD, 1942, Testimony, pp. 1910–11, 1956–57. HD. See also pp. 1869–1964, 1271–1339. (3) Memo, Col W. L. Wilson for Col R. G. Prentiss, Jr. HD: 314 (Correspondence on MS) III.

[9] See below, pp. 63–67, 151–60.

The extent to which The Surgeon General could discharge his responsibility for the health and medical care of the Army depended also upon willingness of commanders of the Ground and Air Forces to admit that the Commanding General, Services of Supply, or one of his subordinates, had any authority—even technical and professional—over matters for which they were responsible and upon which their own surgeons could advise them.

So far as hospitalization in the United States was concerned, this involved mainly the Air Forces. Since the Ground Forces were to occupy and use stations operated by the Services of Supply, AGF headquarters readily accepted the dictum that the "Medical Department under the command of the Commanding General, Services of Supply," would furnish all of its hospitalization and evacuation in the United States except that provided by field medical units operating under tactical control. On the other hand, it will be recalled that the Air Forces already had a separate set of hospitals and the reorganization placed them, along with stations they served, under command of the Commanding General, Army Air Forces.

Several documents issued after the reorganization purported to clarify the respective responsibilities of the commanders of the Air and Service Forces and the relationships of the Air Surgeon and The Surgeon General. A General Staff directive charged all commanders with "command responsibility for the operation of all medical facilities under their control and for future planning in connection therewith." It also charged the Commanding General, Army Air Forces, "with development and operation of air evacuation," and the Commanding General, Services of Supply, with providing "for the evacuation of sick and wounded delivered to his control," and with "administrative responsibility for the coordination of the plans of all commands for evacuation of the sick and wounded to be delivered to his control, and for coordination of plans for hospitalization within the continental United States." An SOS directive on 18 June 1942 charged The Surgeon General with "the initial preparation and the maintenance of basic plans for military hospitalization and evacuation operations, and the coordination of the plans therefor of all commands concerned." An announcement of an agreement between the Air Surgeon and The Surgeon General, approved by G–3, had stated earlier that the "routine conduct of medical activities with the Army Air Forces" was a "responsibility of each local surgeon acting under the Air Surgeon, who is responsible to The Surgeon General for the efficient operation of Medical Department technical activities with the Air Forces." It had also stated that the Air Surgeon would not duplicate activities of the Surgeon General's Office, "with the exception of those procedures necessary for the proper control of Medical Department personnel and activities under the jurisdiction of the Army Air Forces." [10]

None of these documents specifically stated that the Services of Supply was to

[10] (1) Ltr, SG to CG SOS, 25 Mar 42, sub: Med Serv of Army. HD: 321.6–1. (2) Memo, CG SOS for ACofS G–3 WDGS, 26 Mar 42, sub: Med Activities under WD Cir 59, 1942, with Memo for Record. HD: Wilson files, "Book I, 26 Mar 42–26 Sep 42." (3) Ltr, CG SOS to all CA Comdrs and SG, 26 May 42, sub: Med Activities under WD Cir 59, 1942. SG: 020.–1. (4) Ltr AG 704 (6–17–42)MB–D–TS–M, TAG to CGs AGF, AAF, SOS, All Def Comds, All Depts, All Theaters, and All Sep Bases, 18 Jun 42, sub: WD Hosp and Evac Policy. HD: 705.–1. (5) Ltr SPOPM 322.15, CG SOS to CGs and COs of CAs, PEs, and Gen Hosps, and to SG, 18 Jun 42, sub: Opr Plans for Mil Hosp and Evac, with incl. SG: 705.–1.

exercise authority over AAF hospitalization and all of them were sufficiently vague to permit a variety of interpretations. Difficulties that arose from Air Forces' resistance to SOS claims of authority and from the Air Surgeon's strivings for completely separate AAF hospitalization will be discussed later.[11]

The division of responsibility for hospital units being prepared in the United States for overseas service was clearer. This problem involved mainly the Army Ground Forces, for the Air Forces at that time had no such units and made no bid for them.[12] Moreover, in February 1942 General Magee had secured Staff approval of a policy of "providing over-all hospitalization for task forces, instead of attempting to provide separate hospitalization for the air and ground components thereof. . . ." [13] While it was clear that the reorganization placed medical units that were organic elements of air and ground combat forces under AAF and AGF headquarters respectively, responsibility for nonorganic service units, such as hospitals, was left to be "directed by the War Department." [14]

The Ground Surgeon believed that medical units normally used in combat zones in close support of ground troops should be assigned to the Ground Forces and those normally used in communications zones, to the Services of Supply.[15] Mindful of his position as chief medical officer of the Army, The Surgeon General wanted all hospital units—those that served in combat as well as in communications zones—and certain other medical units that normally served as parts of field armies, such as medical laboratories and depots, to be under the jurisdiction of the Services of Supply.[16] On the recommendation of its Hospitalization and Evacuation Branch, SOS headquarters first requested that only general and station hospital units be placed under SOS control but later adopted The Surgeon General's position.[17]

After considerable investigation and study of the larger problem of jurisdiction over service units in general, G–3 took a view that coincided with the Ground Surgeon's. On 30 May 1942 it announced that the three major commands would, in general, train the nondivisional service units which they used.[18] On 8 July 1942 this principle was extended to cover acti-

---

[11] See below, pp. 106–09, 117–20, 173–76, 182–88.

[12] In March 1942 AAF Headquarters concurred in the SOS proposal that SOS have jurisdiction over general and station hospital units and AGF over all other field medical units. Memo, CG SOS for ACofS G–3 WDGS, 26 Mar 42, sub: Med Activities under WD Cir 59, 1942. HD: Wilson files, "Book I, 26 Mar 42–26 Sep 42."

[13] 1st ind SGO 322.4–1, SG to TAG, 5 Feb 42, and 2d ind AG 320.2 (1–29–42) MSC–C, TAG to SG, 18 Feb 42, on Memo, C of Air Staff for SG, 29 Jan 42, sub: Expansion Program of AAF for Calendar Year 1942. HD: 320.3 (Trp Basis).

[14] WD Cir 59, 2 Mar 42.

[15] Cmtee to Study the MD, 1942, Testimony, pp. 409–13. HD.

[16] (1) Memo, SG for CG SOS, 16 Mar 42. SG: 020.–1. (2) Memo, Act SG for Tng Div SOS, 31 Mar 42. SG: 322.3–1. (3) Ltr, SG to CG SOS, 28 Oct 42, sub: Recomds in Regard to Activation, Control, and Tng of Med Units, with 1 incl. SG: 320.3–1.

[17] (1) Memo for Record on Draft Memo, CG SOS for ACofS G–3 WDGS, 26 Mar 42, sub: Med Activities under WD Cir 59, 1942. HD: Wilson files, "Book I, 26 Mar 42–26 Sep 42." (2) Memo SP 020 (3–28–42), CG SOS (init WLW[ilson]) for ACofS G–3 WDGS, 17 Apr 42, same sub. Same file. (3) Memo, CG SOS for ACofS G–3 WDGS, 14 May 42, sub: Responsibility for Tng. HRS: G–3/353 (Only) vol. II. (4) For a discussion of the general problem, see Robert R. Palmer, Bell I. Wiley, and William R. Keast, *The Procurement and Training of Ground Combat Troops* (Washington, 1948), pp. 499–511, in UNITED STATES ARMY IN WORLD WAR II.

[18] Memo WDGCT 353 (5–30–42), ACofS G–3 WDGS for CGs AGF, AAF, and SOS, 30 May 42, sub: Responsibility for Tng. HRS: G–3/320.2 "Activation, vol. I."

vations also.[19] As a result, for the rest of the war the Services of Supply was responsible for activating and training communications zone units. Among them were fixed hospitals, such as general, station, and hospital center units, and certain evacuation units, such as hospital trains and hospital ship companies. The Army Ground Forces was similarly responsible for combat zone units, including surgical and evacuation hospitals as well as such units as medical regiments, medical battalions, medical detachments, and medical supply depots.

With division of responsibility for activating and training service units, AGF headquarters assumed responsibility for recommending the number of mobile units to be included in the troop basis, while The Surgeon General and SOS headquarters concentrated on units for fixed hospitals. Subsequently, responsibility for preparing tables governing the organization and equipment of hospital units was also divided. Since mobile hospitals were designed for use in combat zones, AGF headquarters felt that it should be free to make such changes in personnel and equipment of these hospitals as it found desirable for tactical reasons.

In September 1942 G–4 proposed that AGF headquarters should be given responsibility for the preparation of tables for all AGF service units.[20] General Somervell feared that the chiefs of technical services, including The Surgeon General, might be bypassed if this proposal were adopted. On his recommendation, G–4 amended its original proposal to require AGF to consult with SOS when preparing tables for service units.[21] Thereafter, responsibility for the preparation of tables of organization, tables of equipment, and tables of basic allowances for numbered hospital units was divided, as that for their activation and training had been earlier, between AGF and SOS headquarters.[22]

Even so, The Surgeon General retained considerable authority over the medical equipment and supplies furnished all hospital units, mobile as well as fixed, for one item in each table of equipment was the unit assemblage. It contained all items of medical equipment required for a hospital, was packed according to Medical Department equipment lists, and was issued by Medical Department depots as a single item. While he customarily consulted with the Ground Surgeon when revising equipment lists, The Surgeon General alone was responsible for their preparation and for the packing of unit assemblages.[23]

Further changes affecting the manner in which The Surgeon General could discharge his responsibility for the medical care of the Army occurred as a result of the reorganization of the Services of Supply in the summer of 1942. At that time corps areas were renamed service commands and authority formerly concen-

[19] Memo WDGCT 320.2 (Activation) (7–1–42), ACofS G–3 WDGS for CGs AAF, AGF, and SOS, 8 Jul 42, sub: Responsibility for Activation of Units. HRS: G–3/320.3 "Activation, vol. I."

[20] Memo WDGDS 809, ACofS G–4 WDGS for CG SOS, 21 Sep 42, sub: Prep of T/Os and T/Es. AG: 320.3(3–13–42)(5).

[21] (1) 1st ind SPOPU 320.3(9–21–42), CG SOS to ACofS G–4 WDGS, 25 Sep 42, on Memo WDGDS 809, ACofS G–4 WDGS for CG SOS, 21 Sep 42, sub: Prep of T/Os and T/Es. AG: 320.3(3–13–42) (5). (2) DF WDGDS 867, ACofS G–4 WDGS to ACofS G–3 WDGS, 29 Sep 42, same sub. Same file.

[22] (1) AR 310–60, pars 8 and 16, 12 Oct 42. (2) WD Memo W310–9–43, 22 Mar 43, sub: Policies Governing T/Os and T/Es. HD.

[23] (1) Memo, SG for CG SOS, 5 Nov 42, sub: Make-up of Hosp Unit Assemblies. SG: 475.5–1. (2) Rpt of [SGO] Bd for Determining Possibilities of Deleting Certain Items in a 400-bed Evac Hosp [13 Nov 42]. SG: 475.5–1.

trated in Washington was decentralized to them Thus the control of all general hospitals, except Walter Reed, was transferred from The Surgeon General to commanding generals of service commands. For a while the former retained authority to determine staff allotments for general hospitals, subject to SOS approval; but in April 1943, on the recommendation of the SOS Control Division, that function was also decentralized to commanding generals of service commands.[24] The reorganization also diminished the authority of service command surgeons and altered the Surgeon General's relationship with them. They no longer occupied the position of staff advisers to their commanders but were now subordinated as chiefs of medical branches to the chiefs of personnel or supply divisions of service command headquarters. Moreover, since command responsibilities were emphasized in the field, as in Washington, they could no longer be considered as field representatives of The Surgeon General and could therefore exercise no authority over hospitals not under service command control. Finally, The Surgeon General could—in theory at least—communicate with service command surgeons and hospital commanders only through command channels—that is, through General Somervell and the commanding generals of service commands. This indirect method of intercourse was somewhat offset by the practice of permitting informal direct communication between the Surgeon General's Office and service command surgeons.[25]

Changes in responsibilities for hospital construction and maintenance also occurred, but resulted only partially from the reorganizations discussed above. In December 1941, in conformity with an act of Congress, all of The Quartermaster General's construction and maintenance activities were transferred to the Chief of Engineers.[26] About five months later the War Department concentrated in the latter responsibility which he had previously shared with The Surgeon General for the maintenance of hospital plants.[27] After the War Department reorganization, recommendations of The Surgeon General for construction of new plants and for major alterations of existing plants were subject to review by both the Hospitalization and Evacuation Branch and the Construction Planning Branch of SOS headquarters. The former considered them from the viewpoint of medical needs; the latter, of Army-wide requirements. Both branches were guided by decisions and policies of the General Staff and by directives of the War Production Board. The selection of sites and the internal arrangements of new hospitals, as well as alterations of existing plants, continued to be a joint function of The Surgeon General and the Chief of Engineers. Insistence of the

[24] (1) SvC Orgn Manual, 22 Jul 42, sec 403.02, in WD Hq SOS SvC (formerly CA) Reorgn, 22 Jul 42. HRS. (2) Memo, SG for Dir Control Div SOS, 1 Aug 42. SG: 020.-1. (3) Cmtee to Study the MD, 1942, Testimony, Statement of Col H. D. Offutt, pp. 214-15. HD. (4) AR 170-10, par 6*a*(1)(p), 10 Aug and 24 Dec 42. (5) Memo, Dir Control Div ASF for CofS ASF, 6 Apr 43, sub: Clarification of Prov of AR 170-10. . . . AG: 600.12(10 Mar 42) (1). (6) AR 170-10, C 2, 14 Apr 43.

[25] (1) Edward J. Morgan and Donald O. Wagner, The Organization of the Medical Department in the Zone of the Interior (1946), HD, pp. 97-99. (2) Ltr, SG to CG SOS, 9 May 42, sub: Med Activities under WD Cir 59, 1942. SG: 020.-1. (3) Memo, Chief Professional Servs [SGO] for Mr. Corrington Gill, 2 Oct 42, sub: Supervision and Coord of Professional Care in Mil Hosps in Continental US. SG: 701.-1. (4) SOS Orgn Manual, 10 Aug 42, sec 403.02. (5) For a fuller discussion, see Armfield, *op. cit.*

[26] WD Cir 248, 4 Dec 41.

[27] (1) WD Cir 157, 23 May 42. (2) AR 100-80, 9 Jun 42. (3) See below, pp. 94-96.

latter and of SOS headquarters upon decentralization to the field of as much construction authority and activity as possible, in order to speed construction, resulted by the end of 1942 (as will be seen later) in The Surgeon General's loss of some authority he had previously exercised over the erection and alteration of hospital plants.[28]

The Wadhams Committee

Late in 1942 responsibilities and organization for hospitalization, along with many other aspects of Medical Department work, were the subject of review and comment by a civilian committee appointed by the Secretary of War. This group, which called itself the "Committee to Study the Medical Department" but which will be referred to hereafter for the sake of brevity as the Wadhams Committee (from the name of its chairman, Col. Sanford Wadhams, a retired medical officer), was constituted to "make a thorough survey of professional, administrative, and supply practices of the Medical Department." [29] It probed the relation between the Surgeon General's Office and the SOS Hospitalization and Evacuation Branch, and testimony presented in that connection placed on record information summarized above which might not otherwise have been available.[30] While some of the Committee's recommendations dealt with the position of The Surgeon General in the War Department, they appear to have had little influence on the authority and responsibility of either the Surgeon General's Office or major commands for hospitalization. This subject, along with an account of the Committee's background and investigation as a whole, is discussed fully elsewhere.[31] Recommendations of the Committee on policies and procedures for hospitalization had significant effects and will be discussed at appropriate places in following chapters.[32]

Changes in the Surgeon General's Office

During the early war years changes occurred in the organization of the Surgeon General's Office as well as in higher headquarters, but they affected the divisions most concerned with hospitalization less than others.[33] On 21 February 1942 the Hospital Construction Subdivision was raised in status to a division, reflecting the rapid expansion of construction activities.[34] The next month it was placed, along with the Hospitalization, Planning, and Training Divisions, in a newly formed Operations Service. In August, to describe its functions more accurately, the Hospitalization Division's name was changed to Hospitalization and Evacuation.[35]

The Hospital Construction Division continued to exercise The Surgeon General's advisory supervision over the construction, leasing, and maintenance of all establishments for the care and treatment of the sick and wounded. Colonel Hall remained at its head. To handle wartime

[28] (1) Army Hosp Program in Continental US, extract from sec 6, Analysis, Monthly Progress Rpt, data as of 31 Mar 43. SG: 632.-1. (2) See below, pp. 92-93.

[29] SecWar Memo, 10 Sep 42. AG: 020 SGO (3-30-43)(1).

[30] See above, p. 56, and also Cmtee to Study the MD, 1942, Testimony, pp. 1271-1339, 1690-94, 1869-1964, 1973-2022, 2039-49. HD.

[31] Armfield, *op. cit.*

[32] See below, pp. 93-94, 99, 118, 122-23, 127, 129, for example.

[33] Morgan and Wagner, *op. cit.*, pp. 9-25. These changes will be considered in detail in Armfield, *op. cit.*

[34] (1) See above, pp. 24-26. (2) Memo, unsigned and unaddressed, 1 Dec 42, sub: Rpt on Admin Devs, SGO. HD: 024.-1.

[35] An Rpt, 1943, Oprs Serv SGO. HD.

workloads the number of officers in this Division was increased between December 1941 and December 1942 from 4 to 8; of civilian architects, from 4 to 7; and of civilian clerks, from 7 to 10. During 1943, 1 officer, 1 civilian, and 2 clerks were dropped from the rolls, but a civilian real estate consultant was added, as the hospital construction program neared completion.[36] Changes in the Division's branches reflected shifts in construction policies and problems. In February 1942 there were three branches: Planning and Estimates, Construction and Conversion, and Maintenance and Repairs. In March, when increasing emphasis was placed upon the use of existing buildings, the Construction and Conversion subdivision was separated into two equal branches. Subsequently, the Conversion Branch was likewise subdivided, becoming the Ground Troop Facilities and Air Corps Facilities Branches. This move was perhaps accounted for by the expansion and growing independence of the Air Forces. In the late summer of 1942 the Planning and Estimates Branch was dropped from the Division, foreshadowing the transfer of its activity to the Hospitalization and Evacuation Division. By August, then, the Hospital Construction Division consisted of the Maintenance and Repair, Civilian Facilities Conversion, Ground Troop Facilities, and Air Corps Facilities Branches. This organization continued until July 1943.[37]

The Hospitalization Division, under Col. Harry D. Offutt, limited its activities largely to the development of hospitalization policies, the control of bed credits in general hospitals, and the maintenance of liaison with other divisions of the Office whose activities affected the functioning of hospitals.[38] The names of its subdivisions reflect this fact. In February 1942, they were the following: Hospital Inspection, Bed Credits, and Liaison. In March, the inactive Inspection subdivision was dropped. In August, the two remaining subdivisions became the Bed Credits and Evacuation Branch and the Miscellaneous Branch.[39] During 1942 this Division gradually took on another function, the periodic revision required by SOS headquarters of a basic directive for hospitalization and evacuation operations.[40] In September 1942 it also took over the job of estimating and planning for general hospital beds that would be required in the future.[41] Except for short periods, in December 1942 and again in April 1943, the Division's staff was limited to four officers and four clerks until the latter half of 1943.[42] At that time, the Division was enlarged and reorganized, under a new chief, to enable it to carry out the functions and activities which the war placed upon it.[43]

The Planning and Training Divisions continued to be responsible for numbered hospital units. Col. Howard T. Wickert was chief of the former. It made recommendations for the troop basis, for activation schedules, and for medical support for task forces and overseas theaters. It also prepared and revised tables of organi-

[36] (1) Tynes, Construction Branch, pp. 11-12. (2) Memo, Lt Col Seth O. Craft for Col R.W. Bliss, 8 Jul 43. HD: 319.1-2.

[37] Morgan and Wagner, *op. cit.*, Orgn Charts VI, VII, IX, X, and XI.

[38] An Rpt. FY 1943, Hosp and Evac Div SGO. HD.

[39] Morgan and Wagner, *op. cit.*, Orgn Charts VI, VII, and IX.

[40] An Rpt. FY 1943, Hosp and Evac Div SGO. HD. For this directive, see below, pp. 63-67.

[41] For example, the Hospitalization and Evacuation Division prepared the following document: Memo, SG for CG SOS, 26 Sep 42, sub: Hosp, Gen Hosps. SG: 632.-2.

[42] Memo, Col H. D. Offutt for Chief Oprs Serv SGO, 8 Jul 43. HD: 319.1-2.

[43] See below, pp. 176-78.

zation, tables of equipment, and equipment lists. After separation of responsibility for nonorganic service units between AGF and SOS headquarters, this Division limited itself primarily to SOS medical units but occasionally extended its activities to others when called upon to participate in conferences with the Operations Division of the General Staff on the formation of task forces or the deployment of additional troops to established theaters. After SOS headquarters was given responsibility for training SOS service units, the Training Division (separated from the Operations Service in August 1942) established a Unit Training Branch to discharge its responsibilities in connection with the training of hospital and other medical units.[44]

A Dispute About General Planning for Hospitalization and Evacuation

Closely connected with the War Department reorganization and arising partly from differences of opinion between the Surgeon General's Office and the SOS Hospitalization and Evacuation Branch about their respective responsibilities was a controversy over hospitalization and evacuation planning which developed early in 1942. Within three days after the establishment of the Services of Supply, Colonel Wilson reported to General Lutes on the results of a transcontinental inspection trip which he had undertaken while assigned to G–4 and which he had initiated with a view to having G–4 exercise greater supervision over hospitalization and evacuation. He stated that he had found no definite basic plan for hospitalization and evacuation within the United States, no plan or system of operations for evacuation from theaters, and no basic directive or system for activating, training, equipping, and using numbered hospital units in the United States. He recommended that SOS headquarters give further attention to the problem of numbered hospital units and overseas evacuation and that The Surgeon General be directed to submit basic plans for hospitalization and evacuation operations for the approval of SOS headquarters and subsequent publication "for the guidance of all concerned." [45] General Lutes approved the proposal, and on 14 March 1942 directed The Surgeon General to submit such plans.[46] The Surgeon General's Hospitalization Division conferred with the Office of the Chief of Transportation and on 31 March 1942 submitted a plan for hospitalization and evacuation operations.[47] Considering it unacceptable, Colonel Wilson prepared another which he presented to General Lutes on 18 April 1942 with the statement that its preparation had been necessary "because of the incomplete

[44] (1) An Rpts, SGO, FY 1942 and 1943, and An Rpt, Oprs Serv SGO, FY 1943. HD. (2) Morgan and Wagner, *op. cit.*, pp. 9–23.

[45] (1) Memo G–4/24499–178, Col W. M. Goodman, GSC, Chief Planning Br G–4 (init WLW[ilson]) for Gen Somervell, 20 Jan 42, sub: Current Status of Hosp and Evac. HD: Wilson files, "Vol. I, 15 May 41–20 Jan 42." (2) Memo Old G–4/24499–178, Maj W. L. Wilson for Gen [LeRoy] Lutes, 12 Mar 42, sub: Basic Plans for Hosp and Evac. HD: Wilson files, "No 472, Hosp and Evac, 1941–42." (3) For an earlier interim report see: Memo, same for same, 8 Feb 42, sub: Recent Trip for Study of Hosp and Evac. Same file.

[46] (1) Memo, CG SOS (signed Brig Gen LeRoy Lutes) for SG, 14 Mar 42, sub: Basic Plan for Hosp Oprs. SG: 704.–1. (2) Memo, same for same, 14 Mar 42, sub: Basic Plan for Evac of Sick and Wounded. Same file.

[47] Memo, SG for CG SOS, 31 Mar 42, sub: Basic Plan for Hosp Oprs and Evac of Sick and Wounded, with incl. SG: 704.–1. The first three drafts of this document, as well as proposals submitted by the Chief of Transportation, are on file HD: 705 (Hosp and Evac Planning).

nature and less understandable form of various plans submitted by The Surgeon General."[48] This draft was discussed with the Surgeon General's Office and then was sent to G-4 on 8 May 1942.[49]

On the same day General Lutes charged The Surgeon General with having failed to prepare hospitalization and evacuation plans either before or after he was so directed.[50] This charge, transmitted to The Surgeon General with a statement by General Somervell that it was "of course inexcusable not to have fully matured basic hospitalization plans,"[51] began a controversy which lasted for many months. General Magee defended himself both in writing and in a personal conference with General Somervell. He took the position that all contingencies to be covered by the plan called for, except enemy raids and local disasters, had already arisen and had been actually handled under existing plans. He believed, furthermore, that the document prepared by his Office was not only adequate but also preferable in some respects to the SOS draft.[52] Later, when documents of the SOS Hospitalization and Evacuation Branch emphasizing the lack of plans for hospitalization and evacuation were presented to the Wadhams Committee, General Magee again defended his position, stating that if the allegations were true "it would indeed appear that chaotic conditions prevailed, but these assertions are not supported by facts." Although Colonel Wilson insisted that "there wasn't any planning" early in 1942 he now stated that The Surgeon General had not been "any more negligent than all the rest of the Army," including G-4.[53] In its final report, the Committee implied approval of The Surgeon General's position, but it made no definite statement clearing him of charges of lack of adequate planning.[54]

The real picture was neither as black as SOS headquarters painted it nor as white as the Surgeon General's Office maintained. Plans for meeting normal hospital requirements for the zone of interior and theaters of operations were being made continuously by the Surgeon General's Office. In view of the generous basis on which normal beds were authorized in the United States, together with the possibilities of expansion by setting up wards in barracks (a method that was almost traditional with the Medical Department), it would seem that emergency needs also were being sufficiently provided for. Since

[48] Memo, Maj W. L. Wilson for Gen Lutes, 18 Apr 42, sub: Hosp and Evac Oprs, SOS. HD: Wilson files, "No 472, Hosp and Evac, 1941-42."

[49] (1) Memo, Col H. T. Wickert, SGO for Col [W. L.] Wilson, SOS, 30 Apr 42, with incl Memo, SG for Dir Oprs SOS, 30 Apr 42. HRS: ASF Hosp and Evac Sec file, "Misc Classified Corresp from Off CG ASF to AGO." (2) Memo, CG SOS for ACofS G-4 WDGS, 8 May 42, sub: Hosp and Evac Oprs SOS. HRS: G-4 files, "Hosp and Evac Policy."

[50] Memo, Brig Gen LeRoy Lutes for Gen Somervell, 8 May 42, sub: Activities of SG. SG: 704.-1.

[51] Memo, Gen Somervell for Gen Magee, 8 May 42. SG: 704.-1.

[52] 1st ind, SG to CG SOS, 12 May 42, on Memo, Gen Somervell for Gen Magee, 8 May 42. SG: 704.-1. The following note appears on this indorsement: "Personally delivered by Gen Magee, 12 May 42." General Lutes prepared a reply to General Magee, pointing out errors in the latter's defense and contending that there were no plans. ([2d ind SPOPG 370.05 (Policy), CG ASF (init LL[utes]) to SG, 19 May 42, on Memo, Gen Somervell for Gen Magee, 8 May 42. HRS: ASF Hosp and Evac Sec file, "Misc Classified Corresp from Off CG ASF to AGO."]) Whether or not this reply was sent to General Magee is uncertain. No copy of it has been found in SGO files. An ink note attached to the copy cited states: "This is in reply to a formal indorsement written by Surg. Gen. in which he took exception to criticism of his lack of a suitable plan. He visited Gen Somervell on the subject. Gen S may want to know of this reply. Lutes." In pencil on this copy is the following notation: "Suspend for Jun 3."

[53] Cmtee to Study the MD, Testimony, pp. 1988-89, 1995-98, 1919-23. HD.

[54] Cmtee to Study the MD, Rpt, p. 15, HD.

no enemy attack or severe epidemic occurred, the latter statement can be made with less certainty than the former. Moreover, the Surgeon General's Office was collaborating with the Chief of Transportation in planning facilities, personnel, and equipment for the evacuation of patients from theaters of operations. But the Medical Department had not prepared a basic directive for hospitalization and evacuation such as SOS headquarters required, nor was any one division in the Surgeon General's Office charged with the preparation of comprehensive Army-wide plans for hospitalization and evacuation. Certainly confusion existed as to responsibilities under the new War Department organization, but one may question whether, under the circumstances, it was any more incumbent on The Surgeon General than on higher headquarters to define those responsibilities and to require subordinate commanders to submit plans for hospitalization and evacuation.

The "plan" which Colonel Wilson drafted differed considerably from the one prepared by The Surgeon General's Hospitalization Division.[55] Perhaps this was caused as much by ambiguity of the SOS directive requiring the preparation of a "plan" as by The Surgeon General's lack of officers trained in planning, which SOS headquarters charged. A comparison of the two drafts shows that Colonel Wilson accepted and incorporated most of the information, pertaining chiefly to established policies and procedures, which The Surgeon General's draft contained. Greatest change was the addition of statements outlining the responsibilities of various commanders for hospitalization and evacuation and requiring them to submit plans, in specified forms at specific times, to The Surgeon General, who in turn was to review and co-ordinate them and then submit them along with his own "plan" to SOS headquarters. Reviewing the SOS draft, G–4 called it "an 'omnibus document' which undertakes to do a number of things," and suggested that two documents should be issued in its place: one, a statement of basic policies and procedures for hospitalization and evacuation; the other, a directive calling for "data and sub-plans from the field."[56] Subsequently, after collaboration between G–4 and SOS headquarters, two documents were issued on 18 June 1942. One was a General Staff directive stating in general terms the responsibilities of major commanders for hospitalization and evacuation. This remained unchanged for the balance of the war. The other, revised later on, was an SOS letter with the SOS "plan" as an inclosure.[57] Only the plans which these documents required of subordinate agencies need to be considered here. Responsibilities which they delineated and policies and procedures which the SOS "plan" announced will be discussed elsewhere in this volume.[58]

Subordinate agencies had to include in hospitalization plans tabulations of beds for normal use, along with statements of

[55] (1) Memo, SG for CG SOS, 31 Mar 42, sub: Basic Plan for Hosp Oprs and Evac of Sick and Wounded, with incl 1. SG: 704.-1. (2) Memo, Maj W. L. Wilson for Gen Lutes, 18 Apr 42, sub: Hosp and Evac Oprs SOS, with Tab A, same sub. HD: Wilson files, "No 472, Hosp and Evac, 1941–42."

[56] Memo, ACofS G–4 WDGS for CG SOS attn Oprs Div, 11 May 42, sub: Hosp and Evac Oprs, SOS. HRS: G–4 files, "Hosp and Evac Policy."

[57] (1) Ltr AG 704 (6–17–42) MB–D–TS–M, Sec War to CGs AGF, AAF, SOS, *et al.*, 18 Jun 42, sub: WD Hosp and Evac Policy. HD: 705.-1. (2) Ltr SPOPM 322.15, CG SOS to CGs and COs of CAs, PEs, and Gen Hosps and to SG, 18 Jun 42, sub: Opr Plans for Mil Hosp and Evac. Same file.

[58] See below, pp. 57–58, 81, 88–90, 114, 319–20, for example.

shortages; reports of provisions made to double hospital capacities in emergencies by the use of existing buildings such as apartments, hotels, schools, and dormitories; and reports of relations established with other agencies, such as the Office of Civilian Defense, "under which unilateral or mutual hospitalization support may be planned." Evacuation plans were to include estimates of persons of all types to be evacuated, both normally and in emergencies, along with statements about the status of personnel and equipment required for the transportation and care en route of patients being evacuated.

Hospital, port, and corps area commanders complied with this directive, and on 30 August 1942 The Surgeon General transmitted their plans, along with his own "comprehensive plan," to SOS headquarters.[59] The Surgeon General's "plan" was twofold. It contained a consolidation of the tables presented by corps areas and a draft of a "plan" based largely upon the SOS directive issued on 18 June 1942. The SOS Hospitalization and Evacuation Branch considered this draft acceptable, but revised it before publication, adding statements to bring the compilation of policies and procedures governing hospitalization and evacuation up to date and changing the wording to require The Surgeon General to submit a directive, rather than a "plan," thus making the terminology conform more closely with the fact. The revised edition of the hospitalization-and-evacuation-operations-planning directive was issued by SOS headquarters in November 1942, although it was dated 15 September 1942.[60] To make subsequent revisions as required, The Surgeon General on 7 November 1942 appointed a board of officers, with Colonel Offutt as chairman.[61] Although it submitted a revised version on 12 February 1943, none was published until the end of 1943.[62] That version appeared in the form of a War Department circular.

An evaluation of the importance of the "plan" or directive, as issued in its various versions, is difficult because of the controversial atmosphere in which it was prepared. In April 1943 the director of the ASF Planning Division stated that the 15 September 1942 version was "the first world-wide system for operations in the history of the War Department, under which the sick and wounded might be received from overseas commands and cared for and transported ultimately to a general hospital in the United States."[63] Considered objectively this was undoubtedly an overstatement, but the directive did have certain values which stand out with considerable clarity.

In its initial form the directive helped, at a time when other efforts were being made to achieve the same end, to clarify hospitalization and evacuation responsibilities. It was not strictly applicable to Ground and Air Forces commanders, however, for it was issued in the first two versions as an SOS directive only. When published in later versions as a War Department circular, it became binding upon Ground, Air, and Service Forces alike. In

[59] Memo, SG for CG SOS, 30 Aug 42, sub: Opr Plans for Hosp and Evac. SG: 704.-1.

[60] (1) Memo SPOPH 322.15, CG SOS for CGs and COs of SvCs and PEs and for SG, 15 Sep 42, sub: Mil Hosp and Evac Oprs, with incl 1, same sub. SG: 704.-1. (2) Memo. SG for Chief Oprs SOS, 27 Jan 43. SG: 705.-1.

[61] SG OO 456, 7 Nov 42.

[62] (1) Memo. SG for CG SOS, 12 Feb 43, sub: Opr Plans for Hosp and Evac. SG: 705.-1. (2) WD Cir 316, 6 Dec 43.

[63] Memo SPOPI 370.05, Dir Planning Div ASF for ACofS for Oprs ASF, 23 Apr 43, sub: Hosp and Evac Plans. HD: Wilson files, "Book IV, 16 Mar 43-17 Jan 43."

each version, the directive served as a valuable reference document, for it assembled in one place statements of several policies and procedures that existed only in separate letters, circulars, and regulations. It was not comprehensive in this respect, nor was it always up to date, for many additional policies and procedures had to be established and old ones changed during the periods between revisions. In September 1942 Colonel Offutt stated that his Division could operate effectively under the current version.[64] The following February, when Colonel Wilson visited field installations to evaluate operations under the directive, he found that each headquarters visited, with one exception, thought it clear, understandable, practicable, and of definite benefit.[65]

The value of the subordinate plans submitted in compliance with the basic directive is less clear. Each came to be what The Surgeon General's executive officer, Col. John A. Rogers, called one of them in September 1942—"just a plan to be tucked away." [66] Each was reviewed by the hospitalization and evacuation sections of both the Surgeon General's Office and SOS headquarters. They were then filed for future reference.[67] That no emergency developed to require their use need not detract from the foresightedness of having emergency expansion plans on hand, but whether those on file would have been adequate for a major disaster seems to have been doubted in the fall of 1942.[68] Tabulations of shortages of personnel, equipment, hospital beds, and transportation usually arrived too late to have any appreciable effect upon the supply of those elements, for problems of shortages were handled when they appeared and could not await the submission at periodic intervals of subordinate plans for hospitalization and evacuation. This requirement was dropped from subsequent versions of the directive early in 1944.[69]

In conclusion, one may question whether the benefits derived from the directive counterbalanced the friction and bad feeling which its issuance engendered between SOS headquarters and the Surgeon General's Office. Similar results might have been achieved more harmoniously if the principals in both agencies had been more considerate and understanding in dealing with each other or if relationships and responsibilities of the SOS Hospitalization and Evacuation Branch and the Surgeon General's Office had been more clearly delineated. Such was not the case, however, and the controversy that developed in this instance illustrated dangers and difficulties inherent in the new structure of the War Department and the new position of The Surgeon General.

[64] Diary, Hosp and Evac Br SOS, 22 Sep 42. HD: Wilson files, "Diary."

[65] (1) Résumé of Conf, SvCs and Ports, Feb–Mar 43, incl 1 to Memo SPOPI 337, CG ASF for SG and CofT, 30 Apr 43, same sub. HD: Wilson files, "Book IV, 16 Mar 43–17 Jun 43." (2) Memo, Col W. L. Wilson for Chief Hosp and Evac Br ASF, 17 Feb 43, sub: Visit to 8th SvC and Southern Def Comd. HD: Wilson files, "Book III, 1 Jan 43–15 Mar 43." (Col Robert C. McDonald succeeded Colonel Wilson as Chief, Hospital and Evacuation Branch on 6 February 1943.)

[66] Notes on tel conv between Col E. C. Jones, Surg 5th SvC and Col Rogers, 1 Sep 42. HD: Oprs Div files.

[67] (1) Memo SPOPH 322.15, Chief Hosp and Evac Br SOS for Chief Oprs SOS, 16 Nov 42, sub: SvC and Port Plans for Hosp and Evac Oprs. HD: Wilson files, "Book 2, 26 Sep 42–31 Dec 42." (2) Memo, SG for CG SOS, 30 Aug 42, sub: Oprs Plans for Hosp and Evac. SG: 704.–1. (3) Copies of the subordinate plans are in Wilson files, HD.

[68] See below, pp. 80–84.

[69] (1) For example, see 1st ind SPOPH 322.15 (8–30–42), CG SOS to SG, 26 Sep 42, on Memo, SG for CG SOS, 30 Aug 42, sub: Oprs Plans for Hosp and Evac. CE: 632. (2) WD Cir 140, 11 Apr 44.

CHAPTER V

Hospital Plants in the United States

In December 1941 the Army had a total of approximately 74,250 beds in about 200 station hospitals and 14 general hospitals in the United States.[1] During the next eighteen months it was to build enough additional hospitals to house more than three times the number provided during the fifteen-month period of peacetime mobilization.[2] In addition, it was to have enough hospitals under construction in June 1943 to house over 65,000 more beds.[3] Concurrently, improvements would have to be made in the cantonment-type hospitals already in operation.[4]

Types of Construction

Emphasis on Simplicity

With the country at war, speed in construction and conservation of building materials became factors of paramount consideration. Accordingly the General Staff insisted upon the simplest type of construction. On 29 December 1941 G–4 revoked the authority it had previously granted to construct hospitals on the two-story semipermanent plan,[5] and about a month later revised the War Department construction policy. After 6 February 1942 all construction at new stations, except that already in the advanced planning stage, was to be a modified form of the type designed for theaters of operations.[6] The Engineers interpreted this policy to mean that in station hospitals all warehouses and utility shops, and all buildings used for housing, feeding, and entertaining male members of the hospital staff would be of theater-of-operations-type construction, while those used in the care, treatment, feeding, and recreation of patients and as quarters, messes, and recreation rooms for nurses were to be of cantonment-type construction.[7] General

[1] Bed Status Rpts, end of last week in Dec 41. Off files, Health Rpts Br Med Statistics Div SGO. A few beds were reported in Darnall General Hospital, but they are not included in the number given above because this hospital did not open until March 1942.

[2]

	Gen Hosp	Sta Hosp
Beds Available Sep 40	4,925	7,391
Beds Added Sep 40–Dec 41	10,608	51,345
Beds Added Dec 41–Jun 43	38,226	161,279

Source: Bed Status Rpts. Off file, Health Rpts Br Med Statistics Div SGO.

[3] An Rpt, 1943, Hosp Cons Div SGO. HD.

[4] The even larger program of construction of all types of housing for the Army, of which the hospital expansion program was a part, is discussed in Jesse A. Remington and Lenore Fine, The Corps of Engineers: Construction in the United States, a forthcoming volume in the series UNITED STATES ARMY IN WORLD WAR II.

[5] (1) See above, pp. 23–24. (2) Ltr AG 632(12-27-41), TAG to SG and CofEngrs, 29 Dec 41, sub: Fire-Resistant Type of Cons in Hosps. SG: 632.-1.

[6] Ltr AG 600.12(2-5-42)MO-D-M, TAG to CGs all Depts, CAs, *et al.*, 6 Feb 42, sub: WD Cons Policy. SG: 600.12.

[7] Ltr, CofEngrs to TAG, 14 Feb 42, sub: Hosp in T/O Cantonments, with 1st ind AG 600.12 (2-14-42) MO-D, TAG to CofEngrs, 25 Feb 42. CE: 632 Pt 2.

hospitals, previously expected to be of semipermanent construction, were now to be entirely of cantonment type. This lowering of standards brought quick protests from The Surgeon General.

The decision to abandon two-story semipermanent construction for general hospitals was modified on 31 December 1941. At The Surgeon General's request, G-4 approved its use if neither a loss of time nor a material increase in costs was involved.[8] During the next two months, the Engineers and The Surgeon General's construction officers disagreed on whether semipermanent hospitals could be shown to cost no more than cantonment-type hospitals.[9] In some instances dual bids for the erection of a hospital on either plan were called for, and ten hospitals, including those already begun before the war, were constructed on the semipermanent plan.[10] Subsequently the Engineers found that the initial cost of semipermanent hospitals was "considerably greater," and on 16 April 1942 G-4 returned to its position that only cantonment-type construction be used for general hospitals.[11]

The decision to use theater-of-operations-type construction for buildings in station hospitals remained unchanged. Buildings of this type were of the lightest possible frame construction, with exteriors usually of heavy treated paper or fiberboard. Plumbing was omitted from barracks and placed in separate lavatory buildings. Heat was generally furnished by stoves in each building rather than by a central heating plant.[12] The Surgeon General based his protests against the use of theater-of-operations-type construction for hospitals in the United States on its lower quality. He stated that barracks and quarters of that type were unsuitable for conversion to wards to meet emergency needs for additional beds, that messes lacked comforts desired for officer-patients, and that kitchens had inadequate refrigeration and dishwashing facilities.[13] The Chief of Engineers admitted that it would be difficult to use theater-of-operations-type barracks for emergency wards, but believed it unwise to provide better housing for Medical Department men than for other troops. The General Staff agreed, and on 24 February 1942 reiterated the policy announced earlier that month.[14]

Later in the year, as the shortage of building materials increased, the General Staff proposed an even lower quality of construction for some hospitals. In May

[8] Memo, SG for ACofS G-4 WDGS, 31 Dec 41, with 1st ind, ACofS G-4 WDGS to SG, 31 Dec 41. SG: 632.-1.

[9] (1) Ltr, SG [Col John R. Hall] to TAG 19 Jan 42, sub: Fire-Resistant Type of Hosp Cons. (2) Memo, [Mr] H[arvey] J. H[all] for Col Hall, 5 Feb 42, sub: Comparison Data of the Cantonment-type Cons and the Semipermanent, Fire-Resistant Type, by Bldgs. (3) Ltr, SG (JRH) to CofEngrs, 7 Feb 42, sub: Fire-resistant Type of Hosp. Comparison with Cantonment Types. All in SG: 632.-1.

[10] (1) D/S G-4/33956, ACofS G-4 WDGS to TAG for CofEngrs, 8 Mar 42, sub: Gen Hosp Cons. AG: 322.3 "Gen Hosp." (2) Ltr AG 322.3 Gen Hosp (3-8-42) MO-D, TAG to CofEngrs, 10 Mar 42, same sub. SG: 632.-1. General hospitals of this type were Bushnell, McCloskey, Kennedy, Valley Forge, and Schick; there were also five station hospitals of the same type, located at Camps Atterbury (Indiana), Butner (North Carolina), Carson (Colorado), Campbell (Kentucky), and White (Oregon).

[11] (1) 2nd ind, CofEngrs to TAG, 14 Apr 42, sub: Cons of Hosp, on unknown basic Ltr. CE: 632 Vol. 3. (2) Ltr AG 600.12 (4-15-42) MO-DM, TAG to CGs of AGF, AAF, SOS, *et al.*, 16 Apr 42, sub: WD Cons Policy, ZI. SG: 600.12.

[12] Engineering Manual, OCE, Oct 43, Ch. IX, Pt I, par 10-03*c*.

[13] Memo, SG for CofEngrs, 9 Feb 42, sub: Proposed Hosp at Centerville and Grenada, Miss. SG: 632.-1.

[14] (1) Ltr, CofEngrs to TAG, 14 Feb 42, sub: Hosp in T/O Cantonments, with 1st ind, 25 Feb 42. CE: 632 Pt 2. (2) Ltr AG 600.12 MO-D-M, TAG to CGs, COs, and C of Arms and Servs, 24 Feb 42 sub: WD Cons Policy, ZI. SG: 600.12.

1942 the Secretaries of War and Navy and the Chairman of the War Production Board agreed upon a directive which required construction to be reduced to the minimum in both quantity and quality.[15] In conformity with this directive the General Staff decided to move units in advanced states of training to field tent camps and to use existing cantonments for the training of new units. They proposed to provide hospitalization for field camps in screened and floored tents.[16] The Surgeon General objected and suggested limiting hospitalization in tents to one third of that required for field camps and providing the rest in cantonment-type buildings, erected either in field camps or as additions to near-by station hospitals.[17] The General Staff approved the limitation of hospitalization in tentage but directed the use of theater-of-operations-type buildings for the remainder.[18] This meant that in some places buildings used for the care and treatment of patients, as well as those for housing personnel and storing supplies, were to be of low quality construction. Again The Surgeon General protested the use of "a hospital of a lower grade than the cantonment type unit." [19] While the policy was not changed, the practice of using tentage and theater-of-operations-type construction for entire hospital plants seems to have been limited chiefly to AGF maneuver areas.[20]

Conversion of Existing Buildings

Another method of achieving speed and conservation was to convert existing civilian buildings into Army hospitals. In mobilization plans this method had had high priority and in the fall of 1940 The Surgeon General had considered its use.[21] Soon after war began his construction officers again started looking for civilian buildings suitable for conversion.[22] On 19 March 1942, about the time the decision was being made to construct no more semipermanent hospitals, SOS headquarters suggested the acquisition of civilian buildings to house additional general hospital beds.[23] A little over a month later the Chief of Staff considered the possibility of abandoning entirely the construction of new general hospitals in favor of the civilian-facilities-conversion method. He gave up that idea after The Surgeon General's Construction Division and SOS headquarters pointed out difficulties involved.[24]

---

[15] Directive for Wartime Cons, 20 May 42, incl to Ltr AG 600.12 (5-20-42) MO-SPAD-M, TAG to CGs AAF, Depts, CAs, and C of Tec Servs, 1 Jun 42, same sub. SG: 632.-1.

[16] Draft Memo WDGCT 600.12, ACofS G-4 WDGS for CofS, n d, sub: Housing for 1943 Trp Basis. SG: 632.-1.

[17] Memo SG for Col [Lester D.] Flory, Oprs SOS, 17 Jul 42, sub: Comments on Housing for the 1943 Trp Basis. SG: 632.-1.

[18] (1) WD Cir 278, 21 Aug 42. (2) Mil Hosp and Evac Oprs, 15 Sep 42, par 13*b* (1), incl 1 to Ltr SPOPH 322.15, CG SOS to CGs and COs of SvCs, PEs, and to SG, 15 Sep 42, sub: Mil Hosp and Evac Oprs. HD: 322 (Hosp and Evac).

[19] 1st ind, SG to CofEngrs thru CG SOS, 8 Sep 42, on Memo CE 354 SPEOT, CofEngrs for SG, 27 Aug 42, sub: Hosp Fac for Fld Cp. SG: 632.-1.

[20] (1) See below, pp. 104-06. (2) Tynes, Construction Branch, p. 36.

[21] Memo, Act ACofS G-4 WDGS for CofS, 12 Nov 40, sub: Gen Hosp Program. HRS: G-4/29135-11.

[22] (1) Ltr, Col John R. Hall, SGO to Dr. Morris Fishbein, AMA, 4 Feb 42. SG: 601.-1. (2) Memo, Maj Achilles L. Tynes, SGO for SG, 26 Feb 42, sub: Rpt of Insp Trip to Monroe and Charlotte, NC. SG: 632.-1.

[23] Memo SP 632 (3-19-42), CG SOS for CofEngrs, 19 Mar 42, sub: Add Gen Hosps. SG: 632.-1.

[24] (1) Memo SPEX 632 (5-1-42), [Maj Gen Wilhelm D.] Styer for [Lt Gen Joseph T.] McNarney, 1 May 42, sub: Acquisition of Existing Hosps, . . . in lieu of Cons of New Gen Hosps. (2) Memo, CG SOS for CofSA, 3 May 42. (3) Memo, JTM[cNarney] for CofSA, 5 May 42. (4) D/S 632 (5-3-42), DepCofSA for SG, n d. All in SG: 632.-1. (5) Ltr, SG to CG SOS, 3 May 42. SG: 601.-1.

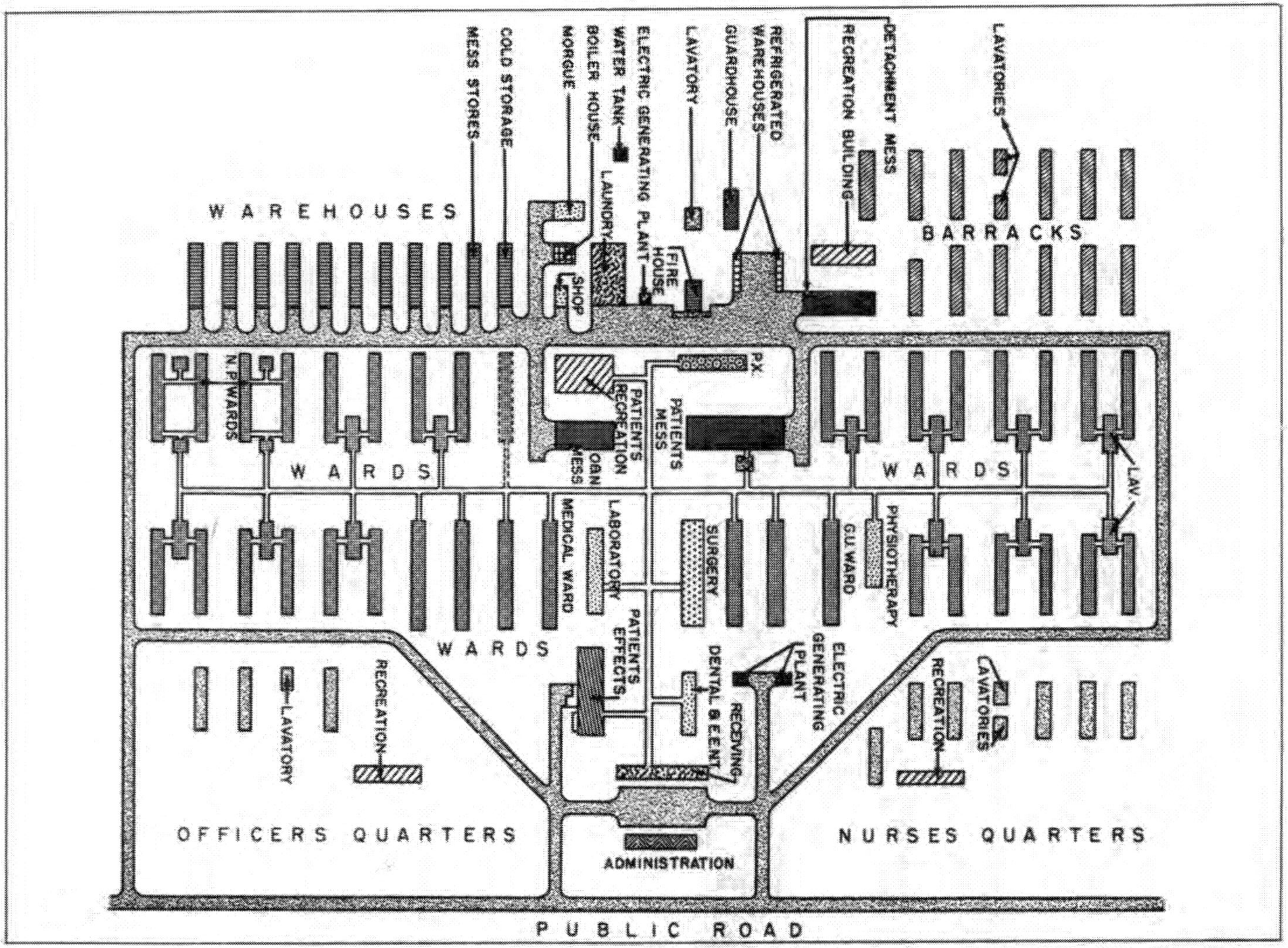

PLAN FOR THEATER-OF-OPERATIONS-TYPE HOSPITAL

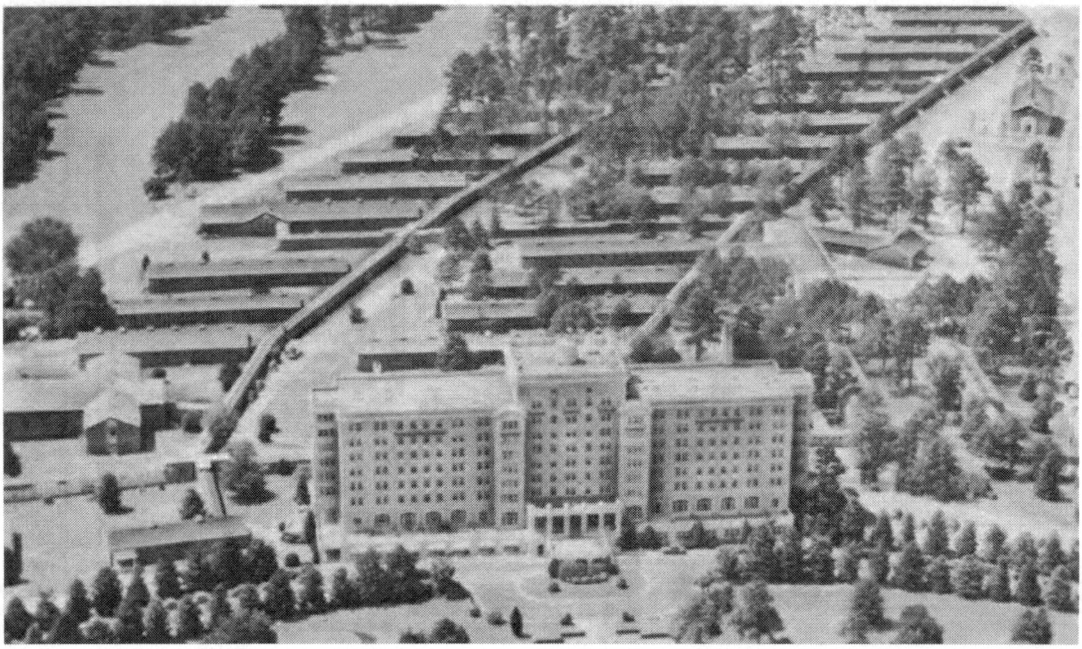

OLIVER GENERAL HOSPITAL *converted from the Forest Hills Hotel.*

A "Directive for Wartime Construction," issued two weeks later, confirmed as policy the practice of converting existing buildings into hospitals whenever practicable and of constructing new buildings otherwise.[25]

Difficulties involved in the civilian-facilities-conversion method restricted its use. Of hundreds of buildings which civilians offered to the Medical Department, not over 3 percent were suitable for use as hospitals.[26] Many were too small. Some had corridors, stairways, and doors that were too narrow to permit the passage of patients on litters. Others that were several stories high lacked adequate elevator service. Still others were in undesirable locations.[27] In some instances, where both the buildings and locations were suitable, local politicians and owners tried to get higher prices than the War Department was willing to pay. In others, local citizens banded together to prevent Army acquisition because they feared a depreciation in neighboring property values.[28] Finally, even after suitable buildings were found and all arrangements for acquisition completed, additions and alterations had to be made before the Medical Depart-

[25] Directive for Wartime Cons, 20 May 42, incl to Ltr AG 600.12 (5-20-42) MO-SPAD-M, TAG to CGs AAF, Depts, CAs, and C of Tec Servs, 1 Jun 42, same sub. SG: 632.-1.

[26] Ltr, Maj Lawrence G. King, SGO to Lt Col Albert Pierson, Off ACofS G-4 WDGS, 18 Jun 42, sub: Util of Existing Bldgs as Hosps. SG: 601.-1.

[27] (1) Ltr, SG to CG SOS, 3 May 42. SG: 601.-1. (2) Memo, SG for CofSA thru CG SOS, 19 May 42, sub: Preliminary Surv of Atlantic City Hotels for Hosp. HD: Hosp Insp Rpts, p. 680.

[28] (1) Pers Ltr, Col Harry D. Offutt to Col Don [G.] Hilldrup, 21 Apr 42. SG: 632.-2 (3d SvC)AA. (2) Notes on Conf, Hosp Cons Div SGO, 26 Mar 42, sub: Gen Hosp Program. HD: 632.-1.

TABLE 2—ARMY HOSPITALS ESTABLISHED IN CONVERTED CIVILIAN BUILDINGS BY END OF 1943

Hospital	Civilian Buildings
AAF Regional Sta Hosp	Miami Biltmore, Floridian, Gulf Stream, King Cole, Nautilus, Pancoast, and Tower Hotels
Army & Navy Gen Hosp Annex	Eastman Hotel
Ashford Gen Hosp	Greenbrier Hotel
Bronx Area Sta Hosp	Lebanon Hosp
Camp Shanks Sta Hosp	Rockland State Hosp
Charlotte, N. C., Sta Hosp	Charlotte Sanatorium
Dante Sta Hosp, San Francisco, Calif. (Later part of Letterman Gen Hosp)	Dante Hosp
Darnall Gen Hosp	Kentucky State Hosp
Deshon Gen Hosp	Butler Hosp
England Gen Hosp (Formerly AAF Sta Hosp, Atlantic City, N. J.)	Haddon Hall, Cedarcraft, Colton-Manor, Dennis, Keystone, New England, Rydal, Traymore, Warwick, and Chalfonte Hotels
Gardiner Gen Hosp (Formerly AAF Sta Hosp, Chicago, Ill.)	Chicago Beach Hotel
Halloran Gen Hosp	Willowbrook School
Hoff Gen Hosp Annex	Jefferson School, Calif.
Los Angeles, Calif., Sta Hosp	Villa Riviera Hotel
Mason Gen Hosp	Pilgrim State Hosp
New Haven, Conn., Sta Hosp	Wm. Wirt Winchester Hosp
Oakland Area Sta Hosp	Oakland Hotel
Oliver Gen Hosp	Forest Hills Hotel
Pasadena Area Sta Hosp	Vista Del Arroyo Hotel
Percy Jones Gen Hosp	Battle Creek Sanitarium
Percy Jones Gen Hosp Annex	Kellogg Estate, Battle Creek, Mich.
Ream Gen Hosp (Formerly AAF Sta Hosp, Palm Beach, Fla.)	Breakers Hotel
Rhodes Gen Hosp Annex	Marcy NYA Facility, N. Y.
St. Petersburg, Fla., Sta Hosp	Don-Ce-Sar Hotel
Seattle Area Sta Hosp	New Richmond Hotel
Staten Island Area Sta Hosp	Seaside Hosp
Torney Gen Hosp	El Mirador Hotel
Walter Reed Gen Hosp Annex	National Park College

Sources: (1) Ltr, SG to Sec War thru CG ASF, 18 May 43, sub: Gen Hosp Program. Use of converted hotels (Air Forces), with 7 nds. HD: 632.–1 (Hosp Expansion). (2) Incl, Record of Expansion and Contraction, Hosp ZI, and Hosp Ships, to Memo, Chief Cons Br SGO for HD SGO, 1 Nov 46, same sub. Same file. (3) Diary Hosp Cons Br SGO, 15 and 20 Jul 44. HD: 024.7–3. (4) An Rpt, 1943, England Gen Hosp, p. 3. HD. (5) An Rpt, 27 Nov 44, Hq AAF Reg Sta Hosp No. 1, pp. 1–6. HD.

ment could move in and set up functioning hospitals. Despite these difficulties and problems, the Army acquired enough civilian buildings by the end of 1943 to house twenty-three hospitals and expand five others. *(Table 2)*

Development of One-Story Semipermanent Type Hospital

Concurrently with increasing emphasis on conservation of building materials, forces were at work during 1942 which

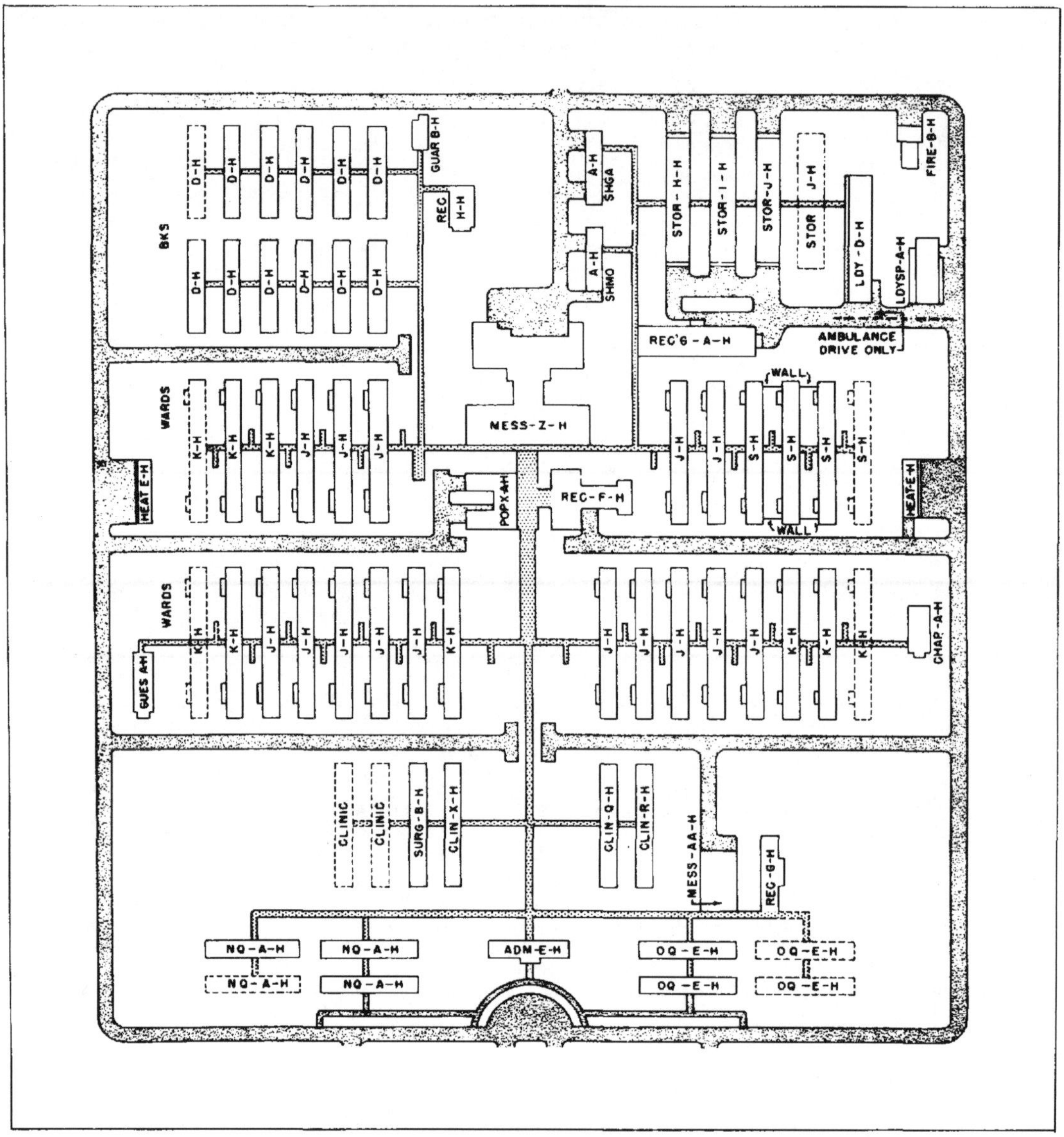

PLAN FOR TYPE A HOSPITAL

were to cause the War Department to turn again to the construction of semipermanent hospitals. As early as February 1942 the Clay Products Association of the Southwest began a campaign for the use of its materials by the Army, at least in hospital construction.[29] In April the Administrator of Veterans Affairs protested against the repetition of a World War I

[29] (1) Ltrs, Norman W. Kelch, Engr-Mgr, Clay Products Assn of the Southwest to UnderSecWar, 13 Feb and 3 Mar 42, sub: Fire-resistive Cons for Cantonment Type Hosps. (2) Ltr, UnderSecWar to Kelch, 19 Mar 42. (3) Ltr, CofEngrs to Kelch, 6 Mar 42. All in CE: 632 Pt 1.

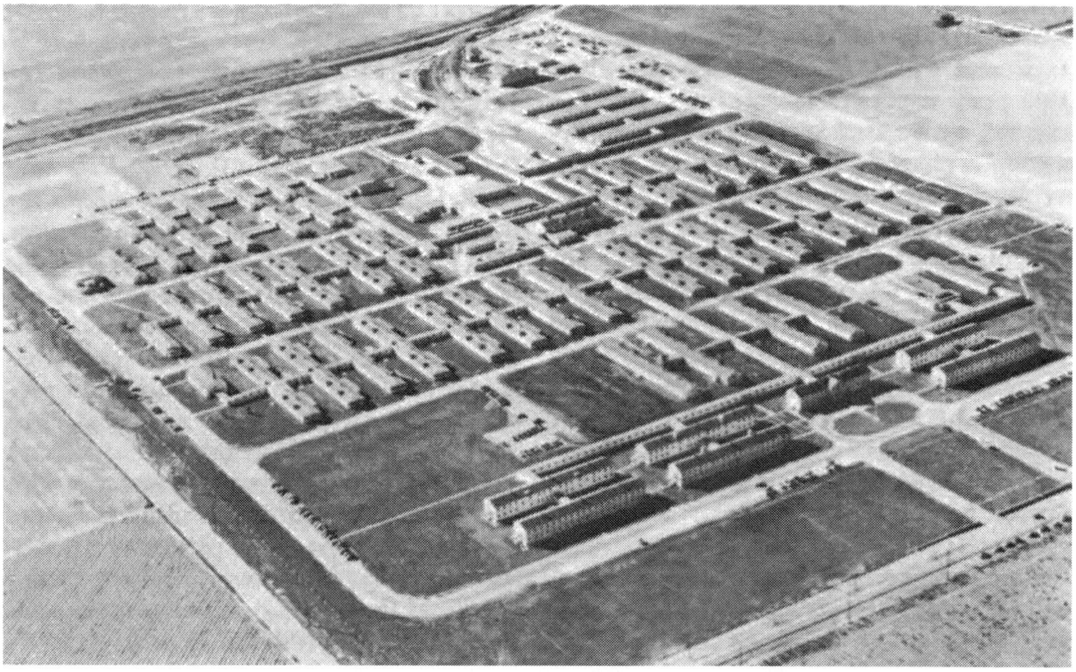

BIRMINGHAM GENERAL, A TYPE A HOSPITAL

mistake—the construction of hospitals that could not be converted to postwar use.[30] By June shortages of lumber had begun to develop in some areas, while surpluses of brick and tile had begun to accumulate. In some places, therefore, the Engineers began to build cantonment-type hospitals of tile and brick instead of lumber.[31] Then, on 10 August 1942, the War Production Board informed The Surgeon General of the availability of tile and brick and urged their use in hospital construction. The Surgeon General replied that he had always preferred noninflammable materials for hospital construction.[32] Soon afterward, his representatives joined the Engineers in work on plans for a new type of hospital.

The chief obstacle to development of plans for a one-story semipermanent hospital, which the Chief of Engineers proposed on 26 August 1942, was a difference of opinion between his Office and The Surgeon General's over the internal characteristics of various buildings. Feeling it necessary to hold the cost of construction as near as possible to that of cantonment-type buildings, the Engineers were prone to limit improvements and refinements to the absolute minimum. On the other hand, Colonel Hall of The Surgeon General's Construction Division saw no reason to

[30] Ltrs, Admin of Vet Affairs to CG SOS and to SecWar, 1 Apr 42. SG: 632.-1.

[31] (1) Ltr, CofEngrs to SG, 11 Jun 42, sub: Use of Structural-Tile Exterior Walls at Ft Des Moines and Cp Dodge Hosps, with 1st ind, SG to CofEngrs, 15 June 42. SG: 632.-1. (2) Exhibit A to Memo, Col John R. Hall for SG, 13 Jun 42, sub: Rpt of Fld Trip covering Insp of 1411-bed Hosp at Cp Atterbury and of the French Lick Hotel Property. HD: Hosp Insp Rpts, p. 726.

[32] (1) Ltr, Chief Bldg Materials Br Oprs WPB to SG, 10 Aug 42. (2) Ltr, SG to WPB, 14 Aug 42, sub: Hosp Cons. Both in SG: 632.-1.

design a third type of hospital if it was not materially better than the cantonment type and equal, in most respects, to the two-story semipermanent type. For example, he wanted larger and more efficiently arranged clinical buildings, stronger and safer neuropsychiatric wards, increased administrative space, and better-equipped messes. After numerous conferences and what must have seemed to the Engineers an uncompromising attitude on the part of the Surgeon General's Office, they composed their differences and during the winter of 1942–43 a civilian architectural firm employed by the Engineers completed drawings for the new type of hospital.[33]

The Type A hospital, as plants constructed according to the new design were called, came to be considered by the Surgeon General's Office as the best for emergency construction in the zone of interior. Basically, it was the two-story semipermanent hospital reduced to one-story form. Being only one story high it was safer for patients and did not require expensive and unhandy two-story ramps. Its clinical facilities were more adequate and more efficiently arranged than those of the two-story hospital. It also cost less to build. Because wards were placed on both sides of corridors and were lengthened from 262 to 287 feet, the Type A hospital covered a smaller area than other one-story plants. Its chief disadvantage was that it was designed on the dispersed-pavilion principle. Before the war's end, twelve hospitals were constructed on this plan.[34] *(Table 3)*

Modification of the Type A Hospital for Postwar Use by the Veterans Administration

In the spring of 1943 plans for the Type A hospital were modified as a result of attempts to co-ordinate wartime hospital construction with postwar needs. On 31 March 1943 the President directed the Federal Board of Hospitalization to review plans for hospital construction of all federal agencies, including the War and Navy Departments.[35] The next month the Board proposed that the Army build some of its hospitals according to standard plans of the Veterans Administration, for use after the war. SOS headquarters raised no objection, but disclaimed any responsibility for justifying and defending this proposal.[36] Anticipating its approval, The Surgeon General's construction officers and the Engineers, in collaboration with the Veterans Administration, prepared layouts for Type A hospitals which substituted five two-story VA-type ward buildings for ordinary wards. In May the President approved the Federal Board's recommendation that two Army general hospitals—McGuire at Richmond, Va., and Vaughan at Hines, Ill.—be constructed on that plan.[37]

Many factors thus shaped the kinds of hospital plants which the Army acquired

[33] (1) Ltr, CofEngrs to SG, sub: One-Story Masonry Wall Gen-Hosp, 26 Aug 42, with 3 inds. (2) Ltr, SG to CofEngrs, 12 Nov 42, sub: One-Story Masonry Cons Hosp, 1100 Series, Drawings by York and Sawyer, with 4 inds. All in SG: 632.-1.

[34] (1) Tynes, Construction Branch, pp. 37, 40–41. (2) The Type A hospitals were Battey, Birmingham, Crile, Cushing, DeWitt, Dibble, Glennan, Madigan, Mayo, Baker, and Northington General Hospitals, and Waltham Regional Hospital.

[35] Ltr, President of US to Sec War, 31 Mar 43. SG: 632.-1.

[36] Memo, CG SOS for SG 17 Apr 43, sub: Completion of Gen Hosp Program in U.S. SG: 632.-1.

[37] (1) Memo, SG for CofEngrs, 3 May 43. SG: 632.-1. (2) Ltr, CofEngrs to CG ASF, 10 May 43, sub: VA Type Ward Bldgs, with 1st ind SPRMC 600.12 (5-10-43), CG ASF to CofEngrs, n d. CE: 632 Vol 4. (3) Ltr, Dir Cons VA to Col John R. Hall, SGO, 19 May 43, with 1st ind, SG to CofEngrs, 1 Jun 43, sub: Hosp Cons. SG: 632.-1. (4) Ltr, SG to CofEngrs, 7 Jun 43, sub: 1785-bed Gen Hosp, Richmond, Va., Area. SG: 632.-1(McGuire Gen Hosp)K.

TABLE 3—BUILDING SCHEDULE FOR TYPE–A HOSPITAL

General Hospital Plan

Building	Type	Title	Number Required	
			For 1727 Beds	For 1515 Beds
ADM	E–H	Administration Building	1	1
ANIM	A–H	Animal House	1	1
BKS	D–H	Med. Det. Adm. & Unit Stores	1	1
BKS	D–H	Med. Det. Barracks	11	10
CHAP	A–H	Chapel	1	1
CLIN	R–H	Clinic, Dental, EEN&T	1	1
CLIN	Q–H	Clinic, Lab. & Prof. Services	1	1
CLIN	X–H	Clinic, X-ray, G. U. & Physiotherapy	1	1
FIRE	B–H	Fire Station	1	1
GUAR	B–H	Guard House	1	1
GUES	A–H	Guest House	1	1
HEAT	G–H	Heating Plant, H. P	As required.	
HEAT	E–H	Heating Plant, L. P	As required.	
HEAT	F–H	Heating Plant, H. P. Annex to L. P	As required.	
INC	A–M	Incinerator—3-ton	1	1
LDY	D–H	Laundry	1	1
LDYSP	A–H	Laundry Steam Plant	1	1
MESS	Z–H	Enl. Patients & Med. Det. Mess	1	1
MESS	AA–H	Officers' & Nurses' Mess	1	1
NQ	A–H	Nurses' Qtrs	4	3
OQ	E–H	Officers' Qtrs	2	2
POPX	A–H	Post Office & Post Exchange	1	1
REC	H–H	Med. Det. Recreation	1	1
REC	G–H	Officers' & Nurses' Recreation	1	1
REC	F–H	Patient's Recreation	1	1
RECG	A–H	Receiving & Evacuation Bldg	1	1
SHGA	A–H	Shops & Garage	1	1
SHMO	A–H	Hospital Shop & Morgue	1	1
STOR	I–H	Med. Storehouse	1	1
STOR	H–H	Med. Storehouse & Offices	1	1
STOR	J–H	Storehouse	2	1
SURG	B–H	Clinic, Surgery	1	1
WARD	K–H	Ward, Combination	9	6
WARD	S–H	Ward, Detention	4	3
WARD	J–H	Ward, Standard	15	15

Covered walks and exit ramps are included in the plan. A number of supplementary buildings may also be added to this type of hospital construction. The basic plan is shown on the opposite page.

Source: Tynes, Construction Branch, p. 49. HD:314.7–2 (Hosp. Const. Br.).

or constructed during World War II. Such forces as necessity for speed in construction, availability of building materials, pressure of civilian groups, and co-ordination of Army wartime construction with postwar needs of other Federal agencies often seemed stronger than medical considerations. The Surgeon General's Office therefore frequently found itself in conflict with higher authorities in attempting to get what it considered to be suitable and satisfactory hospital plants. While undesirable cantonment-type plans drawn before the war were used for most hospitals, better plants were designed and the Army erected 10 two-story and 12 one-story semipermanent hospitals on new plans as well as 2 designed specifically for postwar use by the Veterans Administration.

Estimates of Hospital Capacity Needed

Speed in construction and conservation of materials also affected planning for the expansion of hospitals. During most of 1942 speed was so necessary to keep hospital capacities abreast of the Army's growth that there was little time for re-examining the basis already established for estimating requirements. Hence, conservation of building materials was at first achieved by lowering the quality rather than the quantity of construction. Moreover the need for speed, along with uncertainty about the eventual size of the Army and the rate of its movement overseas, perhaps accounted partially for the fact that until the end of 1942 little attention was given to the co-ordination of station with general hospital requirements, of Army with Navy requirements, and of wartime with postwar requirements. Even disregarding these matters, planning for a rapid and unprecedented expansion was a complicated process. In the first part of 1942 plans had to be made to meet immediate normal requirements. In addition, plans for emergencies were needed because it was feared that sneak attacks, sabotage, or severe epidemics might require hospital beds far in excess of the number normally provided. Later, when emphasis was placed upon reduction in quantity as well as quality of construction, a tendency developed to make long-range plans. All three types of planning—normal, emergency, and long-range—were inevitably interrelated.

Early Plans To Meet Normal Requirements

Plans for station hospitals to house the number of beds authorized by the existing bed ratio were automatically included by the Engineers in general construction plans for each camp, but planning for the expansion of general hospitals was different. Although general hospital beds were authorized for 1 percent of the total strength of the Army, construction of plants to accommodate that number did not automatically follow. Instead The Surgeon General had to request periodically the approval of construction to house specific numbers of general hospital beds. He usually received approval for less than the 1 percent asked for. As a stopgap measure The Surgeon General on 18 December 1941 recommended the construction of four new general hospitals and annexes to two existing hospitals to provide 6,000 additional beds. The next day G–4 approved this recommendation.[38]

[38] (1) Ltr, SG to TAG, 18 Dec 41, sub: Location of 6,000 Add Gen Hosp Beds. SG: 632.-1. (2) Memo, ACofS G–4 WDGS for TAG. 19 Dec 41, sub: Gen Hosps. HRS: G–4/29135–11.

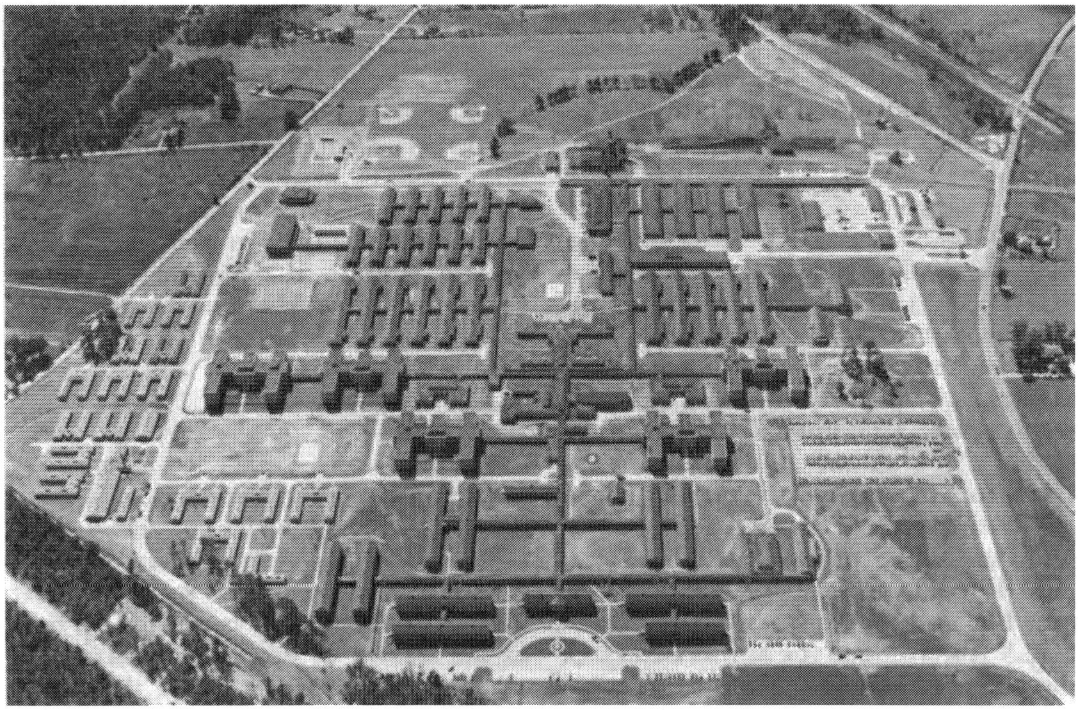

McGUIRE GENERAL, A VA-TYPE HOSPITAL

The following February, after the troop basis for 1942 was published, The Surgeon General recommended enough additional beds (18,600) to make a total by the end of 1942 of 39,600, 1 percent of the planned strength of the Army.[39] Of these, G–4 authorized only 14,000, to be completed by 30 September 1942, advising The Surgeon General informally to include further requirements in longer-range planning.[40] By June 1942 it was possible to project requirements to the end of 1943. Informed that the strength of the Army by that time would be 6,600,000 men The Surgeon General recommended 30,026 beds in addition to those already available or authorized, to make a total of 66,000.[41] Although the SOS Hospitalization and Evacuation Branch agreed to this number for planning purposes, the SOS Construction Planning Branch directed the Engineers a few weeks later to construct only 23,500.[42]

When The Surgeon General estimated total general hospital bed requirements, he planned also their distribution among different hospitals. Before the war all new

[39] Ltr, SG to CofEngrs, 3 Feb 42, sub: Add Gen Hosp Beds. SG: 632.-1.

[40] Memo for Record, on Memo, ACofS WDGS G-4 for TAG, 9 Feb 42, sub: Add Gen Hosp Beds. HRS: G-4/29135-11.

[41] Ltr, SG to CG SOS, 6 Jun 42, sub: Add Gen Hosp Beds. SG: 632.-2.

[42] Memo SPOPM 632, Dir Oprs Div SOS (init WLW[ilson]) for Dir Reqmts Div SOS, 17 Jun 42, sub: Add Gen Hosp Beds. HD: Wilson files, "Book I, 26 May 42-26 Sep 42." (2) Memos SPRMC 601.1, CG SOS for CofEngrs, 4 and 7 Jul 42, same sub. HD: 632.-1.

general hospitals had been constructed on a 1,000-bed plan. Larger hospitals could be operated with a lower ratio of personnel to beds, and after Pearl Harbor he began to recommend the construction of 1,500-bed hospitals.[43] During 1942 hospitals of this size gradually superseded those of 1,000-bed capacity.[44] With this beginning, the tendency to enlarge general hospital capacities was to grow until some of them would reach 6,000 by 1945.

When the Army began to emphasize reductions in quantity as well as quality of construction, attention centered momentarily on the authorized bed ratio. The Inspector General and the director of the SOS Requirements Division believed that it was too high.[45] In June 1942 there were 96,291 beds in general and station hospitals, but only about 73,285 were occupied.[46] According to the authorized ratio, there should have been 129,640 beds.[47] Referring to reports on the occupancy of beds and to directives limiting construction to the essential minimum, SOS headquarters called upon The Surgeon General for an analytical study of bed requirements based on the experience of the previous ten years, rather than World War I, with a view to a possible reduction in authorized ratios.[48] Although tables he submitted showed the ratio of occupied beds to Army strength from 1932 to 1941 to have been nearer 3.5 percent than the authorized ratio, The Surgeon General urged that the latter not be reduced. He pointed out that only 80 percent of the beds provided should be considered available, since approximately 20 percent of the total was lost through "dispersion"—the separation of patients into wards according to disease, rank, and sex. He believed that a higher proportion of men would require beds during war than during peacetime, because battle casualties would need extended periods of hospital care, recruits would have higher sick rates than seasoned soldiers, and accidents would occur more frequently under strenuous training programs.[49] By the time of this reply higher authorities were considering double bunking in barracks and this was to lead to a temporary increase, rather than a reduction, in the authorized bed ratios.

Planning for Emergencies

Hospital construction for normal use was so urgent in the first hectic months of the war that planning for emergencies was left largely to local commanders. The Surgeon General expected them to meet needs that might arise by setting up beds in the solaria of hospital buildings, by placing more beds in wards than were usually considered desirable, and by using as wards the barracks of enlisted hospital-complements and, if necessary, of other troops. These methods were prescribed in

[43] (1) Ltr, SG to TAG, 18 Dec 41, sub: Location of 6,000 Add Gen Hosp Beds. SG: 632.-1.

[44] Ltr, SG to CG SOS, 6 Jun 42, sub: Add Gen Hosp Beds. SG: 632.-2.

[45] Memo for Record, on Memo SPOPM 323.7 Hosp, CG SOS for SG, 22 Jun 42, sub: Reqmts and Distr of Hosp Beds. HD: Wilson files, "Book I, 26 Mar 42–26 Sep 42."

[46] Bed Status Rpts, end of last week in Jun 42. Off file, Health Rpts Br Med Statistics Div SGO.

[47] This figure was arrived at by multiplying the strength of the Army in the United States by 4 percent and the total strength of the Army by 1 percent and adding the results. Of a total strength in June 1942 of 3,074,184, there were in the United States 2,472,407 officers and men. Figures furnished by Strength Accounting Branch AGO, 25 Oct 47.

[48] Memo SPOPM 323.7 Hosp, CG SOS for SG, 22 Jun 42, sub: Reqmts and Distr of Hosp Beds. SG: 632.-2.

[49] 1st ind, SG to Dir of Oprs SOS, 25 Jul 42, on Memo 323.7 Hosp, CG SOS for SG, 22 Jun 42, sub: Reqmts and Distr of Hosp Beds. SG: 632.-2.

Army regulations and, upon The Surgeon General's recommendation, the use of barracks to expand hospital capacities was required by the SOS directive on hospitalization and evacuation issued on 18 June 1942. Included in the same directive by the SOS Hospitalization and Evacuation Branch was another provision which The Surgeon General considered unnecessary—the requirement that subordinate commanders plan to double hospital capacities in emergencies by using civilian buildings such as apartments, hotels, schools, and dormitories.[50]

In the late summer and fall of 1942 a combination of circumstances focused attention upon the question of emergency hospitalization. Plans were being made for the North African invasion and for the reception in the United States of large numbers of casualties. Concurrently, as a means of reducing general construction requirements, the Chief of Staff and the commanding general, Services of Supply, decided to require the double bunking of troops in existing barracks. The Surgeon General warned them that the resultant reduction in per capita air space might lead to severe epidemics of respiratory diseases.[51] General Marshall believed that this risk had to be taken, but feared that existing beds might be insufficient if an epidemic should occur at the same time casualties began to flow back from North Africa. On 10 August 1942 he verbally directed The Surgeon General, through the latter's executive officer, to plan to take over hotels in an emergency for use as Army hospitals and to arrange with local physicians for civilian groups to man them. The next day General Marshall's deputy referred to this directive in a meeting of the General Council (a group of representatives of the General Staff, and of AGF, AAF, and SOS headquarters) and the SOS Chief of Staff afterward directed The Surgeon General "to take immediate" steps to enlarge hospital capacities in the event of an emergency.[52]

The Office of Civilian Defense was making plans for the emergency hospitalization of civilians, earmarking hotels and organizing "affiliated units" of civilian physicians and nurses to staff them if needed.[53] Realizing the possibility of conflict between OCD plans and General Marshall's directive, General Magee discussed the problem with General Lutes and with Dr. George Baehr, who was in charge of OCD medical activities. He then presented it to the Office of Defense Health and Welfare Services' Health and Medical Committee, whose function was to co-ordinate all health and medical activities relating to national defense.

Meanwhile, on 27 and 28 August 1942, General Magee transmitted General Marshall's directive to service commands. They were already listing hotels that could

[50] (1) AR 40–1080, C 2, 16 Mar 40. (2) The Surgeon General's Plan for Hosp (ZI) and Evac, incl to Memo, SG for CG SOS, 31 Mar 42, sub: Basic Plan for Hosp Oprs and Evac of Sick and Wounded. HRS: ASF Hosp and Evac Sec file, "Misc Classified Corresp from Off CG ASF to AGO." (3) Memo, Col H. T. Wickert, SGO, for Col [W. L.] Wilson, SOS, 30 Apr 42, with incl Memo, SG for Dir Oprs SOS, 30 Apr 42. Same file. (4) See above, pp. 65–66.

[51] (1) 1st ind, SG to CG SOS, 11 Jul 42, on Memo, CG SOS for SG, 9 Jul 42, sub: Capacity of Bks. (2) Memo, SG for CG SOS, 25 Aug 42, sub: Double Bunking. All in SG: 632.–1.

[52] (1) Extract from Mins of Gen Council, 11 Aug 42. HD: Wilson files, 600.13 "Hosp Policy and Plans." (2) Memo, CofSA for President of US, 21 Sep 42, sub: Reply to your Memo of Sep 14th Conc Util of Hotels as Mil Hosps. WDCofSA: 632 (14 Aug 42). (3) Memo, Brig Gen Larry B. McAfee for SG, 31 Oct 42. HD: 632.–1 "Hosp Expansion." (4) Statements of SG and his Exec Off, Cmtee to Study the MD, Testimony, pp. 1309ff and 1669ff. HD.

[53] Cmtee to Study the MD, 1942, Testimony, pp. 984ff. HD.

be taken over in emergencies, in accordance with the SOS directive of 18 June 1942. To comply with the new directive, they had merely to review those lists, itemize the medical property that would be required, and arrange with a local physician to build up a staff for each emergency hospital.[54]

The Office of Civilian Defense and the Health and Medical Committee objected to this action because it threatened to interfere with plans for emergency hospitalization for civilians and posed the danger of transferring epidemics from Army camps into cities. The Office of Defense Health and Welfare Services then informed the President of the Army's plan, suggesting that the War Department rescind its directive and plan to provide emergency hospitalization for military personnel entirely within the confines of Army camps and with military professional staffs only.

Meanwhile the plan called for by the Chief of Staff was misinterpreted by the President, who understood that the Army intended to take over hotels and develop them into stand-by hospitals in advance of an emergency. When asked for an explanation, General Marshall assured him that this was not so, but assumed full responsibility for having directed the earmarking of hotels and the organization of civilian staffs for emergency use. The President apparently considered this explanation satisfactory, for he passed General Marshall's letter on to the Office of Defense Health and Welfare Services with the single comment, "for your information."[55]

After General Marshall's explanation to the President it was still necessary to solve the problem of simultaneous planning by the Army and the Office of Civilian Defense to use civilian staffs in emergency hospitals. At first SOS headquarters took the position that "any plan to utilize civilian medical personnel for military hospitalization is entirely a planning matter to establish a potential means to meet major emergencies. . . ."[56] When this assurance failed to satisfy the Office of Civilian Defense, SOS headquarters changed its position and, strangely enough, required The Surgeon General to inform the Health and Medical Committee that it had never been War Department policy to use civilian staffs to care for military patients.[57] Meanwhile General Magee had conferred with General Marshall and with Dr. Baehr. He then proposed a compro-

[54] (1) Memo, SG for Brig Gen LeRoy Lutes, 21 Aug 42, sub: Over-All Plan for Emergency Med Care, Civ and Mil. HD: 632.-1 "Hosp Expansion." (2) Statements by Baehr and Magee, Cmtee to Study the MD, 1942, Testimony, pp. 984ff and 1669ff. HD. (3) Ltrs, CG SOS per SG to CGs of SvCs, 27 and 28 Aug 42, sub: Hosp Expansion. HD: 632.-1.

[55] (1) Ltr, Exec Sec, Health and Med Cmtee to Dir Off of Def Health and Welfare Servs, 5 Sep 42. HD: 632.-1 "Hosp Expansion." (2) Ltr, Dir Off of Civ Def to same, 12 Sep 42. Same file. (3) Ltr, Dir Off of Def Health and Welfare Servs to the President, 10 Sep 42. Natl Archives: Record Group 215, Off of Community War Servs, 922.3. (4) Memo, FDR[oosevelt] for Gen Marshall, 14 Sep 42. WDCofSA: 632 (14 Aug 42). (5) Memo, CofSA for the President, 21 Sep 42, sub: Reply to your Memo. . . . Same file. (6) Memo, FDR[oosevelt] for Hon Paul McNutt, [Dir Off of Def Health and Welfare Servs], 3 Oct 42. Natl Archives: Record Group 215, Off of Community War Servs, 922.3.

[56] (1) Memo SPOPH 701, Lt Col W. L. Wilson, Chief Hosp and Evac Br SOS for Gen Lutes, 17 Sep 42, sub: Current Program for Mil Hosp, with 2 incls. HD: Wilson files, "Book I, 26 Mar 42–26 Sep 42." (2) Ltr SPAAC 601, Chief Admin Serv SOS for Dir OCD, 9 Oct 42. Natl Archives: Record Group 215, Off of Community War Servs, 922.3.

[57] (1) Memo, SG for CG SOS, 8 Oct 42, sub: Planning for Expansion, Army Med Fac. HD: 632.-1 "Hosp Expansion." (2) Ltr, Dir OCD to Maj Gen George Grunert, Chief Admin Serv SOS, 23 Oct 42. Natl Archives: Record Group 215, Off of Community War Servs, 922.3. (3) Memo SPAAC 632 (10-20-42), CG SOS for SG, 26 Oct 42, same sub, with 4 inds. SG: 632.-1. (4) Memo SPOPH 632 (10-10-42), Dep for ACofS for Oprs SOS (init WLW[ilson]) for Chief

mise which in his opinion embodied the wishes of General Marshall and met the approval of Dr. Baehr. According to its terms the Army would plan to use in an emergency only those hotels which it could reasonably expect to staff with military personnel. If civilian doctors and nurses should be needed temporarily the Army would borrow staffs organized by the Office of Civilian Defense and the United States Public Health Service. Although SOS headquarters had disavowed the use of civilian staffs shortly before, it now approved a letter to service commands on 11 January 1943 explaining the compromise just mentioned.[58] On 22 February Dr. Baehr sent a similar explanation to regional medical officers of OCD.[59] Since the contemplated emergency never developed, the Army had no occasion either to take over the hotels earmarked or to call upon the Office of Civilian Defense for emergency staffs.

SOS planning for the emergency expansion of Army hospitals went on concurrently with that directed by General Marshall. On 25 August 1942 the Chief of the Hospitalization and Evacuation Branch informed General Lutes that no plan existed for assuring the availability of beds in case of an epidemic and requested authority to prepare one.[60] Given the go-ahead signal, he proposed on 9 September 1942 that the station hospital bed ratio be raised from 4 percent to 5 percent for the winter of 1942–43 and that housing for additional beds thus authorized should be provided either by converting cantonment-type hospital barracks into wards and constructing theater-of-operations-type barracks for the displaced enlisted personnel or by constructing additional cantonment-type wards wherever a medical detachment already lived in theater-of-operations-type barracks.[61] This plan was approved, and on 19 September 1942 the commanding general, Services of Supply, ordered the Chief of Engineers to put it into effect.[62] As further provision for an emergency, the SOS Hospitalization and Evacuation Branch inserted in the revised version of the hospitalization and evacuation directive dated 15 September 1942 a requirement that each hospital plan to provide additional beds in barracks for 10 percent of the troops served.[63] Thus each hospital would be prepared to care for 15 percent of its station's strength. The 5 percent authorization proved sufficient for the winter's needs.

In the course of the Army's controversy with the Office of Civilian Defense, General Marshall directed General Snyder, the medical officer on The Inspector General's staff, to investigate means of meeting requirements that might develop in an emergency. General Snyder reported that enough beds existed, on the 4 percent

Admin Serv SOS, 20 Oct 42, same sub. HD: Wilson files, "Book 2, 26 Sep 42–31 Dec 42." (5) Memo SPOPH 632 (11–17–42), ACofS for Oprs SOS (init WLW[ilson]) for same, 22 Nov 42, same sub. Same file. (6) Ltr, Act SG to Exec Sec, Health and Med Cmtee, 14 Dec 42. SG: 632.-1.

[58] (1) 3d ind, Act SG to Chief of Admin Serv SOS, 14 Dec 42, on Memo SPAAC 632 (10–20–42), CG SOS for SG, 26 Oct 42, sub: Planning for Expansion, Army Med Fac. SG: 632.–1. (2) Ltr SPX 632 (1–8–43) OB-S-SPOPH-M, CG SOS to CGs all SvCs, 11 Jan 43, same sub. HD: 632.–1.

[59] Ltr, Chief Med Off OCD to Regional Med Offs OCD, 22 Feb 43, sub: Cooperation with the Army in the Care of Mil Casualties. HD: 632.–1.

[60] Memo SPOPH 620 (7–4–42) Bks, Col Wilson for Gen Lutes, 25 Aug 42, sub: Capacity of Bks. HD: Wilson files, "Book 1, 26 Mar–26 Sep 42."

[61] Memo SPOPH 322.15, ACofS for Oprs SOS (init WLW[ilson]) for Cons Br Reqmts Div SOS, 9 Sep 42, sub: Opr Plans for Hosp and Evac. HD: Wilson files, "Book I, 26 Mar–26 Sep 42."

[62] Memo SPRMC 632 (9–9–42), CG SOS for CofEngrs, 19 Sep 42, sub: Add Hosps. SG: 632.–1.

[63] Mil Hosp and Evac Oprs, sec I, par 3*b* (3), incl 1 to Ltr SPOPH 322.15, CG SOS to CGs of SvCs and PEs and to SG, 15 Sep 42, sub: Mil Hosp and Evac Oprs. HD: 322.

basis, to meet ordinary requirements plus those of a minor epidemic. He estimated that 7,500 additional beds could be made available by treating minor cases in quarters; 6,000, by treating uncomplicated cases of venereal disease on a duty status; 97,000, by caring for convalescent patients in barracks; 25,000, by reducing the floor area per bed in existing wards; and a substantial number, by improving administrative procedures and limiting the performance of elective operations. In case of an unusually severe epidemic, all barracks, he believed, could be converted into hospitals and troops could be moved into warehouses, regimental recreation buildings, and chapels.[64] Under an SOS directive, The Surgeon General attempted later to carry out some of General Snyder's recommendations for more effective bed utilization.[65] His recommendations for meeting the needs of an epidemic never had to be put into effect.

Long-Range Planning

Late in 1942 the Army began to try to co-ordinate hospital construction with other requirements and with postwar needs. To this end SOS headquarters insisted that each service forecast its normal needs as far ahead as possible.[66] The Surgeon General found it difficult to anticipate station hospital requirements because they depended, as always, upon troop distributions unknown by him. In addition, records of existing station hospitals were unreliable, those of the divisions of the Surgeon General's Office differing among themselves and with records of the Engineers.[67] But projection into the future of general hospital bed requirements was less difficult.

In forecasting the need for general hospital beds in the fall of 1942, The Surgeon General adopted a new basis for estimates. Plans for the invasion of North Africa were being made and it was expected that large numbers of combat casualties would be returned to the United States. From World War I experience it appeared that beds would be needed in general hospitals in the United States for 1.7 percent of all overseas forces if patients requiring 120 or more days of hospitalization were evacuated from theaters of operations.[68] The Surgeon General therefore added .7 percent of the strength of overseas forces to the 1 percent of the total strength of the Army already established as the basis for estimating general hospital bed requirements. On 26 September 1942 he recommended that a total of 96,000 general hospital beds be provided by the end of 1943 and of 124,800 by the middle of 1944. About two months later, when the projected Army strength was changed, he proposed that the mid-1944 figure be cut to 103,500. SOS headquarters approved his recommendations, and until the early part of 1943 this figure stood as the number of beds authorized for planning purposes, but not for construction.[69] *(Chart 4)*

[64] Ltr, IG per Brig Gen Howard McC. Snyder to CofSA, 10 Nov 42, sub: Surv of Hosp Fac and their Util. HRS: WDCSA 632.

[65] See below, pp. 127, 130–31.

[66] (1) Memo, CofEngrs for SG, 10 Oct 42, sub: Prep of Sec V of Army Sup Program. SG: 632.-1. (2) Memo for Record, on 3d ind SPOPH 632 (9-26-42), CG SOS to SG, 29 Oct 42, on Memo, SG for CG SOS, 26 Sep 42, sub: Hosp, Gen Hosps. HD: Wilson files, "Book 2, 26 Sep 42–31 Dec 42."

[67] (1) Cmtee to Study the MD, 1942, Rpt, p. 8. HD. (2) Memo, Dir Control Div SGO for SG, 8 Feb 43, sub: Statistics on Hosp Beds. SG: 632.-2.

[68] Statistics of World War I were analyzed in *Army Medical Bulletin*, No. 24 (1931).

[69] (1) Memo, SG for CG SOS, 26 Sep 42, sub: Hosp, Gen Hosps, with 4 inds. SG: 632.-2. (2) Memo, Chief Hosp Cons Div SGO for Asst Dir Fiscal Div SGO, 19 Jan 43, sub: Bed Reqmts for FY 1944. Same file. (3) Ltr, SG to CG SOS, 11 Mar 43, sub: Hosp, Gen Hosps. SG: 323.7-5.

CHART 4—THE SURGEON GENERAL'S ESTIMATES IN 1941–42 OF BED REQUIREMENTS IN GENERAL HOSPITALS IN CONTINENTAL UNITED STATES AND ACTUAL BEDS REPORTED JANUARY 1942–JULY 1944

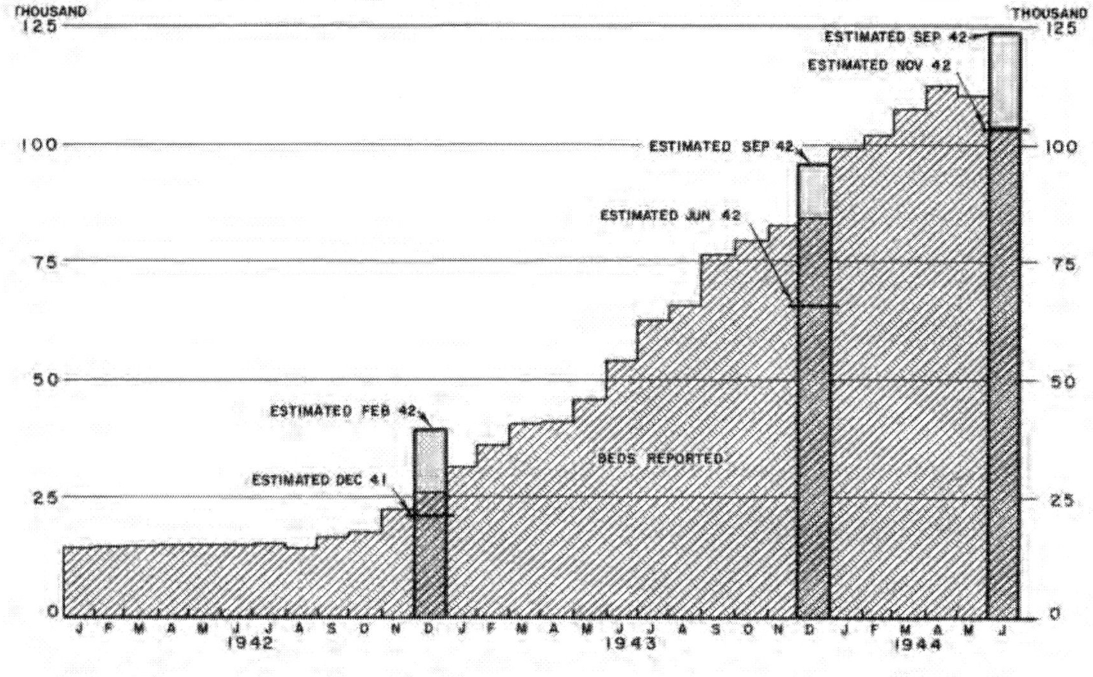

Source: (1) Documents referred to in Chap V, sec "Estimates of Hospital Capacity Needed."
(2) Bed Status Reports, Health Reports Br, Med Statistics Div, SGO.

Early in 1943 a combination of circumstances pointed toward intensified efforts by the General Staff and SOS headquarters to limit construction. In January a study of hospital bed occupancy, prepared by the Surgeon General's Office for inclusion in the SOS Monthly Progress Report, showed that estimated requirements had been higher than actual needs. While there was a close correlation between estimated requirements and occupied beds in station hospitals, a discrepancy between estimated requirements and occupied beds in general hospitals had grown from 11,000 to 45,000 during 1942. The Surgeon General explained that this resulted from better health and fewer combat casualties than anticipated.[70] In March 1943 certain members of Congress threatened to investigate the use of all hospital beds, both civilian and military, in the United States.[71] Soon afterward the Secretary of the Navy proposed that the Army and Navy consider the possibility of making joint use of their hospitals.[72] Furthermore, the Surgeon General of the

[70] (1) SOS Monthly Progress Rpt, Sec 5, Pt IV, *Health*, pp. 44–45, 31 Jan 43.

[71] *Establishing a Select Committee to Investigate Hospital Facilities Within the United States of America, 78th Cong, 1st sess on* H. Res. 146, 3 March 1943.

[72] Memo WDGDS 2857, ACofS G–4 WDGS for CofSA, 15 Mar 43, sub: Joint Army-Navy Use of Available Hosp Accommodations. HRS: G–4 files, "Hosp and Evac Policy."

United States Public Health Service, calling attention to the interest of Congress and of the War Production Board in the matter, suggested to Brig. Gen. Frank T. Hines, Administrator of Veterans Affairs and Chairman of the Federal Board of Hospitalization, the desirability of co-ordinating the hospital construction planning of all Government agencies.[73] As a result, the President on 31 March 1943 ordered the War and Navy Departments, the Federal Security Administration, and the Veterans Administration to submit all plans for additional hospital construction to the Federal Board of Hospitalization for co-ordination and submission to him, through the Bureau of the Budget, for approval.[74]

Meanwhile, despite a discrepancy between estimated and actual requirements in 1942 and in the face of growing interest in limiting hospital construction, The Surgeon General again raised his estimates. On the basis of new troop strength figures from the Bureau of the Budget, he asked SOS headquarters on 11 March 1943 to approve an increase in authorized general hospital beds from 96,000 to 102,882 for December 1943 and from 103,500 to 110,693 for July 1944. He also asked approval of the higher bed ratio which he had been using since September 1942.[75] Apparently the Services of Supply, renamed Army Service Forces on 12 March 1943, was in no mood to approve either additional beds or a higher ratio. Instead, its Requirements Division directed The Surgeon General to review the proposed ratio in the light of recent war experience and to consider a reduction of construction requirements by the joint use of Army and Navy facilities, the expansion of existing general hospitals, and the conversion of station to general hospitals.[76]

Methods which ASF headquarters suggested for reducing hospital construction proved practicable only in part. A study of the possibilities of joint Army-Navy hospitalization promised little in the way of additional beds for Army use.[77] The proposal to reduce the bed ratio got nowhere. The director of the ASF Control Division agreed with The Surgeon General that information on World War II casualty rates was insufficient to warrant a reduction, and the ASF Hospitalization and Evacuation Branch interpreted the 15 September 1942 directive on hospitalization and evacuation as giving The Surgeon General alone the authority to estimate bed requirements for overseas casualties.[78] Hence, the ASF Requirements Division accepted The Surgeon General's estimate of requirements and turned to the remaining means of reducing general hospital construction—the use of station hospital beds and the expansion of existing general hospitals.

In a conference attended by representatives of the Surgeon General's Office on 8 April 1943, the ASF Requirements Divi-

[73] Ltr, SG USPHS to Brig Gen Frank T. Hines, 18 Mar 43. SG: 632.-1.

[74] (1) Ltrs, Franklin D. Roosevelt to SecWar and to Dir Bu of Budget, 31 Mar 43. SG: 632.-1. (2) Ltr, Dir Bu of Budget to Chm Fed Board of Hosp, 2 Apr 43. Same file.

[75] Ltr, SG to CG SOS, 11 Mar 43, sub: Hosp, Gen Hosps. SG: 323.7-5.

[76] 1st ind, CG ASF to SG, n d, on Ltr, SG to CG SOS, 11 Mar43, sub: Hosp, Gen Hosps. SG: 323.7-5.

[77] (1) 2d ind, SG to CG ASF, 31 Mar 43, on Ltr, SG to CG SOS, 11 Mar 43, sub: Hosp, Gen Hosps. SG: 323.7-5. (2) 1st ind, SG to CG ASF, 12 Jun 43, on Memo, CG ASF for SG, 19 Mar 43, sub: Joint Army-Navy Use of Available Hosp Accommodations. SG: 705.-1.

[78] (1) Memo SPOPH 632 (5 Apr 43), ACofS for Oprs ASF (init WLW[ilson]) for ACofS for Mat ASF, 7 Apr 43, sub: Hosp, Gen Hosps. HD: Wilson files, "Book IV, 16 Mar 43-17 Jun 43." (2) Memo, Dir Control Div ASF for CG ASF, 2 Apr 43, sub: Situation with Respect to Army Hosps. SG: 322.15.

sion pointed out that the construction or acquisition of general hospitals to provide a total of 83,000 beds had already been approved. To provide approximately 103,500 beds by December 1943, about 20,500 additional beds would be required. On the basis of projected overseas movements, 5,400 station hospital beds would be surplus by that time. If they should be converted to general hospital use, housing for only 15,100 additional general hospital beds would need to be constructed. Additional general hospital requirements during 1944 could be met by using increasingly large numbers of surplus station hospitals for that purpose. ASF headquarters therefore approved the expansion of thirteen existing general hospitals by 250 beds each, the construction of seven new general hospitals, and the acquisition of Pilgrim State Hospital, Brentwood (Long Island), New York, in order to provide the total number of beds required by December 1943.[79]

Reviewing this plan as the President had directed, the Federal Board approved the construction of the thirteen 250-bed annexes, the acquisition of Pilgrim State Hospital, and the construction of two new general hospitals.[80] Before it acted on the five other general hospitals, the Air Forces gave up certain buildings it had been using, including the Chicago Beach Hotel at Chicago and the Haddon Hall Hotel at Atlantic City. Furthermore, ASF headquarters decided that adjustments in the military program would make possible a reducion in authorized beds by approximately 7,000. Accordingly on 22 June 1943 the commanding general, Army Service Forces, directed The Surgeon General to withdraw from the Federal Board requests for approval of 8,750 additional beds and to provide, instead, 1,810 beds in the two hotels being vacated by the Air Forces. In the opinion of ASF, this would complete the general hospital building program in the United States.[81]

The events just described reveal a pattern that was to be repeated later in the war—increases in estimated bed requirements by The Surgeon General, publication of statistics showing relatively low occupancy of beds already provided, and subsequent efforts by higher headquarters to limit or reduce the number authorized. In this instance, such efforts resulted from attempts to reduce construction costs and save building materials but later from a need to conserve personnel. Earlier, as already noted, the urgent necessity for additional hospitals precluded doubts about estimated requirements as well as co-ordination of hospital construction programs of various federal agencies, both military and civilian. When such co-ordination was finally undertaken, the Army program had been virtually completed. Experiences encountered in planning for emergency hospitalization revealed the difficulties involved in co-ordinating plans of the Army with those of other agencies and in permitting several War Department agencies to work independently on a single problem.

---

[79] (1) Memo, "Basis used by Gen Wood at Conf on Hosp, ZI, SOS, 8 Apr 43, attended by Hall, Offutt, Wickert, Welsh," undated and unsigned. HD: SGO Oprs Div files. (2) Memo, CG ASF for SG, 9 Apr 43, sub: Completion of Gen Hosp Program in US. HRS: Hq ASF Somervell files, "SG 1943." (3) Memo, CG ASF for SG, 10 Apr 43, same sub. SG: 632.-1.

[80] Photostat copy, Res adopted by Fed Bd Hosp, 21 May 43. SG: 632.-1 (McGuire Gen Hosp)K. See also pp. 000, above.

[81] (1) Ltr, SG to SecWar thru CG ASF, 18 May 43, sub: Gen Hosp Program, Use of Converted Hotels (AF), and 6 inds. SG: 632.-1. (2) Memo, CG ASF for SG, 22 Jun 43, sub: Completion of Gen Hosp Program. Same file.

Location, Siting, and Internal Arrangement of Hospital Plants

In the hospital construction program attention had to be given not only to types of construction and estimates of the capacity needed but also to the location, siting, and internal arrangements of hospital buildings. After war was declared the selection of locations and sites, especially for general hospitals, became more complicated, while the need for speed in construction raised again the question of control over the internal arrangements of hospitals.

Selection of Locations and Sites

Station hospitals had to be located at camps whose situation was chosen by higher authority than the Surgeon General's Office, but selection of sites within those camps was a joint enterprise of The Surgeon General and the Chief of Engineers. In selecting locations for general hospitals The Surgeon General had more authority but not a free hand. He set up criteria of his own but was also subject to policies established by higher authority, to review of ASF headquarters, and to the Engineers' opinion of the suitability of available sites within general areas.

After war began The Surgeon General continued to regard as important such factors as climate, terrain, utilities connections, transportation systems, and communications networks. Moreover the growth of war industries and military installations necessitated more careful investigation than before of available labor, housing, and commodity markets. Furthermore there was the well-established policy of locating general hospitals in areas near large training camps, in order to simplify the transfer of patients from station to general hospitals. Occasionally these factors conflicted with each other. For example, cities with adequate housing, labor, and commodity markets were scarce in the South and Southwest, where most troops were concentrated.[82] A policy of hospitalizing war casualties near their homes was not established until the general hospital construction program had been virtually completed.[83] It therefore had little effect upon hospital locations. If it had been established earlier, more general hospitals might have been located in centers of population rather than in centers of troop density and the problem of finding areas with adequate markets might have been less difficult.

Early in 1942 G-4 ordered all new general hospitals to be located between the Atlantic and Pacific coast ranges as a safety masure.[84] It was immediately evident that this policy conflicted with the necessity of placing hospitals near ports of debarkation where they could readily receive patients returning from overseas theaters.[85] In June 1942, therefore, SOS headquarters permitted the construction of some general hospitals near the coasts to support ports of debarkation, but it made even more restrictive the area for the location of others by moving its boundaries inland to a line running from

[82] The above information was taken from numerous reports of inspection of areas for hospital locations. They are filed in SG: 632.-1 and in HD: Hosp Insp Rpts.

[83] See below, pp. 116-17.

[84] (1) Rpt on SGO Staff Conf, 17 Feb 42, in Diary of SGO Hist Subdiv, HD. (2) Info furnished by Col John R. Hall (Ret), 2 Dec 50. HD: 314 (Correspondence on MS) III.

[85] Ltr, SG to TAG, 14 Feb 42, sub: Add Gen Hosp Beds. SG: 632.-1.

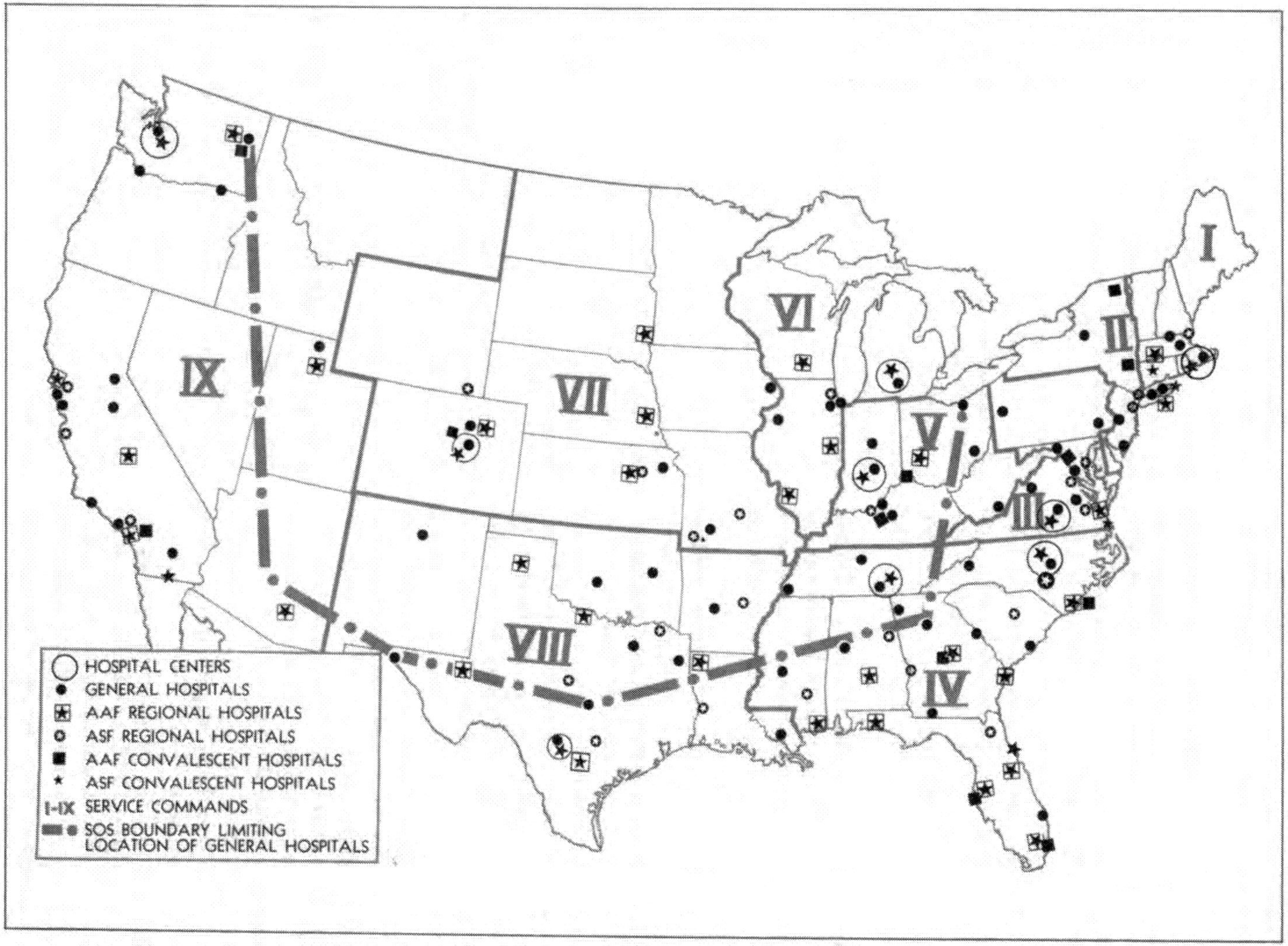

LOCATION OF GENERAL, CONVALESCENT, AND REGIONAL HOSPITALS DURING WORLD WAR II

Spokane to Phoenix to El Paso to Temple (Texas) to Atlanta to Cleveland.[86] This limitation was not strictly observed and toward the end of 1942 General Marshall in a conference with General Magee verbally abrogated both the G-4 and SOS restrictions.[87] Of the 51 general hospitals authorized, acquired, or constructed between the beginning and end of the war, 28 were outside the area prescribed by SOS headquarters, 4 were on its edge and 19 were within it.[88] Of the 28 outside the area, 9 were in the populous northeastern section of the country and 7 were in the Pacific Coast area.

Increasing emphasis during 1942 upon the use of existing civilian buildings for Army hospitals complicated the process of site selection and sometimes interfered with proper location. In some instances several buildings, such as hotels or civilian hospitals, had to be surveyed for engineering features and potential bed capacities before a decision could be made either to use one of them or to erect a new Army plant in the same general area. In the latter case a satisfactory site still had to be selected. Existing buildings were sometimes chosen simply because they were suitable for conversion into Army hospitals, even though they were in towns that were smaller than The Surgeon General considered desirable or were outside the area prescribed by SOS headquarters.[89]

The Surgeon General's selection of locations for general hospitals had to be reviewed by SOS headquarters before the Engineers could investigate specific sites for their construction. Of eighteen locations which The Surgeon General proposed in June 1942, the SOS Hospitalization and Evacuation Branch changed almost a third because its chief considered them too near the coast or other general hospitals and too far from adequate rail facilities and large towns.[90] During the winter of 1942 that Branch urged The Surgeon General rather unsuccessfully to locate more hospitals in the West, to care for possible increases in troop concentrations and evacuee loads in that area.[91] About the same time, the SOS Requirements Division became involved, insisting upon the speedy selection of locations for all hospitals to be constructed by June 1944. This made selection more difficult, according to both The Surgeon General and the Chief of Engineers, and in some instances The Surgeon General found it expedient to agree to sites which, although

[86] Opr Plans for Hosp and Evac, sec I, par 5 *c*, incl 1 to Ltr SPOPM 322.15, CG SOS to CGs and COs of CAs, PEs and Gen Hosps, and to SG, 18 Jun 42, same sub. HD: 705.-1.

[87] 1st ind, SG to CG SOS, 15 Jan 43, on Memo SPRMC 632, CG SOS for SG, 18 Dec 42, sub: Hosp, Gen Hosps. SG: 632.-1.

[88] General Hospitals established outside the area were: Ashford, Newton D. Baker, Birmingham, Brooke, Butner, Cushing, Dibble, Deshon, DeWitt, Edwards, England, Finney, Fletcher, Foster, Hammond, Halloran, Madigan, Mason, McCaw, McGuire, Moore, Oliver, Pickett, Ream, Rhoads, Torney, Valley Forge, and Woodrow Wilson; those inside the area were: Ashburn, Battey, Borden, Bruns, Bushnell, Carson, Gardiner, Glennan, Harmon, Kennedy, Mayo, Nichols, Percy Jones, Prisoner-of-War General Hospital No. 2, Schick, Thayer, Vaughan, Wakeman, and Winter; those on the edge were Baxter, Crile, McCloskey, and Northington.

[89] (1) Ltr, SG to CG SOS, 3 May 42. SG: 601.-1. (2) Memo CE 632 (Hosps) SPEOT, CofEngrs for CG SOS, 19 Dec 42, sub: Adv Planning for Add Gen Hosp Fac. SG: 632.-1.

[90] Memo SPOPM 632, ACofS for Oprs SOS (init WLW[ilson]) for Dir Reqmts Div SOS, 17 Jun 42, sub: Add Gen Hosps. HD: Wilson files, "Book I, 26 Mar 42-26 Sep 42."

[91] (1) 3d ind SPOPH 632 (9-26-42), CG SOS (Oprs SOS) to SG, 29 Oct 42, with n. for record, on Memo, SG for CG SOS, 26 Sep 42, sub: Hosp, Gen Hosps. HD: Wilson files, "Book 2, 26 Sep 42-31 Dec 42." (2) 5th ind SPOPH 632 (9-26-42), ACofS Oprs SOS for ACofS Mat SOS, 5 Dec 42, on same memo. Same file.

less desirable in his opinion, were superior for construction purposes.[92]

Throughout the early war years, local pressure on the War Department sometimes complicated the process of selecting hospital locations and sites but apparently did not often sway the judgment of those responsible for making the choice. In their attempts to lure additional wartime activities, many communities and cities made attractive offers, including the presentation of lands for general hospitals and the extension of utilities lines to the edges of those areas. In some instances there seemed to be a buyers' market. For example, after The Surgeon General planned to establish a general hospital in the Fort Worth–Waco (Texas) area, six cities offered valuable inducements. From the sites offered, The Surgeon General selected the one which, in the opinion of his representative and that of the Chief of Engineers, seemed best suited for hospital purposes.[93] In other instances local authorities banded together to prevent the establishment of hospitals in their areas.[94] Sometimes United States Senators and Representatives also attempted to influence the selection of certain locations. Generally they seem to have met with little success. For example, Sens. Charles L. McNary and Rufus C. Holman and Rep. Walter M. Pierce were particularly insistent upon the establishment of hospitals near LeGrande and Hot Lake, Oreg., rather than at Spokane and Walla Walla, Wash., but after appropriate investigations the latter locations were approved.[95] Likewise, Sen. John H. Bankhead and Rep. Carter Manasco sought a hospital for Jaspar, Ala., a mining town suffering from a lack of war projects, but The Surgeon General's representative recommended that Jaspar not be selected, and the place finally chosen for the one hospital in Alabama was Tuscaloosa.[96] On the other hand, a hospital was located at Martinsburg, W. Va., a city commended for that purpose by Rep. Jennings Randolph;[97] and, as a rule, after The Surgeon General's Construction Division made tentative selections of locations and sites, it discussed them with appropriate Senators and Representatives and secured their co-operation and help in dealing with local authorities.[98]

In view of the many factors involved, it is not surprising that the process of site selection was slow and gave rise to considerable criticism later in the war. Much of this criticism sprang from the fact that there were too few hospitals in densely populated areas to enable all patients

[92] (1) Memo, CG SOS (Dir Reqmts Div) for SG, 18 Dec 42, sub: Hosp, Gen Hosps, with 1st ind, SG to CG SOS, 15 Jan 43. SG: 632.-1. (2) Memo CE 632 (Hospitals) SPEOT, CofEngrs for CG SOS, 19 Dec 42, sub: Adv Planning for Add Gen Hosp Fac. Same file. (3) Ltr, Col John R. Hall to Lt Col Don J. Leehey, Off Div Engr, Portland, Oreg, 23 Mar 42. SG: 601.-1.

[93] (1) Memo, Col John R. Hall for SG, 31 Dec 41, sub: Rpt of Insp Trip Made for the Purpose of Locating Add Gen Hosp . . . in North Texas Area, with 12 incls. SG: 632.-1. (2) D/S, ACofS G-4 WDGS to TAG, SG, and CG 8th CA, 19 Jan 42, sub: Site for Gen Hosp, Temple, Tex. HRS: G-4/29135-11.

[94] Notes on Conf, 26 Mar 42, Hosp Cons Div SGO, atchd to Ltr, SG to TAG, 14 Feb 42, sub: Add Gen Hosp Beds. HD: 632.-1.

[95] (1) Ltr, SG to Hon Rufus C. Holman, US Sen, 21 Apr 42. SG: 601.-1. (2) Memo, Col John R. Hall for SG, 3 Jun 42, sub: Insp Trip to Oreg, Wash, and Calif. Same file.

[96] (1) Memo, Maj Lee C. Gammill for Col John R. Hall, 6 Jul 42, sub: Jaspar, Ala, Hosp Sites. HD: Hosp Insp Rpts. (2) Memo, Lt Col Achilles L. Tynes for SG, 22 Aug 42, sub: Rpt on Site Bd Surv for Location of Gen Hosp at Greeneville (sic), SC and Jaspar, Ala. SG: 601.-1.

[97] Memo, Col John R. Hall for SG, 15 Jun 42, sub: Insp of Proposed Sites Offered by City of Martinsburg, W. Va. HD: Hosp Insp Rpts.

[98] Info furnished by Col Hall (Ret), 2 Dec 50. HD: 314 (Correspondence on MS) III.

evacuated from overseas theaters to be cared for near their homes. It was generally forgotten—or ignored—that most of the general hospitals were located to facilitate the transfer of patients from station hospitals in training camps and that the War Department did not establish a policy of hospitalizing overseas evacuees near their homes until most of the general hospitals had been established.

Control over Internal Arrangement of Hospitals

The Surgeon General continued to insist that building schedules, hospital layouts, and floor plans of all new hospitals, plans for all "major" alterations to existing buildings, and all subsequent changes in such plans should be referred to his Office for approval.[99] On the other hand, the Chief of Engineers attempted, as did The Quartermaster General before him, to decentralize as much authority as possible in order to save time. Beginning in February 1942, he again raised the question of having The Surgeon General approve standard building schedules and layouts for use in the field, without further reference to the latter's Office, but apparently neither the Chief of Engineers nor SOS headquarters wished to challenge The Surgeon General's position. While official construction policy letters did not require the reference of layouts and plans to his Office, the Engineers generally followed that practice.[100]

The extent of The Surgeon General's authority over hospital construction was discussed but not defined after reorganization of the Services of Supply in the late summer of 1942. On 5 August General Magee requested that certain functions be "retained" in his Office, not decentralized to the field. Among them were the approval of hospital floor plans and layouts, plans for the conversion of civilian buildings into Army hospitals, and all major alterations to existing hospital buildings.[101] General Somervell's reply was inconclusive. He stated that the approval of floor plans and layouts had been and was at that time a responsibility of the Chief of Engineers, but that it was the practice to secure concurrence of the Surgeon General's Office in them. Plans for the conversion of civilian buildings, he stated, fell in a "twilight zone" that was not well defined either before or after the reorganization. As for alterations to existing hospitals, General Somervell stated that there was no clear definition of the word "major." He implied that The Surgeon General should agree with the Chief of Engineers to decentralize authority for alterations to service commands. If The Surgeon General could not trust service command surgeons to supervise alterations properly, General Somervell concluded, he should replace the surgeons.[102]

---

[99] (1) Ltr, SG to CofEngrs, 9 Feb 42, sub: Hosp Bldg Schedules. (2) 1st ind, SG to CofEngrs, 1 May 43, on Ltr 600.92 (Gen) SPEEG, CofEngrs to SG, 25 Apr 42, sub: Typical Hosp Layouts. (3) 1st ind, SG to CofEngrs, 2 Aug 42, on Synopsis Ltr, CofEngrs to SG, 28 Jul 42, sub: Auth of Div Engr to Auth Cons. All in SG: 632.-1.

[100] (1) Ltr, SG to CofEngrs, 9 Feb 42, sub: Hosp Bldg Schedules. SG: 632.-1. (2) Ltr 600.92 (Gen) SPEEG, CofEngrs to SG, 25 Apr 42, sub: Typical Hosp Layouts. Same file. (3) Ltr AG 600.12 (2-19-42) MO-D-M, TAG to CGs of all Depts and CAs, COs of Exempted Stas, and C of Arms and Servs, 24 Feb 42, sub: WD Cons Policy, ZI. HRS: G-4/31751. (4) 1st ind, CofEngrs to CG AAF, 25 Aug 42, on Ltr, CG AAF to CofEngrs, 19 Aug 42, sub: Hosp Cons. AAF: 632 "B Hosp and Infirmaries."

[101] Ltr, SG to CG SOS, 5 Aug 42, sub: Liaison in Reorgn of SvCs. SG: 020.-1.

[102] 1st ind, CG SOS to SG, 15 Aug 42, on Ltr, SG to CG SOS, 5 Aug 42, sub: Liaison in Reorgn of SvCs. SG: 020.-1.

Within the same month it became apparent that local changes in approved plans for converting civilian buildings into hospitals needed to be more strictly controlled. Aware of the difficulties of such conversions, The Surgeon General asked authority on 2 August 1942 to commission five civilian architects to serve as advisers on the spot in the alterations required. The commanding general, Services of Supply, disapproved this request because the Chief of Engineers considered it an encroachment upon his responsibility.[103] Meanwhile word reached Washington that local engineer and medical officers had made unnecessary and expensive changes in plans for one of the conversions. After a conference on this problem on 14 August 1942 among representatives of the Services of Supply, the Chief of Engineers, The Surgeon General, and the War Production Board, General Somervell directed that no changes should be made in approved plans for altering hotels or other buildings without the written consent of both The Surgeon General and the Chief of Engineers.[104]

In following months The Surgeon General and the Chief of Engineers agreed upon a partial decentralization of authority to approve alterations of existing hospitals. On 5 October 1942 the War Department delegated to service commanders the authority to approve alterations costing up to $10,000 on any building, at any one time and place.[105] On 13 November 1942 The Surgeon General suggested, as he had before, that all "major" alterations to hospital buildings, regardless of cost, be sent to his Office for approval. He defined "major" alterations as those requiring structural changes to convert sections of buildings or entire buildings from one use to another, to convert ward to office space or vice versa, or to extend buildings into areas expected to be kept vacant. The Chief of Engineers insisted that the term "major" changes would be misleading and suggested that the phrase "changes involving more than $10,000" be used instead. Undoubtedly aware of the War Department's action of 5 October 1942, The Surgeon General reluctantly agreed and on 3 December 1942 the Chief of Engineers issued a letter authorizing local alterations costing up to $10,000 on hospital buildings, without prior approval of The Surgeon General.[106]

In November 1942 the Wadhams Committee attributed what it considered to be shortcomings in hospital construction partially to the limited extent of The Surgeon General's authority but also to the inadequacy of his own construction staff. Stating that the division of responsibility between the Chief of Engineers and The Surgeon General had permitted "passing the buck," it recommended that the latter be given more authority over construction. At the same time the committee proposed that The Surgeon General strengthen his construction staff by adding to it outstanding civilian hospital architects and by placing at its head a nonmedical man

[103] (1) Memo for Record, on DF, CG SOS to SG, 17 Sep 42, sub: Increase in Procurement Objective, AUS. AG: SPGA 210.1 Med 1-20.

[104] (1) Memo 323.7 Hosp SPPDX, Mr. L. G. Woodford for Gen Harrison, 14 Aug 42, sub: Conversion of Hotels to Army Hosps. SG: 632.-2. (2) SOS Memo S100-2-42, 27 Aug 42, sub: Limitation on Alterations to Hosps. CE: 632, Pt 2.

[105] AR 100-80, C 3, 5 Oct 42.

[106] (1) Memo, SG for CofEngrs, 13 Nov 42, sub: Routing of Project Ests Affecting Hosp Bldgs, with 1st ind CE 600.94 (Surg Gen) SPEUU, CofEngrs to SG, n d; 2d ind, SG to CofEngrs, 25 Nov 42, and 3d ind CE 600.94 (Surg Gen) SPEUU, CofEngrs to SG, 7 Dec 42. SG: 632.-1. (2) Ltr, CofEngrs to CGs of SvCs, 3 Dec 42, sub: Nonrecurrent Project Ests Involving Hosp Bldgs. CE: 632, Pt 2.

experienced in hospital planning. The Surgeon General naturally agreed that he should have more authority, but he concurred with the chief of his Hospital Construction Division in defending the practice of placing a doctor at its head and ascribed the division's shortage of trained architects to the disapproval of his request to commission five to assist in the conversion program.[107]

Maintenance of Hospital Plants

Responsibility for Maintenance

Even before The Surgeon General lost control over hospital alterations costing less than $10,000, he had also lost authority over the expenditure of funds for hospital repair and maintenance. At the beginning of 1942 funds from three appropriations were used for hospital maintenance. Two of them, the Barracks and Quarters (B&Q) appropriation and the Construction and Repair of Hospitals (C&RofH) appropriation, were Engineer appropriations; the third, the Medical and Hospital Department (M&HD) appropriation, was made to the Medical Department. Funds from the B&Q appropriation and from the M&HD appropriation were controlled exclusively by the Engineers and the Medical Department respectively. Those from the C&RofH appropriation were controlled jointly by the Chief of Engineers and The Surgeon General. B&Q funds paid for such things as firing boiler plants of hospitals and repairing certain buildings occupied and used by operational personnel. C&RofH funds provided for the maintenance of buildings occupied and used by patients and for the upkeep of installed equipment. M&HD funds were used to maintain noninstalled Medical Department equipment and to meet expenses connected with the purchase of medical supplies.[108]

The use of three funds for hospital maintenance produced complications. One was confusion about the fund to which various expenditures should be charged. In January and February 1942 questions arose over whether repairs to hospital barracks should be charged to B&Q or to C&RofH funds.[109] Fine distinctions sometimes had to be made in applying the C&RofH fund rather than the M&HD fund and vice versa. For example, carpenters were employed from both. Those paid with M&HD funds could repair hospital furniture and noninstalled equipment, but not buildings and installed equipment; those paid with C&RofH funds had to do that.[110] Another problem arose in the joint administration of C&RofH funds. Although they were Engineer funds, their appropriation was based on estimates prepared by The Surgeon General and they were allotted to hospitals on his recommendation. Corps area and post surgeons controlled their expenditure and reported on it to The Surgeon General, but post engineer officers performed the work.[111]

---

[107] (1) Cmtee to Study the MD, 1942, Rpt. HD. (2) Cmtee to Study the MD, 1942–43, Actions on Recomd, Recomd No 31. HD. (3) Memo, Col John R. Hall for Exec Off SGO, 3 Dec 42. SG: 632.–1.

[108] Tynes, Construction Branch, p. 54. Also see the language of the appropriations acts.

[109] (1) Ltr CE 121.2 (Funds) CU, CofEngrs to SG, 7 Jan 42, sub: Policy for Div of B&QA Funds and C&RofHA Funds, with 1st ind, SG to CofEngrs, 1 Mar 42. (2) Ltr CE 121.2 (Funds) CUC, CofEngrs to SG, 25 Feb 42, sub: Policy for Div of B&QA, C&RofHA and Air Corps Tec Funds, and 1st ind, SG to CofEngrs, 1 Mar 42. Both in SG: 632.–1.

[110] Memo, Col F[rancis] C. Tyng for Budget Off WD, 22 Mar 42, sub: Trf of Approp C&RofH from a Sep Approp to M&HD, A. SG: 632.–1.

[111] (1) Memo, Col F. C. Tyng for Budget Off WD, 22 Mar 42, sub: Trf of Approp C&RofH from a Sep Approp to M&HD, A. SG: 632.–1. (2) AR 40–585, par 3 and 4, 16 Jul 31.

Early in 1942 the Chief of Engineers began to simplify the administration of the C&RofH fund. In order to reduce bookkeeping, he proposed on 31 January 1942 the abandonment of a practice of subdividing the fund into several smaller project-funds.[112] He also began to make allotments directly to district engineers, without securing The Surgeon General's and corps area surgeons' recommendations.[113] Then he directed district engineers to prepare estimates of C&RofH funds in the same way they did those of B&Q funds.[114] The Surgeon General went along with these changes, but insisted that corps area surgeons be informed of allotments made to hospitals and that they continue to report to him on all expenditures made from such allotments.[115]

The next month the merger of the C&RofH appropriation with either the B&Q or the M&HD appropriation came up for consideration. The Chief of Engineers wanted the C&RofH fund merged with the B&Q fund under his control. Hearing of pending legislation to that effect, The Surgeon General recommended to the Budget Officer of the War Department on 22 March 1942 that the C&RofH and the M&HD appropriations be combined into one, under Medical Department control. In support of this recommendation he pointed out unsatisfactory features of having a fund controlled jointly by the Engineers and the Medical Department.[116] This action came too late, because the merger of C&RofH with B&Q funds under a single appropriation called Engineer Service, Army, had already occurred on 5 March 1942.[117] The Surgeon General protested against this "radical departure" from accepted practices, maintaining now that joint control of the C&RofH fund had been satisfactory, that only doctors could determine the maintenance required for hospitals, and that Congress had always been, and might be expected to continue to be, more liberal in appropriating funds for hospital maintenance than for the routine maintenance of Army posts.[118] He failed, however, to keep control over funds expended for hospital maintenance, for on 23 May 1942 the War Department charged the Chief of Engineers with responsibility for repairs and utilities at general hospitals and on 9 June 1942 rescinded the Army regulation which had outlined The Surgeon General's former authority over hospital maintenance.[119] With the reorganization of the Services of Supply, the Chief of Engineers requested The Surgeon General on 17 August 1942 to close out all fiscal transactions pertaining to hospital

[112] Memo CE 121.2 (Projects) CUC, CofEngrs for SG, 31 Jan 42, sub: Project Revision. SG: 632.-1.

[113] Ltr, Surg 4th CA to SG, 19 Jan 42, sub: C&RofH Funds, with 2d ind, CofEngrs to SG, 13 Feb 42. SG: 632.-1 (4th CA) AA.

[114] Ltr CE 315 (Forms) CUC, CofEngrs to SG, 27 Jan 42, sub: Application of OCE Forms No 395 and 395-A to An Est of Funds Req of C&RofH, A. SG: 632.-1.

[115] (1) 1st ind, SG to CofEngrs, 23 Jan 42, on Ltr, Surg 4th CA to SG, 19 Jan 42, sub: C&RofH Funds. SG: 632.-1 (4th CA)AA. (2) Ltr, Maj Seth [O.] Craft to Surg 2d CA, 7 Mar 42. SG: 632.-1 (2d CA)AA. (3) Ltr, same to Capt Joe [E.] McKnight, MAC, Off of Surg 1st CA, 4 Feb 42. SG: 632.-1 (1st CA)AA.

[116] (1) Ltr, SG to CofEngrs, 25 Feb 42, sub: C&RofH Funds, as Affected by Pending Legislation, H. Res. 6611. SG: 632.-1. (2) Memo, SG for Budget Off WD, 22 Mar 42, sub: Trf of Approp C&RofH . . . to M&HD, A, for FY 1943. SG: 632.-1.

[117] (1) 5th Supp Nat Def Approp Act, 1942, Public Law 474, apvd 5 Mar 42. (2) GAO Acts and Procedures Ltr 4236, 7 Mar 42. HD: 121.2.

[118] (1) Ltr CE 121.2 (Funds) CUC, CofEngrs to SG, 24 Mar 42, sub: Maintenance of Hosp Structures. (2) Memo, SG for Maj Gen T[homas] M. Robins, Asst CofEngrs, 26 Mar 42, sub: Maintenance and Repair of Hosps. (3) Memo CE 600.3 (Gen)-CU, CofEngrs for SG, 10 Apr 42, sub: Repairs and Util Functions at MD Fac, with 1st ind, SG to CofEngrs, 23 Apr 42. All in SG: 632.-1.

[119] (1) WD Cir 157, 23 May 42. (2) AR 100-80, 9 Jun 42.

maintenance and to plan to transfer the funds, personnel, and equipment used in that work to the Engineers as of the close of business on 31 August 1942.[120]

After responsibility was concentrated in the Chief of Engineers, the maintenance and repair of hospitals failed to suffer as the Surgeon General's Office had anticipated. The surgeons of several service commands reported favorably on the performance of maintenance work under the new system.[121] As late as 1945, Col. Achilles L. Tynes, of the Hospital Construction Division, pointed out that hospitals had experienced no difficulty in getting repairs during the war and that it could not be proved that retention of control of funds by theMedical Department would have been more satisfactory than control by the Engineers.[122]

Reflooring and Reroofing

Throughout the war, maintenance programs of magnitude had to be carried on concurrently with new construction programs, largely as the result of the use of cantonment-type construction in the majority of hospitals built both before and after the war began. Green pine lumber, the only type available in many cases, was frequently used for both flooring and roofing. As it dried and warped, it pulled the nails through tar-paper roofing, tearing it and producing leaks, and caused floors to shrink and splinter, leaving them unsightly, insanitary, and dangerous. Beginning late in 1941 and continuing through 1942, The Surgeon General and the Chief of Engineers initiated and carried through extensive programs of reroofing and reflooring. Asphalt strip shingles gradually replaced tar-paper roofs, and old floors were covered with layers, first of plywood and then of linoleum or similar material. In corridors, imitation-rubber strip-runners were laid to protect floors, to reduce noise, and to increase patients' safety. These costly programs might have been avoided had better materials been available and authorized for initial hospital construction.[123]

Efforts to Increase the Safety and Comfort of Patients

Despite the War Department's policy of "Spartan simplicity" in construction and maintenance during 1942 and 1943, the Engineers and the Medical Department tried to increase the safety and comfort of patients in hospitals. The practice of installing automatic sprinkler systems as protection against fire in cantonment-type wards was continued and extended to include recreation, mess, post exchange, and clinic buildings as well.[124] Numerous requests from separate hospitals for heat in corridors, to protect patients as well as the pipes of sprinkler systems from extreme cold, had prompted The Surgeon General

[120] Ltr, Asst CofEngrs to SG, 17 Aug 42, sub: Trf of Repairs and Util Functions. SG: 632.-1.

[121] An Rpts, 1942, Surg 5th, 7th, and 9th SvCs. HD.

[122] Tynes, Construction Branch, p. 64.

[123] Correspondence among The Surgeon General, The Quartermaster General, and the Chief of Engineers on these programs is on file in SG: 632.-1; SG: 632.-1 (1st thru 9th CAs)AA; and CE: 632 Vol. 3. Also see Speech, Lessons Learned from Planning and Constructing Army Hospitals, by Col Hall, 16 Sep 43 (HD: 632.-1), and Tynes, Construction Branch, pp. 65-67.

[124] (1) 2d ind, SG to TAG, 19 Jan 42, and 3d ind AG 671.7 (31 Dec 42) MO-D, TAG to CofEngrs, 26 Jan 42, on Synopsis Ltr, Div Engr Carib Div to CofEngrs, 31 Dec 41, sub: Automatic Sprinkler Systs. SG: 671.-2. (2) OCE Cir Ltr 1665, 2 Jun 42, sub: Automatic Sprinkler and Fire Alarm Systs in Small Hosps. CE: 671.3, Pt 1. (3) SOS Memo S30-2-42, sub: Policy Governing Instl of Automatic Sprinkler Systs and Fire Alarm Systs. SG: 671.2.

in October 1941 to reverse an earlier decision and request the installation of heating facilities.[125] On 4 February 1942 the Secretary of War authorized their installation in the corridors of all cantonment-type hospitals then under construction or planned.[126] Getting approval for the installation of air-cooling systems in hospitals in hot southern areas was considerably more complicated.

During the first summer that the Army began to use cantonment-type hospitals on a wide scale, hospital commanders and corps area surgeons, especially in areas with high temperatures, had complained that patients suffered from heat in wards and that the temperature in operating rooms and clinics was frequently unbearable.[127] The attic space above the low-ceilinged cantonment-type buildings collected and held heated air, raising the temperature in the buildings higher than on the outside. Dust in new camps often made it necessary to close all windows, and use of sterilizers and developing tanks in clinics and dark rooms increased humidity in those sections of hospitals.[128] Colonel Offutt, Chief of The Surgeon General's Hospitalization Division, promised in September 1941 that attempts would be made to correct this situation by the summer of 1942.[129]

During the next spring the Surgeon General's Office collaborated with local surgeons and representatives from manufacturing concerns in working out systems employing mechanical air conditioners, evaporative coolers, and forced-air ventilation. The mechanical air conditioners were self-contained package-type coolers, like those used in restaurants and offices. Outside air was drawn into buildings over coils containing a refrigerating gas, and air-duct installation was not required. Evaporative coolers were useful in dry areas of the Southwest, where the humidity was extremely low. These devices drew hot outside air into buildings through wet, porous substances; as the moisture evaporated, the air cooled. In the hot and humid climate of the South and Southeast, where evaporative cooling was not practicable, forced ventilation was used. Exhaust fans in attics blew out hot air, producing a condition in the wards below similar to that found outside in the shade with a light breeze.[130] Using C&RofH funds allocated by The Surgeon General, local hospital commanders and utilities officers began to install such systems during the spring of 1942.[131]

Before this program had gotten very far it encountered a directive, on 20 May

[125] Ltr, SG to QMG, 29 Oct 41, sub: Heating of Enclosed Corridors. CE: 632, Pt I.

[126] Ltr SGO 674.-1, SG to CofEngrs, 7 Jan 42, sub: Instl of Heating Fac in Corridors of Cantonment-type Hosps, with 1st ind, CofEngrs to TAG, 27 Jan 42, and 2d ind, TAG to CofEngrs, 4 Feb 42. CE: 632, Pt I.

[127] For example, see: (1) Synopsis Ltr, AF Combat Comd Hq to CofAC, 5 Jul 41. SG: 632.-1. (2) 1st wrapper ind, Surg 9th CA to SG, 3 Jul 41. SG: 673.-4 (9th CA)AA. (3) Ltr, Surg 4th CA to SG, 6 Sep 41, sub: Comfort and Welfare of Pnts in Cantonment Hosps. SG: 632.-1 (4th CA)AA.

[128] Speech, Lessons Learned from Planning and Constructing Army Hospitals, by Col Hall, 16 Sep 43. HD: 632.-1.

[129] Ltr, SG (per Col H. D. Offutt) to Surg 4th CA, 10 Sep 41, sub: Comfort and Welfare of Pnts in Cantonment Hosps. SG: 632.-1 (4th CA)AA.

[130] (1) Speech, Lessons Learned from Planning and Constructing Army Hospitals, by Col Hall, 16 Sep 43. HD: 632.-1. (2) Memo, Col John R. Hall for SG, 16 Jun 43, sub: Résumé of Procurement of Air-Conditioning and Ventilative Equip for Cantonment-Type Hosps. SG: 673.-4.

[131] (1) 1st ind, SG to CofEngrs, 14 Feb 42, on Ltr, Carrier Corp to SG, 12 Feb 42. (2) Ltr, SG to CofEngrs, 6 Apr 42, sub: Special Features for Ventilation of Hosps. (3) Ltr, SG to Various Sta and Gen Hosps, 3d, 4th, 5th, 6th, 7th, and 8th CAs, 6 May 42, sub: Air Conditioning of Operating Rms, X-ray Rms, and Recovery Rms. All in SG: 673.-4.

1942, severely restricting the use of mechanical and electrical equipment in Army construction.[132] The Chief of Engineers, who by now controlled funds for the purchase of cooling equipment and was responsible for its installation, sought approval of the War Production Board for installing the apparatus recommended by The Surgeon General.[133] The Board approved the use of air conditioners in operating rooms, X-ray clinics, and recovery wards, but failed to deal with The Surgeon General's proposal to install exhaust fans or evaporative coolers in other hospital buildings.[134] The supply of fans and coolers already on hand was believed to be limited, but no Government agency actually knew its extent.[135] Consequently the SOS Resources Division wanted to limit installation to cases of greatest need and in August 1942 approved only a limited program.[136] Early in 1943 a practice of transferring equipment from nonessential to military uses developed and the War Production Board ascertained that dealers had considerable stocks of air-conditioning and mechanical-ventilating equipment on hand.[137] When The Surgeon General resubmitted his proposal in January and February,[138] therefore, the War Department issued a policy letter on the subject.

Under the new policy the installation of cooling equipment from existing inventories or from recaptured stocks was permitted in areas where the average July temperature exceeded 75° Fahrenheit. Depending upon humidity of the area in which a hospital was located, either evaporative coolers or exhaust fans were permitted in operating rooms, wards, X-ray rooms, clinics, dispensaries where minor operations were performed, and patients' mess halls. Where neither of these types served the purpose, air conditioners might be installed in operating rooms, X-ray rooms, flight surgeons' clinics, and recovery wards. In desert areas, evaporative coolers might also be used in quarters occupied by personnel on night duty.[139]

Installation of the long-desired equipment now began. Since authority to approve jobs amounting to $10,000 or less had been decentralized to service commands, the installation of air-conditioning and mechanical-ventilating systems was a responsibility of local engineers. The Chief of Engineers and The Surgeon General developed guides for their use, and on 15 April 1943 the Chief of Engineers informed service command engineers of procedures to follow in processing requests

[132] Directive for Wartime Cons, 20 May 42, incl to Ltr AG 600.12 (5–20–42) MO–SPAD–M, TAG to CGs of AAF, Depts, and CAs and to C of Tec Servs, 1 Jun 42, same sub. SG: 632.–1.

[133] (1) Ltr, CofEngrs to Refrigeration Sec and Fan and Blower Sec WPB, 20 Jun 42. CE: 673, Pt 3. (2) Ltr, SG to CofEngrs, sub: Ventilation and Air Conditioning for Cantonment-type Hosp Bldgs, 13 Jun 42. SG: 673.–4.

[134] Ltr, WPB to CofEngrs, 23 Jun 42. CE: 673, Pt 3.

[135] (1) Memo, 1st Lt James J. Souder for Col John R. Hall, 2 Aug 42, sub: Conf on Evaporative Cooling for Hosp Bldgs. SG: 673.–4. (2) Notes on tel conv between Lt Col Norris G. Kenny and Col John R. Hall, 29 Jun 42. Same file.

[136] (1) Memo, Dir Resources Div SOS for SG, 30 Jun 42, sub: Exception from 'List of Prohibited Items for Cons Work' of Ventilation Fans for Hosps. SG: 673.–4. (2) Memo SPRMC 674.4(8–11–42), CG SOS for CofEngrs, 16 Aug 42, sub: Policy Determining Instl of Humidifying Coolers. CE: 673, Pt 3.

[137] Memo, Capt James J. Souder for Col John R. Hall, 15 Feb 43, sub: Conf on Air Conditioning and Ventilation for Hosps. SG: 673.–4.

[138] (1) Memo, SG for Maj Frank Seeter, Resources Div SOS, 23 Jan 42, sub: Ventilative Treatment in Cantonment-Type Hosps. SG: 673.–4. (2) Memo, SG for Production Div SOS, 22 Feb 43, same sub. Same file.

[139] WD Memo W100–4–43, 24 Mar 43, sub: Policy for Air-Conditioning, Cooling, and Ventilation of Army Instls, Continental US. SG: 673.–4.

for that work.[140] Although delivery of units was delayed in some cases until the fall of 1943, many hospitals had air-cooling systems in time for both patients and operational personnel to benefit from reduced temperatures during the summer of that year.[141]

Correction of Errors in Cantonment-Type Hospitals

While improvements already mentioned were being made, the Engineers and the Medical Department worked to correct inadequacies of space for various functions, especially in cantonment-type hospitals. The prewar practice of providing more room for administrative and service activities, X-ray work, storage, and recreation was continued.[142] Action was also taken to furnish ear, eye, nose, and throat (EENT) clinics with more space than that originally planned. This occurred after the War Department established a policy of giving eye examinations and spectacles to all soldiers who required them. Existing EENT clinics were enlarged or were abandoned in favor of new ones set up in ward buildings.[143]

In the fall of 1942 the Wadhams Committee found fault particularly with shortage of occupational therapy facilities, inadequacy of space for post exchange and recreational activities, and lack of safety features in neuropsychiatric wards.[144] The chief of The Surgeon General's Hospital Construction Division, Colonel Hall, agreed that post exchanges and recreational facilities were too small but stated that War Department construction policies were responsible for that fault. He believed that it was unnecessary and impractical to have occupational therapy facilities in station hospitals, because in his opinion all patients needing occupational therapy should be sent to general hospitals.[145] Nevertheless, in compliance with an SOS directive, The Surgeon General submitted a comprehensive program on 17 January 1943 for the construction of additional occupational therapy buildings, recreation buildings, detachment dayrooms, post exchanges, libraries, chapels, officers' and nurses' recreation buildings, and theaters in all hospitals of two hundred or more beds.[146] SOS headquarters apparently considered this program as one going beyond the bounds of War Department construction policies, and returned it for reconsideration. After

[140] (1) Memo, SG for CofEngrs, 27 Apr 43, sub: Instl Plans for Air Conditioning, Evaporative Cooling, and Mechanical Ventilation. SG: 673.-4. (2) Ltr, CofEngrs to CG 2d SvC attn Dir of Real Estate, Repairs, and Utils, 15 Apr 43, same sub. Same file.

[141] For example, see: An Rpts, 1943, of Kennedy and Ashburn Gen Hosps and of Sta Hosps at Scott Fld and Cps Bowie, Beale, and Maxey. HD.

[142] (1) Ltr, SG to CofEngrs, 27 Jan 42, sub: Request for Urgent Emergency Cons. SG: 632.-1. (2) Ltr, SG to CofEngrs, 6 Jul 42, sub: Request for Working Drawings for Admin Bldg, Type HA-1 and HA-2, with 4 inds. Same file. (3) An Rpts, 1942, Sta Hosps at Cps Dodge and Forrest and 1943, Sta Hosps at Cps Beale, Hale, and Hood. HD.

[143] (1) Memo, Col John R. Hall for Chief Professional Serv SGO, 30 Jul 42, sub: Conversion of Ward Bldg into an Enlarged EENT Clinic. SG: 632.-1. (2) Ltr, SG to CofEngrs, 7 Aug 42, sub: Plans for Conversion of a Ward Bldg into an EENT Clinic. Same file. (3) An Rpt, 1942, Sta Hosp at Cp Forrest and 1943, Sta Hosps at Cps Beale, Ellis, Hale, and Hood. HD.

[144] (1) Cmtee to Study the MD, 1942-43, Actions on Recomd, Recomd Nos 10, 15, and 47. HD. (2) Cmtee to Study the MD, 1942, Rpt, pp. 6, 7, 12, and 24. HD.

[145] (1) Memo, Col John R. Hall for Exec Off SGO, 3 Dec 42. SG: 632.-1. (2) Extract from 1st ind, SG to CG SOS, 15 Dec 42, on extract from Memo, CG SOS for SG, 26 Nov 42, in Cmtee to Study the MD, 1942-43, Actions on Recomd, Recomd Nos 10 and 15. HD.

[146] Extracts from Ltr, SG to CG SOS, 17 Jan 43, sub: Recreational Fac in Army Hosps, in Cmtee to Study the MD, 1942-43, Actions on Recomd, Recomd No 10. HD.

that, it seems to have passed for some months among the offices of The Surgeon General, the Chief of Engineers, and the SOS Requirements Division,[147] and improvements of the kind asked for were not approved until the latter half of the war.

With regard to neuropsychiatric wards, Colonel Hall pointed out that plans for their construction had been completely revised during 1941. Faults that continued to exist, he said, resulted either from failure of construction officers to follow specifications closely or from the difficulty of constructing wards in wooden buildings so that patients could not escape or commit suicide yet at the same time could be easily removed in case of fire.[148] On his advice, The Surgeon General recommended on 31 December 1942 that the Engineers be instructed to provide all neuropsychiatric wards, including those already constructed, with the features called for in revised plans.[149] During the first half of 1943 the Engineers undertook a program of improving neuropsychiatric wards in compliance with this recommendation.[150]

In the spring of 1943, in order to eliminate the need for alterations and additions to hospitals after completion, plans for some cantonment-type buildings were redrawn. This may have resulted from a report made by the Seventh Service Command's Inspector General. Investigating construction projects at hospitals in his area, he concluded on 9 March 1943 that similar alterations could be avoided in the future by a revision of construction plans.[151] Soon after his report reached Washington, the Engineers began to collaborate with the Surgeon General's Office in revising plans for cantonment-type administration buildings, clinics, and messes. By the middle of 1943 this project had apparently been completed,[152] but this was too late to effect significant savings in hospital alterations, for the major portion of the hospital construction program had already been completed.

Conformity of Hospital Construction to Needs

As hospitals were constructed to meet wartime needs experiences encountered in the period of peacetime mobilization were repeated in individual instances. With the Army growing by leaps and bounds troops sometimes moved into new camps before hospitals were completed, and old camps were expanded before existing hospitals could be enlarged. In some areas there were unexpected delays in construction. For these there were numerous causes. Among them were unfavorable weather conditions; shortages of equipment such as electric cables, pumps, motors, and especially high pressure boilers; and labor troubles, including scarcity of laborers and disputes between employers and em-

[147] Cmtee to Study the MD, 1942–43, Actions on Recomd, Recomd No 10. HD.

[148] (1) Memo, Col John R. Hall for Exec Off SGO, 3 Dec 42. SG: 632.-1. (2) Extract from 1st ind SG to CG SOS, 14 Dec 42, on Memo, CG SOS for SG, 26 Nov 42, in Cmtee to Study the MD, 1942–43, Actions on Recomd, Recomd No 47. HD.

[149] Ltr SPMCC 632.-1, SG (init JRH[all]) to CG SOS, 31 Dec 42, sub: NP Wards. CE: 632, Vol. 3.

[150] Ink note, "All items referred to have been taken care of by revised drawings and specifications and by circular letter and informal conference with SGO, 7/29/43," on Ltr, SG to CG SOS, 31 Dec 42, sub: NP Wards. CE: 632, Vol. 3.

[151] Ltr, IG 7th SvC to IG, 9 Mar 43, sub: Cons Plans, Gen Hosps, with 2 inds. SG: 333.1-1 (7th SvC)AA.

[152] (1) Memo, CofEngrs for SG, 24 Mar 43, sub: Hosp Bldg Plans, with 1st ind, SG to CofEngrs, 2 Apr 43. SG: 632.-1. (2) Ltr CE 600.13 (Hosp) SPEEW, CofEngrs to SG, 31 Mar 43, sub: Proposed Hosp Messes, with 3 inds. Same file.

ployees. For posts where actual needs outstripped hospital construction, The Surgeon General set aside additional beds in general hospitals and local medical officers resorted to expedients used before the war to provide adequate hospital care.[153]

As a whole, construction kept up with actual needs even though it lagged considerably behind estimated requirements. During the first year and a half of the war the number of station hospitals increased from about 200 to more than 425; and the number of normal beds (that is, those for which 100 square feet of space each was provided in ward buildings) rose from about 58,725 to over 220,000. During the entire period the total number of station hospital beds that were occupied throughout the United States was continuously lower than the total number of normal beds provided. From December 1942 to March 1943, when the incidence of respiratory diseases increased and the transfer of patients from station to general hospitals was restricted to save places for anticipated casualties, the number of patients in station hospitals exceeded the number of normal beds available but not of normal beds provided. (Only 80 percent of the beds provided were considered available, because the necessity of segregating patients into separate wards according to disease, sex, and grade meant that empty beds in "wrong" wards, amounting as a rule to 20 percent of the total, could not be used.) During the entire period, however, emergency and expansion beds (that is, those set up on the basis of 72 square feet each not only in wards but also in porches, solaria, halls, etc.) made the number of all beds available greater than the number of beds occupied.[154]

The number of general hospitals in operation increased from 14 in December 1941 to 40 by June 1943; of beds in them, from about 15,500 to more than 53,750. The total number of occupied beds never reached the total of normal beds provided, but from April through September 1942 in general hospitals the number of occupied beds exceeded the number of normal beds available. This overcrowding resulted largely from the policy of giving the station hospital program priority over that for general hospitals because of the more immediate need for station hospital beds. General hospitals, as did station hospitals, set up emergency and expansion beds when they were needed. Older and better-established hospitals, such as Walter Reed and the Army and Navy General Hospital, tended to be more crowded than newer ones, because the latter had to await the presence of supplies and equipment as well as full complements of personnel before patients could be transferred to them in large numbers. By June 1943, as more new general hospitals opened, the number of available normal beds outnumbered by a comfortable margin the number of occupied beds.[155] *(Chart 5)*

---

[153] (1) An Rpts, 1942, Surg 1st, 3d, and 4th SvCs. HD. (2) An Rpts, 1942, Sta Hosps at Cps McCoy and Adair and Borden Gen Hosp. HD. (3) Memo CE 600.914 (WWGH) SPEOT, CofEngrs for SG, 15 Dec 42, sub: Progress at Woodrow Wilson Gen Hosp. SG: 632.-1 (WWGH)K. (4) Ltr, CO Valley Forge Gen Hosp to SG, 17 Oct 42, sub: Completion Date. SG: 632.-1 (VFGH)K. (5) Ltr, Col E[rnest] R. Gentry to Col H. D. Offutt, 24 Oct 42. SG: 323.7-5 (Borden GH)K. (6) Rpts on Status of Hosp in US, 1 and 6 Feb 43. SG: 632.-1. (7) Memo, SG for CG ASF, 31 Mar 43. HD: 632.-2.

[154] The above is based on: (1) Bed Status Rpts. Off file, Health Rpts Br Med Statistics Div SGO. (2) ASF Monthly Progress Rpt, Sec 7, *Health*, pp. 13-16, 28 Feb 43.

[155] The above is based on: (1) Bed Status Rpts. Off file, Health Rpts Br Med Statistics Div SGO. (2) ASF Monthly Progress Rpts, Sec 7, *Health*, 28 Feb and 31 May 43.

Chart 5—Status of Station and General Hospital Beds in Continental United States: December 1941–June 1943

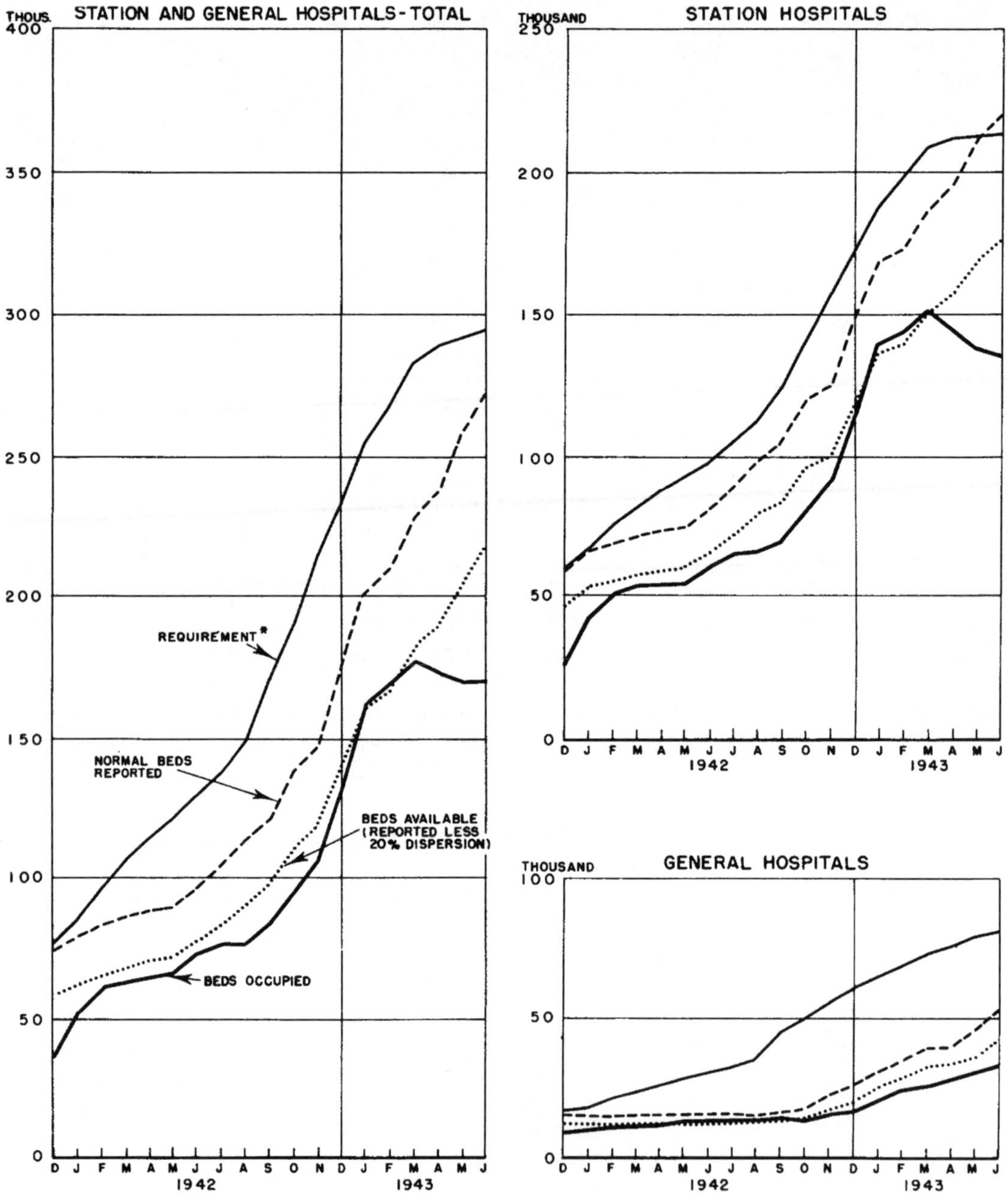

* Based on War Department determined percentage of troop strength.

Source: Figures for normal beds reported, beds available, and beds occupied, as of the end of the last full week of the month (except Nov 1941, the figure for which is as of 14 Nov), shown in Bed Status Reports, Health Reports Br, Med Statistics Div, SGO.

CHAPTER VI

Early Adjustments in the Zone of Interior Hospital System

As the number of hospitals in the United States increased, changes occurred in the hospital system—that is, the combination of hospitals of different types operating under and serving different major commands. It will be recalled that there were only two types of zone-of-interior hospitals at the beginning of the war—station and general hospitals. As the Army's needs changed with its wartime expansion and combat experience, some of these installations developed characteristics or were given functions which made them differ from the normal. For example, special hospitals were required for prisoners of war and others had to be prepared to receive combat casualties from theaters of operations. Moreover the desirability of establishing a new type of hospital to care for convalescent patients was considered. Expansion of the Army, along with reorganization of the War Department, also raised questions as to which commands should be served by and should operate hospitals of different types. Therefore, before discussing the development of special characteristics and functions of some hospitals, an explanation of the command relationships of station and general hospitals with higher headquarters is in order.

Command Relationships of Hospitals

Station Hospitals

Classified according to major commands under which they operated, station hospitals with few exceptions were either Army Service Forces (called Services of Supply until March 1943) or Army Air Forces hospitals. ASF station hospitals furnished hospitalization not only for men and women of the Service Forces but also for those of the Army Ground Forces. Hence, large camps such as Fort Bragg (North Carolina) and Fort Jackson (South Carolina), with several infantry divisions each, were served by ASF station hospitals. By August 1942 there were 133 ASF station hospitals; by February 1943, 166. In February they ranged in size from 18 to 3,017 beds and had an average capacity of 643 beds each. AAF station hospitals were as numerous as ASF station hospitals, but were generally smaller. Located at AAF bases and fields and normally serving only AAF personnel, they numbered 103 in August 1942 and 169 in February 1943. On the latter date they ranged in size from 19 to 1,471 beds and had an average capacity of 233 beds each.[1] Since troops of the Ground Forces and of defense commands were usually hospitalized in ASF hospitals, these commands had no "named" station hospitals under their jurisdiction, but in a few cases they established what amounted to hospitals of that type in the United States.

Defense command troops were generally dispersed over extensive areas to guard the coasts of the United States. Receiving only emergency medical care in their own installations, they were ordinarily treated in ASF hospitals, or in near-by Air Forces, Navy, and civilian hospitals. In general, this system seems to have worked well,[2] but in the Western Defense Command where troops were concentrated to ward off a sneak Japanese attack, difficulties arose. Delays in the Defense Command's decision on troop distributions, as well as overlapping jurisdictions of the Defense Command, the Ninth Service Command, and the Army Air Forces, impeded attempts of The Surgeon General, the Service Command, and SOS headquarters to provide adequate facilities.[3] In April 1942, to meet an immediate need for beds in the Los Angeles area, the Western Defense Command arranged with the Veterans Administration to take over its buildings at Sawtelle, Los Angeles, Calif., from which neuropsychiatric patients were being evacuated inland. The 73d Evacuation Hospital, a Western Defense Command unit, then moved in and established a 750-bed hospital, which became the station hospital for all troops, Service Forces as well as Defense Command, in the area. In the fall of 1942, at the request of the Western Defense Command, the Ninth Service Command took over the operation of this hospital. Although a Defense Command unit, it had actually served as a named station hospital for approximately six months.[4]

The hospitalization of AGF troops on maneuvers continued to be provided during the early war years essentially as before the war. Ground Forces units, such as evacuation hospitals, furnished immediate care for patients with minor illnesses and injuries, but transferred those requiring major surgery and long-term treatment to near-by ASF hospitals. This sufficed for a situation in which maneuvers shifted from place to place and lasted for a comparatively short time, but The Surgeon General considered different arrangements necessary when in the fall of 1942 the Ground Forces began almost year-round use of two areas, the A. P. Hill Military Reservation in Virginia and the Desert Training Center in California and Arizona.

---

[1] Annex B to Memos, SG for CG SOS, 30 Aug 42 and 12 Feb 43, sub: Opr Plan for Hosp and Evac. SG: 705.-1.

[2] (1) An Rpt, 1943, Surg, Northwestern Sector WDC. HD. (2) An Rpt, 1943, Surg WDC. HD. (3) Incl 1 to Ltr, CG WDC to SG, 21 Dec 43, sub: Opr Plans for Mil Hosp and Evac. HD: Wilson files, "Hosp and Evac Plans." (4) Ltr, CG SDC to SG, 30 Mar 44, sub: Plans for Mil Hosp and Evac. Same file.

[3] (1) Memo, Chief Misc Br Oprs SOS for Chief Oprs SOS, 14 Apr 42, sub: Add Hosp Cons, WDC. HD: Wilson files, "Book I, 26 Mar 42-26 Sep 42." (2) 1st ind, CG WDC to TAG, 9 Oct 42, on basic Ltr not located. HD: Wilson files, "Book 2, 26 Sep 42-31 Dec 42." (3) SG: 632,-1(Cp Haan)C and 632.-1(Cp Callan)C. (4) See also Memo SPOPH 632, ACofS for Oprs SOS for ACofS OPD WDGS, 26 Sep 42, sub: Hosp Fac for Eastern and Western Def Comds. HD: Wilson files, "Book 2, 26 Sep 42-31 Dec 42."

[4] (1) Ltr, Surg III Corps to SG thru Mil Channels, 3 Feb 43, sub: An Rpt Med Activities III Corps, 1942. Ground Med files: 319.1-2. (2) Ltr, CG WDC to TAG thru CG 9th SvC, 2 Sep 42, sub: Hosp at Sawtelle, Calif, and 4 inds. SG: 632.-1 (Sawtelle, Calif)F. (3) An Rpt, 1942, 73d Evac Hosp. HD.

Although the Ground Forces operated a numbered evacuation hospital on the A. P. Hill Military Reservation for a short time, the Third Service Command was responsible for providing fixed hospitalization for troops in that area. AGF headquarters maintained that the reservation was being used only temporarily. The Ground Surgeon believed that it was satisfactory to give emergency care in a temporary hospital, operated by personnel of numbered units under service command control, and to evacuate patients with serious illnesses and injuries to the Fort Belvoir Station Hospital fifty miles away. Supporting the Service Command Surgeon, The Surgeon General maintained that adequate hospitals should be provided in the immediate area in which troops were quartered, in order to avoid long ambulance hauls, and that any facilities less than those provided in cantonment-type buildings were unsatisfactory for the hospitalization of troops in the United States. The War Department General Staff supported the position of the Ground Forces, while SOS headquarters gave wavering support to the Medical Department, alternately approving and disapproving recommendations of The Surgeon General. The upshot of the whole matter was that the Third Service Command, failing to secure War Department approval of its plans, continued for a period of almost two years to operate in this area a temporary hospital located in winterized tents and manned by numbered station hospital units without nurses.[5]

When the War Department decided to operate the Desert Training Center (later called the California-Arizona Maneuver Area) as a simulated theater of operations under the jurisdiction of the Army Ground Forces, the Ground Surgeon agreed with other officers from AGF and ASF headquarters that hospitalization should be provided for it in the same manner as for an actual theater. As a result, engineer units of the communications zone erected theater-of-operations-type buildings for hospitals, and beginning in February 1943, communications zone headquarters moved in numbered station and general hospital units to relieve the Ninth Service Command of all responsibility for hospitalization within the area. By June 1943 the communications zone had either in operation or in the planning stage eight 250-bed and one 150-bed station hospitals and three 1,000-bed general hospitals. Until these were all in operation, the Desert Training Center continued to send large numbers of patients to neighboring ASF hospitals. Later, as communications zone general hospitals began to offer definitive medical care, the number of patients evacuated to ASF hospitals decreased. Supplied with equipment authorized by tables of basic allowances and manned by numbered hospital units which had their own nurses with them, these communications zone hospitals continued to provide station and general hospital types of care until the California-Arizona Maneuver Area closed in the spring of 1944. This plan of hospitalization not only gave participating units invaluable practical experience but also demonstrated the possibility of using num-

[5] Documents dealing with this extended controversy may be found in the following files: SG: 701.-1 (Cp A. P. Hill)C; SG: 632.-1 (Cp A. P. Hill)C; AG: 632(9-18-42) (1); HRS: MID files 600-659, "Vol. I, Jan 42-Jul 44," and HD: Wilson files, 354.1 "Cp A. P. Hill." See also An Rpts, 1943, 66th, 108th, 222d, and 230th Sta Hosps (HD) and Comment by Brig Gen Frederick A. Blesse, 5 Dec 50. (HD: 314 [Correspondence on MS] III.)

bered hospital units in the zone of interior medical service.[6]

General Hospitals

All general hospitals in the United States were operated by the Army Service Forces but were planned to care for patients from the Ground, Air, and Service Forces alike. This arrangement was seriously threatened in the fall of 1942 by an attempt of the Air Forces to establish its own general hospitals. Although unsuccessful at the time, this attempt was a forerunner of others which later in the war had significant effects upon the hospital system. It deserves consideration here not only for that reason but also because it illustrates difficulties created by the War Department reorganization of 1942.

Until the fall of that year only fifteen general hospitals were in operation but beginning in September this number grew until it reached thirty-one by January 1943.[7] While new general hospitals were opening, the Air Forces began to establish in effect—though not in name—separate general hospitals for AAF personnel. Having received authority to recruit its own physicians, the Air Forces manned some of its station hospitals with specialists normally assigned only to general hospitals. In the winter of 1942–43 smaller AAF station hospitals began to transfer patients to these instead of general hospitals. The Air Forces also began to transfer to AAF station hospitals patients returned from theaters by airplane. With the development of such practices certain AAF station hospitals requested the Surgeon General's Office to reduce drastically—if not eliminate altogether—the number of beds in general hospitals set aside for AAF patients. Later the Air Surgeon's Office asked for specialized equipment with which to establish fifty-four specialty centers in neurosurgery, orthopedic surgery, thoracic surgery, and deep X-ray therapy in AAF station hospitals.[8]

The Air Surgeon found legal justification for such actions in the reorganization of the War Department, which in his opinion established the Air Forces as a "command of equal authority" with the Service Forces, as well as in the indefinite terms of current directives governing the transfer of patients to general hospitals. His attempt to set up separate general hospitals for the Air Forces was prompted in part by a desire to establish a separate medical department, but it also sprang from professional considerations. The Air Surgeon contended that Air Forces men, especially combat crew members, required specialized care which only AAF hospitals could give. He believed that fliers were often lost to further combat duty because general hospitals unnecessarily reclassified them for limited service. Furthermore, he insisted that Air Forces hospitals were more efficiently operated

[6] (1) History of Medical Section, C–AMA. HD. (2) Draft Memo for Record, undated and unsigned. HRS: ASF Planning Div files, 353 DTC 1942–43. (3) Memo, Col William E. Shambora for ACofS G–3 AGF, 11 Mar 43, sub: Insp of La and DTC Maneuvers. Ground Med files: 354.2 "Maneuvers." (4) Interv, MD Historian with Col Shambora, 18 Apr 49. HD: 000.71. (5) An Rpts, 1943, 13th, 22d, 34th, and 297th Gen Hosps, and 37th, 59th, 94th, 107th, 127th, and 181st Sta Hosps. HD. (6) Sidney L. Meller, The Desert Training Center and C–AMA, Study No 15 (1946). AG.

[7] See below, *Table 15*, pp. 304–13.

[8] (1) See Tabs F, G, I, K, and L of Memo SPOPI 020, CG ASF for CofSA, 30 Apr 43, sub: Unification of Med Serv of Army by SG. AG: 020 SGO (3–30–43)(1). (2) Memo, Brig Gen C[harles] C. Hillman for SG, 15 Mar 43, sub: Rpt of Observation Trip. HD: 333. (3) Memo, Chief Professional Serv Br Air Surg Off for Chief Sup Div Air Surg Off, 5 May 43. SG: 323.7–5.

than Service Forces hospitals and should therefore, in the interest of economy, give the highest type of medical care for which they were equipped and staffed.[9]

The Surgeon General disapproved the Air Forces' establishment of separate general hospitals under any guise, for he wished to maintain a unified medical service under his direction as chief medical officer of the Army. Stating that men of the Air Forces were not different from those of other arms and services, who also suffered from occupational diseases and hazards, he insisted that general hospitals were adequately staffed and equipped to care for them as well as for the sick and wounded of the rest of the Army. Permitting AAF hospitals to perform the functions of general hospitals would make it more difficult, he stated, to supervise and co-ordinate professional practices and procedures. It would also result in duplication of hospital buildings (since general hospitals were already planned to care for the patients of all major commands) and in an uneconomical use of personnel and equipment. Finally, he argued, having separate sets of hospitals for patients evacuated from theaters of operations would complicate the evacuation process and would cause confusion in the submission of medical reports.[10]

The question of whether the Air Forces would be permitted to establish separate general hospitals came to a head early in 1943 in connection with a movement initiated by the ASF Chief of Staff to reaffirm The Surgeon General's authority as chief medical officer of the Army.[11] It reached the General Staff first, and finally the Secretary of War. G-4 tended to favor the Air Forces, and while conceding that opposing contentions of The Surgeon General and the Air Surgeon were both just, he accepted the latter's view that AAF hospitals were more efficient than those of the Service Forces. He recommended, therefore, that the Air Forces be granted "additional authority" to treat all of their own combat personnel, including evacuees, in AAF hospitals.[12] The Office of the Deputy Chief of Staff went a step further, publishing a directive on 20 June 1943 which gave the Air Forces authority not only to treat its own combat personnel but also to operate whatever general hospitals were necessary for that purpose.[13] Within a week the Air Surgeon's Office recommended the establishment of five AAF general hospitals: three by the conversion of AAF station hospitals and two

[9] (1) Memo, Air Surg for CG AAF, n d, sub: [Comments on Gen Somervell's Memo of 30 Apr 43 for CofSA], with 2 incls. Asst SecWar for Air: 632(AAF Hosp). (2) Brief and Discussion, Tab B, to Memo, C of Air Staff for CofSA, 7 Oct 42, sub: Specialized Hosp and Recuperative Fac for AAF Pers. AAF: 354.1 "Rest Ctrs and Conv Homes." (3) Hubert A. Coleman, Organization and Administration, AAF Medical Services in the Zone of the Interior (1948), pp. 93-94. HD.

[10] (1) Memo SPMCB 701.-1, SG for CG SOS, 13 Oct 42, sub: Specialized Hosp and Recuperative Fac for AAF Pers. AAF: 354.-1 "Rest Ctrs and Conv Homes"(1). (2) 1st ind, SG to CG ASF, 12 Apr 43, on Memo SPOPH 020(3-30-43), CG ASF for SG, 30 Mar 43, sub: Relationship between SG and Air Surg. SG: 024.-1.

[11] For more details on this movement, see John D. Millett, *The Organization and Role of the Army Service Forces* (Washington, 1954), pp. 132-37, in UNITED STATES ARMY IN WORLD WAR II; Blanche B. Armfield, Organization and Administration (MS for companion vol. in Medical Dept. series), HD., and Coleman, *op. cit.*, pp. 93-107. Documents concerning it are on file as follows: AG: 020 SGO (3-30-42) (1); HRS: G-4 file, "Hosp and Evac Policy"; SG: 024.-1; and HRS: Hq ASF, Gen Styer's files, "Med Dept."

[12] Memo WDGDS 4440, ACofS G-4 WDGS for CofSA, 15 Jun 43, sub: Med Serv of Army, with incl. HRS: G-4 file, "Hosp and Evac Policy."

[13] Memo WDCSA/320(5-26-43), DepCofSA for CGs AAF, AGF, ASF, 20 Jun 43, sub: Med Serv of Army. HRS: G-4 file, "Hosp and Evac Policy." The Deputy Chief of Staff, Lt. Gen. Joseph T. McNarney, was an AAF officer.

by the transfer of the Borden (Oklahoma) and Torney (California) General Hospitals to Air Forces' jurisdiction.[14] By this time a new Surgeon General, Maj. Gen. Norman T. Kirk, was in office.[15] He attacked the problem vigorously, and the entire matter reached the Secretary of War, who called representatives of the General Staff, the commanding generals of the Air and Service Forces, and others into conference. General Kirk then proposed a compromise which the commanders of both the Air and Service Forces accepted.[16]

General Kirk admitted that Air Forces combat crews needed special treatment and consideration and offered to place flight surgeons in his Office and in general hospitals to serve as advisers in that field. He agreed also to the Air Forces' establishment of convalescent centers. The Air Forces for its part agreed that all general hospitals would continue to operate under The Surgeon General and the commanding general, Army Service Forces, and that patients evacuated from theaters of operations would be sent to general hospitals. The only exception to the latter point was that combat crew members suffering from operational fatigue alone would be sent directly to AAF convalescent centers. These centers were to be equipped and staffed as station hospitals, but one of them, located at Coral Gables, Fla., was authorized to perform a function of general hospitals—the reclassification of officers for limited service and the recommendation for their appearance before retiring boards. These terms of agreement were issued on 9 July 1943, with a statement that they had been personally approved by the Secretary of War.[17] On the same day, the authority which had been granted to the Air Forces to establish separate general hospitals was revoked.[18]

This agreement did not dispose of the question of whether or not AAF station hospitals would give general-hospital-type treatment to zone of interior patients. At the time General Kirk drafted its terms, he had also drafted a statement of policy on the transfer of patients to general hospitals, defining more specifically the types of cases to be transferred. He had intended to have it included in the 9 July 1943 agreement,[19] but instead, on 14 July 1943, he requested its publication as a War Department circular.[20] While maintaining the traditional responsibility of station hospital commanders for the selection of patients for transfer to general hospitals,

[14] Memo [Air Surg] (init R[ichard] L. M[eiling]) for CofSA, 26 Jun 43, sub: Med Serv of AAF. Asst SecWar for Air: 632 (AAF).

[15] Gen Kirk assumed office on 1 June 1943.

[16] (1) Draft memo, prepared by SG, dated 3 Jul 43, sub: Hosp, with pencil note, "7/3/43 Personally delivered by Gen Kirk to Gen Somervell." SG: 705.-1 and SecWar: SP 632 (3 Jul 43). (2) Memo, CG AAF for DepCofSA, 5 Jul 43, sub: Hosp. Same files. (3) Memo, [Col] F. M. S[mith] for Gen Somervell, 5 Jul 43. HRS: Hq ASF Gen Styer's files, "Med Dept." How the matter reached the Secretary of War is not clear. On 19 November 1950 General Kirk wrote: "A conference was called in his [Secretary of War's] office one morning. I was called in ahead of time and Mr. Stimson told me that Secretary of Air, Mr. Lovett, had been to him that morning and told him about the memorandum. That the Air Force couldn't blame me for bringing it to his attention." Ltr, Maj Gen Norman T. Kirk to Col Roger G. Prentiss, Jr, 19 Nov 50, with incl. HD: 314 (Correspondence on MS) I.

[17] (1) Memo WDCSA/632 (9 Jul 43), DepCofSA for CGs AAF, ASF, AGF, 9 Jul 43, sub: Hosps. HRS: G-4 file, "Hosp and Evac Policy." (2) Memo, CG AAF for CG ASF, 5 Jul 43, sub: Hosps. AAF: 354.-1 "Rest Ctrs and Conv Homes." (3) Memo, CG ASF for CG AAF, 5 Jul 43. HRS: Hq ASF Gen Styer's files, "Med Dept."

[18] (1) Memo, DepCofSA for CG AAF, ASF, AGF, 9 Jul 43, sub: Med Serv of the Army. HRS: G-4 file, "Hosp and Evac Policy."

[19] Draft memo prepared by SG, 3 Jul 43, sub: Hosps, with incl 1, sub: Policy regarding Trf of Pnts to Named Gen Hosps. SG: 705.-1.

[20] Memo SPMCM 300.5-5, SG for Publications Div AGO, 14 Jul 43. AG: 704.11 (14 Jul 43)(1).

the revised policy left them less discretion in the matter than they had previously exercised. Its language was directive rather than advisory. The following categories of patients must be transferred to general hospitals: those needing specialized treatment of the types for which general hospitals had been designated; those who would be hospitalized for ninety days or more; those upon whom elective surgery of a formidable type would be performed; those with specific types of fractures, and, with one exception, those evacuated from overseas theaters. Only Air Forces patients on a flying status, evacuated because of operational fatigue alone, were to bypass general hospitals and go direct to Air Forces convalescent centers.[21] This directive combined with the agreement already discussed to resolve for a time in The Surgeon General's favor the question of the Air Forces' establishment of separate general hospitals.

Special Types of ASF Station Hospitals

Although all ASF station hospitals were essentially alike in the work they did and the way they operated, a few established in the early war years differed in some respects from the normal. Among them were WAAC hospitals, all-Negro hospitals, and hospitals for civilians and prisoners of war.

Hospitals for Waacs

Formation of the Women's Army Auxiliary Corps in May 1942 emphasized certain problems such as the segregation of women from men in hospitals, the establishment of services not ordinarily found in Army hospitals, and the procurement of nonstandard drugs (that is, those not formally standardized for Army use) for the treatment of women. The law establishing the WAAC directed the Secretary of War to provide hospitalization for its members "to conform as nearly as practicable to similar services rendered to the personnel of the Army" and permitted the use of "facilities and personnel of the Army" for this purpose.[22] The Surgeon General approved of this policy. He believed that additional wards should be constructed at established hospitals to supply enough beds to permit the segregation of men from women and of women according to disease and rank. Because he expected women to have a higher sick rate, he recommended the provision of beds for 5 percent of the strength of the WAAC, rather than for 4 percent, as was the case with men. He proposed the procurement of a limited number of female physicians, first as contract surgeons and later as commissioned members of the Medical Corps, to serve in hospitals where the WAAC patient load was high. Otherwise, he planned to give Waacs the same medical care as men. As experience with the hospitalization of Waacs accumulated and statistics showed their noneffective rate to be only slightly higher than that for men, the Army provided hospital beds for them in the same ratio as for men and sent them to the same hospitals, though to segregated wards. Nevertheless, three Army hospitals were occupied chiefly by female patients.[23]

---

[21] WD Cir 165, 19 Jul 43.

[22] Public Law 554, 77th Cong., 2d sess., sec 10.

[23] (1) Rpt, SGs Conf with CA and Army Surgs, 25–28 May 42. HD: 337. (2) Memo, SG to CofEngrs, 6 May 43, sub: Med Fac for WAAC. SG: 632.-1. (3) AG Memo W 100-9-43, 3 Jul 43, sub: Housing for WAAC Pers. HD: 322.5-1 (WAC). (4) Memo, Maj Margaret D. Craighill, MC, Liaison Off for WAC for Col [Raymond W.] Bliss, 25 Aug 43, sub: Hosp for WAAC. Same file. (5) Memo, SG for CG SOS, 4 Jan 43, sub: Util of Women Doctors. HRS: Hq ASF Gen Styer's files, "Med Dept 1943."

At the WAAC training centers—Fort Des Moines (Iowa), Daytona Beach (Florida), and Fort Oglethorpe (Georgia)—the station hospitals became predominantly WAAC hospitals, staffed largely by women and caring mainly for women. This was especially true at Daytona Beach. By the end of 1943 its 601-bed hospital had an enlisted complement made up almost entirely of women, only fifty men being assigned for duty in and around the hospital. At Fort Des Moines, female doctors engaged as contract surgeons were assigned for duty with the Waacs. At first the development and supervision of special professional services for women were left largely to local hospital commanders. Station hospitals at training centers developed gynecologic and obstetric services and procured locally special drugs required for the medical care of women. In May 1943, approximately a year after the WAAC was established and a month after Congress authorized the commissioning of women physicians in the Army, The Surgeon General assigned a female Medical Corps officer to his Office to supervise the handling of medical problems peculiar to female personnel.[24]

All-Negro Hospitals

The establishment of two all-Negro station hospitals in the United States came not as a result of any policy of The Surgeon General to segregate patients racially for medical care and treatment, but rather as a result of The Surgeon General's opposition to the integration of Negro doctors and nurses with white professional personnel in the operation of hospitals caring for white patients.[25] This consideration had already resulted in the establishment in May 1941 of groups of all-Negro wards in the hospitals at Fort Bragg (North Carolina) and Camp Livingston (Louisiana). Perhaps because of unencouraging reports from these experiments, the Army had not extended the practice to other hospitals. After war started, The Surgeon General revived a recommendation, previously disapproved by the General Staff, that all-Negro hospitals be established to employ additional Negro doctors and nurses. The Staff reversed its earlier decision, and during 1942 an all-Negro station hospital was organized at Fort Huachuca (Arizona), a post at which Negro troops were being trained. A separate hospital, manned by white doctors and nurses, continued in operation to care for white patients. The year before, the Army Air Forces had established an all-Negro hospital at Tuskegee, Ala.

Establishment of all-Negro hospitals and wards did not signify a general abandonment of the Army's long-established policy of nonsegregated treatment. Other hospitals manned by white doctors and nurses continued to treat patients of both races on a nonsegregated basis throughout the war.[26] Nor did it mean that the Medical

[24] (1) An Rpts, 1943, Sta Hosps, Daytona Beach and Ft Oglethorpe. HD. (2) Memos, Dr Paul Titus, Consultant, to SG, [27 Sep 43] and 1 Nov 43, sub: Rpts on Surg (Obstetrics-Gynecology) as an Army Serv. HD: 210.01. (3) Memo, SG for CG SOS, 4 Jan 43, sub: Util of Women Doctors. HRS: Hq ASF Gen Styer's files, "Med Dept 1943." (4) Mattie E. Treadwell, *The Women's Army Corps* (Washington, 1954), Ch. XXXI, in UNITED STATES ARMY IN WORLD WAR II. (5) Margaret D. Craighill, History of Women's Medical Unit (1946). HD.

[25] For a full discussion of the question of the use of Negro professional personnel by the Medical Department, see John H. McMinn and Max Levin, Personnel (MS for companion Vol. in Medical Department series). HD. Also see Ulysses Lee, The Employment of Negro Troops, a forthcoming volume in the series UNITED STATES ARMY IN WORLD WAR II.

[26] (1) Ltr, SG to TAG, 25 Oct 40, sub: Plan for Util of Negro Offs, Nurses, and EM in MD, and 3 inds. (2) Memo, SG for ACofS G-1 WDGS, 7 Jul 41, sub: Rpts on Util of Negro Med Pers. (3) Memo, Maj

Department would fail to use Negro enlisted personnel and civilians in other hospitals. As early as December 1941, for example, Negro enlisted men were assigned to the medical detachment of at least one station hospital—that at Chanute Field (Illinois).[27] Later Negro enlisted men and women were assigned to other Army hospitals. While many were employed in housekeeping and maintenance operations, some were assigned to technical and administrative duties.[28]

Before leaving this subject one needs to look ahead to the later war years. At that time the practice of using Negro doctors and nurses on a segregated basis was modified. Such civilian groups as the National Association of Colored Graduate Nurses, certain segments of the press, some members of Congress, the Negro civilian aide to the Secretary of War, and the President's wife (Mrs. Franklin D. Roosevelt) urged The Surgeon General, ASF headquarters, and the Secretary of War to use more Negro nurses and to use them on a nonsegregated basis.[29] In December 1943 and again in May 1944 ASF headquarters directed The Surgeon General to procure and use additional Negro nurses.[30] Accordingly, Negro nurses on duty with the Army increased from 218 in December 1943 to 512 by July 1945. Although some continued to serve with all-Negro hospitals in this country and in theaters of operations, others were used on a nonsegregated basis in 4 general hospitals, 3 regional hospitals, and at least 9 station hospitals in the United States.[31] During 1945 nonsegregated use of Negro doctors occurred in at least one instance. When the troop strength of Fort Huachuca declined, the patient load decreased and professional staffs of the two station hospitals at that post were reduced accordingly. Services of the two then gradually merged and both doctors and nurses of the two races served together to care for white as well as Negro personnel.[32] Thus the primary reason for the establishment of separate all-Negro wards and hospi-

Arthur B. Welsh for [Brig] Gen [Larry B.] McAfee, 17 Jan 42. (4) Memo, SG for ACofS G-3 WDGS, 30 Jan 42. (5) Memo, SG for TAG, 16 Mar 42, sub: SecWar's Press Conf on Use of Negro Doctors. All in HD: 291.2. (6) Memo, ACofS G-1 WDGS for CofSA, 4 Aug 41, sub: Almt of Negro MD Res Offs and Female Nurses. HRS: G-1/15640-46. (7) Memo, P. W. Clarkson, Off ACofS G-1 WDGS for Record, 8 Aug 41. Same file. (8) An Rpt, 1942, Post Surg Ft Huachuca. HD.

[27] An Rpt, 1941, Sta Hosp, Chanute Field. HD.

[28] (1) An Rpts, 1942, Sta Hosps, Cps Shelby and Forrest, and An Rpts, 1942, 702d, 720th, 721st, and 730th Med Sanitary Cos. HD. (2) McMinn and Levin, *op. cit.*

[29] Letters to this effect may be found in the following files: SG: 211 "Nurses, Negro"; OSW: Civ Aide to SecWar, "Nurses"; and AG: 211 "Nurses, Negro." See also Florence A. Blanchfield and Mary W. Standlee, The Army Nurse Corps in World War II (1950), pp. 161-205. HD.

[30] (1) Memo, CG ASF for SG, 14 Dec 43, sub: Utilization of Negro Nurses. SG: 291.2-1. (2) Memo, CofS ASF for SG, 6 May 44, same sub. ASF: 210.31.

[31] (1) Memo, Col Florence A. Blanchfield (SGO) for Col Arthur B. Welsh (SGO), 17 Dec 43, sub: Distr of Colored Nurses. SG: 291.2-1. (2) Memo, SG for Civ Aide to SecWar, 26 Jul 45. SG: 211 "Nurses, Negro." (3) Facts about Negro Nurses and the War, prepared jointly by the National Association of Colored Graduate Nurses and the National Nursing Council for War Service, ca. Jan 45. OSW: Civ Aide to SecWar, "Nurses."

[32] (1) Memo, Asst Aide to SecWar for SG, 29 Mar 45, sub: Staff of Sta Hosp No 1, Ft Huachuca, Ariz. (2) Memo, Dep Chief [of Oprs Serv] for Hosp and Domestic Oprs [SGO] for SG, 8 Jun 45, sub: Rpt of Visit to Sta Hosp, Ft Huachuca, Ariz. (3) Ltr, CO Sta Hosp Ft Huachuca to Maj Gen G[eorge] F. Lull, SGO, 16 Aug 45. All in OSW: Civ Aide to SecWar, "Huachuca." There was some question during the war whether the two hospitals at Huachuca were ever in fact two separate hospitals or merely two sections of one hospital. This arose apparently from the fact that the post surgeon, a white Medical Corps officer, served in addition as commander of the white hospital and exercised at the same time considerable authority over the commanding officer of the all-Negro hospital. Failure to settle this question resulted in dissatisfaction on the part of the latter. See letters in the file just cited and in SG: 323.3 (Ft Huachuca)N.

tals—opposition to the integrated use of Negro and white professional personnel in the care of both white and Negro patients—had begun to lose some of its force by the end of the war.

Army Hospitals for Civilians

By the end of 1942 a situation developed which required the establishment in the United States of several hospitals for civilian employees and their families. During 1941 the Army had initiated industrial hygiene programs in Army-owned plants and depots. Under Medical Department supervision, these programs expanded rapidly during 1942 to keep pace with wartime industrial growth. Designed to give only emergency medical care, industrial hygiene facilities were adequate in areas where civilian hospitals were available. Toward the end of 1942, when the Ordnance Department established storage depots for explosives in isolated regions, lack of hospitals retarded employee procurement and increased absenteeism. Workers were reluctant to move with their families to such areas and failure to receive prompt medical care often resulted in prolonged illnesses. To help maintain depot production levels, The Surgeon General proposed in December 1942 that the Army construct and operate hospitals in remote areas which lacked adequate medical facilities. In February 1943 the Secretary of War authorized the construction of hospitals at the Sierra (California), Umatilla (Oregon), Black Hills (South Dakota), Tooele (Utah), Sioux (Nebraska), and Navajo (Arizona) Ordnance Depots. Constructed during 1943, these hospitals operated under service command supervision until after the end of the war. They differed from other Army station hospitals in having a minimum of military personnel assigned to them, in providing family medical care, including gynecologic and obstetric services, and in requiring payment for services rendered. Despite recommendations of The Surgeon General, similar hospitals were not established in other places. In one instance, permission was granted to establish an Army hospital but was withdrawn partly on account of political pressure and partly because the community itself, after an extended period of time, provided additional hospital accommodations. In another, authority was granted to hospitalize civilian employees and their families in a near-by Army station hospital.[33]

Hospitals for Prisoners of War

Early in 1942, when prospective combat operations demanded preparation for the internment of prisoners of war, The Provost Marshal General and The Surgeon General agreed upon basic policies for their hospitalization. In compliance with the Geneva Convention,[34] hospital accommodations and medical care for prisoners of war were to be equal to those for United States troops, and prisoners

[33] (1) Ltr, SG to SecWar thru CG SOS, 11 Dec 42, sub: Med Care for Civ Employees of Army-Operated Plants, and their Families, with 4 inds. (2) Ltr, SG to CofS SOS, 21 Jan 43, same sub. (3) Memo WDGDS-2172, SecWar for CG SOS, 9 Feb 43, same sub. All in AG: 701(9-17-41)(1). (4) W. L. Cooke, Jr, Organization and Administration of Preventive Medicine Program, pp. 53-59. HD. (5) An Rpts, 1943, Sta Hosp Black Hills and Tooele Ord Depots. HD. (6) An Rpts, 1942 and 43, Surg, 1st thru 9th SvC. HD. (7) Memo, Capt J[ames] J. Souder for Col J[ohn] R. Hall, 8 Apr 43, sub: Conf on Prov of Hosp Fac for Instls in Ogden, Utah, Area. SG: 632.-1.

[34] Article I, Chapter I, Conventions of 1906 and 1929. See *Army Medical Bulletin,* No. 62 (1942), pp. 88 and 105.

were to assist in the care of their compatriots. Promulgated in tentative regulations published in April 1942 and reiterated in September 1943, these policies governed the hospitalization of prisoners throughout the war. For separate prisoner-of-war camps, the Army constructed hospitals with beds for 4 percent of the inmates. For prisoners at Army posts, wards surrounded by wire fences were added to existing station hospitals. Whether in separate camps or on Army posts, such hospitals operated under service command supervision and, except for the use of captured enemy personnel and civilian registered nurses, were similar to other service command hospitals. Prisoners requiring more specialized care than offered in station hospitals were transferred to general hospitals.[35]

Port and Debarkation Hospitals

Hospitals were needed near ports for large numbers of transients—troops awaiting shipment overseas as well as patients being returned to general hospitals in the United States. In accord with SOS directives, hospitals for ports and staging areas were exempt from service command jurisdiction and operated directly under port commanders who in turn were subject to control by the Chief of Transportation.[36] For most of 1942, many ports lacked adequate staging area hospitals and therefore sent patients to others located near by. At Los Angeles, for example, patients from the port were cared for in the Western Defense Command's 73d Evacuation Hospital at Sawtelle. The ports at Charleston, New Orleans, and San Francisco used Stark, LaGarde, and Letterman General Hospitals, respectively, while those at Boston and Hampton Roads sent patients to near-by service command station hospitals. During 1942 and 1943 special port and staging area hospitals were constructed and opened to care for port personnel and transient troops. They differed from other station hospitals primarily in that their surgical services were considerably smaller and less important than their medical services, because they normally performed only emergency surgery for the thousands of troops who passed through ports.[37]

The kind of hospitals that would be used to receive transient patients returning from theaters of operations remained uncertain until the latter part of 1942. Special debarkation hospitals under port control might be established in existing buildings with only the personnel and equipment needed to "process" returning patients—that is, replace their missing records, make partial payments of the

[35] (1) Memo, Capt Charles M. Huey, Mil Intel Aliens Div OPMG for Chief Aliens Div OPMG, 26 Dec 41, sub: Conf Regarding the Estab of Hosp . . . in PW Cps. SG: 255.-1. (2) Tentative Regulations: Interned Alien Enemies and Prisoners of War. AG: 383.6(8-9-42)(1). (3) PW Cir 1, 24 Sep 43. PW Off OPMG. (4) Memo, CofS ASF for SG and QMG, 26 May 43, sub: Hosp Fac for PW Cps, and 1st ind. SG: 632.-1. (5) An Rpts, 1943, Surg, 7th and 8th SvCs. HD. (6) An Rpts, 1943, Sta Hosp PW Cps at Florence, Ariz; Cp Clark, Mo; and Como, Miss. HD. (7) See also: Rene H. Juchli, Record of Events in the Treatment of Prisoners of War, World War II (1945). HD.

[36] Mil Hosp and Evac Oprs, incl 1 to Ltr SPOPH 322.15, CG SOS to CGs and COs of SvCs and PEs and to SG, 15 Sep 42, sub: Mil Hosp and Evac Oprs. HD: 322(Hosp and Evac).

[37] (1) An Rpts, 1942 and 43, Surg, Boston, New York, Hampton Roads, Charleston, New Orleans, Seattle, and Portland PEs, and An Rpts, 1943, Surg, Cps Myles Standish, Kilmer, and Plauche. HD. (2) Opr Plan for Mil Hosp and Evac, Boston, 30 Nov 42; New York, 10 Dec 42; Hampton Roads, 15 Dec 42; Charleston, 24 Nov 42; New Orleans, 12 Dec 42; San Francisco, 9 Jul and 1 Dec 42; and Seattle, 27 Nov 42. HD: Wilson files. (3) SG: 632.-2, 1942 and 43, (LaGarde GH)K, (Letterman GH)K, and (Stark GH)K.

money due them, classify them according to disease or injury, and prepare them for further travel to general hospitals. Such hospitals had been used during World War I,[38] and for a while in 1942 it seemed as if SOS headquarters and certain port commanders expected their revival. One SOS directive implied that ports might establish special debarkation hospitals,[39] and Charleston, Seattle, and San Francisco expressed a desire for them.[40]

The Surgeon General had other plans. During the emergency period he had used general hospitals near ports—Tilton for New York, Stark for Charleston, LaGarde for New Orleans, and Letterman for San Francisco—to receive and care for patients brought in on ships. After war began he continued this system, granting unlimited bed credits in near-by general hospitals to ports receiving overseas casualties.[41] He also located some of the general hospitals planned early in 1942 in coastal areas, though not in close proximity to ports,[42] with the expectation that they would process patients arriving from theaters.

A final decision to this effect came in the fall of 1942 in connection with plans for the reception of casualties from the North African invasion. At that time whole trainloads of patients with a variety of ills could be sent to a single general hospital, because hospitals had not yet been designated for the specialized treatment of certain types of cases nor had the policy of hospitalizing casualties near their homes been established.[43] Two alternatives therefore presented themselves, namely, ship-to-train movements, in which patients would be transferred directly from ships to trains for transfer to distant general hospitals, and ship-to-hospital movements, in which they would be moved from ships to near-by hospitals before undertaking further travel.[44] The possibility of using ship-to-train movements exclusively, thereby eliminating the need for a debarkation hospital at or near the port, arose at Hampton Roads. Piers at that port had ample trackage to accommodate hospital trains, making it possible to move patients under cover directly from ships to trains. The port commander preferred this procedure, his surgeon explaining that it would maintain the port as an agency of movement, its primary purpose.[45] While The Surgeon General and the chief of the SOS Hospitalization and Evacuation Branch recognized the merits of this position, both felt that some ship-to-hospital movement would be unavoidable. Some patients would require immediate hospital care before further travel; in some instances ship-to-train evacuation might

[38] *The Medical Department . . . in the World War* (1923), vol. V, pp. 426–33, 786, 791, 800.

[39] Mil Hosp and Evac Oprs, par 5 *d* (3) (d), incl 1, to Ltr SPOPM 322.15, CG SOS to CGs and COs, CAs, PEs, GHs and SG, 18 Jun 42, sub: Opr Plans for Mil Hosp and Evac. HD: 705.-1.

[40] Opr Plans for Mil Hosp and Evac, Jul 42, Charleston, Seattle, San Francisco, New Orleans, and Boston. HD: Wilson files.

[41] For example, see: (1) Ltr, SG to CG NYPE, 18 Feb 42, sub: Bed Almts in Gen Hosps. Same file. (2) Ltr, SG to CG 9th CA, 5 Jan 42, sub: Bed Almts in Barnes Gen Hosp. SG: 632.2 (Barnes GH)K. (3) 2d ind, SG to CG NYPE, 9 Mar 42, on Ltr, Port Surg Sub-Port of Boston to Port Surg NYPE, 5 Mar 42, sub: Bed Credits. SG: 632.-2 (NYPE)N. (4) 1st ind, CG SOS (SG) to CO CPE, 29 Aug 42, on Ltr, CO CPE to CG SOS, 21 Aug 42, sub: Bed Credits. SG: 632.-2 (Stark GH)K.

[42] For example, Valley Forge, Woodrow Wilson, Moore, Torney, Hammond, Baxter, and McCaw General Hospitals. Also see above, pp. 88–90.

[43] See below, pp. 116–17.

[44] Rpt, Conf, CofT, SG, SOS, NYPE, and HRPE, 23 Oct 42. TC: 370.05 (Plans, Policies, Procedures).

[45] (1) Ltr, CG HRPE to SG, 10 Nov 42. SG: 705.-1 (HRPE)N. (2) Ltr, Port Surg HRPE to SG, 15 Dec 42, sub: Opr Plans for Mil Hosp and Evac. HD: Wilson files.

interfere with troop movements; in others, casualties might arrive unexpectedly when trains were unavailable.[46] For these reasons they overruled the port commander. Since the housing shortage in Norfolk made impracticable a proposal to take over a hotel for hospital use, arrangements were made to use the station hospital at Fort Monroe and five hundred beds in the Veterans Administration hospital at Kecoughtan, Va., for debarkation purposes.[47] This action made it clear that some hospital, whatever its kind, would be established to receive casualties at every port of debarkation.

Unlike his counterpart at Hampton Roads, the port commander at New York wanted Halloran General Hospital, being opened on Staten Island, to serve solely as a debarkation hospital under port control.[48] The Chief of Transportation, on the other hand, wished to keep ports free of the burden of administering large hospitals and on 9 November 1942 announced that SOS directives authorized ports to operate hospitals for assigned personnel and transient troops only, not for patients being returned from theaters.[49] Concurrence of the SOS Hospitalization and Evacuation Branch in this interpretation placed an official stamp of approval on The Surgeon General's plan to use general hospitals under service command control, rather than special hospitals under port control, for debarkation activities.

Most general hospitals located near ports performed dual functions—providing definitive treatment for some patients and processing others for further travel—until late in the war. This created complications. Ports were granted unlimited bed credits in such hospitals, but near-by station hospitals also continued to receive bed credits in them. This overlapping caused some concern in SOS headquarters.[50] Investigation showed that Halloran General Hospital kept a list of patients earmarked for transfer to other general hospitals when the evacuation load required it.[51] Stark, LaGarde, and Barnes General Hospitals simply waited until the necessity arose and then transferred patients receiving definitive care to other general hospitals located farther away from ports. Others, notably Letterman and Lovell, kept beds vacant while awaiting the arrival of evacuated casualties. This system occasionally caused the transfer of patients needing general hospital care to station hospitals. In the opinion of some hospital commanders, it was also wasteful of both professional personnel and highly specialized equipment.[52] Later, when the evacuation load reached its peak, The Surgeon General partially shared their view, for in 1945, as will be seen later, he proposed the conversion of

[46] (1) 1st ind, Chief Hosp and Evac Br SOS to CofT, 18 Nov 42, sub: Evac, on unknown basic Ltr. TC: 370.05(Plans, Policies, Procedures). (2) Ltr, CG HRPE to SG, 10 Nov 42. SG: 705.-1 (HRPE)N.

[47] (1) Off memo, signed by Col H. D. Offutt, 9 Nov 42. HD: 370.05 "Spec Oprs." (2) Ltr, Act SG to CG HRPE, 14 Nov 42. SG: 705.-1 (HRPE)N.

[48] (1) Diary, Chief Hosp and Evac Br SOS, 2 Nov 42. HD: Wilson files, "Diary." (2) Ltr, Port Surg NYPE to Col H. D. Offutt, 12 Nov 42. SG: 705(NYPE)N. (3) An Rpt, 1942, Halloran Gen Hosp. HD.

[49] (1) Diary, Chief Hosp and Evac Br SOS, 3 Nov 42. HD: Wilson files, "Diary." (2) Ltr, CofT to CGs of PEs, 9 Nov 42, sub: Mil Hosp and Evac. TC: 370.05 (Plans, Policies, Procedures).

[50] Diary, Chief Hosp and Evac Br SOS, 14 Dec 42. HD: Wilson files, "Diary."

[51] Memo SPOPH 701, Chief Hosp and Evac Br SOS for ACofS for Oprs SOS, 27 Dec 42, sub: Availability of Hosp Beds for Port of NY. HD: Wilson files, "Book 2, 26 Sep 42–31 Dec 42."

[52] An Rpts, 1942 and 43, Halloran, Stark, LaGarde, Barnes, Letterman, and Lovell Gen Hosps. HD.

staging area station hospitals into debarkation hospitals.[53]

Designation of General Hospitals for Specialized Treatment

Early in 1943 The Surgeon General initiated a formal program of specialization in general hospitals. During World War I the Medical Department had manned and equipped certain hospitals for the care of particular types of cases.[54] In the interval between wars specialization had continued on a limited scale. By January 1942, for example, deep X-ray therapy had been established as a specialty in the Army and Navy, Fitzsimons, Lawson, Letterman, Walter Reed, and William Beaumont General Hospitals.[55] In March 1942 Darnall General Hospital opened to receive psychotic patients who needed closed ward treatment.[56] Other specialty centers gradually developed at hospitals where eminent specialists were assigned,[57] and toward the end of 1942 The Surgeon General made it known that he intended to formalize and extend existing specialization. Apparently he awaited only the development of circumstances warranting such action.[58]

In the winter of 1942 that development occurred. Beginning in September new general hospitals opened in increasing numbers.[59] It was soon evident that a limited supply of specialists would prohibit the staffing of each one for all kinds of surgical and medical work. Referring to this problem, the surgeon of the Fourth Service Command suggested in January 1943 that certain general hospitals in his area be equipped and manned to give specialized care in different branches of surgery.[60] Simultaneously with the opening of the new general hospitals, a transition from defensive to offensive warfare presaged the arrival of large numbers of combat casualties requiring complicated surgery. Moreover, public insistence upon hospitalization of casualties near their homes grew until The Adjutant General in December 1942 proposed establishment of a policy to conform with the demand.[61] If adopted and applied too rigidly, such a policy would conflict with The Surgeon General's unpublished plan to transfer casualties to hospitals specializing in particular diseases or injuries. He therefore made a counterproposal: patients needing specialized treatment would be sent to general hospitals designated for such, while those requiring prolonged but not specialized treatment would be transferred to hospitals in the vicinity of their homes.[62]

---

[53] See below, p. 192.

[54] *The Medical Department . . . in the World War* (1923), vol. V, pp. 171–73.

[55] SG Ltr 44, 15 May 41, and SG Ltr 1, 2 Jan 42.

[56] An Rpt, 1942, Darnall Gen Hosp. HD.

[57] An example of this development was found in Tilton General Hospital which established a special neurosurgical section during 1942 and was designated a neurosurgical center in March 1943. An Rpts, 1942 and 43, Tilton Gen Hosp. HD.

[58] (1) Memo, SG for Dir Control Div SOS, 1 Aug 42. SG: 020.-1. (2) Memo, Chief Pers Serv SGO for Dir Mil Pers SOS, 2 Dec 42. SG: 323.7-5.

[59]

Month	*Number of General Hospitals Reporting Patients Weekly*
August 1942	15
September 1942	17
October 1942	19
November 1942	22
December 1942	26
January 1943	31

[60] Ltr, CG 4th SvC (Chief Med Br) to SG, 23 Jan 43, sub: Surg Serv, Gen Hosps, with 1st ind, CG SOS (SG) to CG 4th SvC attn Chief Med Br, 8 Feb 43. SG: 323.7-5 (4th SvC)AA.

[61] (1) Draft memo, TAG for CofS SOS, 29 Dec 42, sub: Hosp of Casuals Returned to the US as Battle Casualties. AG: 701(12-29-42)(1). (2) IAS, TAG to SG, 29 Dec 42, same sub. Same file.

[62] (1) 1st memo ind, SG to TAG, 7 Jan 43, on IAS, TAG to SG, 29 Dec 42, sub: Hosp of Casualties. AG: 701(12-29-42)(1). (2) Memo SPOPH 701(1-16-43), ACofS for Oprs SOS for TAG, 19 Jan 43, same sub. Same file.

Approval and publication of this policy on 1 February 1943 [63] required the formal designation of specialty centers. For several weeks afterward The Surgeon General's Hospitalization and Evacuation Division worked on this problem,[64] and on 6 March 1943 the War Department designated nineteen general hospitals for the following specialties: chest surgery, maxillofacial and plastic surgery, ophthalmic surgery and the treatment of the blind, neurosurgery, and the performance of amputations.[65] About two months later, two additional specialties—vascular surgery and the treatment of the deaf—were announced and another general hospital was placed on the list.[66] Further extension of specialization occurred during the later war years.

The Question of Establishing Convalescent Hospitals

During the latter part of 1942 the opinion gained favor both in civilian and military circles that special accommodations for convalescent patients should be provided either as separate hospitals or as annexes to existing hospitals. Among civilians it developed apparently from a desire either to "do something for the boys" or, in some instances, to dispose of large estates with questionable market values.[67] In the Army it arose from the need to save both manpower and hospital beds. The idea was not new, for during World War I the Medical Department had conducted "reconstruction" programs in general hospitals and convalescent centers both in the United States and France.[68] In the latter half of 1942 several widely separated hospitals—the Fort Bliss Station Hospital in Texas, the Jefferson Barracks Station Hospital in Missouri, and the Lovell General Hospital in Massachusetts—established programs to harden patients for return to duty, to reduce the period of their convalescence, and to salvage for full field duty those who might otherwise be either discharged from the Army or placed in the limited service category.[69] In January 1943 the surgeon of the Eighth Service Command recommended the organization of casual detachments to recondition convalescent patients and salvage psychoneurotic soldiers for full duty.[70] The surgeon of the Ninth Service Command proposed the establishment of "overflow installations" to free hospital beds of patients no longer needing hospital care but not yet ready for full military duty.[71] In this connection, General Snyder, a medical officer on the staff of The Inspector General, found in a survey in November 1942 that approximately 67 percent of the patients

[63] WD Cir 34, 1 Feb 43.

[64] (1) Memo, SG for TAG, 24 Feb 43, sub: Cir Ltr 50, Spec Hosps. AG: 705(2-24-43)(1). (2) Ltr, Col Arden Freer, SGO to Col S[anford] W. French, Hq 4th SvC, 8 Feb 43. SG: 323.7-5 (4th SvC)AA.

[65] WD Memo W40-9-43, 6 Mar 43, sub: Gen Hosps for Spec Surg Treatment. AG: 705(2-24-43)(1).

[66] WD Memo W40-14-43, 28 May 43, sub: Gen Hosp, Specialized Treatment. AG: 323.7-5(W40-9-43)(3-6-43).

[67] The Surgeon General received numerous offers. For some of the replies he made, see: (1) Ltr SPMCC, SG to Mr. W. K. Kellogg, 4 Aug 42. (2) Ltr, Act SG to Hon Joseph F. Guffey, US Sen, 20 Nov 42. (3) Ltr, Act SG to Hon Lex Green, H. R., 12 Dec 42. All in HD: 601.-1.

[68] (1) *The Medical Department . . . in the World War* (1927), vol. XIII, pp. 79-222. (2) Charles E. Remy, The History of a Convalescent Camp of the American Expeditionary Forces in France (1942). HD.

[69] An Rpts, 1942, Sta Hosps at Ft Bliss and Jefferson Bks, and Lovell Gen Hosp. HD. Similar action was being taken in the European Theater of Operations at the same time. See Memo, Consultant in Surg ETO to Dir Professional Serv ETO, 28 Sep 42, sub: Rpt on Visit to Med Instls in Northern Ireland. HD: ETO file, "Col Elliott C. Cutler, Rpts Jul 42-Dec 42."

[70] An Rpt, 1942, Chief Med Br 8th SvC. HD.

[71] An Rpt, 1942, Chief Med Br 9th SvC. HD.

in Army hospitals were convalescent and could be cared for in barracks, if necessary, to release hospital beds for patients requiring close medical supervision.[72]

While medical officers in the field were becoming aware of the convalescent problem, it was also receiving attention in Washington. In September 1942 it came up in the hearings of the Wadhams Committee.[73] A month later the Air Forces requested authority "to establish and operate specialized hospital and recuperative centers for individualized treatment, rehabilitation, and classification of Air Forces personnel."[74] The Air Surgeon believed that special hospitals should be established under Air Forces' control to treat and rehabilitate Air Forces patients suffering from such conditions as staleness, anoxia, operational fatigue, aeroneurosis, and aero-embolism.[75] Surgeon General Magee, on the other hand, strongly disapproved the establishment by the Air Forces not only of general hospitals, as discussed earlier, but also of any hospitals other than the station hospitals which they already operated. Moreover, he preferred to carry on reconditioning programs in existing hospitals. He argued that convalescent patients often needed observation and sometimes "active therapeutic management" by doctors fully acquainted with their cases and should therefore not be moved far from hospitals where they received definitive care. He contended furthermore that the establishment of convalescent hospitals would lead to duplication of buildings and a waste of personnel and equipment. Hence, he refused to concur in the Air Forces' proposal, but gave his approval instead to the establishment of nonmedical AAF rest camps. To the Wadhams Committee's recommendation for the establishment of separate convalescent accommodations free of the hospital atmosphere, The Surgeon General replied on 15 December 1942: "It is the opinion of this office that convalescent sections may be more advantageously operated as integral parts of military hospitals. . . ."[76]

Before final action was taken on the Air Forces' request, both the Air Surgeon and The Surgeon General began to initiate reconditioning programs in existing hospitals. In November 1942 the Wadhams Committee recommended this step as well as the establishment of convalescent hospitals.[77] The next month, the commanding general, Army Air Forces, published a directive, prepared by the Air Surgeon, requiring all Air Forces hospitals "to institute recreation and reconditioning programs for convalescent patients."[78] In January 1943 The Surgeon General pro-

[72] Ltr, Asst to IG (Brig Gen Howard McC. Snyder) to IG, 10 Nov 42, sub: Surv of Hosp Fac and their Util. IG: 705-Hosp(A).

[73] Cmtee to Study the MD, 1942, Testimony, pp. 205, 383-84, 441-42, and 460. HD.

[74] Memo, C of Air Staff for CofSA, 7 Oct 42, sub: Specialized Hosp and Recuperative Fac for AAF Pers. AAF: 354.1 "Rest Ctrs and Conv Homes."

[75] (1) Cmtee to Study the MD, 1942, Testimony of Brig Gen David N. W. Grant, pp. 383-84. HD. (2) Brief and Consideration of Non-Concurrence [of SG], Tab B and par IV of Memo, C of Air Staff for CofSA, 7 Oct 42, sub: Specialized Hosp and Recuperative Fac for AAF Pers. AAF: 354.1 "Rest Ctrs and Conv Homes."

[76] (1) Cmtee to Study the MD, 1942, Testimony of Offs of SGO, pp. 163-66, 441-42, 460, HD. (2) Memo SPMCB 701.-1, SG for CG SOS, 13 Oct 42, sub: Specialized Hosp and Recuperative Fac for AAF Pers. AAF: 354.1 "Rest Ctrs and Conv Homes" (1). (3) Extract from 1st ind, SG to CG SOS, 15 Dec 42, on extract from Memo, CG SOS for SG, 26 Nov 42, in Cmtee to Study the MD, 1942-43, Actions on Recomd, Recomd No 24. HD.

[77] Cmtee to Study the MD, 1942-43, Actions on Recomd, Recomd No 14. HD.

[78] (1) AAF Memo 25-9, 14 Dec 42, sub: Recreation and Reconditioning for Conv Pnts in AAF Hosps. AAF: 300.6. (2) Howard A. Rusk, "Convalescence and Rehabilitation," *Doctors at War,* Morris Fishbein, ed. (New York, 1945), pp. 303-04.

posed a War Department circular to require all fixed hospitals, overseas as well as in the United States, to inaugurate reconditioning programs. Fearing that such programs would require additional personnel and construction and doubting its own authority to order their establishment, SOS headquarters delayed publication of this directive until 11 February 1943.[79] Both the Air Forces and War Department directives provided for programs of recreation, graded exercises, and drills; the former, for a program of education as well. Until late 1943 only a few hospitals, among them the station hospitals at Camp Crowder (Missouri), Fort Benning (Georgia), Jefferson Barracks (Missouri), and the O'Reilly General Hospital, developed effective programs.[80]

Meanwhile the Air Forces' persistence in demanding separate convalescent facilities led the General Staff to consider that problem. At first G-4 was reluctant to permit the Air Forces to establish even rest centers, proposing instead that they "farm out" convalescents in civilian resort hotels. G-4 felt that the convalescent problem was one for the future, since the immediate needs of combat zones could be met by the organization of rest camps in theaters and patients returned to the United States either would be ready for sick leaves at home or would need definitive care in general hospitals.[81] Both the Ground and Service Forces agreed with this viewpoint[82] but the Air Surgeon was striving for authority to establish "specialized hospital and recuperative centers."[83] Tending to agree with the Air Forces on the need, G-1 on 16 March 1943 recommended the provision of such facilities not only for the Air Forces but for the Ground and Service Forces as well.[84] Because of conflicting opinions, G-4 called the commanding generals of the Ground, Service, and Air Forces into conference with the General Staff on 7 May 1943.[85] The viewpoint of G-1 prevailed and on 14 June 1943 G-4 directed ASF headquarters to investigate the proposal to establish convalescent facilities, to determine the requirements of the Army as a whole, and to take whatever action appeared desirable.[86]

Two days before this directive was issued Surgeon General Kirk had instructed his Hospital Construction Division to prepare a program for the establishment of convalescent annexes at general hospitals. On

[79] (1) Ltr SPMCB 300.5-1, SG to TAG, 7 Jan 43, sub: WD Cir, with atchd corresp from various offs in SOS. AG: 701(1-7-43)(1). (2) AG Memo W40-6-43, 11 Feb 43, sub: Conv and Reconditioning in Hosps. Same file.

[80] An Rpts, 1942 and 43, Sta Hosps at Jefferson Bks, and 1943-44, Reconditioning Div SGO. HD.

[81] Memo WDGDS 2317, ACofS G-4 WDGS for ACofS G-1 WDGS, 6 Feb 43, sub: Rest and Recuperation of Mil Pers. AAF: 354.1 "Rest Ctrs and Conv Homes."

[82] (1) Memo 720 GNGAP-A, CG AGF for ACofS G-1 WDGS, 25 Feb 43, sub: Rest Cps for AGF Pers. AAF: 354.1 "Rest Ctrs and Conv Homes." (2) DF SPGAM/720/Gen(2-8-43)-16, CG SOS for ACofS G-1 WDGS, 27 Feb 43, sub: Rest and Recuperation of Mil Pers. HRS: G-1/354.7(2-8-43).

[83] (1) Comment No 2, Air Surg to Dir Base Serv AAF, 10 Feb 43, on R&R Sheet, Dir Base Serv AAF to Air Surg, 2 Feb 43, sub: Renaming of Pers Rest Ctr Projects. AAF: 354.1 "Rest Ctrs and Conv Homes." (2) R&R Sheet, Dep C of Air Staff to Air Surg, 18 Feb 43, sub: Specialized Hosp and Recuperative Fac for AAF Pers, with atchd draft Memo, CG AAF for AsstSecWar for Air, 10 Feb 43, and draft Memo, AsstSecWar for Air for SecWar, 15 Feb 43. Same file.

[84] Memo, ACofS G-1 WDGS for CofSA, 24 May 43, sub: Specialized Treatment for Aircraft Combat Crew Pers. HRS: G-1/354.7(2-8-43).

[85] Coleman, *op. cit.*, pp. 384-86, citing Memo, ACofS G-4 WDGS for ACofS G-1, G-3, OPD WDGS, and CGs AGF, AAF, ASF, n d, and Memo WDGAP/354.7(3-8-43), ACofS G-1 WDGS for CofSA, 25 May 43.

[86] Memo WDGDS 4588, ACofS G-4 WDGS for CG ASF, 14 Jun 43, sub: Recuperation Ctrs for Conv Pnts. Filed as incl to ind dated 29 Jul 43. HD: Wilson files, "Day File, Jul 43."

21 June 1943 ASF headquarters approved the program The Surgeon General presented.[87] Neither mentioned separate facilities for the Air Forces, hoping apparently to keep the convalescent care of all patients under their own control. The day before, however, a short-lived memorandum (already discussed) had granted the Air Forces authority to hospitalize combat crew members returned from theaters of operations and to operate whatever general hospitals were necessary for that purpose.[88] As a part of the compromise settlement of this question, it will be recalled, Surgeon General Kirk agreed to the Air Forces' establishment of convalescent centers for the care of both combat crew members suffering solely from operational fatigue and other Air Forces patients whose medical care had been completed in general hospitals, while the Air Surgeon agreed to the continued operation of all general hospitals by the Service Forces. The Air Forces therefore activated eight convalescent centers in the latter half of 1943,[89] while the Service Forces established convalescent annexes at each general hospital. Convalescent hospitals as such were not authorized until the spring of 1944.[90]

[87] (1) Memo, Col John R. Hall for SG, 12 Jun 43. (2) 1st ind SPRMC 322 (18 Jun 43), CG SOS to SG, 22 Jun 43, on unknown basic Ltr. Both in SG: 632.-1.

[88] See above, pp. 107–08.

[89] AAF Memo 20–12, 18 Sep 43.

[90] See below, pp. 188–90.

CHAPTER VII

Minor Changes in Hospital Administration

The outbreak of war and expansion of the hospital system produced few changes of consequence in hospital administration. In fact, as in prewar mobilization planning, greatest attention seemed to be devoted to physical plants, while the internal organization and administration of hospitals remained largely under peacetime policies and procedures. The Surgeon General's Office continued to consider such matters as belonging properly within the province of hospital commanders and concerned itself, as before the war, with attempts to modify administrative procedures outside Army hospitals that affected the length of time patients occupied hospital beds. In some instances it seemed loath to break with the past, opposing altogether or accepting reluctantly suggestions for changes in the organization of hospitals and in the manner in which they were staffed. Although it took constructive steps to eliminate problems involved in supplying and equipping new and expanded hospitals, a shortage of many items continued to plague hospital commanders until early in 1943.

Question of Simplified Organization and Internal Administrative Procedures

The practice of leaving the organization and administration of hospitals largely, within broad limits already established by Army regulations and technical manuals, to the discretion of local hospital commanders continued to result in variations as numerous as the hospitals themselves, both in the number of services supplied and in the relation of such services to one another and to the commanding officer.[1] In some instances hospital commanders took advantage of the freedom permitted them and increased the efficiency of their installations by organizing services not ordinarily found in military hospitals. For example, the Camp Maxey (Texas) and Fort Bliss (Texas) Station Hospitals, adopting a practice of civilian medicine, established diagnostic clinics to expedite the "work-up" of cases and weed out those not requiring immediate hospitalization. The clinic at Camp Maxey, the hospital commander estimated, saved at least 600 hospital admissions during 1942.[2] Other commanding officers showed less initiative, organizing and arranging customary services in numbers and relations which they considered desirable. Thus, in the absence of specific organizational directives and standard administrative proce-

[1] An Rpts, 1942, Sta Hosps at Cps Butner, Maxey, Howze, Cooke, Bowie, and Ft Bliss, and An Rpts, 1943, Sta Hosps at Cps Carson, Beale, Lee, Maxey, and Ft Bliss. HD.

[2] An Rpt, 1942, Sta Hosp at Cp Maxey, and An Rpts, 1942 and 1943, Sta Hosp at Ft Bliss. HD.

dures, efficient organization and smooth functioning depended largely upon the administrative capabilities of hospital commanders and their staffs and upon the supervision and advice they received from higher authorities.[3]

In the fall of 1942 the Wadhams Committee had stated that Army hospital organization and administration needed improvement. It recommended the procurement of trained hospital administrators for assignment to key positions on the staffs of hospital commanders and as consultants to The Surgeon General and service command surgeons. It also recommended that hospital organization be simplified. Citing a hospital in which thirty-three sections or services operated directly under the commanding officer as proof of need for such action, the Committee suggested a "model organization" in which all functions of a hospital would be grouped under the chiefs of three divisions: the Medical, Administrative, and Service Divisions.[4]

The Surgeon General took issue with these recommendations. He expressed doubt that any hospital commander had thirty-three section or division chiefs reporting directly to him and asserted that the hospital organization outlined in Technical Manual 8–260 was the result of many years of medico-military hospital administration and represented the opinion of able officers of the Medical Department. "No advantage would appear to accrue," he stated, "for [from?] any major change at this time." He was equally opposed to the proposal to assign special hospital administrators to key positions in station and general hospitals. "Lay" administrators were used in civilian hospitals, he stated, only because doctors did not have time for administrative duties. He asserted that Medical Corps officers could administer Army hospitals best, since some functions found in civilian hospitals either were lacking in military hospitals or were handled by other Army agencies, such as the Corps of Engineers. He admitted that specialists in hospital administration were useful in some positions, pointing out that approximately one hundred had already been commissioned in the Medical Administrative Corps for administrative work in hospitals. As to the assignment of hospital administrators to his own Office or to those of service command surgeons, he made no comment.[5]

Later, after the commanding general, Services of Supply, directed him to take immediate action on the Committee's recommendation, The Surgeon General modified his position. On 16 January 1943 he informed General Somervell that he was negotiating with Dr. Basil C. MacLean, Superintendent of Strong Memorial Hospital, Rochester, N. Y., regarding a commission and assignment to his Office to make a comprehensive survey of military hospital organization and administration and to advise him on the procurement and assignment of additional hospital administrators from civilian life.[6] Dr. MacLean was unable to accept a commission immediately, but on 23 April 1943 he was made a lieutenant colonel and assigned to The Surgeon General's Hospitalization and Evacuation Division.

---

[3] See An Rpt, 1942, Chief Med Br 8th SvC. HD.

[4] (1) Cmtee to Study the MD, 1942, Rpt, HD. (2) Extract from Memo, CG SOS for SG, 26 Nov 42, in Cmtee to study the MD, 1942–43, Actions on Recomd, Recomd Nos 26 and 27. HD.

[5] Extract from 1st ind, SG to CG SOS, 15 Dec 42, in Cmtee to Study the MD, 1942–43, Actions on Recomd, Recomd No 27. HD.

[6] Extracts from 3d ind, SG to CG SOS, 16 Jan 43, in Cmtee to Study the MD, 1942–43, Actions on Recomd, Recomd Nos 26 and 27. HD.

The Surgeon General's reaction to another of the Wadhams Committee's recommendations further exemplified his reluctance to interfere with the internal administration of hospitals. Finding that some diagnostic procedures which required only forty-eight hours in civilian hospitals sometimes took as much as ten days in Army hospitals, the Committee recommended that "a centralized system of control of the length of patients' stay be instituted to record currently the length of stay by major professional classifications for each hospital, to study the causes of abnormal occupancy, and to institute action to correct undesirable conditions."[7] Such a system was already operating effectively in the Second Service Command and The Surgeon General agreed that information on the time patients stayed in hospitals would be "highly desirable from a statistical point of view." Nevertheless, he believed it "impracticable" to establish such a system for all Army hospitals because of the paper work involved, and indicated that he preferred to depend upon professional consultants "inquiring into unnecessarily long periods of hospitalization with a view to corrective action."[8] To supplement their efforts The Surgeon General issued a circular letter on 9 November 1942, urging hospital commanders to prevent the padding of records by "repetition, verbosity, and inclusion of extraneous historical material and forms" and to reduce "irrelevant, routine, and repetitive requests" for laboratory examinations.[9]

Certain changes in the organization of general hospitals did occur as a result of their transfer from control of The Surgeon General to that of service commands in the fall of 1942. Since few were located on Army posts, most had post as well as hospital functions, and their commanding officers were both post and hospital commanders. Duties of such officers as post commanders were relatively unimportant compared with their duties as hospital commanders, for post functions of a general hospital existed only to serve the hospital. Nevertheless, after general hospitals became service command installations the organization of their post function was expected to conform with the standard post organization outlined in the SOS Organization Manual, 30 September 1942. It grouped post activities functionally in seven divisions: Administrative, Personnel, Operations and Training, Supply, Repairs and Utilities, Internal Security and Intelligence, and Medical. The result was that relatively minor post functions, previously organized as administrative sections or services, were raised to division status, equal on paper at least to the Medical Division. The latter usually comprised all hospital functions, administrative—such as medical supply, the registrar's office, and the enlisted complement—as well as professional. The commanding officer's double role meant that while only some seven division chiefs reported to him directly as post commander, in most instances the original number of section or branch chiefs of the Medical Division also reported to him directly as chief of that

[7] (1) Extract from Memo, CG SOS for SG, 26 Nov 42, in Cmtee to Study the MD, 1942–43, Actions on Recomd, Recomd No 25. HD. (2) Cmtee to Study the MD, Rpt, pp. 5, 7, 10, 13. HD.

[8] (1) Extract from 1st ind, SG to CG SOS, 15 Dec 42, on extract from Memo, CG SOS for SG, 26 Nov 42, in Cmtee to Study the MD, 1942–43, Actions on Recomd, Recomd No 25. HD. (2) History, Office of the Surgeon, Second Corps Area and Second Service Command from 9 September 1940 to 2 September 1945, pp. 8 and 102. HD.

[9] SG Ltr 148, 9 Nov 42, sub: Hosp Admin and Professional Servs.

division—that is, as commander of the hospital.[10] *(Chart 6)*

Efforts To Shorten the Average Period of Hospitalization

As the number of hospitals increased and the patient load became heavier, the Surgeon General's Office along with other agencies of the War Department devoted attention to administrative procedures outside Army hospitals which affected the occupancy of hospital beds. For the most part such procedures were those that governed the disposition of patients after completion of treatment—either by return to duty or separation from the Army—and were hence essentially personnel procedures.

Attempts To Speed the Disposition of Officer-Patients

Two problems arose during the early war years in the disposition of officer-patients after hospitalization. The first resulted from keeping on active duty, rather than retiring, officers qualified for limited service only; the other, from loss of touch with units and organizations to which officers qualified for full duty should return.[11]

The procedure for the assignment of officers qualified for limited service only, in effect in January 1942, required hospital commanders to hold officers after completion of treatment while reports of their cases were sent through military channels to The Adjutant General in Washington for instructions on assignments.[12] On 21 March 1942 a revision of this procedure cut out some of the correspondence and time involved by permitting post and corps area commanders to assign all limited service officers except those under the jurisdiction of the Army Air Forces. The latter still had to be reported to the commanding general, Army Air Forces, for assignment.[13]

The normal procedure for returning general service officers to their "proper" stations also needed modification. In many cases organizations to which they belonged either had left for overseas service or had moved to some other location in the United States, without informing the hospital or officer concerned. New assignments had to be made in such cases. On 6 October 1942 the War Department issued instructions permitting corps area commanders to make assignments of all officers in this category except those belonging to the Air Forces. The latter, like AAF limited service officers, could be assigned only by the commanding general, Army Air Forces.[14] These changes reduced but did not eliminate entirely difficulties of hospital commanders in procuring assignments for officer-patients.[15]

A further revision of directives governing the disposition of officers was issued the last day of 1942. It tended to expedite the process. Under the new procedure, all officers needing hospitalization who belonged to troop units in the United States,

[10] (1) SOS Orgn Manual, 1942, sec 402.02 and 406.01. HD. (2) Rpt, Conf of CGs SvCs [SOS], 2d sess, 17 Dec 42, p. 41. HD: 337. (3) An Rpts of the following Gen Hosps: Hoff, Baxter, Billings, Tilton (1942), and Ashburn, Baxter, Percy Jones, Kennedy, and Hoff (1943). HD.

[11] (1) Ltr, TAG to CGs Armies, Army Corps, Divs, CAs, and Depts; CofS GHQ; C of Arms and Servs; CG AF Combat Comd; C of Armored Force; COs of Exempted Stas, 21 Jan 42, sub: Physical Fitness of Offs. AG: 201.6 (1-17-42)(3). (2) AR 40-600, par 5 *a*, 31 Dec 34. (3) WD Cir 24, sec III, 27 Jan 42.

[12] (1) AR 40-600, par 5 *a*, 31 Dec 34. (2) WD Cir 24, sec III, 27 Jan 42.

[13] WD Cir 83, 21 Mar 42.

[14] AR 40-600, par 5 *a*, 6 Oct 42.

[15] For example, see An Rpt, 1942, Tilton Gen Hosp. HD.

CHART 6—ORGANIZATION OF BAXTER GENERAL HOSPITAL COMPARED WITH STANDARD PLAN FOR SOS POST ORGANIZATION, 1942–43

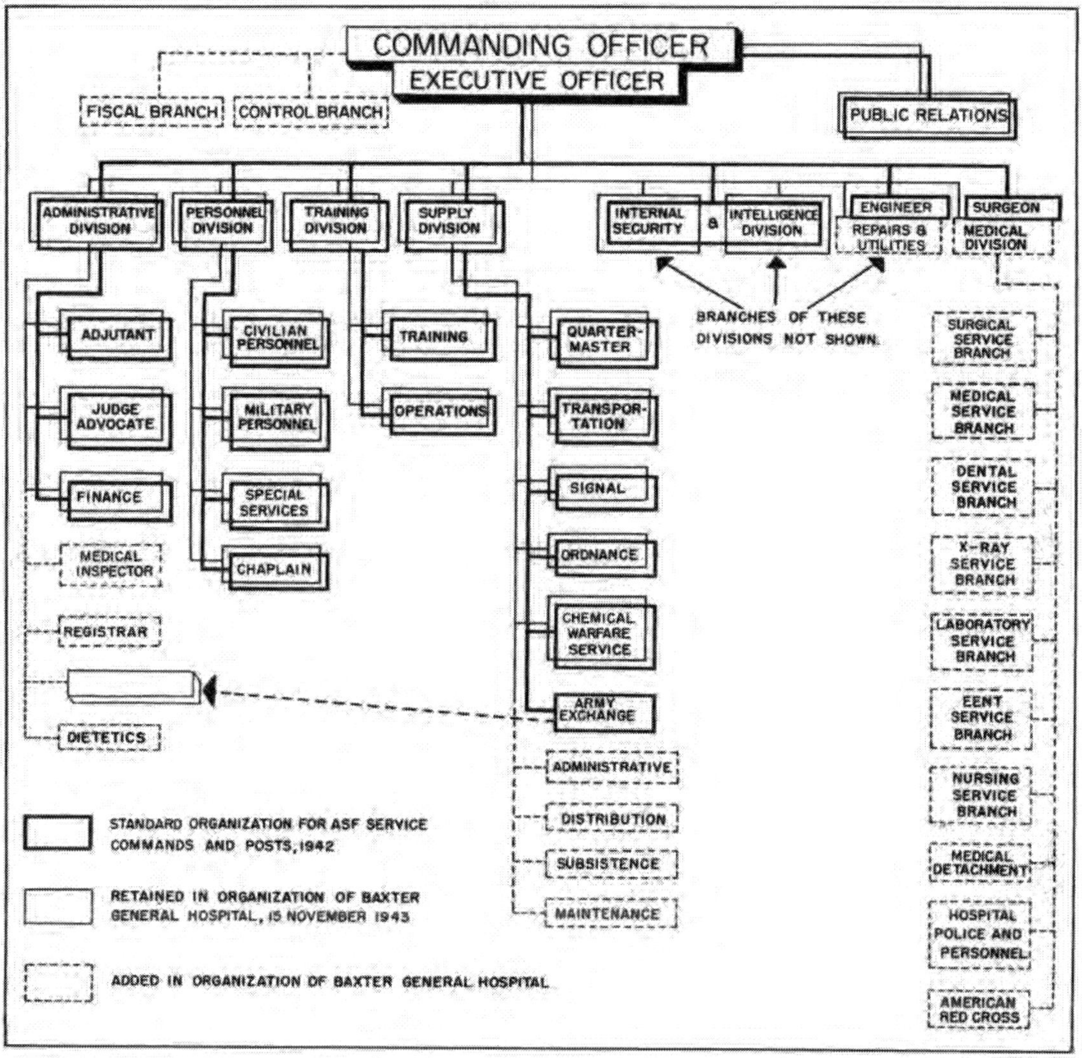

who had returned from theaters, or who were en route to overseas destinations, were transferred at the time they entered general hospitals to replacement pools of their respective arms and services. Upon completion of hospital treatment, whether qualified for general or limited service, they could be returned to pools to await permanent reassignment. Other officers, for example those of station complements, were not assigned to such pools and had to be returned to their proper stations. In either case, hospitals might dispose of patients as soon as their medical treatment had been completed, without waiting for higher headquarters to make assignments.[16] Nevertheless, some hospital commanders continued to hold officer-patients until higher headquarters had acted upon the recommendations of hospital disposition boards.[17]

Attempts To Speed the Disposition of Enlisted Men

Delays in the disposition of enlisted men, both those being discharged from the Army on certificates of disability and those being returned to duty for limited service, also caused the Medical Department concern. As in the case of officers, such delays resulted in part from administrative actions required of headquarters outside hospitals. Attempts were made to remove this cause of delay during the early war years. Later, emphasis was to be placed upon simplifying procedures within the hospitals themselves.

Failure to receive service records and allied papers, such as individual clothing and equipment records, of enlisted patients transferred to general hospitals was one cause of delay. Without such records hospitals could not release men entitled to discharge from the Army. As early as December 1941 some hospitals complained about this situation.[18] To correct it The Surgeon General secured the issuance of a War Department letter requiring "the immediate transfer of such papers to a general hospital when a member of the command is transferred thereto." [19] This of course did not solve the problem of patients whose records had been lost or destroyed. Several officers, including the commanding general of Lovell General Hospital, the director of training of the Services of Supply, the finance officer of the New York Port of Embarkation, and representatives of the Surgeon General's Office, became interested in it almost simultaneously.[20] On 6 June 1942, therefore, the War Department published a directive permitting hospital personnel officers to prepare payrolls, final pay statements, and new service records on the basis of affidavits of men whose records had been lost in disasters either at sea or on land.[21] Within a month, both SOS headquarters and the Chief of Finance decided that this policy should be broadened to include all lost records, whether or not they had disappeared as a result of military action.[22] This was done by a new War Department directive published on 24 July 1942.[23] Its provisions helped to speed

[16] WD Cir 424, 31 Dec 42.

[17] (1) An Rpts, 1943, Tilton, LaGarde, Ashburn, and O'Reilly Gen Hosps. HD. (2) Memo, Lt Col Basil C. MacLean, MC for [Brig] Gen [Raymond W.] Bliss thru Col [Albert H.] Schwichtenberg, 6 Nov 43, sub: Observations Based on Recent Visits of Varying Periods to 9 Gen Hosps. SG: Gen Bliss's Off files, "Util of MCs in ZI" (19) #1. In this letter, Colonel MacLean stated: "The wastage in days and dollars is scandalous and can be attributed directly to the stupidities of a cumbersome and complex procedure which is not easily adaptable to a war time load."

[18] (1) Statement of CO Lawson Gen Hosp, Agenda of SGO Conf with COs Gen Hosps, 15 Dec 41. HD: 337.-1. (2) Inf memo, SG for TAG [Dec 41], sub: Trf of Pnts. AG: 201.3 (1-23-42)(8).

[19] Ltr, TAG to CGs Armies, Army Corps, *et al.*, 29 Jan 42, sub: Delay in Trf of S/R. AG: 201.3 (1-23-42)(8).

[20] (1) Ltr, CG Lovell Gen Hosp to TAG, 21 May 42, sub: Lost S/R. HRS: G-1/10381. (2) Memo SPTRU 333.1 (5-12-42), Dep Dir Tng SOS for Dir MPD SOS, 12 May 42; sub: EM. Same file.

[21] (1) 2d ind, CofF to TAG, 2 Jun 42, on Ltr, Fin Off, Brooklyn, NY to CofF, thru Fin Off 2d CA, 24 May 42, sub: Pay of EM without S/R. AG: 240 (5-24-42)(1). (2) WD Cir 177, sec I, 6 Jun 42.

[22] (1) Memo, CG SOS for CofSA, 27 Jul 42, sub: Prompt Discharge of EM on CDD from Gen Hosp. HRS: G-1/10381. (2) Memo SPFDR 300.3/360354 (WD Cir), CofF for C of Admin Servs SOS, 21 Jul 42, sub: Proposed WD Cir. AG: 240 (1-3-42)(1).

[23] WD Cir 244, 24 Jul 42.

the discharge of enlisted men on certificates of disability by making it unnecessary to hold patients in hospitals while missing records were located or until new ones were issued by The Adjutant General.[24]

At station hospitals a serious cause for delay in discharging patients for disability was that officials outside hospitals had both to initiate and to consummate the action. Under existing regulations an enlisted man's immediate commanding officer had to initiate the certificate required for this purpose (WD AGO Form 40), and an authority higher than the station hospital commander, either the post commander or the service commander, had to approve the certificate and the recommendations of the medical board who examined the man.[25] When members of the Wadhams Committee visited Army hospitals in the fall of 1942, they found that complaints on this score were general.[26] The Committee recommended that authority to approve disability discharges be vested in all commanders of camps having a strength of 20,000 or more.[27] About the same time, General Snyder found in a survey which he was making that approximately 12 percent of all patients were awaiting disability discharges. To free beds for other patients, he recommended that measures be taken to require organization commanders to initiate disability certificates promptly and to permit commanders of all posts having a strength of 5,000 or more to approve disability discharges.[28] Accordingly, The Surgeon General prepared a memorandum, published by the War Department on 30 November 1942, requiring "all concerned" to insure prompt action by unit commanders in initiating disability certificates. In December he also secured a modification of Army regulations to permit commanders of all stations with housing capacities of 5,000 or more to grant disability discharges.[29] These actions, particularly the latter, simplified the disposition of such patients and in at least one hospital reduced the average period of their stay by almost two thirds, from fifty-eight to twenty-one days.[30] Causes for delay still existed for papers still had to be transmitted between unit and hospital commanders and between hospital and post commanders.

Early in 1943 G-1 directed SOS to make a study of War Department regulations governing disability discharges "with a view to their clarification and the speedy consummation of discharges under this authority."[31] The revision of regulations which SOS headquarters subsequently proposed seemed to The Surgeon General

[24] (1) Ltr, CO Tilton Gen Hosp to TAG, 31 Jul 42, sub: Discharge of EM, with 1st ind, TAG to CG Tilton Gen Hosp, 25 Aug 42. AG: 220.8 (8-1-34)(1). (2) An Rpts, 1942, Torney Gen Hosp, and 1943, LaGarde Gen Hosp. HD.

[25] AR 615-360, sec II, par 5, 8, 9, 11, 14, and 16, 4 Apr 35 and 26 Nov 42.

[26] (1) Memo by Dr J. H. Musser, n d, sub: Visit to Louisiana Hosp Instls. Pers files of Dr Lewis H. Weed, Mem of the Wadhams Cmtee. (2) Memo by Dr Arthur H. Ruggles, n d, sub: Visit with Mr. James Hamilton to Cp Devens, Mass. Same file.

[27] (1) Extract from Memo, CG SOS for SG, 26 Nov 42, in Cmtee to Study the MD, 1942-43, Actions on Recomd, Recomd No 12. HD. (2) Cmtee to Study the MD, 1942, Rpt, p. 5. HD.

[28] Ltr, Asst IG to IG, 10 Nov 42, sub: Surv of Hosp Fac and their Util. IG: 705-Hosp (A).

[29] (1) 3d ind, SG to CG SOS, 24 Nov 42, on Ltr, Asst IG to IG, 10 Nov 42, sub: Surv of Hosp Fac and their Util. IG: 705-Hosp (A). (2) WD Memo W40-9-42, 30 Nov 42, sub: Delays in Processing WD AGO Form 40. Same file. (3) WD Cir 404, sec III, 14 Dec 42.

[30] An Rpts, 1942, Sta Hosp at Sheppard Fld, and Surg 7th SvC. HD.

[31] Memo, ACofS G-1 WDGS for Dir MPD SOS, 9 Feb 43, sub: Discharge of EM on CDD. AG:220.8 (2 Jun 42)(2) Sec 1.

likely to retard rather than to speed discharges. He therefore requested a conference of representatives of his own Office and of The Adjutant General, The Judge Advocate General, the commanding general of Services of Supply, and the Veterans Administration, to consider the entire question.[32] As a result a revision was worked out which eliminated some channels of communication and placed time limits upon the transfer of papers required for disability discharges.[33]

Under the new procedure, published on 16 April 1943, patients were to be transferred (on paper) from their own units to the station complement of the post on which the hospital treating them was located within forty-eight hours after hospitals decided to discharge them. Thus, all steps leading up to discharges for disability were to be under the control of post commanders, independent of any action by unit commanders. Station complement commanders were required to forward disability certificates to station hospitals within twenty-four hours after they were requested, and hospital commanders had to forward all papers, with recommendations, to post commanders within forty-eight hours after action by medical boards examining patients. In addition, discharge of patients was not to be delayed until all records of previous medical examinations had been received. Furthermore, hospital commanders were charged with the responsibility, under post commanders, for processing all records within the time limits allowed.[34]

Under the revised regulation the amount of time needed to process the papers required for disability discharges was reduced appreciably. In the station hospital at Camp Chaffee (Arkansas) for example, the time was cut from approximately eighteen to five days.[35] Here, as in other instances, the post commander eliminated even the transmission of records from station complement headquarters to hospitals and from hospitals to post headquarters. He accomplished this by placing detachments to which patients were transferred to await discharge under the command of members of the hospital staff and by permitting hospital commanders to exercise the authority of post commanders to approve disability discharges. In this way, the entire process of granting discharges on certificates of disability was centralized under station hospital commanders.[36] Such was already the case in general hospitals, because enlisted men treated in them belonged to detachments of patients, rather than to the units to which they had been assigned previously, and general hospital commanders had had authority since September 1941 to grant discharges on certificates of disability. Further simplification of procedures within hospitals themselves remained to be done during the later war years.

The disposition of psychotic patients involved problems not ordinarily encountered in other disability discharges. Until the spring of 1943 patients who became mentally deranged within six months after induction and required institutional care after discharge from the Army had to be

[32] Memo SPMCH 300.3-1, SG for TAG, 7 Mar 43. AG: 220.8 (2 Jun 42)(2) Sec I.

[33] Memo, CG SOS for ACofS G-1 WDGS, 17 Mar 43, sub: Discharge of EM on CDD. AG:220.8 (2 Jun 42)(2) Sec I.

[34] AR 615-360, C 4, 16 Apr 43.

[35] An Rpt, 1943, Sta Hosp at Cp Chaffee. HD.

[36] (1) Comments of Surg, 1st, 2d, and 7th SvCs, Rpt, SGs Conf with Chiefs Med Br SvCs, 14-17 Jun 43, pp. 56-58. HD: 337. (2) An Rpts, 1943, Sta Hosps at Cp Chaffee, and Fts Custer, Bragg, and Riley. HD.

sent to State mental institutions or to St. Elizabeth's Hospital in Washington, D. C. Only patients with more than six months' service were "line-of-duty" cases and therefore eligible for care by the Veterans Administration. To arrange for State care of mental patients frequently required several weeks or else turned out to be impossible altogether.[37] To relieve other hospitals of the accumulation of such patients awaiting discharge, The Surgeon General opened Darnall General Hospital on 1 March 1942, established additional closed ward facilities at Valley Forge and Bushnell (Utah) General Hospitals in the fall of 1942, and on 12 June 1943 activated Mason General Hospital in buildings acquired from the State of New York.[38] In March 1943 Congress authorized the Veterans Administration to care for patients regardless of their "line-of-duty" status.[39] Thereafter, Army hospitals encountered less difficulty in disposing of psychotic patients, since they could transfer any of them to the Veterans Administration.

More than a year before this Congress had taken action which might have resulted in delaying the disposition of patients. On 12 December 1941 Congress authorized the Army to retain in its hospitals, rather than transfer to the Veterans Administration, patients whose terms of service had expired but who needed continuing hospitalization.[40] The extension of all terms of service, on the following day, for "the duration plus six months," reduced the importance of this authorization considerably.[41] The question remained of how long the Army would keep patients who could not be returned eventually to active duty.

Wishing to free as many beds as possible, The Surgeon General appealed to a policy which the Federal Board of Hospitalization had established in 1940: the early transfer to the Veterans Administration of patients who could not be salvaged for further service.[42] The Wadhams Committee, on the other hand, responsive perhaps to a feeling among the public that the Army should do everything possible for its sick and wounded men, recommended that the Army keep all patients, except those who were neuropsychiatric, until they had received maximum therapeutic benefits.[43] This might have proved embarrassing for The Surgeon General had not the Federal Board ruled, in February 1943, that under its 1940 resolution the decision as to when patients should be transferred to the Veterans Administration rested with The Surgeon General.[44] This ruling left him free either to transfer patients as soon as it was determined that they could not be returned to duty, thus saving beds for other Army patients, or to keep them for extended periods of Army hospitalization as increasing emphasis

[37] (1) SG Ltrs 99, 4 Sep 42; 1, 1 Jan 43; and 6, 2 Jan 43. (2) An Rpts, 1942, Darnall, Stark, and Tilton Gen Hosps, and Sta Hosp at Cp Roberts. HD.

[38] An Rpts, Hosps named above, 1942 and 1943. HD. (2) Rpt, SGs Conf with CA and Army Surgs, 25–28 May 42. HD: 337. (3) Memo, Col H. D. Offutt for Col J. R. Hall, 22 Sep 42. SG: 632.-2. (4) Extract from 1st ind, SG to CG SOS, 15 Dec 42, on extract from Memo, CG SOS for SG, 26 Nov 42, in Cmtee to Study the MD, 1942–43, Actions on Recomd, Recomd No. 22. HD.

[39] (1) Public Law 10, 78th Cong, 17 Mar 43, 57 Stat 10. (2) AR 615-360, C 4, 16 Apr 43.

[40] (1) Public Law 333, 77th Cong., 12 Dec 41, 55 Stat 333. (2) Ltr, Franklin D. Roosevelt to SecWar, 12 Dec 41. AG: 322.8 (9–1–34) Case 1.

[41] Public Law 338, 13 Dec 41, 55 Stat 338.

[42] 2d ind, SG to TAG, 19 Mar 42, on Ltr 220.811–1, SG to TAG, 31 Jan 42, sub: Policy Conc Discharge of Disabled EM. AG: 200.8 (8–1–34) Case 1.

[43] Cmtee to Study the MD, 1942, Rpt, p. 12. HD.

[44] Ltr, Chm Fed Board of Hosp to SG, 4 Feb 43, in Cmtee to Study the MD, 1942–43, Actions on Recomd, Recomd No 29. HD.

came to be placed on Army reconditioning and rehabilitation during the later war years.

Delays in the disposition of enlisted patients occurred also, as in the case of officers, when their organizations had moved to undisclosed destinations or when men were physically fit for only limited service at the end of treatment. Such patients were found less in station than in general hospitals, since the latter treated those who had the more serious illnesses or injuries and required longer periods of medical care. Both the men whose organizations had moved and those qualified for only limited service required new assignments. To prevent their being held in hospitals awaiting assignment by higher headquarters, meanwhile occupying beds needed for other patients, The Surgeon General's Hospitalization Division recommended on 22 January 1942 that casual detachments be set up near all general hospitals for the immediate assignment, on a temporary basis, of all enlisted patients whose hospitalization had been completed.[45] Instead of approving this recommendation, the Secretary of War, on the advice of the General Staff, directed that Air Corps (after March 1942, Air Forces) enlisted patients be reassigned by the chief of the Air Corps; others, by corps area commanders.[46] Two days later, after Colonel Offutt protested that this failed to solve the problem, the War Department suggested that corps area commanders furnish hospitals with blocks of available assignments or that they designate stations to which enlisted men might be sent temporarily, pending permanent assignments.[47] This procedure worked well in some corps areas. In others, where corps area commanders failed to establish casual detachments under such "permissive regulation," it was less successful in enabling hospitals to speed the disposition of patients.[48]

Other Efforts To Shorten the Period of Hospitalization

The speed-up of dispositions was not the only way by which beds could be saved for patients who really needed them. The same result could be accomplished by limiting the treatment given in hospitals. During the winter of 1942–43 The Surgeon General instituted measures of that type. Among them were the treatment of patients with uncomplicated cases of gonorrhea on a duty status and the curtailment of elective operations.

Although the majority of patients with gonorrhea in civilian life were treated on an out-patient basis, the Army had customarily hospitalized soldiers with that disease.[49] In the fall of 1942 such patients often remained in hospitals for more than a month and, according to General Snyder, occupied approximately 6,000 beds. During 1942, some posts in the Fourth Service Command had begun to use sulfonamide compounds to treat patients with gonorrhea on a duty status, thus avoiding long periods of hospitalization. On 10 November 1942 General Snyder recommended the immediate considera-

[45] Ltr, SG to TAG, 22 Jan 42, sub: Disposition of Pnts. SG: 705.-1.

[46] (1) 1st ind AG 220.31 (1-22-42)EA, TAG to SG, 30 Jan 42, on Ltr, SG to TAG, 22 Jan 42, sub: Disposition of Pnts. SG: 705.-1. (2) WD Cir 24, 27 Jan 42.

[47] Ltr, TAG to CGs of all CAs, 29 Jan 42, sub: Disposition of Pnts in Gen Hosps. AG: 322.3 Gen Hosp (1-28-42)(1).

[48] (1) Ltr, Col Harry D. Offutt to Col W. H. Smith, 9 Mar 42. SG: 323.7-5 (LaGarde GH)K. (2) Rpt, SGs Conf with CA and Army Surgs, 25-28 May 42, p. 2. HD: 337.

[49] Paul Padgett, The Diagnosis and Treatment of the Venereal Diseases (1948). HD.

tion of standardizing this practice throughout the Army.[50] The Surgeon General then requested the appointment of a board of medical officers to review accumulated experience to determine the wisdom of extending on-duty treatment of gonorrhea patients.[51] By January 1943 the board had completed its work. It recommended that the policy of treating patients with uncomplicated cases of gonorrhea on a duty status be encouraged, but not required.[52] Adoption of this policy reduced the number of patients in hospitals and thereby lessened both construction and personnel requirements.[53]

At the same time, to achieve the same end, General Snyder also recommended the curtailment of elective operations, such as the repair of hernias, the removal of pilonidal cysts, and the correction of internal derangements of knee joints and other preinduction disabilities.[54] In conformity with this recommendation, The Surgeon General directed hospitals to consider for elective operations only men who might be of definite value to the Army afterwards.[55] Although this directive did not require a curtailing of elective operations, some hospitals reduced the number performed.[56] Later during 1943, when the manpower shortage demanded maximum use of available men, it was necessary to relax this policy.[57]

Early Changes in the Size and Composition of Hospital Staffs

With the war making increasingly heavy demands upon the Nation's available manpower, zone of interior hospitals faced the prospect of having to function with staffs that had progressively lower proportions of Medical Corps officers and able-bodied enlisted men. Although reductions were carried to greater lengths during the latter part of the war, they started during its early years and the practice of replacing physicians and able-bodied enlisted men by personnel in other categories began at that time.

Throughout 1942 the personnel guide that had been issued in April 1941 remained effective for station hospitals, and the Surgeon General's Office instructed general hospitals to use tables of organization of corresponding numbered units as their guide.[58] During the year, his Office not only revised such tables but in December presented for Staff approval new guides for manning both station and general hospitals in the zone of interior.[59] Made partly at the instance of the General Staff as a means of reducing the Army's requirements for physicians,[60]

[50] Ltr, Asst IG to IG, 10 Nov 42, sub: Surv of Hosp Fac and their Util. IG: 705-Hosp (A).

[51] (1) 3d ind, SG to CG SOS, 24 Nov 42, on Ltr, Asst IG to IG, 10 Nov 42, sub: Surv of Hosp Fac and their Util. IG: 705-Hosp (A). (2) Ltr, SG to CG SOS, 19 Nov 42, sub: Apmt of Bd for Investigation of Treatment of VD on Duty Status. Same file.

[52] WD AGO Memo W40-2-43, 19 Jan 43, sub: Treatment of Individuals with Uncomplicated Gonorrhea on a Duty Status. HD: 726.1-1.

[53] An Rpts, 1942, Sta Hosps at Cp Butner and Ft Bragg. HD.

[54] Ltr, Asst IG to IG, 10 Nov 42, sub: Surv of Hosp Fac and their Util. IG: 705-Hosp (A).

[55] SG Ltr 167, 30 Nov 42, sub: Performance of Elective Oprs for Pre-Induction Disabilities.

[56] An Rpts, 1943, Fletcher Gen Hosp and Sta Hosp at Cp Chaffee. HD.

[57] SG Ltr 190, 17 Nov 43, sub: Sel of Cases for Elective Opr for Pre-Induction Disability.

[58] Ltr, Col H. D. Offutt to Col E. R. Gentry, Borden Gen Hosp, 4 Nov 42. SG: 323.7-5 (Borden GH)K.

[59] Incl 1, Annexes A and B, to Memo, Act SG for DepCofS WDGS thru Mil Pers Div SOS, 14 Dec 42, sub: Availability of Physicians. SG: 322.051-1.

[60] Memo, ACofS G-1 WDGS for SG thru Pers Div SOS, 1 Apr 42, sub: Availability of Physicians. HRS: G-1/16331-16335. For a full treatment of the question of the Army's requirements and the availability of physicians, see John H. McMinn and Max Levin, Personnel (MS for companion vol. in Medical Dept. series), HD.

TABLE 4—POSITIONS AND RANKS IN ZONE OF INTERIOR HOSPITALS PERMITTED BUT NOT REQUIRED TO BE FILLED BY MEDICAL ADMINISTRATIVE CORPS OFFICERS, 9 APRIL 1941

Size of Hospital	Adjutant	Medical Supply Officer	CO Enlisted Detachment	Mess Officer	Assistant Registrar [a]	Assistant Adjutant	Assistant Medical Supply Officer	Assistant CO Enlisted Detachment	Assistant Mess Officer
50 & 75 Beds	....	2d Lt	....	....	....	....	....	....	....
100, 150, & 200 Beds	1st Lt	2d Lt	1st Lt	....	....	....	....	....	....
250, 300, 350, & 400 Beds	1st Lt	1st Lt	1st Lt	Capt	....	....	....	....	....
450 Beds	1st Lt	Capt	1st Lt	Capt	....	....	....	....	....
500, 600, & 700 Beds	Capt	Capt	Capt	Capt	....	2d Lt	....	....	2d Lt
750, 800, & 900 Beds	Capt	Capt	Capt	Capt	....	2d Lt	....	1st Lt	2d Lt
1,000 Beds	Capt	Capt	Capt	([b])	....	2d Lt	....	1st Lt	2d Lt
1,500 & 2,000 Beds	Capt	Capt	Capt	([b])	1st Lt	2d Lt	2d Lt	1st Lt	2d Lt

[a] The registrar was required in all hospitals to be a Medical Corps officer.
[b] The mess officer of hospitals with 1,000 or more beds was required to be a Major, Medical Corps.

Source: Guide for Determination of Medical Department Personnel, C 1, MR 4–2, Hospitals, 9 April 1941.

these changes were expected to lower the number of Medical Corps officers authorized for hospitals of various sizes and to increase the use of Medical Administrative Corps officers in administrative positions.

Throughout 1942 allowances of Medical Corps officers for zone of interior hospitals were considerably higher than those later prescribed in the guides. For example, on 21 October 1942 the Surgeon General's Office informed the commander of a 1,500-bed general hospital that his allotment should consist of eighty officers of the Medical Corps, ten of the Medical Administrative Corps, and additional members of other corps.[61] An allotment based on the revised table of organization for numbered general hospitals would have had 23 fewer Medical Corps officers, and one based on the December 1942 guide for named hospitals would have had 34 fewer Medical Corps officers and 13 more Medical Administrative Corps officers. High allotments were somewhat offset by the fact that in most cases the number of Medical Corps officers actually assigned failed to equal the allowance. Hospital commanders therefore complained of shortages, but their complaints seem to have been based on this discrepancy alone and not on a consideration of all their resources. In addition to assigned physicians, many hospital commanders had at their disposal medical officers of units attached for training as well as those awaiting assignment in Medical Department pools. Moreover, later in the war hospitals had to get along with even fewer assigned Medical Corps officers, and as commanders continued to assert that their hospitals provided a high standard of medical care their complaints of shortages of physicians during this period should be taken at something less than face value.[62]

[61] Ltr, Lt Col Paul A. Paden to Brig Gen R[oyal] Reynolds, Kennedy Gen Hosp, 21 Oct 42. SG: 323.7-5 (Kennedy GH)K.

[62] (1) An Rpts, 1942, Chiefs Med Br SvCs, 1st–9th SvCs. HD. (2) An Rpts, 1942, Lovell, Hoff, Billings, Kennedy, and Ashburn Gen Hosps, and Sta Hosps at Fts Benning and Belvoir, and Cps Adair, Lee, Blanding, and Chaffee. HD.

Replacement of physicians in administrative jobs by Medical Administrative Corps officers began in 1942. At the beginning of the war the personnel guide for named hospitals permitted but did not require the use of Medical Administrative Corps officers in certain positions. *(Table 4)* At that time the Surgeon General's Office apparently considered them primarily as assistants to Medical Corps officers in the more responsible administrative positions.[63] Early in 1942, therefore, physicians, sometimes with Medical Administrative Corps assistants, held such positions as executive officer, registrar, adjutant, mess officer, medical detachment commander, and medical supply officer in many hospitals in the zone of interior. In compliance with General Staff and SOS directives,[64] The Surgeon General made plans during 1942 to use Medical Administrative Corps officers more widely. First he proposed to increase the supply by opening a second Medical Administrative Corps officer candidate school.[65] Then in June he requested certain hospital commanders to make studies of the positions which administrative officers could fill.[66] Before such studies could be completed, a War Department directive, issued on the recommendation of SOS headquarters, ordered the commanding generals of the Air and Ground Forces and of corps areas to relieve Medical Corps officers of all duties not requiring professional medical training and to replace them with Medical Administrative Corps or Branch Immaterial officers.[67] This action left to individual commanders the decision as to which positions were suitable for administrative officers. Generally they were considered to be those of detachment commander, medical supply officer, adjutant, and registrar.[68] By the end of 1942 service commands reported that administrative officers had replaced physicians in administrative positions to the extent which supply of the former permitted.[69] The qualifying phrase was important, for a shortage of Medical Administrative Corps officers for use in the zone of interior existed throughout 1942 [70] and their widespread substitu-

[63] (1) Ltr, Act SG to the Hon D. Lane Powers, Mem of Cong, 29 Mar 41. SG: 210.2–1. (2) Ltr, Lt Col John M. Welch to Dr Wilburt C. Davison, Dean, Sch of Med, Duke Univ, 31 Jan 42. SG: 210.1–1. (3) Ltr, Col George F. Lull to Col C[harles] M. Walson, 5 Jun 42. Same file. (4) Ltr, Brig Gen W[illiam] L. Sheep, CG Lawson Gen Hosp to Col H. D. Offutt, 12 Feb 42. SG: 323.7–5 (Lawson GH)K.

[64] (1) Memo, ACofS G–1 WDGS for SG thru Pers Div SOS, 1 Apr 42, sub: Availability of Physicians. (2) Memo, ACofS G–1 WDGS for Pers Div SOS, 9 May 42, same sub. (3) Memo, CG SOS for SG, 22 May 42, same sub. All in HRS: G–1/16331–16335.

[65] (1) Ltr, SG to Pers Sec SOS, 26 May 42, sub: Procurement Objective, MAC. (2) Memo, CG SOS for CofSA, 29 May 42, sub: Increase in Procurement Objective, MAC, with 2d ind, SG to Chief Pers Serv SOS, 6 Jun 42. (3) Memo, CG SOS for CofSA, 5 Jun 42, same sub. (4) Ltr, TAG to SG, 13 Jun 42, same sub. All in AG: 210.1(1–14–42)(2) Sec 2A.

[66] Memo, SG for COs Sta Hosps at Sheppard Fld, Fts Lewis, Ord, Sam Houston, Leonard Wood, Devens, Indiantown Gap Mil Res, Cp Lee, and Fitzsimons, Army and Navy, Wm. Beaumont, Walter Reed, and Lawson Gen Hosps, 29 Jun 42, sub: Conservation of Available MC Offs. SG: 322.051–1.

[67] Ltr, TAG to CGs AGF, AAF, all CAs, 13 Jul 42, sub: Relief of MC Offs from Duties Which Do Not Require Professional Med Tng. AG: 210.31(7–10–42)(4).

[68] (1) Ltr, CG 8th CA to TAG, 22 Jul 42, sub: Relief of MC Offs. AG: 210.31(7–10–42)(4). (2) Memo, SG for Dir Mil Pers SOS, [10 Oct 42]. SG: 322.051–1. (3) Ltr, Lt Col J[ames] R. Hudnall, SGO to Lt Col Arthur J. Redland, 5th SvC, 10 Aug 42. SG: 320.3–1 (5th SvC).

[69] (1) Rpt, Conf of CGs SvCs [SOS], 2d sess, 17 Dec 42, pp. 19, 33, 96. HD: 337. (2) An Rpts, 1942, Chief Med Br (Surg) 3d and 9th SvCs. HD.

[70] (1) Ltr SPMCQ 322.056.–1, SG to TAG, 28 Sep 42, sub: Increase in Procurement Objective AUS for Duty with MAC (SG). AG: SPGA 210.1 Med 1–20. (2) Memo, SG for Dir Mil Pers SOS [10 Oct 42]. SG: 322.051–1. (3) Ltr SPMCM 210.1–1, SG to Dir Mil Pers SOS, 13 Oct 42, sub: Procurement Objective, MD. AG: SPGA 210.1 Med 1–20. (4) Memo, Lt Col

tion for Medical Corps officers remained to be carried out during the later war years.

Changes in the composition of the enlisted staffs of hospitals were more general. Experience in the employment of civilians had already demonstrated that able-bodied enlisted men could be replaced by personnel of other types. During the first year and a half of the war the practice of substitution was extended. Limited service enlisted men (that is, those with physical defects which disqualified them for service with the field forces) and Women's Army Auxiliary Corps enlisted women were added to civilians as replacements for enlisted men who were physically qualified for general service.

Early in 1942 hospital commanders often had fewer enlisted men than they considered desirable, and the Surgeon General's Office reported continual shortages for Medical Department activities. Large numbers were needed for the many new hospitals opening in the zone of interior. Units going overseas had to have full complements and hospitals called upon to supply them often had difficulty securing replacements.[71] In July SOS headquarters issued a directive, recommended by the Surgeon General's Office, to give such hospitals priorities on replacement requisitions.[72] About the same time it announced that the Army would begin in August to induct limited service men and assign them directly to hospitals and other zone of interior installations.[73] These measures were apparently helpful, for by the end of 1942 many hospitals reported that their allotments were full.[74] Even so, a few commanders complained of shortages,[75] but generally, complaints were less of shortages than of difficulties in using limited service men and civilians.

Hospitals had had experience with limited service enlisted men as early as December 1941, when the War Department began to transfer physically unfit men from field force units to zone of interior installations.[76] At first hospitals absorbed men of this type readily because they were few in number and were used to fill vacancies, supplementing existing forces of able-bodied men. Gradually it became the practice to withdraw able-bodied men from hospital staffs for service with field forces and to use limited service men not as supplements but as substitutes for them.[77] As this happened hospital commanders encountered difficulties. The

Basil C. MacLean for Gen Bliss thru Col Schwichtenberg, 6 Nov 43, sub: Observations Based on Recent Visits for Varying Periods to Nine Gen Hosps. SG: Gen Bliss's Off files, "Util of MCs in the ZI" (19) #1.

[71] (1) Memo, SG for Dir Mil Pers SOS [10 Oct 42]. SG: 322.051-1. (2) DF WDGAP 322.051, ACofS G-1 WDGS to SG thru Mil Pers Div SOS, 28 Oct 42. Same file. (3) Rpt, SGs Conf with CA and Army Surgs, 25-28 May 42, pp. 20, 31. HD: 337. (4) An Rpts, 1942, Chief Med Br 2d and 5th SvCs. HD.

[72] Ltr SPX 220.31 (7-11-42)EC-SPMCP-PS-M, CG SOS to CGs SvCs and CGs Gen Hosps, 28 Jul 42, sub: Filler Repls for Units Ordered Overseas. SG: 220.31-1.

[73] SOS Cir Ltr 25, 10 Jul 42, sub: Asgmt of Limited Serv EM. SG: 220.31-1.

[74] An Rpts, 1942, Hoff, Ashford, Billings, Lovell, Tilton, Hammond, Bushnell, Torney, O'Reilly, and Lawson Gen Hosps and Sta Hosps at Cps Wheeler, Murphy, Young, Croft, Roberts, Chaffee, McCoy, Sheppard Fld, and Fts Knox and Riley. HD.

[75] An Rpts, 1942, Sta Hosps at Jefferson Bks and Cp Lee. HD.

[76] Ltr AG 220.31 (12-18-41)EA-A, TAG to all Army, CA, and Exempted Sta Comdrs other than AC and C of Armored Force, 23 Dec 41, sub: Clearing Fld Force Units of Pers not Physically Qualified for Fld Serv. SG: 220.31-1.

[77] (1) SOS Cir 13, 12 May 42, sub: Absorption of Limited Serv Pers in Overhead Instls of SOS. AG: 220.3(12 May 42)(2). (2) WD Memo W615-3-42, 17 Aug 42, sub: Asgmt of Limited Serv Pers. HD: 220.31-1. (3) Ltr AG 220.31(4-5-43)PE-A-SPOA, CG ASF to C of Tec Servs, 7 Apr 43, sub: Util of Limited Serv Pers. Same file.

field forces tended to place "problem" men in the limited service category and to promote others just before transfer—actions bound to create morale problems for receiving hospitals.[78] Moreover, limited service men were often unable to do a full day of hard work, and hospitals—operating around the clock—found it difficult to assign all of them to special jobs within their physical limitations. Of equal importance, such men had often had no Medical Department training. Hospitals therefore had to maintain continuous training programs for newcomers. Even so they could not always train enough technicians, for in many instances physical incapacity happened to be coupled with low mentality and little education.[79] By the end of 1942 this problem had become so serious that The Surgeon General sought a commitment from SOS headquarters to assign to the Medical Department greater numbers of limited service men of good caliber.[80] Failing in this, he resorted to the establishment in April 1943 of special regiments to train whatever limited service men the Medical Department might receive.[81]

As limited service men came to constitute a larger part of the enlisted force, hospitals gradually began to think of civilians as supplementing rather than replacing enlisted men. By the end of 1942 many hospitals with full complements of enlisted men also had sizable numbers of civilian employees. In recruiting civilians, hospital commanders encountered the same problems they had experienced in 1941. In addition, they found it increasingly difficult to maintain stable civilian forces. As able-bodied civilian employees were inducted into the armed services, they had to be replaced by women and elderly or physically-handicapped men. Even the widespread use of civilians of these types failed to bring stability, for they left hospitals in growing numbers to take better paying jobs elsewhere. Competition with war industries and other government agencies was keen and hospital wage-scales were frequently lower than those prevailing in surrounding areas. As a result, hospital commanders found the use of civilians "very vexatious, time consuming, and expensive," [82] and by the end of 1942 some of them began to think it would be better to replace civilians with limited service men, however unsatisfactory, or with members of the Women's Army Auxiliary Corps.[83]

When the question of using Waacs in Army hospitals was first raised in the spring of 1942, The Surgeon General expressed opposition because, he said, their use would conflict with civilian personnel employment, would interfere with training of enlisted men, and would create diffi-

[78] (1) Ltr AG 220.31(4-1-42)EA-A, TAG to CG AGF, CGs Eastern, Western, Southern, and Central Def Comds, and all CA Comdrs, 2 Apr 42, sub: Clearing Fld Force Units of Pers Not Physically Qualified for Fld Serv. SG: 220.31-1. (2) Ltr AG 220.31(7-2-42), TAG to CGs AGF, AAF, SOS, etc., 14 Jul 42, same sub. Same file.

[79] (1) An Rpts, 1942, Sta Hosps at Ft Knox, Cps Roberts, Bowie, Maxey, Chaffee, Atterbury, Lee, Wolters, Forrest, and Hoff and Tilton Gen Hosps. HD. (2) An Rpts, 1942, Chiefs Med Br 1st, 2d, 3d, and 7th SvCs. HD.

[80] (1) Memo, SG for Dir Mil Pers SOS thru Dir Tng SOS, 3 Dec 42, sub: Asgmt of Class I and Class II Limited Serv Pers to MRTCs. SG: 220.31-1. (2) Memo SPGAE/220.3(12-3-42)-132, Dir Mil Pers SOS for SG, 10 Dec 42, same sub. Same file.

[81] Ltr, CG ASF per SG to CGs MRTCs, MDETS, etc., 16 Apr 43, sub: Util of Limited Serv Pers. HD: 220.31-1.

[82] Ltr, CO LaGarde Gen Hosp to Col G[eorge] F. Lull, SGO, 28 Dec 42. SG: 323.7-5(LaGarde GH)K.

[83] The above paragraph is based on: An Rpts, 1942, Ashford, Billings, Bushnell, Hoff, Percy Jones, Tilton, and Torney Gen Hosps, and Sta Hosps at Ft Riley, and Cps Atterbury, Blanding, Chaffee, Croft, Howze, Lee, Maxey, Roberts, Wheeler, Wolters, and Young. HD.

culties centering around housing and recreation.[84] During 1942, as civilians became increasingly hard to get and keep and as limited service men replaced those qualified for overseas service in growing numbers, the idea gradually gained currency among hospital commanders, service command surgeons, and members of the Surgeon General's Office that Waacs, who could not leave their jobs and who had sufficient ability and education to absorb technical training, were a "better bet" than either civilians or limited service enlisted men.[85] Meanwhile, as plans were made to expand the women's corps, both the War Department General Staff and SOS headquarters put pressure on all of the services, including the Medical Department, to use Waacs extensively to release men for combat duty.[86] About the same time, the Wadhams Committee recommended their employment in hospitals.[87] Accordingly, early in 1943 the Surgeon General's Office began to plan for their assignment to Medical Department installations.

At first The Surgeon General decided to conduct experiments at Halloran (New York) and Valley Forge (Pennsylvania) General Hospitals to see what jobs Waacs could fill.[88] Failing to obtain WAAC units for this purpose, on 26 January 1943 he appointed a board of officers, composed of the chief of his Hospitalization Division and members of the Personnel and Training Divisions, to study the problem. Soon afterward he requested reports from service commands, the Air Forces, the Transportation Corps, and the Army Medical Center on hospital jobs which Waacs could fill, the numbers needed, and the construction required to house them.[89] From these surveys The Surgeon General's board found that the Air Forces planned to use Waacs in all hospitals having 200 or more beds and that the commanders of SOS hospitals having 500 or more beds felt that they could use them to replace from 30 to 50 percent of their enlisted men. Not all hospital commanders, it should be noted, were enthusiastic about using Waacs, their attitudes depending to a large extent upon what General Grant, the Air Surgeon, called the "personal equation."[90] The board estimated that

[84] Memo, Lt Col Gilman C. Mudgett, SOS for SG, 31 Mar 42, sub: Possible Use of Mems of the WAAC in Army Hosps, with 1st ind, SG to CG SOS, 14 Apr 42; and 2d ind SPTRS 290 (WAAC)(3-21-42), CG SOS to SG, 29 Apr 42. SG: 322.5-1 (WAC).

[85] (1) Ltrs, CO LaGarde Gen Hosp to Col H. D. Offutt, SGO, 21 and 29 Sep 42, and to Col G. F. Lull, SGO, 28 Dec 42. SG: 323.7-5 (LaGarde GH)K. (2) An Rpts, 1942, Cp Howze and Sheppard Fld Sta Hosps, and Chief Med Br 3d SvC. HD. (3) Ltr, CO Valley Forge Gen Hosp to SG, 19 Jan 43, sub: Request Allocation and Asgmt of a WAAC Unit, with 1st ind. SG: 322.5-1. (4) Ltr, Col G. F. Lull, SGO to Col W. H. Smith, LaGarde Gen Hosp, 5 Jan 43. SG: 323.7-5(LaGarde GH)K. (5) Ltr, Lt Col D[aniel] J. Sheehan, SGO to Brig Gen James E. Baylis, CG MRTC, Cp J. T. Robinson, Ark, 22 Feb 43. HD: 220.31-1.

[86] (1) Memo S635-2-42, 22 Oct 42, sub: Asgmt of WAAC. AG: 320.2(10-1-32)(3) Sec 16. (2) Memo, CG SOS for C of Sup and Admin Servs, 22 Oct 42, sub: Data for Study on Use of WAAC. Same file.

[87] Extracts from Memo, CG SOS for SG, 26 Nov 42, and from 2d ind, CG SOS to SG, 21 Dec 42, in Cmtee to Study the MD, 1942-43, Actions on Recomd, Recomd No 88. HD.

[88] (1) Extract from 3d ind, SG to CG SOS, 16 Jan 43, on extract from Memo, CG SOS for SG, 26 Nov 42. (2) Extract from 1st ind, SG to CG SOS, 8 Mar 43, on extract from Memo, CofS SOS for SG, 26 Feb 43. Both in Cmtee to Study the MD, 1942-43, Actions on Recomd, Recomd No 88. HD.

[89] (1) SG OO 41, 26 Jan 43. (2) Memo, CG SOS per SG for CG 1st SvC, attn Chief Med Br, 29 Jan 43, sub: Employment of WAAC in Sta and Gen Hosps, ZI. HD: 322.5-1. The same letter was sent to all Service Commands. (3) Memos, SG for CG AAF, MDW and AMC, and for CofT, 3 Feb 43, same sub. Same file.

[90] 1st ind, CG AAF per Air Surg to SG, 26 Feb 43, on Memo, SG for CG AAF attn AF Surg, 3 Feb 43, sub: Employment of WAAC in Sta and Gen Hosps, ZI. SG: 322.5-1.

more than ten thousand Waacs would be needed for hospitals and in March 1943 recommended that WAAC headquarters be asked what number they could supply.[91] The Surgeon General then sent each service commander a tabulation of Waac requirements for hospitals in his command, for inclusion in the Waac requisition which it was anticipated SOS headquarters would require each to submit.[92] Soon afterward, Waac recruiting collapsed and WAAC headquarters could promise The Surgeon General, on 2 June 1943, only 150 to 170 women for training each month, beginning in September 1943.[93] The extensive use of Waacs in hospitals therefore had to wait.

Problem of Furnishing Supplies and Equipment for Hospitals

Providing sufficient medical supplies and equipment for large numbers of new station and general hospitals, and for old hospitals that were expanding with unprecedented rapidity, as well as for dispensaries, infirmaries, induction stations, and medical units destined for overseas service, presented the Medical Department a problem of great magnitude.[94] It was partially simplified by the practice of issuing hospital assemblages as single items. Using equipment lists prepared during the emergency period, medical depots packed assemblages which included, within the limits of supplies and equipment available, all items needed to establish hospitals of various sizes and kinds, ranging from 25-bed station hospitals to 1,000-bed general hospitals. As new hospital plants were constructed the Surgeon General's Office had assemblages of appropriate sizes shipped to them. As established hospitals were expanded, local medical supply officers requisitioned standard assemblages to fit their needs.[95] This system not only saved time and personnel that would have been required to list the manifold items required for each hospital but also relieved local supply officers, many of whom were unacquainted with tables of equipment and inexperienced in estimating hospital needs, of the necessity of determining what items would be required for hospital expansions.

Changes in the requisitioning procedure used by hospitals to meet recurrent operational needs became imperative as soon as the wartime expansion began. Before the war, hospitals were permitted to make only quarterly and emergency requisitions, all of which had to be reviewed by corps area surgeons before being sent to depots for filling. To enable hospitals to meet urgent needs that resulted from rapid expansions, as contrasted with emergency needs that could not be foreseen, The Surgeon General early in January 1942 permitted the submission of "special" requisitions at any time.[96] To eliminate an unnecessary step and thus speed the requisitioning process, he began a system of

[91] Rpt of Proceedings of Bd of Offs, n d, incl 4 to Memo, SG for Planning Serv WAAC Hq, 13 Mar 43, sub: Util of WAAC in MD. HD: 322.5-1.

[92] Memo, CG SOS per SG for CG 3d SvC, 27 Mar 43, sub: Employment of WAAC in Sta and Gen Hosps, ZI. HD: 322.5-1.

[93] (1) Memo, SG for CG ASF, 2 Jun 43, sub; Tec Tng for WAAC Pers. HD: 322.5-1. (2) Mattie E. Treadwell, *The Women's Army Corps*, Ch. XIX.

[94] Except where otherwise noted, this section is based on Richard E. Yates, The Procurement and Distribution of Medical Supplies in the Zone of the Interior during World War II (1946), pp. 169-87. HD.

[95] (1) Ltr, SG to MD Depots, 2 Feb 42, sub: Med Depot Program for 1942. SG: 475.5-1. (2) SG Ltr 141, 2 Nov 42, sub: MD Equip Lists. (3) SG Ltr 156, 24 Nov 42, sub: Sup Policies and Procedures, ZI Instls.

[96] SG Ltr 2, 8 Jan 42, sub: Requisitions.

direct supply on 10 February 1942. After that date hospital medical supply officers could submit requisitions directly to depots, without corps area intervention.[97]

In the early months of the war, the Medical Department continued to be handicapped by a shortage of many items. As a result, depots found it necessary to ship incomplete assemblages and partially filled requisitions. Missing items were placed on back order, to be shipped when available. Among the items which hospitals most frequently failed to receive were dental supplies and equipment, surgical instruments and operating room equipment, laboratory equipment, X-ray developing-tanks and cassettes, hospital furniture including beds, and food carts. New hospitals suffered most from these shortages. In a few instances the receipt of incomplete assemblages delayed their opening or the opening of some of their clinics and wards. When hospitals opened with incomplete equipment they usually had to send surgical patients to near-by hospitals and have dental, laboratory, and X-ray work done elsewhere. To make up for shortages that continued to exist, they resorted to borrowing, improvising, and purchasing in the open market. Some borrowed beds from the local quartermaster and such items as X-ray developing-tanks, cassettes, and food carts from other Army hospitals or from Veterans Administration facilities. Others improvised X-ray developing-tanks and food carts. Many had their own "utilities" personnel build missing items of hospital furniture. Sometimes, when money was available, hospitals purchased necessary supplies on the local market. In some instances, officers used their own instruments and in one case, where there was a shortage of typewriters, civilian typists were required to provide their own. While these shortages undoubtedly taxed the ingenuity of hospital commanders and operating personnel, they failed, apparently, to affect medical care adversely, for hospital commanders seemed able to arrange for the use of local civilian or near-by Army facilities without undue difficulty.[98]

In the latter part of 1942 The Surgeon General intensified his efforts to solve medical supply problems. Most measures taken toward that end, such as the improvement of depot operations, are outside the scope of this study. Two deserve consideration here. The requisition system was completely revised and placed on a monthly basis, effective 1 January 1943. After that date hospitals submitted separate monthly requisitions for standard-expendable, standard - nonexpendable, and nonstandard items. They could still submit "special" and emergency requisitions.[99] Concurrently, the stock-control system was revised. The system formerly in effect had permitted hospitals to keep large stocks on hand and had not required accurate "due in" records. As a result some hospitals held in storage items that were needed by others, and medical supply officers often did not know which items of their requisitions remained to be shipped by depots. In the fall of 1942, therefore, the Surgeon General's Office established lower stock levels and devised a new stock-

[97] SG Ltr 11, 10 Feb 42, sub: Direct System of Sup for Posts, Cps, and Stas.

[98] The above paragraph is based on information in the following: An Rpts, 1942, Chiefs Med Br 1st, 3d, 4th, 5th, 6th, 7th, and 9th SvCs; Ashford, Bushnell, Billings, Deshon, Harmon, Hoff, and Percy Jones Gen Hosps; and Sta Hosps at Fts Belvoir and Bliss, Sheppard Fld, and Cps Adair, Atterbury, Butner, Cooke, Howze, Maxey, and McCoy. HD.

[99] SG Ltr 156, 24 Nov 42, sub: Sup Policies and Procedures, ZI Instls.

record card for posts and general hospitals. These changes not only produced better supply administration but also released large amounts of supplies and equipment for redistribution to hospitals suffering from shortages.[100] The combination of measures begun in 1942, along with completion of the hospital expansion program during 1943, resulted in a greatly improved supply situation. During the rest of the war hospitals and service command surgeons reported generally that requisitions were promptly filled and that the supplies and equipment which they received were of good quality and of sufficient quantity to meet their needs.[101]

[100] For example, see the following: An Rpts, 1943, Surg 7th SvC, and Sta Hosps at Cps Lee and Maxey. HD.

[101] (1) Memo, Dir Sup Planning Div SGO for Act Chief, Sup Serv SGO, 22 Dec 43, sub: Rpt of Visits to Hosp Instls. SG: 333.1-1. (2) Memo, Dir Distr and Reqmts Div SGO for Mr. Edward R. Reynolds, 20 Jan 44, sub: Data for Inclusion in . . . Rpt on Accomplishments of SGO. SG: 024.-1. (3) An Rpts at random; for example, An Rpts, 1943, Hoff, Percy Jones, Ashford, and Dibble Gen Hosps; An Rpts, 1944, Surg 2d, 5th, and 9th SvCs, and Beaumont, Baker, Birmingham, and Lovell Gen Hosps; An Rpts, 1945, Surg 2d SvC, and Beaumont and Birmingham Gen Hosps. HD.

CHAPTER VIII

Providing Hospitalization for Theaters of Operations

In the first year and a half of the war the Medical Department had to provide hospitalization for reinforced garrisons in overseas departments and bases, for new forces sent to hold lines of supply and communication throughout the world, and for task forces engaged in the first defensive-offensive operations against the enemy. Meanwhile it had to organize, train, and equip other units for use when the Army should become engaged in full-scale offensives. Early in 1942 the Pacific held first claim on hospital units sent overseas. In the summer emphasis shifted to Europe and North Africa, and thereafter hospitals went to those theaters in increasing numbers. By the latter part of the year, after emergency shipments had been made, it was possible to take stock of hospitalization already furnished to theaters with a view to establishing a basis for further planning.

Meeting Early Emergency Needs

Status of Hospital Units and Assemblages

When the Japanese struck Pearl Harbor the Medical Department had 22 general, 24 station, 17 evacuation, and 8 surgical hospital units that had been activated as training units. Of these, 3 station hospitals were already overseas and 9 station, 12 general, 4 evacuation, and 3 surgical hospital units included in the War Department pool of task force units were authorized almost 100 percent of their table-of-organization enlisted strength and from 50 to 75 percent of their commissioned strength. The rest had half or less than half of their enlisted strength and from three to five officers each. In addition to the training units, affiliated hospital units consisting chiefly of professional commissioned personnel—doctors and nurses—had been organized (but not activated) as follows: 41 general, 11 evacuation, and 4 surgical hospitals. Under prewar plans, it will be recalled, affiliated units were to be called to active duty as needed immediately upon the outbreak of war, were to be supplied with enlisted personnel, and were then to go into service without further ado.[1] According to a report of The Surgeon General in November 1941, hospital assemblages had already been issued to 3 station and 2 evacuation hospital units; while assemblages for 2 general, 11 station, 4 evacuation, and 3 surgical hospital units were packed and ready for immediate issue from depots, and those for 10 general, 9

[1] See above, pp. 5–6, 40.

station, 17 evacuation, and 5 surgical hospital units were being packed but were not yet ready for issuance.[2]

Plans for Meeting Emergency Needs

Early in January 1942 The Surgeon General outlined to G–3 the system he wished to use in meeting emergency needs. Affiliated units would be called to active duty and each would receive approximately one half of its authorized enlisted strength from a training unit. The rest of its personnel would be supplied by reception centers, zone of interior installations, and other medical units. Each training unit which transferred personnel to an affiliated unit would retain a cadre, in order to train additional "fillers" for other affiliated units. Some training units, especially station hospital units, would be sent overseas as needed, having first been brought to authorized strength with both enlisted and commissioned personnel transferred from other medical units or installations. Each unit would draw individual equipment, clothing, and motor transport at its home station. Only those going overseas would receive hospital assemblages, preferably at ports of embarkation.[3]

Soon after he had proposed this system The Surgeon General realized that modifications would be necessary. The activation of training units at reduced strength, a policy adopted on his recommendation in 1941, resulted in the hurried assembly, often at ports of embarkation, of additional personnel to make up the other half of a unit. Members of units going overseas therefore frequently had little time to become acquainted with one another's capabilities before embarkation. Installations from which "fillers" were drawn suffered from resulting personnel and training problems. To obviate these difficulties The Surgeon General recommended in February 1942 that all training units be activated at full table-of-organization enlisted strength.[4] He received the support in March 1942 of the SOS Hospitalization and Evacuation Branch and in April of AGF headquarters. In May G–3 approved the proposal.[5]

The Surgeon General secured only partial approval of his stand in opposition to the issuance of hospital assemblages before the departure of units for theaters. After completing a survey of storage space in corps areas, G–4 in December 1941 disapproved a request that General Magee had made in November to hold assemblages in depots until units were assigned missions involving medical care.[6] General Magee then sought approval of his position in a personal conference with General Somervell, who was at that time the Assistant Chief of Staff, G–4. On the basis of his understanding of the agreement reached then, General Magee resubmitted his request.[7] Instead of approving it,

[2] Ltr, SG to TAG, 5 Nov 41, sub: Equip for Med Units in WD Pool of Task Forces. SG: 475.5–1.

[3] Memo, SG for AcofS G–3 WDGS, 13 Jan 42, sub: Activation . . . Med Units, with incls. HD: 326.01–1.

[4] (1) Memo, Act SG for ACofS G–3 WDGS, 28 Feb 42, sub: Orgn and Dispatch of MD TofOpns Units. SG: 322.3. (2) An Rpts, 1942, of following Gen Hosps: 2d, 30th, 42d, 105th, 118th, and 210th, and of following Sta Hosps: 10th, 12th, 13th, 17th, 151st, 166th, and 172d. HD.

[5] (1) Memo G–4/24499–178, Maj William L. Wilson for [Lt] Gen [LeRoy] Lutes, 12 Mar 42, sub: Basic Plans for Hosp and Evac. HD: Wilson files, "No 472, Hosp and Evac, 1941–42." (2) Ltr, CG AGF for CG SOS, 23 Apr 42, sub: Auth of Grades and Ratings for MD Tactical Hosp. AG: 221(7–1–41) Sec 1H, Pt 1. (3) Ltr, TAG to CGs AGF, AAF, SOS, Armored Force, etc., 6 May 42, same sub. Same file.

[6] D/S G–4/31793, ACofS G–4 WDGS to SG, 31 Dec 41, sub: Comments on Draft of Ltr, 'Current Policies and Procedures for . . . Sups.' HD: 475.5–1.

[7] Memo, SG for ACofS G–4 WDGS, 10 Jan 42, sub: Equip for Numbered Hosps. HD: 475.5–1.

as The Surgeon General had expected, G-4 now proposed a compromise. Unit assemblages would be declared controlled items. As such, they would not be issued through corps areas to units upon requisition but would be issued directly as the War Department determined. Meanwhile, The Surgeon General would make fractional issues of unit equipment for training purposes.[8]

Although he concurred in this compromise, officially published on 21 January 1942,[9] The Surgeon General did not give up hope that he could continue to hold unit assemblages in medical depots until numbered hospitals were assigned operational missions. Once they were declared controlled items, the most practical method of achieving this end would be to secure War Department agreement not to require their issuance prior to that time. This might be done indirectly. Consequently, on 24 January 1942 The Surgeon General requested G-4 to include in movement orders for numbered hospital units ordered overseas a paragraph directing The Surgeon General to ship appropriate assemblages to ports of embarkation or staging areas. On 6 February 1942 G-4 approved this recommendation.[10] As will be seen later, neither the 21 January 1942 compromise nor the approval of the inclusion of a paragraph in movement orders settled the controversy over the issuance of equipment.

Methods of Meeting Emergency Needs

In defense areas—the Atlantic bases, the Panama Canal Zone, Alaska, and Hawaii—where hospitals already existed, the hospital situation was serious though not critical. To meet emergency needs existing facilities could be expanded and additional "provisional" hospitals could be established by spreading thin the personnel and equipment already available. Army patients could also be hospitalized in civilian institutions wherever they were available.[11] Hence few hospital units went to those areas in the first few months following Pearl Harbor. Between 1 January and 30 June 1942, 2 general hospitals were sent to the Panama Canal Zone and 3 general and 4 station hospitals to Hawaii to supplement existing and improvised hospitals in those areas.[12] In addition, troops sent to garrison new bases included medical detachments to operate the hospitals needed for their care,[13] but the more pressing needs of other areas generally took precedence in the shipment both of numbered hospitals and supplementary personnel and equipment.[14]

Troops deployed to protect shipping lanes and to hold the enemy while preparations for the offensive went forward re-

[8] Memo for Record on D/S, ACofS G-4 WDGS for TAG, 16 Jan 42, sub: Equip for MD Units, and on Memo, Chief Planning Br G-4 WDGS for Brig Gen B. B. Somervell, 16 Jan 42, same sub. HRS: G-4/33344.

[9] (1) Memo, SG for ACofS G-4 WDGS, 17 Jan 42. SG: 475.5-1. (2) Ltr AG 400 (1-16-42)MD-D-M, TAG to SG, 21 Jan 42, sub: Equip for MD Units. HRS: G-4/33344.

[10] (1) Memo, SG for ACofS G-4 WDGS, 24 Jan 42, sub: Proposed Modification of Mvmt Orders. SG: 475.5-1. (2) D/S, ACofS G-4 WDGS for TAG, 6 Feb 43, same sub. HRS: G-4/33344.

[11] An Rpt, Med Activities Newfoundland Base Comd, 1942; An Rpt, Med Activities Surg Trinidad Sector and Base Comd, 1942; An Rpt, Dept Surg Panama Canal Dept, 1942; An Rpt, MD Activities Hawaiian Dept, 1942, sec I. HD.

[12] Ltr AG 221(1-31-42)EA-C, TAG to CG Hawaiian Dept, 18 Feb 42, sub: Grades and Ratings, MD, Hawaii. SG: 320.2-1 (Hawaiian Dept) AA.

[13] An Rpt, Med Activities US Army Force, Aruba, NWI, 1942, and Hist Record, US Army MD in Greenland, Jul 41-Feb 43. HD.

[14] Paraphrase of Rad AG 320.2(1-12-42) MSC-A, TAG to CG Hawaiian Dept, 14 Jan 42. SG: 320.2-1(Hawaiian Dept)AA.

quired hospitalization in areas that had no American facilities. The greatest immediate need was in the South and Southwest Pacific. During the period from 1 January to 1 July 1942, inclusive, 2 evacuation, 2 surgical, 4 general, and 14 station hospitals were sent to Australia; 2 evacuation, 2 general, and 2 station hospitals to islands in the South Pacific; and 2 station hospitals to islands other than the Hawaiian group in the Central Pacific. During the same period, 1 general and 1 station hospital went to Northern Ireland, a general hospital to Iceland, and 2 general and 3 station hospitals to England. In May and June 1942, hospitals were sent also to India, to care for troops engaged in supply and service activities there, and to Northwest Canada, to care for those who were helping to build the Alcan highway. Meanwhile other hospital units were being earmarked for task forces, especially for the GYMNAST (North Africa), MAGNET (Northern Ireland), and BOLERO (England) operations. These demands drew heavily upon available units and assemblages and sometimes made it impossible for The Surgeon General and OPD to meet without modification requests of theater commanders.[15] *(Table 5)*

In sending numbered hospital units overseas, The Surgeon General departed from prewar plans, using training units as well as affiliated units. This was caused in part by the character of the war. Station hospitals, for which no affiliated units had been organized, were needed for defense forces sent out early in 1942 more than were surgical, evacuation, and general hospitals. Moreover, the earmarking of some affiliated hospitals for task forces that were formed early but sent out later, or not at all, may have tied up enough affiliated units to require the use of training units in meeting overseas needs between Pearl Harbor and 2 July 1942. At any rate, all station hospitals and the two surgical hospitals dispatched during this period were nonaffiliated units. Of the thirty-seven station hospitals sent out, seventeen had been activated during 1941 and the rest after war began. Both surgical hospitals were nonaffiliated units that had been activated in 1941. Of the fifteen general hospitals shipped, nine were affiliated units supplied (except for one) with enlisted personnel from training units activated during 1941. The remainder were nonaffiliated training units activated in 1941. Of the 4 evacuation hospital units sent out, 2 were affiliated units and 2 were nonaffiliated units activated in 1940 and 1941. Thus the prior activation and training of normal Army units proved more valuable in meeting emergency hospital needs than did the formation and organization of units affiliated with civilian hospitals or schools.

Modification of Hospitals for Overseas Areas

Development of New Types of Units

Early in the war it was necessary to develop new types of hospitals to meet the needs of island-type warfare and of motorized operations on land. Experience in planning hospitalization for the earliest task forces and garrisons for islands in the

[15] (1) Memo, Lt Col A[rthur] B. Welsh for Brig Gen L[arry] B. McAfee, 1 Apr 42. HD: Welsh Planning file. (2) Memo for Record on IAS, 5 Apr 42, sub: Hosp Units for SUMAC [Australia] and SPOONER [New Zealand]. HRS: WPD 704.2(3-9-42). (3) Memo, Maj A. B. Welsh for Gen Magee, 23 Jan 42, sub: Status of Hosp Units. HD: 320.2 (Trp Basis).

TABLE 5—HOSPITAL UNITS SHIPPED OVERSEAS, 7 DECEMBER 1941 TO 1 JULY 1942

Unit	No. of Beds	Date of Activation	Date of Embarkation	Destination
	General Hospitals			
[a] 2d	1,000	31 Jan 42	1 Jul 42	England
[a] 4th	1,000	13 Jan 42	23 Jan 42	Australia
[a] 5th	500	3 Jan 42	19 Feb 42	N. Ireland [b]
[a] 18th	500	20 Apr 42	26 May 42	New Zealand
[a] 30th	1,000	15 May 42	4 Jun 42	England
[a] 42d	500	20 Apr 42	19 May 42	Australia
[a] 105th	1,000	20 Apr 42	19 May 42	Australia
[a] 118th	500	21 Apr 42	19 May 42	Australia
[a] 142d	500	20 Apr 42	26 May 42	New Zealand
147th	1,000	1 May 41	16 Jun 42	Hawaii
148th	1,000	10 Feb 41	21 Mar 42	Hawaii
204th	1,000	10 Feb 41	8 Apr 42	Hawaii
208th	500	1 Jun 41	18 Feb 42	Iceland
210th	1,000	1 Jun 41	8 Jan 42	Panama, C. Z.
218th	750	6 Jun 41	8 Jan 42	Panama, C. Z.
	Station Hospitals			
1st	150	10 Feb 41	30 Jan 42	Christmas Island
2d	250	16 Mar 42	18 May 42	Australia
3d	250	18 Mar 42	30 Jun 42	England
5th	250	7 Jan 41	17 Feb 42	Australia
8th	250	10 Feb 41	17 Jan 42	Bora Bora
9th	250	11 Feb 41	23 Jan 42	Australia
10th	350	10 Feb 41	14 Jan 42	N. Ireland
12th	250	10 Feb 41	18 Feb 42	Australia
13th	250	16 Mar 42	18 May 42	Australia
16th	150	16 Mar 42	3 Jun 42	England
17th	250	16 Mar 42	18 May 42	Australia
18th	250	16 Mar 42	18 May 42	Australia
22d	250	10 Feb 41	27 Feb 42	Hawaii
25th	250	24 Mar 42	28 May 42	Liberia
26th	150	10 Feb 41	31 Jan 42	Canton Island
44th	50	4 Jun 42	14 Jun 42	Canada
45th	50	29 May 42	12 Jun 42	Canada
46th	25	2 Jun 42	17 Jun 42	Canada
47th	250	18 Jun 41	18 Feb 42	Australia
71st	250	14 Apr 42	9 May 42	Fiji Islands
95th	50	30 Apr 42	27 May 42	India
97th	50	28 Apr 42	27 May 42	India
98th	50	28 Apr 42	27 May 42	India
99th	50	28 Apr 42	27 May 42	India
100th	50	1 May 42	27 May 42	India
109th	250	1 Jun 41	23 Jan 42	New Caledonia
151st	250	1 Jun 41	30 Jun 42	England
153d	250	1 Jun 41	18 Feb 42	Australia
155th	500	1 Jun 41	18 May 42	Australia
156th	250	3 Jun 41	11 Mar 42	Hawaii
159th	750	1 Jun 41	19 Mar 42	India
165th	250	1 Jun 41	27 Feb 42	Hawaii
166th	250	1 Jun 41	19 May 42	Australia
171st	250	3 Apr 42	18 May 42	Australia
172d	250	20 Mar 42	19 May 42	Australia
174th	250	29 Mar 42	18 May 42	Australia
175th	150	17 Feb 42	14 Mar 42	Ascension Island
	Evacuation Hospitals			
1st	750	1 Aug 40	4 Mar 42	Australia
[a] 7th	750	22 Jan 42	7 Apr 42	Tongatabu
10th	750	10 Feb 41	4 Mar 42	Australia
[a] 52d	750	12 Jan 42	23 Jan 42	New Caledonia
	Surgical Hospitals			
28th	400	10 Feb 41	4 Mar 42	Australia
33d	400	25 Jan 41	4 Mar 42	Australia

[a] Affiliated units.

[b] This unit returned from Nova Scotia to Boston on 4 March 1942, and embarked again at New York on 12 May 1942.

Sources: Unit cards filed in Orgn and Directory Section, Oprs Br, AGO, and annual reports filed in HD

Pacific revealed the need for hospitals that were smaller and more mobile than the only hospital available for that purpose—the 250-bed station hospital. As a result, the Surgeon General's Office and the medical section of General Headquarters collaborated in developing a new type of hospital, called the field hospital, in the first months of 1942. When G–4 called upon the Surgeon General's Office to develop an "island-type hospital," the latter submitted the table of organization for this unit. The General Staff approved the table and it was published on 28 February 1942.[16]

The field hospital had a headquarters and three hospitalization units. Each of the latter could operate independently with a capacity of 100 beds. As a single unit the hospital could care for 380 patients. Staffed to care for minor ills and injuries and equipped to function in the field under tents, the field hospital or any one of its hospitalization units could serve as a fixed hospital on islands, in other isolated areas, or at air bases distant from other facilities. Having sufficient transportation to move its own personnel and equipment, any unit of the hospital, when reinforced with surgical personnel, could be used as a mobile hospital to support ground troops in combat or task forces in landing operations. In addition, the field hospital or any of its units, The Surgeon General asserted, could be readily transported by air—an assertion supported by

[16] (1) Interv, MD Historian with Brig Gen Alvin L. Gorby, 21 Feb 52. HD: 000.71. (2) Ltr AG 400(1–19–42)MSC–D, TAG to SG, 22 Jan 42, sub: Equip for Island Type Hosp. SG: 475.5–1. (3) DF G–3/42108, ACofS G–3 WDGS to ACofS G–1 and G–4 WDGS, 17 Feb 42, sub: T/O and E for a Fld Hosp Unit, with incl. AG: 320.2(10–30–41)(2). (4) History of Organization and Equipment Allowance Branch [SGO], 1939–44, p. 5. HD.

loading and flight tests during the latter part of 1942.[17]

The field hospital thus surpassed in flexibility any other hospital which the Medical Department had. In order to make units of that type available, SOS headquarters arranged for the activation of five in April 1942.[18] A few months later, when the troop basis was revised, authority was granted for the activation of twenty-two by the end of 1942.

During the months following the development of the field hospital, the Surgeon General's Office revised the table of organization for station hospital units to provide, in effect, additional types of fixed hospitals. At the beginning of the war the station hospital table of organization provided only for those of 250-, 500-, and 750-bed capacities.[19] When station hospital units of smaller capacities were needed, The Surgeon General had to prepare special tables for their activation. In May 1942, for example, a special table of organization for a 150-bed station hospital was issued.[20] Two months later the revised version of the regular table was ready for publication. It provided for station hospitals of seventeen different sizes, ranging in capacity from 25 to 900 beds.[21] The inclusion of station hospital units of various sizes in the 1943 troop basis simplified The Surgeon General's problem of recommending hospital support for small garrison forces.

At the same time that small fixed-hospital units were being supplied for garrison forces scattered throughout the world, the Surgeon General's Office was developing a combat zone hospital that was more mobile and required less personnel than either the 400-bed surgical hospital or the 750-bed evacuation hospital. The latter had no motor transport for its own movement and could be used only in relatively stable situations. The surgical hospital, developed in 1940, was only partially mobile. Its surgical unit was authorized enough transport to move itself but its two hospital units had only "utility" vehicles.[22]

In order to provide a more mobile combat zone hospital, The Surgeon General developed a 400-bed motorized evacuation hospital. Its table of organization, concurred in by the Ground Surgeon and approved by G-3, was published on 2 July 1942.[23] This unit, unlike the surgical and 750-bed evacuation hospitals, at first had enough motor transport to move all of its personnel and equipment at one time. It differed from the surgical hospital in organization also. It will be recalled that the latter had three independent units with separate headquarters—a surgical unit and two ward units. The motorized evacuation hospital, on the other hand, had no separate units and only one headquarters, but it could be split into two self-contained 200-bed surgical hospitals. This change in organization resulted

[17] (1) Memo, SG for TAG, 1 Feb 42, incl to DF G-3/42108, ACofS G-3 WDGS to ACofS G-1 and G-4 WDGS, 17 Feb 42, sub: T/O and E for Fld Hosp Unit. AG: 320.2(10-30-41)(2). (2) Ltr, SG to CG USAFIA, 26 Jun 42, sub: Fld Hosp, T/O 8-510. HD: Wilson files, 400 "Med Equip and Sups." (3) Memo, SG for CG SOS, 3 Oct 42, with 2d, 5th, and 6th inds. SG: 704.-1.

[18] Memo, SG for CG SOS, 22 Mar 42, sub: Activation of Fld Hosp Units, with 1st ind, CG SOS to SG, 1 Apr 42. SG: 322.3-33.

[19] T/O 8-508, Sta Hosp, ComZ, 25 Jul 40.

[20] T/O 8-560S, Sta Hosp (150-bed), 23 May 42.

[21] T/O 8-560, Sta Hosp, ComZ, 22 Jul 42.

[22] T/O 8-232, Evac Hosp, 1 Oct 40, and T/O 8-231, Surg Hosp, 1 Dec 40.

[23] (1) History of Organization and Equipment Allowance Branch [SGO], 1939-44, p. 4. HD. (2) Memo for Record on Memo, CG SOS for TAG, 1 Jul 42, sub: T/O for Evac Hosp (Motorized). AG: 320.3(10-30-41)(2) Sec 8D. (3) T/O 8-581, Evac Hosp, Motorized, 2 Jul 42.

in a saving of both enlisted and commissioned personnel—a factor of importance in the development of the new unit.[24]

The motorized evacuation hospital soon superseded the surgical hospital in the troop basis, although the table of organization of the latter was not rescinded until August 1944.[25] In August 1942 AGF headquarters, with the concurrence of The Surgeon General and the Ground Surgeon, had surgical hospitals, only three of which were used as such during the war, redesignated and converted into motorized evacuation hospitals. In November 1942 units of the new type were included, along with 750-bed evacuation hospitals, as mobile units in the 1943 troop basis.[26]

Since none of the hospital units available at the beginning of the war or developed in Washington in the following year met the needs of small combat forces fighting in Pacific jungles, the Southwest Pacific Area attempted during 1942 to solve its own problem. To provide surgical support for task forces employed in areas where the only practicable means of transportation was by foot, the chief surgeon of that area developed a 25-bed portable surgical hospital. It was designed to permit its equipment and supplies to be carried in 35- to 40-pound packs by its own personnel or by native bearers. It could therefore move along with combat troops through jungle trails, either to prepare casualties for the long litter-haul to the rear or to care for them until more adequate hospitals could be established. In September 1942 SWPA headquarters activated twenty-six such "provisional" units with personnel taken from other hospitals. Receiving reports of this development, The Surgeon General soon afterward adopted the portable surgical hospital as a regular unit. In November 1942, forty-eight were included in the 1943 troop basis. In May 1943 ASF headquarters ordered the activation of twenty under a special table of organization which was published the following month.[27]

Changes Affecting the Mobility of Hospitals

By the fall of 1942 circumstances developed which tended to cancel some of the results of earlier attempts of The Surgeon General to increase the mobility of hospitals. Shortages of motor equipment and of shipping space prompted the General Staff, on 2 October 1942, to direct the three major commands to reduce the motor vehicles authorized for their respective units.[28] In compliance with this order AGF headquarters reduced the transport of the motorized evacuation hospital (making it a semimobile unit) and the Surgeon General's Office reduced that of the field hospital. These hospitals were

[24] (1) Comparison of T/O 8-231, 1 Dec 40, and T/O 8-581, 2 Jul 42. (2) See also Off Diary of Col Albert G. Love, Chief HD, SGO, 8 Sep and 9 Oct 42. HD.

[25] (1) Memo, Col Arthur B. Welsh for Gen Kirk, 2 Dec 43. SG: 322.15-1-MEDC. (2) WD Cir 333, 15 Aug 44.

[26] (1) Memo 32.02/29(Med)(R)-GNGCT/(1 Aug 42), CG AGF for ACofS G-3 WDGS, 1 Aug 42, sub: Redesignation of Surg Hosp as Evac Hosp, with Memo for Record. Ground Med files: "Maneuvers, 1942." (2) Ltr, SG to CG ASF, 26 Apr 43, sub: Status of Surg Hosps. SG: 322.15-1.

[27] (1) An Rpt, Chief Surg SWPA, 1942. HD. (2) Ltr, Comdr-in-Chief SWPA to CG SOS, 21 Nov 42, sub: Improvement of Equip and Orgn, with 2 inds. SG: 322.15-10. (3) Memo, CG ASF for TAG, 26 May 43, sub: Constitution and Activation of Ptbl Surg Hosp. AG: 322(5-26-43). (4) T/O & E 8-572S, Ptbl Surg Hosp, 4 Jun 43.

[28] Ltr, TAG to CGs AGF, AAF, and SOS, 2 Oct 42, sub: Review of Orgn and Equip Reqmts. AG: 400(8-10-42)(1) sec 22.

left with enough transport for partial movements only. Each had to employ its vehicles in shuttle fashion or supplement them with "pool" vehicles in order to move from one location to another.[29] Reductions in allotments of motor vehicles to other hospital units had insignificant effects upon mobility, because their vehicles were used for administrative purposes only.[30]

Other ways of increasing the mobility of hospitals than by the formation of new units were reductions in the size and weight of equipment and improvements in methods of packing it. When war began, equipment lists of all hospitals contained types and quantities of items such as office desks, armchairs, and kitchen equipment which were ordinarily used only in hospitals in the United States.[31] In view of shortage of shipping space and the need for mobility in overseas hospitals, SOS headquarters directed The Surgeon General on 12 March 1942 to eliminate all unnecessary equipment and to reduce the gross weight and cubic displacement of station and general hospital assemblages by at least 40 percent.[32] The Surgeon General replied that his Office had already begun that process. On 30 June 1942 he reported that the required reduction had been made in station hospital assemblages and that it would be made in others at an early date.[33] During the following summer special boards appointed by The Surgeon General reviewed equipment lists of all hospitals, making reductions as they could, and sent the revised lists to medical depots for use in making up hospital assemblages. By November 1942 The Surgeon General reported to the Wadhams Committee that the gross weight and cubic displacement of all hospitals designed for overseas service had been reduced by an average of 40 to 42 percent.[34] By that time many hospitals with heavy bulky equipment were already in operation in overseas theaters.[35]

Shortly before The Surgeon General reported reductions in the size and weight of hospital equipment, the Ground Surgeon raised the question of its packing. He informed the Surgeon General's Office that equipment of evacuation hospitals was so packed that it did not lend itself readily to manual handling and speedy unpacking for setups. Meanwhile the 15th Evacuation Hospital, stationed at Fort George G. Meade, Maryland, conducted experiments in packing under the supervision of the Ground Surgeon.[36] The Surgeon General learned that this hospital

[29] (1) T/O 8-510, Fld Hosp, 28 Feb 42 and 8 Apr 43; T/O 8-581, Evac Hosp, Motorized, 2 Jul 42; and T/O 8-581, Evac Hosp, Semimobile, 8 Jan 43. (2) 1st ind 323.3 GNRQT-1/18390 (10-2-42), CG AGF to TAG, 1 Dec 42, on Ltr, TAG to CGs AGF, AAF, and SOS, 2 Oct 42, sub: Review of Orgn and Equip Reqmts. AG: 400 (8-10-42)(1) sec 22. (3) Ltr, SG to CG SOS, 14 Dec 42, sub: Changes in Fld Hosp. SG: 322.15-10. (4) 2d ind, SG to CG SOS, 10 Feb 43, on Ltr, Comdr-in-Chief SWPA to CG SOS, 21 Nov 42, sub: Improvement of Equip and Orgn. Same file.

[30] For example, see T/O 8-550, Gen Hosp, 1 Apr 42, and T/E 8-550, Gen Hosp, 19 Mar 43.

[31] Memo entitled "Correcting Info as to Confidential Document Submitted by Mr. [Corrington] Gill, Entitled 'Rpt to Cmtee on Data from Files of Hosp and Evac Br, Plans Div, SOS,' " submitted as incl to Ltr, SG to Col Sanford Wadhams, Chm, Cmtee to Study the MD, 7 Nov 42. HD: 321.6.

[32] Memo, Oprs Div SOS for SG, 12 Mar 42, sub: Increase in Mobility of Fld Force Hosps. SG: 475.5-1.

[33] Memos, SG for Oprs Div SOS, 21 Mar and 30 Jun 42. SG: 475.5-1.

[34] Memo cited, n. 31.

[35] (1) Memo SPOPH 701, CG SOS for SG, 19 Oct 42, sub: Info Submitted by Chief Surg SWPA. HD: Wilson files, "Book IV, 16 Mar 43-17 Jun 43." (2) Ltr, Med Insp NATO to SG, 27 Jan 43, sub: Observations on Med Serv in NATO. HD: Wilson files, "Experience in Med Matters from Overseas Forces."

[36] Comment by Brig Gen Frederick A. Blesse on first draft of this chapter. HD: 314 (Correspondence on MS) III, Incl 1.

had developed a method of packing its equipment so that each crate or package could be handled by two men and contained items used in one particular section of a hospital only.[37] In November 1942 General Magee appointed a board of officers to study this accomplishment and submit recommendations for more practical methods of packing and assembling equipment than those being used by medical depots.[38] As a result of this investigation, The Surgeon General's Supply Service drew up specifications for the standardized packing and crating of equipment of motorized evacuation hospitals.[39]

Subsequently, during 1943, the system found satisfactory for evacuation hospitals was adopted for other units. Each box, properly marked, now contained supplies and equipment for use in a particular section of a hospital only. This system speeded unpacking and repacking for movement in the field by making it possible to assemble at a particular spot all supplies and equipment needed for a ward, an operating room, or an office, and by making it unnecessary to unpack equipment not required when only part of a hospital was being established.[40]

Reductions in the Personnel of Hospital Units

Modifications in tables of organization of existing hospitals, like changes in equipment and motor transport, were required by other than medical considerations. During the early part of 1942 both G-1 and SOS headquarters put considerable pressure on The Surgeon General to save commissioned personnel, especially Medical Corps officers, lest there be insufficient numbers to go around, on the scale already planned, in a 7,500,000-man Army. Among the steps they directed him to take was the revision of tables of organization, both to reduce the number of officers authorized and to substitute Medical Administrative Corps for Medical Corps officers.[41] Having already begun the process of revision, The Surgeon General replied that he would continue it.[42] In April the revised tables for general, surgical, and convalescent hospitals and hospital centers were published; in July, those for evacuation and station hospitals.[43]

These revisions resulted in the saving of Medical Corps officers more by cuts in the number of such officers in each unit than by the substitution of Medical Administrative for Medical Corps officers. The reason lay perhaps in the fact that tables of organization for numbered hospitals, unlike personnel guides for zone of interior

[37] (1) Ltr, SG to CG SOS, 7 Oct 42, sub: Evac Hosp Equip. SG: 475.5-1. (2) An Rpt, 15th Evac Hosp Motorized, 1942. HD.

[38] (1) 1st ind, CG SOS to SG, 15 Oct 42, on Ltr, SG to CG SOS, 7 Oct 42, sub: Evac Hosp Equip. SG: 475.5-1. (2) SG OO 462, 11 Nov 42, sub: Bd of Offs to Study Equip of New 400-Bed Motorized Evac Hosp.

[39] (1) Rpt of Bd for . . . a 400-bed Evac Hosp [13 Nov 42]. SG: 475.5-1. (2) Memo, Lt Col R[euel] E. Hewitt for Col F[rancis] C. Tyng, 19 Dec 42. Same file.

[40] (1) Richard E. Yates, The procurement and Distribution of Medical Supplies in the Zone of the Interior during World War II (1946), p. 146. HD. (2) An Rpt, Med Assembly Unit Atlanta ASF Depot, 1943. HD.

[41] (1) Memo, ACofS G-1 WDGS for SG thru Pers Div SOS, 1 Apr 42, sub: Availability of Physicians. HRS: G-1/16331-16335. (2) Memo, CG SOS for SG, 22 May 42, sub: Availability of Physicians. Same file.

[42] (1) Memo, SG for Pers Div SOS, 27 Apr 42. HRS: G-1/16331-16335. (2) Memo, SG for Dir Mil Pers SOS, 5 Jun 42, sub: Availability of Physicians. Same file.

[43] T/O 8-550, Gen Hosp, 1 Apr 42; T/O 8-570, Surg Hosp, 1 Apr 42; T/O 8-590, Conv Hosp, 1 Apr 42; T/O 8-540, Hosp Ctr, 1 Apr 42; T/O 8-580, Evac Hosp, 750-bed, 2 Jul 42; T/O 8-560, Sta Hosp, 22 Jul 42.

installations,[44] already required the use of Medical Administrative Corps officers in a considerable proportion of administrative positions. The revised tables also reduced the number of nurses authorized for some hospitals. In general, greatest changes were made in large communications zone units, such as 1,000-bed general and 750-bed station hospitals. In the former, 17 Medical Corps officers and 15 nurses were eliminated; in the latter, 13 Medical Corps officers and 15 nurses. In each, one Medical Administrative Corps officer, one Sanitary Corps officer, and one warrant officer were added as replacements for some of the Medical Corps officers eliminated. In smaller communications zone units, such as the 250-bed station hospital, and in combat zone units, such as the 750-bed evacuation and the 400-bed surgical hospital, no personnel reductions were made, but from one to three Medical Administrative or Dental Corps officers were substituted for a like number of Medical Corps officers. The development of the 400-bed motorized evacuation hospital for use in the combat zone resulted in a considerable saving of both Medical and Nurse Corps personnel, because the new unit required fifteen physicians and twelve nurses fewer than did the surgical hospital which it replaced in the troop basis.[45]

In the fall of 1942 emphasis shifted from reductions in the numbers of officers and nurses to those of enlisted men. With a growing need for manpower economy in the Army, the General Staff in October directed the three major commands to revise downward their tables of organization.[46] By then responsible for tables of combat zone hospital units, AGF headquarters revised the tables of both the 400-bed and 750-bed evacuation hospitals. With The Surgeon General's concurrence, the number of enlisted men in a motorized evacuation hospital was reduced from 248 to 217; in a 750-bed unit, from 318 to 308. The revised tables reflected, incidentally, as did others published later, the militarization of hospital dietitians and physical therapists, who until December 1942 had served as civilian employees.[47] Cuts in the personnel of communications zone hospital units did not occur at this time, because SOS headquarters considered it "inadvisable," in view of revisions of tables within the preceding year, to direct any further "arbitrary reduction."[48]

Hospital Units in the Troop Basis

Throughout 1942 and 1943 the number of hospital units in the troop basis increased significantly with each of its revisions but always remained smaller than The Surgeon General considered adequate for the Army being mobilized. Using World War I casualty and evacuation experiences as a basis, The Surgeon General estimated that fixed beds should be

[44] See above, p. 133.

[45] T/O 8-508, Sta Hosp, 25 Jul 40; T/O 8-560, Sta Hosp. 22 Jul 42; T/O 8-507, Gen Hosp, 25 Jul 40; T/O 8-550, Gen Hosp, 1 Apr 42; T/O 8-232, Evac Hosp, 1 Oct 40; T/O 8-580, Evac Hosp, 2 Jul 42; T/O 8-231, Surg Hosp, 1 Dec 40; T/O 8-570, Surg Hosp, 1 Apr 42; T/O 8-581, Evac Hosp, Motorized, 2 Jul 42.

[46] Ltr, TAG to CGs AGF, AAF, and SOS, 2 Oct 42, sub: Review of Orgn and Equip Reqmts. AG: 400(8-10-42)(1) sec 22.

[47] (1) T/O 8-580, Evac Hosp, 750-bed, 23 Apr 43, and T/O 8-581, Evac Hosp, Semimobile, 8 Jan 43. (2) Memo 320.2/53(Med) GNRQT-3/26660 (11-18-42), CG AGF for ACofS G-3 WDGS, 1 Jan 43, sub: T/O and T/E 8-581, Evac Hosp, Semimobile. AG: 320.3 (10-30-41)(1) sec 8D. (3) Memo 321/732(Med) GNRQT-3/37444, CG AGF for ACofS G-3 WDGS, 16 Apr 43, sub: T/O and T/E, Evac Hosp (750 pnts). Same file.

[48] Memo SPGAE 011.1 (10-14-42), CG SOS for ACofS G-3 WDGS, 7 Dec 42, sub: Review of Orgn and Equip Reqmts. AG: 400(8-10-42)(1) sec 22.

provided for 10 to 15 percent of the strength of each theater of operations.[49] He calculated mobile bed requirements in the early part of 1942 on the basis of 1 convalescent, 4 surgical, and 10 evacuation hospitals for each type-army. The time when these units should be activated depended upon such factors as the amount of training required by each, the rate of troop movement to overseas areas, and the amount of combat action which might be encountered.

At the beginning of 1942 both G–3 and the Chief of Staff believed that the mobilization of service units should be delayed because the training of divisions required more time than that of nondivisional units and a lack of shipping limited forces that could be sent overseas during 1942.[50] Hence, in the troop basis issued on 17 January 1942, which provided for a 71-division, 3,600,000-man Army by the end of the year, there were included only 2 convalescent, 28 evacuation, 8 surgical, 45 general, and 40 station hospital units.[51] The Surgeon General urged that additional units be authorized, but the General Staff disapproved. In its opinion the 55,000 beds provided for in 45 general and 40 station hospitals would be adequate for the 550,000 troops which, it was expected, could be sent overseas during 1942.[52]

In the spring of 1942 plans were made to send a larger number of troops overseas during the rest of the year. Under the BOLERO plan, thirty divisions, or 1,000,000 men, were to be sent to the United Kingdom for an operation against the continent either late in 1942 or early in 1943. In May the President raised the size of the Army to be mobilized by the end of 1942 to 4,350,000.[53] The number of units originally thought requisite in view of these changes was reduced considerably in the course of discussions among representatives of SOS and AGF headquarters and the Surgeon General's Office, and on 23 May 1942 SOS headquarters recommended to G–3 that 2 convalescent, 6 evacuation, 8 surgical, 62 general, 103 station, 22 field hospitals and 9 hospital centers should be included in the revised troop basis, in addition to the units already authorized.[54] G–3 considered the recommended number of fixed-hospital units too large, but approved it when The Surgeon General explained that BOLERO alone would require 100,000 beds, or more than the number authorized in the additional units.[55]

---

[49] (1) Albert G. Love, "War Casualties," *Army Medical Bulletin* No. 24 (1931), pp. 53–68. (2) Off Diary of Col Albert G. Love, Chief HD SGO, 6 Mar 42. HD.

[50] Kent R. Greenfield, Robert R. Palmer and Bell I. Wiley, *The Organization of Ground Combat Troops* (Washington, 1947), p. 199, in UNITED STATES ARMY IN WORLD WAR II.

[51] Ltr, TAG to C of Arms and Servs, etc., 17 Jan 42, sub: Mob and Tng Plan, 1942. AG: 381(12–27–41)(2).

[52] (1) Memo, Act SG for ACofS G–3 WDGS, 28 Feb 42, sub: Orgn and Dispatch of MD TofOpns Units. SG: 322.3–1. (2) 2d ind AG 320.2(1–29–42) MSC–C, TAG to SG, 18 Feb 42, on Memo, C of Air Staff for SG, 29 Jan 42, sub: Expansion Program of AAF for Calendar Year 1942. HD: 320.2(Trp Basis).

[53] Greenfield *et al.*, *op. cit.*, pp. 201–06. Also see Ray S. Cline, *Washington Command Post: The Operations Division* (Washington, 1951), pp. 143–63, in UNITED STATES ARMY IN WORLD WAR II; and Maurice Matloff and Edwin M. Snell, *Strategic Planning for Coalition Warfare, 1941–42* (Washington, 1953), pp. 190–96, in UNITED STATES ARMY IN WORLD WAR II, for more information on BOLERO.

[54] (1) Memo, Lt Col A. B. Welsh for the Record, 13 Apr 42. HD: 320.2(Trp Basis). (2) Memo SPOPP 320.2 Serv Units (5–23–42), Dep Dir Oprs SOS for ACofS G–3 WDGS, 23 May 42, sub: Reqmts of Serv Units. . . . SG: 475.5–1.

[55] (1)Memo WDGCT 320.2(5–23–42), ACofS G–3 WDGS for CGs AGF and SOS, 25 May 42, sub: Reqmts of Serv Units. . . . SG: 475.5–1. (2) Memo, SG for Oprs Div SOS, 30 May 42, same sub. SG: 320.3–1. (3) Memo, ACofS G–3 WDGS for CG SOS, 5 Jun 42, same sub. Same file.

During the late summer and fall of 1942 plans for the 1943 troop basis, through which a 7,500,000-man Army was to be mobilized by the end of 1943,[56] called for sizable increases in the numbers of hospital units of all types. For the support of ground troops in combat, 7 convalescent, 20 evacuation, 52 semimobile evacuation, and 48 portable surgical hospitals were authorized for activation by December 1943. The number of fixed-hospital units which G–3 authorized—52 field, 192 general, and 327 station hospital units—was less than The Surgeon General recommended.[57] G–3's authorization of the smaller number apparently resulted from a shortage of physicians to staff more. The Surgeon General believed that enough beds and other equipment to care for the maximum estimate of sick and wounded men would have to be provided in any event. He therefore recommended again an increase in authorized units and urged that he be permitted, if his recommendation should be disapproved, to procure adequate equipment for overseas hospitals regardless of the troop basis.[58] Both G–3 and OPD agreed to the latter proposition and SOS headquarters arranged to assure the procurement of equipment which The Surgeon General considered necessary.[59]

The Question of Equipping and Using Numbered Hospitals in the Zone of Interior

Throughout 1942 and most of 1943 the Surgeon General's Office and SOS headquarters were engaged in an inconclusive dispute over the issuance of equipment to numbered hospital units and the use of such units on a functional basis in the United States. This dispute, like the one over planning for zone of interior hospitalization already discussed, exemplified difficulties resulting from misunderstanding about the respective responsibilities of the Surgeon General's Office and the SOS Hospitalization and Evacuation Branch. Of more significance, it involved the following problems: the method of training hospital units in the United States, the contribution of such units to the medical service during training periods, and whether or not such units should receive full issues of equipment in the United States.

After war began most hospital units in the zone of interior continued primarily as schools for tactical training. A few were issued full assemblages and operated hospitals on maneuvers. As a rule, though, under a policy announced in January 1942 and already discussed, hospital units received only field training equipment, soldiers' individual equipment, and motor transport, for use in unit field training. The Surgeon General expected them to receive technical training and experience with professional supplies and equipment in zone of interior hospitals. This "parallel" method of training seemed satisfactory when only one or two units were located on a particular post, but delay in construction of housing for a hospital unit near each of twenty-two general hospitals and

[56] Greenfield *et al.*, *op. cit.*, pp. 212–17.

[57] (1) Diary, Hosp and Evac Br SOS, 28 Oct 42. HD: Wilson files, "Diary." (2) Memo, SG for CG SOS, 25 Jan 43. HD: 632.–2. (3) Table, Auth Units (Hosp Type) in 1942 and 43 Trp Basis. HD: 320.2 (Trp Basis).

[58] (1) Memo, SG for CG SOS, 25 Jan 43. HD: 632.–2. (2) Ltr, SG for CG SOS, 6 Mar 43, sub: Adequacy of Plans for Overseas Hosp. SG: 322.15–1.

[59] (1) Memo SPOPH 701(3–6–42), Dir Plans Div ASF for Gen [LeRoy] Lutes, 15 Mar 43, sub: Adequacy of Plans for Overseas Hosp. HD: Wilson files, "Book III, 1 Jan 43–15 Mar 43." (2) 1st ind, ACofS for Oprs SOS to SG, 16 Mar 43, on Ltr, SG to CG SOS, 6 Mar 43, same sub. SG: 322.15–1.

thirty-four station hospitals in the United States, as The Surgeon General requested,[60] caused units to be grouped on posts wherever troop housing was available. Whenever this happened there were so many officers and men of numbered units in each named hospital concerned that they had to take turns serving alongside of, or "parallel" to, their opposite numbers.[61]

This entire system was challenged early in 1942. By March Colonel Wilson was convinced that hospital units could be best prepared for overseas service by being issued complete equipment and by being required to function as hospitals in the United States.[62] Moreover AGF headquarters wanted to train unit personnel in the storage, maintenance, and repair of hospital equipment and to have hospital units self-sufficient in so far as messing and administration were concerned. In May, therefore, AGF headquarters recommended that all hospital units scheduled for maneuvers and all newly activated units be given full issues of equipment for permanent retention.[63] The Surgeon General was willing to make some concessions to the Ground Forces but not to issue complete assemblages as SOS headquarters directed in June and again in August 1942. In a paper duel which his Office fought with SOS headquarters over this matter, The Surgeon General reached a point by 7 September 1942 of agreeing to the issuance of housekeeping equipment, but he requested approval of a policy of withholding all other equipment in assemblages until units were assigned to operational missions.[64]

By this time SOS headquarters had decided not only to force The Surgeon General to issue complete assemblages to all units but also to require him to employ units under SOS control in the zone of interior medical service. There seem to have been several reasons for this decision. In September 1942 a report from the Southwest Pacific Area emphasized the desirability of issuing equipment to units in training to permit them to learn to pack and move it easily and to reduce its size and weight by eliminating unnecessary items.[65] Moreover, many units were becoming restless from long periods of training without opportunities either to function as hospitals or to assist in zone of interior hospital operations; and stories of doctors being called from civilian practice only to sit and wait around Army camps

[60] Memo, Act SG for ACofS G-3 WDGS, 28 Feb 42, sub: Orgn and Dispatch of MD TofOpns Units. SG: 322.3-1.

[61] (1) For example, see the An Rpts, 1942 and/or 1943 of 3d, 6th, 23d, 50th, 79th, and 108th Gen Hosps and An Rpt, 1943, 36th Sta Hosp. HD. (2) Consolidated Rpt, SGs Observers for 1942 Maneuvers, transmitted to ASF Hq by Memo, SG for Dir Tng ASF, 16 Jun 43. Ground Med files: "Rpt of Maneuver Observers, SGO, 1942." (3) Memo, Dir Planning Div ASF for Gen Lutes, 4 Aug 43, sub: Sta Hosp in Maneuver Areas. Ground Med files: 354.2 "Maneuvers."

[62] Memo G-4/24499-178, Maj W. L. Wilson for Gen Lutes, 12 Mar 42, sub: Basic Plans for Hosp and Evac. HD: Wilson files, "No 472, Hosp and Evac, 1941-42."

[63] Ltr 475.5/49-GNSPL (5-26-42), CG AGF to Dir Oprs SOS, 26 May 42, sub: Equip for Med Units. HD: Wilson files, 400 "Med Equip and Sups."

[64] (1) 2d ind, SG to Dir Oprs SOS, 29 May 42; 3d ind, CG SOS to SG, 22 Jun 42; 4th ind, SG to Dir Oprs SOS, 30 Jun 42; 5th ind, CG SOS to SG, 9 Jul 42; 6th ind, SG to Dir Oprs SOS, 20 Jul 42; 7th ind, CG SOS to SG, 6 Aug 42; and 8th ind, SG to CG SOS, 7 Sep 42, on Memo 475/826-GNSPL(5-22-42), CG AGF for Dir Oprs SOS, 22 May 42, sub: Equip for MD Units. SG: 475.5-1. (2) Memo, Lt Col A[rthur] B. Welsh for Gen [Larry B.] McAfee, 11 Jun 42. HD: 320.2(Trp Basis). (3) Diary, Hosp and Evac Br SOS, 13 Aug 42. HD: Wilson files, "Diary."

[65] Ltr, Col P[ercy] J. Carroll to ACofS G-4 USASOS SWPA, 19 Sep 42, sub: Data for Lt Col [Willard S.] Wadelton. HD: Wilson files, "Experience in Med Matters from Overseas Forces." Colonel Wilson had asked Colonel Wadelton to get information for him on a visit of the latter to SWPA.

began to reach the public and the Army Inspector General.[66]

At the same time, it appeared that there would be insufficient Medical Department enlisted men and Medical Corps officers to supply both zone of interior installations and numbered units with their authorized numbers, and the General Staff began a drive for more efficient personnel utilization.[67] The chief of the SOS Hospitalization and Evacuation Branch believed that personnel required for zone of interior hospitals could be reduced by using numbered hospital units to help operate such installations. Furthermore, he believed that a reserve of hospital beds for emergencies could be provided by issuing equipment to numbered units.[68] In addition, some of the obstacles to assemblage-issuance and unit-use were being removed. Although equipment was still in short supply, the Surgeon General's Office and SOS headquarters were making renewed efforts to increase its availability. Housing, including warehouse space for equipment which had been authorized in the spring of 1942, was expected to be available for occupancy between September 1942 and January 1943.[69] Finally the Wadhams Committee was appointed early in September 1942, and SOS headquarters may have expected its support in this instance.[70] Whether because of one, some, or all of these reasons, SOS headquarters on 16 September and again on 12 October 1942 directed The Surgeon General to prepare a plan for the use of numbered hospital units in the zone of interior medical service and on 17 September 1942 requested his comments on the draft of a policy requiring the issuance of assemblages to all hospital units in training.[71]

Receipt of these communications caused confusion and consternation in the Surgeon General's Office. The Operations Service called for comments from other sections—the Supply, Professional, and Personnel Services and the Hospital Construction, Hospitalization, and Training Divisions. After several conferences to discuss the action that should be taken, final decision was to request no change in the policy on the issuance of equipment and to submit no plan for the use of numbered units. To support this decision, the Surgeon General's Office marshaled an array of arguments. The most important seem to have been lack of sufficient equipment to permit the issuance of assemblages to all

[66] (1) Memo for Record on Memo SPOPH 320.2, ACofS Oprs SOS (init WLW[ilson]) for SG, 16 Sep 42, sub: Asgmt, Tng, and Util of TofOpns Med Units. HD: Wilson files, "Book I, 26 Mar 42–26 Sep 42." (2) Diary, Hosp and Evac Br SOS, 25 Sep 42. HD: Wilson files, "Diary." (3) Memo, Dir Mil Pers Div SGO for Dir HD SGO, 14 Apr 44. HD: 326.1–1.

[67] See above, pp. 131–37, and Memo, DepCofSA for SG thru CG SOS, 17 Oct 42, sub: Availability of Physicians. SG: 322.05–1.

[68] Memo SPOPM 322.15, Chief Hosp and Evac Br SOS for Gen Lutes, 15 Sep 42, sub: Directive for Hosp and Evac Oprs. HD: Wilson files, "Book I, 26 Mar 42–26 Sep 42."

[69] (1) Memo, Chief Hosp and Evac Br SOS for Gen Lutes, 23 Aug 42, sub: Status of Procurement of Med Supplies. HD: Wilson files, 440 "Med Sups." (2) Memo, CofEngrs for SG, 19 Sep 42, sub: Fld Hosp Units. HD: 632 "Housing."

[70] Colonel Wilson stated to the Committee that one of the problems of the Medical Department was the development of a system for training medical units with their equipment before going overseas. Ltr, Chief Hosp and Evac Br Plans Div Oprs SOS for Chm, Cmtee to Study the MD, 21 Oct 42, sub: Med Problems. HD: Wilson files, "Book 2, 26 Sep 42–31 Dec 42."

[71] (1) Memo SPOPH 320.2, ACofS Oprs SOS (init WLW[ilson]) for SG, 16 Sep 42, sub: Asgmt, Tng, and Util of TofOpns Med Units. HD: Wilson files, "Book I, 26 Mar 42–26 Sep 42." (2) 1st ind SPOPH 320.2 (9-26-42), ACofS Oprs SOS (same init) to SG, 12 Oct 42, on Memo, SG for Oprs Div SOS, 26 Sep 42, same sub. HD: 632 "Hosp-Housing." (3) Draft Ltr SPOPP 475, CG SOS to SG, 17 Sep 42, sub: Equip for MD Units. SG: 475.5–1.

units and fear that the zone of interior medical service would be left in the lurch if numbered units were used to furnish it and were then sent overseas. To these were added other arguments. According to the Surgeon General's Office, units needed equipment neither for training nor for emergency hospitalization. Those in training could get experience with equipment in zone of interior hospitals and equipment required for emergencies could be shipped from depots when needed. Units were not qualified either to repack equipment for overseas shipment or to determine deletions and substitutions to reduce total weight. The former should be done by depots to prevent breakage and the latter could be done properly only by qualified boards and representatives of The Surgeon General. Units could not replace regularly assigned personnel in zone of interior hospitals without interrupting care of the sick and lowering the standard of professional work. Their mere presence near such hospitals constituted an adequate reserve of hospital facilities for emergencies; and their use as units would not reduce zone of interior personnel requirements because their members were already assisting in the medical service under the system of parallel training. Finally, The Surgeon General stated that he had no reason to believe that unit training was deficient. In requesting that existing policy on assemblage-issuance not be changed, The Surgeon General's supply representative explained personally to SOS headquarters the shortage of medical equipment. In refusing to submit a plan for the use of numbered units, The Surgeon General called attention to a plan for providing an effective medical service for a 7,500,000-man Army with 48,000 to 50,000 physicians which he was submitting at the request of the Deputy Chief of Staff of the Army.[72]

In this instance, SOS headquarters adopted a more lenient attitude toward The Surgeon General's action than might have been expected. Perhaps this resulted from an awareness of the critical aspect of the medical supply situation and from some hesitancy to push The Surgeon General when he had orders from the Deputy Chief of Staff of the Army to present a "plan." Perhaps it resulted from the apparent inclination of the Wadhams Committee toward The Surgeon General's position rather than that of the SOS Hospitalization and Evacuation Branch.[73] At any rate, SOS headquarters tabled the directive requiring a plan for the use of numbered units,[74] and the chief of its Hospitalization and Evacuation Branch worked out a compromise on the assemblage-issuance question. He adopted a new definition of assemblages, proposed by the SOS Plans Branch: henceforth assemblages would contain only Medical Department items. Items needed by hospitals but supplied by other services, such

[72] (1) Memo, SG for Oprs Div SOS, 26 Sep 42, sub: Med Unit Assemblages. SG: 475.5-1. (2) Memo, SG for Oprs Div SOS, 26 Sep 42, sub: Asgmt, Tng, and Util of TofOpns Med Units, with 2d ind, Act SG to Chief Oprs Div SOS, 14 Nov 42. SG: 320.2. Numerous memos from chiefs of various sections of SGO giving these arguments are in HD: 632 "Hosp-Housing."

[73] Cmtee to Study the MD, 1942, Testimony, pp. 1869ff. HD. After the war General Lutes stated that General Somervell personally directed a "lenient attitude" toward the Surgeon General's Office because of the Wadhams Committee's report. He was proceeding cautiously, General Lutes stated, to determine who was correct. Ltr, Lt Gen LeRoy Lutes to Col R[oger] G. Prentiss, Jr, 8 Nov 50. HD: 314 (Correspondence on MS) III.

[74] 3d ind SPOPH 320.2 (9-26-42), CG SOS to SG, 22 Nov 42, on Memo, SG for Oprs Div SOS, 26 Sep 42, sub: Asgmt, Tng, and Util of TofOpns Med Units. SG: 320.2.

as the Quartermaster Corps, would not be included in assemblages and would be issued whenever units requested them. The Surgeon General would determine the time when enough Medical Department equipment was available to issue complete assemblages to all units. Until that time he would make partial issues. Afterward, he would issue complete assemblages to all hospital units under AGF control. Assemblages for station and general hospitals under SOS control would be located in Medical Department depots so that delivery could be made in emergencies within seven days and so that units in training might readily inspect and study them.[75] When the Surgeon General's Office found even this policy unsatisfactory, SOS headquarters delayed announcing it officially until the medical supply situation had improved. Then, on 18 January 1943, SOS headquarters had the new policy published.[76]

At the beginning of the new year a combination of circumstances caused a revival of the question of using numbered units in the zone of interior. Contrary to what might have been expected, the "plan" which The Surgeon General submitted to the Deputy Chief of Staff on 14 December 1942 did not deal with this question, but only with the bulk allotment of Medical Corps officers to the three major commands.[77]

Soon afterward, in January 1943, the SOS Director of Training received criticism from at least one service command of deficiencies in unit training. About the same time the chief of the SOS Hospitalization and Evacuation Branch reported that failure to use units while in the United States was being criticized publicly. He then requested and received authority from his superior officer in SOS headquarters to collaborate with the SOS Training Director and the Surgeon General's Office in working out a plan to answer such criticism.[78] In a subsequent conference of representatives of the Surgeon General's Office AGF headquarters, and SOS headquarters, it was "unanimously agreed," the last reported, that The Surgeon General would estimate the amount of medical personnel required for hospital service at each camp of 10,000 or greater population, would determine the minimum permanent staff required for each hospital at those camps, and would make a definite plan, based upon OPD shipment schedules, for the use of numbered units to operate such hospitals under the supervision of permanent staffs.[79] The chief of the SOS Hospitalization and Evacuation Branch then took a trip around the country and found, he reported, that each service command surgeon agreed that he could operate a satis-

[75] (1) Draft memo SPOPH 475(9-26-42), CG SOS for SG, 23 Oct 42, sub: Equip for Fld Med Units. HD: Wilson files, "Book 2, 26 Sep 42-31 Dec 42." (2) Diary, Hosp and Evac Br SOS, 1 Nov 42. HD: Wilson files, "Diary." (3) Memo SPOPH 475(9-26-42), Chief Hosp and Evac Br SOS for Chief Plans Br SOS, 2 Nov 42, sub: Med Unit Assemblages. HD: Wilson files, "Book 2, 26 Sep 42-31 Dec 42."

[76] (1) WD Memo W700-4-43, 18 Jan 43, sub: Equip for Fld Med Units. HD: Wilson files, "Book III, 1 Jan 43-15 Mar 43." (2) Memo SPOPH 440, Chief Hosp and Evac Br SOS for Gen Lutes, 27 Jan 43, sub: Status of Procurement of Med Sups. Same file.

[77] Memo, Act SG for DepCofSA thru Mil Pers Div SOS, 14 Dec 42, sub: Availability of Physicians. SG: 322.051-1.

[78] (1) Memo, CG SOS (Tng Div) for SG, 5 Jan 43, sub: Tng of MC Pers. SG: 353.-1. (2) Memo SPOPH 320.2, Chief Hosp and Evac Br SOS for Gen Lutes, 16 Jan 43, sub: Asgmt, Tng, and Util of TofOpns Med Units. HD: Wilson files, "Book III, 1 Jan 43-15 Mar 43."

[79] (1) Diary, Hosp and Evac Br SOS, 20 Jan 43. HD: Wilson files, "Diary." (2) Memo, Maj J[ohn] S. Poe for the Record, 21 Jan 43, sub: Conf 4A526 Pentagon Bldg, 20 Jan 43. HD: 632 "Hosp-Housing."

factory hospital service under the proposed plan.[80]

The plan which The Surgeon General presented on 14 April 1943 indicated that agreement on the subject had not been unanimous. Instead of providing for the use of numbered units to operate zone of interior hospitals, it called for the use of members of such units, on a two-for-one basis, to make up deficits in personnel—that is, differences between assigned and authorized strength in zone of interior hospitals. "This was done," The Surgeon General stated, "because the primary function of the T/O unit is TRAINING."[81]

By this time seventy-eight general hospitals were reported "back-logged" in the United States, with no immediate prospect of employment overseas. Both the chief of the ASF Hospitalization and Evacuation Branch and the ASF Director of Training feared that the General Staff would reduce the number of Medical Department units in the troop basis if they were not fully used.[82] Before he could take further action toward that end Colonel Wilson was succeeded in his position in SOS headquarters by Col. (later Brig. Gen.) Robert C. McDonald, and for a time the question remained in abeyance.

Meanwhile changes occurred in the training and use of some hospital units. Completion of housing near zone of interior hospitals made it possible to train more personnel than before on a "parallel" basis;[83] and year-round use by the Ground Forces of the A. P. Hill Military Reservation and the Desert Training Center provided opportunities for several units to function as hospitals, furnishing medical and surgical care for patients in those areas.[84] The issuance of assemblages to evacuation hospital units under the revised policy permitted them to train with full equipment and work out a system of functional packing to increase unit mobility.[85] Yet as a rule general and station hospital units still lacked assemblages in the United States and had infrequent opportunities to function as hospitals before going overseas. Meanwhile, the time which some of them spent in training lengthened considerably. For example, although affiliated units had been intended for prompt shipment overseas, the fifty-one affiliated general hospital units that were eventually sent out remained in the United States for an average of eight months. One, the 27th General Hospital unit, stayed in this country seventeen months. *(Tables 6, 7)*

The unsolved problems of assemblage-issuance and unit-use faced Surgeon General Kirk when he succeeded General Magee in June 1943. Soon afterward he took them up with Colonel McDonald. Perhaps the entry of new participants made solution easier, for neither was unalterably committed to the position of his predecessor. In addition, despite his ASF position, Colonel McDonald identified himself closely with the Medical Department and held personal views of these

---

[80] Memo SPOPI 337, CG SOS (init WLW[ilson]) for SG and CofT, 30 Apr 43, sub: Resume of Confs. HD: Wilson files, "Book IV, 16 Mar 43–17 Jun 43."

[81] Ltr, SG to CG ASF, 14 Apr 43, sub: Asgmt of TofOpns Units for Tng. SG: 632.-1.

[82] (1) Memo SPOPI 322(4-14-43), ACofS Oprs SOS (init WLW[ilson]) for Dir Tng ASF, 19 Apr 43, sub: Asgmt of TofOpns Units. HD: Wilson files, "Book IV, 16 Mar 43–17 Jun 43." (2) Memo SPTRU 370.5 (4-19-43), Dir Tng ASF for ACofS Oprs ASF, 27 Apr 43, same sub. SG: 353.-1.

[83] 1st ind, SG to Dir Tng SOS, 9 Jan 43, on Memo, CG SOS for SG, 5 Jan 43, sub: Tng of MC Pers. SG: 353.-1.

[84] See above, pp. 104–06.

[85] An Rpts, 1943, of following Evac Hosps: 27th, 32d, 39th, 51st, 99th, 103d, 106th, 110th, and 145th. HD.

Number of Unit	Affiliation	Date of Activation	Date of Embarkation	Initial Destination
1st	Bellevue Hospital, New York, N. Y.	10 Jun 43	28 Dec 43	England
2d	Presbyterian Hospital, New York, N. Y.	31 Jan 42	1 Jul 42	England
3d	Mt. Sinai Hospital, New York, N. Y.	1 Sep 42	4 May 43	N. Africa
4th	Western Reserve University, Cleveland, Ohio	13 Jan 42	23 Jan 42	Australia
5th	Harvard University, Boston, Mass.	3 Jan 42	19 Feb 42	N. Ireland [a]
6th	Massachusetts General Hospital, Boston, Mass.	15 May 42	7 Feb 43	N. Africa
7th	Boston City Hospital, Boston, Mass.	10 Jun 43	5 Dec 43	England
9th	Society of the New York Hospital, New York, N. Y.	15 Jul 42	31 Jul 43	Guadalcanal
12th	Northwestern University, Chicago, Ill.	28 Jan 42	12 Dec 42	N. Africa
13th	Presbyterian Hospital, Chicago, Ill.	15 Jan 43	5 Jan 44	New Guinea
17th	Harper Hospital, Detroit, Mich.	15 Jul 42	30 Jul 43	N. Africa
18th	The Johns Hopkins Hospital, Baltimore, Md.	20 Apr 42	26 May 42	New Zealand
19th	Rochester General Hospital, Rochester, N. Y.	24 Jul 42	5 Sep 43	England
20th	University of Pennsylvania, Philadelphia, Pa.	15 May 42	19 Jan 43	India
21st	Washington University, St. Louis, Mo.	12 Jan 42	20 Oct 42	England
23d	Buffalo General Hospital, Buffalo, N. Y.	15 Jul 42	29 Jul 43	N. Africa
24th	Tulane University, New Orleans, La.	15 Jul 42	21 Aug 43	N. Africa
25th	Cincinnati General Hospital and University of Cincinnati, Ohio	10 Jun 43	23 Dec 43	England
26th	University of Minnesota, Minneapolis, Minn.	1 Feb 42	20 Oct 42	England
27th	University of Pittsburgh, Pittsburgh, Pa.	15 Jul 42	5 Jan 44	Australia
29th	University of Colorado, Denver, Colo.	1 Sep 42	3 Nov 43	New Caledonia
30th	University of California, San Francisco, Calif.	15 May 42	4 Jun 42	England
31st	Denver General Hospital, Denver, Colo.	1 Jun 43	18 Oct 43	Espiritu Santo
32d	University of Indiana, Indianapolis, Ind.	15 Jan 43	5 Sep 43	England
33d	Albany Hospital, Albany, N. Y.	15 Jul 42	7 Jul 43	N. Africa
36th	Wayne University, Detroit, Mich.	28 May 43	20 Aug 43	N. Africa
37th	Kings County Hospital, Brooklyn, N. Y.	15 Jan 43	7 Jul 43	N. Africa
38th	Jefferson Medical College, Philadelphia, Pa.	15 May 42	21 Sep 42	Egypt (Suez)
39th	Yale University, New Haven, Conn.	15 Jul 42	3 Nov 42	New Zealand
42d	University of Maryland, Baltimore, Md.	20 Apr 42	19 May 42	Australia
43d	Emory University, Atlanta, Ga.	1 Sep 42	21 Aug 43	N. Africa
44th	University of Wisconsin, Madison, Wis.	15 Jan 43	25 Sep 43	Australia
45th	Medical College of Virginia, Richmond, Va.	15 May 42	21 Mar 43	N. Africa
46th	University of Oregon, Portland, Oreg.	15 Jul 42	21 Aug 43	N. Africa
47th	College of Medical Evangelists, Loma Linda, Calif.	10 Jun 43	11 Jan 44	New Guinea
50th	Seattle College, Seattle, Wash.	4 Sep 42	29 Dec 43	England
52d	Syracuse University, Syracuse, N. Y.	1 Sep 42	6 Jan 43	England
58th	Western Pennsylvania Hospital, Pittsburgh, Pa.	15 Jan 43	8 Oct 43	England
64th	Louisiana State University, New Orleans, La.	15 Jul 42	21 Aug 43	N. Africa
65th	Duke University, Durham, N. C.	15 Jul 42	13 Oct 43	England
67th	Maine General Hospital, Portland, Maine	1 Sep 42	24 Nov 42	England
70th	St. Louis University, St. Louis, Mo.	1 Jun 43	21 Aug 43	N. Africa
71st	Mayo Foundation of University of Minnesota, Rochester, Minn.	10 Jun 43	Disbanded 24 Jun 43 [b]	
79th	Long Island College of Medicine, Brooklyn, N. Y.	21 Sep 42	9 Oct 43	N. Ireland
105th	Harvard University, Boston, Mass.	20 Apr 42	19 May 42	Australia
108th	Loyola University, Chicago, Ill.	10 Jun 43	8 Oct 43	England
118th	The Johns Hopkins Hospital, Baltimore, Md.	21 Apr 42	19 May 42	Australia
127th	University of Texas, Galveston, Tex.	15 Jan 43	8 Oct 43	England
142d	University of Maryland, Baltimore, Md.	20 Apr 42	26 May 42	New Zealand
297th	Cook County Hospital, Chicago, Ill.	10 Jun 43	30 May 44	England
298th	University of Michigan, Ann Arbor, Mich.	27 Jun 42	20 Oct 42	England
300th	Vanderbilt University, Nashville, Tenn.	17 Jul 42	21 Aug 43	N. Africa

[a] This unit returned from Nova Scotia to Boston on 4 March 1942 and embarked again at New York on 12 May 1942.

[b] The professional and enlisted personnel of this unit was used to staff the 233d and 237th Station Hospitals, which embarked for Australia on 5 January 1944. The 233d Station Hospital was reorganized and redesignated the 247th General Hospital on 15 October 1944. After the war, on 7 February 1947, the 237th Station Hospital and the 247th General Hospital were consolidated to form again the 71st General Hospital, an inactive unit, to preserve its affiliation with the Mayo Foundation.

Sources: Unit cards filed in Orgn and Directory Section, Oprs Br, AGO; from annual reports filed in HD; and miscellaneous AG and SG files pertaining to individual units.

problems similar to those advocated by the Surgeon General's Office.[86]

General Kirk believed that the current policy on assemblage-issuance might be partly responsible for a problem which theaters had reported and complained of—the receipt of equipment for a single hospital on several vessels at widely separated ports.[87] In July 1943, therefore, he requested its reconsideration. First he proposed a return to the policy advocated by

[86] Interv, MD Historian with Brig Gen Robert C. McDonald, Ret, USA, 5 Mar 51. HD: 000.71.

[87] An Rpt, Issue Br Sup Serv SGO, FY 1944. HD.

TABLE 7—AFFILIATED EVACUATION HOSPITAL UNITS

Number of Unit	Affiliation	Date of Activation	Date of Embarkation	Initial Destination
2d	St. Luke's Hospital, New York, N. Y.	22 Jan 42	4 Sep 42	N. Ireland
7th	New York Post-Graduate Medical School, New York, N. Y.	22 Jan 42	7 Apr 42	Tongatabu
8th	University of Virginia, Charlottesville, Va.	8 Aug 42	2 Nov 42	N. Africa
9th	Roosevelt Hospital, New York, N. Y.	24 Aug 42	26 Sep 42	England
12th	Lenox Hill Hospital, New York, N. Y.	12 Aug 42	6 Jan 43	England
14th	City Hospital, New York, N. Y.	15 Aug 42	10 Jul 43	India
16th	Michael Reese Hospital, Chicago, Ill.	15 Oct 42	14 Apr 43	N. Africa
21st	Oklahoma School of Medicine, Oklahoma City, Okla.	17 Aug 42	29 Aug 43	Guadalcanal
25th	West Suburban Hospital, Oak Park, Ill.	18 Aug 42	19 Oct 42	New Zealand
27th	University of Illinois, Chicago, Ill.	15 Oct 42	3 Apr 44	N. Africa
30th	University of Texas, Galveston, Tex.[a]	15 Jul 42	7 Sep 43	Australia
38th	Charlotte Memorial Hospital, Charlotte, N. C.	16 Apr 42	5 Aug 42	England
48th	Rhode Island Hospital, Providence, R. I.	13 Aug 42	18 Jan 43	India
51st	Sacramento County Hospital, Sacramento, Calif.	24 Oct 42	3 Apr 44	N. Africa
52d	Pennsylvania Hospital, Philadelphia, Pa.	12 Jan 42	23 Jan 42	New Caledonia
56th	Baylor University, Dallas, Tex.	4 Apr 42	16 Apr 43	N. Africa
59th	San Francisco Hospital, San Francisco, Calif.	6 Apr 42	12 Dec 42	N. Africa
73d	Los Angeles County General Hospital, Los Angeles, Calif.	2 Jan 42	20 Jan 43	India
77th	University of Kansas, Kansas City, Kans.	10 May 42	5 Aug 42	England
92d	St. Mary's Hospital, Pueblo, Colo.[b]	25 Aug 42	28 Jun 43	Australia

[a] The 30th Evacuation Hospital was supplied with professional personnel from the 30th Surgical Hospital, a unit affiliated with the University of Texas but never activated. On 13 September 1942 the 30th Evacuation Hospital was redesignated the 30th Evacuation Hospital (Motorized); early in January 1943 it was changed to the 30th Evacuation Hospital, Semimobile.

[b] The 7th Surgical Hospital, a nonaffiliated unit activated on 1 August 1940, was redesignated the 92d Evacuation Hospital (Motorized) on 25 August 1942. Early in 1943 it was renamed the 92d Evacuation Hospital, Semimobile. Officers and nurses of the 64th Surgical Hospital, a unit affiliated with St. Mary's Hospital, Pueblo, Colo., and never activated, had been assigned to the 7th Surgical Hospital. In July 1945 the 64th Surgical Hospital was reconstituted on the inactive list of the Army to preserve its identity and its affiliation with St. Mary's Hospital.

Sources: Unit cards filed in Orgn and Directory Section, Oprs Br, AGO; from annual reports filed in HD; and miscellaneous AG and SG files pertaining to individual units.

his predecessor—withholding all equipment for hospital units until they reached ports of embarkation—and then a compromise between that and the existing policy. Ultimately he withdrew both proposals. After an investigation of split shipments, Colonel McDonald reported that the current policy seemed to have little effect in causing such a problem. Furthermore, representatives of The Surgeon General agreed that a change in policy might produce a six-to-twelve month period of confusion in supply matters.[88] Thus the policy on the issuance of equipment to

[88] (1) Ltr, SG to CG ASF, 10 Jul 43, sub: Equip for Fld Med Units. SG: 475.5-1. (2) 1st ind SPOPI 008 (7-10-43), CG ASF to SG, 9 Aug 43, on basic Ltr just cited. HD: Wilson files, "Day File, Aug 43." (3) Ltr, SG to CG ASF, 6 Aug 43, sub: Equip for Fld Med Units. HRS: ASF Control Div, 334 "Procedure Cmtee, G-58." (4) Diary, Hosp and Evac Br ASF, 27 Aug 43. HD: Wilson files, 400 "Med Equip and Sups." (5) Memo for Record, 7 Sep 43, on Memo, SG for Col R. C. McDonald, Plans Div Oprs ASF, 7 Sep 43. SG: 475.5-1. (6) 1st ind SPOPI 440 (6 Aug 43), CG ASF to SG, 28 Aug 43, on basic Ltr cited in (3) above. HD: Wilson files, "Day File, Aug 43."

numbered medical units, which the Surgeon General's Office had formerly opposed, remained in effect for the rest of the war.[89]

General Kirk called for a full discussion of the question of using numbered hospital units in the zone of interior medical service in his first conference with service command surgeons. They agreed that the existing situation was deplorable. For example, one stated that it was difficult, when several units were located on a single post, to schedule their personnel for "parallel training" without having men "falling all over each other." Another, stressing morale, stated that one unit had been in his command "so long that they've worn out all of their films showing them over and over, and they've worn out all their shoes doing the same hikes. . . ."

In general, service command surgeons seemed favorably inclined toward the proposal to use numbered units in the operation of zone of interior hospitals, but several feared that administrative difficulties might arise unless units and their commanding officers were placed under the control of station surgeons. Others believed that professional problems might develop if numbered units were withdrawn from named hospitals either for field training or for overseas service without adequate personnel being left behind to operate zone of interior hospitals.[90] To avoid such a situation, the Surgeon General's Office announced that the adoption of any plan for the use of numbered units to operate zone of interior hospitals was contingent upon two conditions: first, the assignment of two hospital units to the named hospital in which they were to serve, and second, the existence of suitable barracks to house such units. Colonel McDonald agreed to these conditions and suggested that the Surgeon General's Office prepare a plan for trial on one post The chief of The Surgeon General's Training Division lacked enthusiasm for this proposal but agreed to investigate its possibilities.[91] Accordingly he drafted a plan by November 1943 for consideration by other officers of the Surgeon General's Office, but their comments indicated no diminution of opposition to the basic idea.[92]

By that time events were taking place which were to cause the whole matter to be dropped. In September 1943 the General Staff forbade the use of War Department funds to build more housing for numbered hospitals in the United States, thereby denying quarters for the two units per named hospital which The Surgeon General had recommended.[93] The next month the ASF Hospitalization and Evacuation Branch, which had initiated

[89] (1) See above, pp. 45–46, 141–42. (2) Rpt of Subcmtee on Employment of Med Resources, Cmtee on Med and Hosp Serv of Armed Forces, Off SecDef, 25 May 48, pp. 394–95. HD.

[90] (1) Rpt, SGs Conf with Chiefs Med Br SvCs, 14–17 Jun 43, pp. 242, 244, 245, 259, 260. HD: 337. (2) Memo, CG SOS (SG) for CGs of SvCs, 12 Jul 43, sub: Asgmt of TofOpns Units for Tng . . . , with inds from SvCs in reply. SG: 353.-1.

[91] Rpt, SGs Conf with Chiefs Med Br SvCs, 14–17 Jun 43, pp. 253–64. HD: 337. (2) Diary, Hosp and Evac Br ASF, 16 Jun 43. HD: Wilson files, "Diary."

[92] (1) Memo, Maj C[arl] C. Sox for Col A. B. Welsh, 10 Nov 43, sub: Comments on Tentative Plan for the Functional Employment of Numbered ASF Med Units. (2) Memo, Maj John S. Poe for no addressee, 10 Nov 43, sub: Comments on Col Wakeman's Proposal. (3) Memo, Col A. B. Welsh for Gen R. W. Bliss, 12 Nov 43. (4) Memo, Col A. H. Schwichtenberg for Gen R. W. Bliss, 13 Nov 43, sub: Comments on Tentative Plan. . . . All in SG: 322.3-1.

[93] (1) Memo, Maj J. S. Poe for Col H[oward] T. Wickert, 7 Jul 43. HD: 632 "Hosp Housing." (2) Memo Maj J. S. Poe for Col A. B. Welsh, 16 Sep 43. Same file.

and pushed the proposal, was abolished. Of greater importance was the change in conditions that had prompted the proposal in the first place. From the middle of 1943 onward the pressing need for hospitals overseas caused the departure of most units which had been held back as well as the prompt shipment of others after brief periods of training.[94] This disposed of the argument that services of personnel, especially doctors, were being wasted. It meant also that fewer and fewer units were left for use in hospitals at home. Finally, during the latter half of 1943 the troop population of the United States began to shrink so rapidly that the general employment of numbered hospital units to assist with medical care in the zone of interior perhaps no longer seemed useful. As a result, the long and tedious controversy between the Surgeon General's Office and ASF headquarters over the equipment and use in the United States of numbered hospital units reached an inconclusive end.

Preparing for the Support of Offensive Warfare

Shift of Emphasis Away From the Pacific

By about the middle of 1942, when emphasis in providing hospitalization for theaters shifted from the Pacific to other areas of the world, emergency needs resulting from the Japanese attack had been met and preparations for the invasion of North Africa were under way. To support the build-up of troops in the United Kingdom and subsequent successful North African operations, hospitals went in increasing numbers to both the European and the North African theaters in the last half of 1942 and the early months of 1943. During the same period other units were sent to scattered areas throughout the world to care for troops engaged in service functions in support of more active theaters. Since combat on a large scale had not yet begun, fixed hospitals were needed more than mobile ones, and station more than general hospitals. For example, by 15 March 1943 the War Department had shipped overseas, according to The Surgeon General's records, 140 station hospitals, ranging in size from 25- to 750-bed capacity, 27 general hospitals, and 14 field hospitals, but only 2 convalescent, 3 surgical, 17 750-bed evacuation, and 6 400-bed evacuation hospitals.[95]

Of those shipped after 30 June 1942, the major portions were units that had been activated and trained after the war began. A few of the units that were activated during 1941 and were still in the United States in mid-1942 were sent overseas in the following months, but the majority of the older units continued during the early war years as training units, furnishing filler personnel for others activated during 1942 and 1943 or for affiliated units previously organized. *(Tables 8, 9, 10, 11.)* As in the first six months of the war, although affiliated units continued to come on active duty on The Surgeon General's recommendation, many did not go overseas immediately. For example, although forty-two affiliated general hospital units had been activated by the middle of January 1943, only nineteen of them had been shipped by 15 March 1943. The remain-

[94] (1) See below, pp. 218–23. (2) Memo, Dep Chief Oprs Serv SGO for Dir Hosp Div SGO, 17 Feb 44, with incl. SG: 323.3.

[95] Table entitled Medical SOS Units as of 15 March 1943. SG: 322.05–1.

TABLE 8—USE OF NONAFFILIATED GENERAL HOSPITAL UNITS ACTIVATED DURING 1941

Unit Designation	Date of Activation	Supplied Enlisted Personnel for Affiliated Units that Embarked January–July 1942			Went to Theaters of Operations January–July 1942		Supplied Cadres for Other Units and Later Went Overseas	Supplied Cadres for Other Units and Later Were Inactivated	
		Unit Designation	Date of Embarkation	Destination	Date of Embarkation	Destination	Date of Embarkation	Date of Inactivation	Date of Disbandment
53d	10 Feb 41						29 Dec 43		
56th	1 Feb 41	4th	23 Jan 42	Australia			12 Oct 43		
63d	10 Feb 41						15 Jan 43		
66th	10 Feb 41	5th	19 Feb 42	N. Ireland				15 Apr 43	11 Nov 44
147th	1 May 41				16 Jun 42	Hawaii			
148th	10 Feb 41				21 Mar 42	Hawaii			
183d	10 Feb 41							14 Jan 43	11 Nov 44
203d	10 Feb 41	105th	19 May 42	Australia			29 Dec 43		
204th	10 Feb 41				8 Apr 42	Hawaii			
207th	10 Feb 41	30th	4 Jun 42	England				15 Jan 43	11 Nov 44
208th	1 Jun 41				18 Feb 42	Iceland			
209th	1 Jun 41	2d	1 Jul 42	England				10 Jun 43	11 Nov 44
210th	1 Jun 41				8 Jan 42	Panama Canal Zone			
212th	1 Jun 41							15 Jan 43	11 Nov 44
213th	27 Jun 41							15 Jan 43	11 Nov 44
214th	1 Jun 41							15 Jan 43	11 Nov 44
215th	16 May 41	42d	19 May 42	Australia				15 Apr 43	11 Nov 44
216th	1 Jun 41						13 Mar 44		
217th	1 Jun 41	142d	26 May 42	New Zealand			28 Feb 44		
218th	6 Jun 41				8 Jan 42	Panama Canal Zone			
222d	16 Jun 41	18th	26 May 42	New Zealand			1 Apr 44[a]		
223d	17 Jun 41							15 Apr 43	11 Nov 44

[a] As 134th General Hospital.

Sources: Unit cards filed in Orgn and Directory Section, Oprs Br, AGO, and annual reports filed in HD.

der stayed in this country in a training status until later in 1943 or early in 1944. *(See Table 6)*

Negro Hospital Units

Among the hospital units prepared early in the war for overseas service were two with Negro personnel. Their activation and use, like the establishment of all-Negro wards and hospitals in the United States,[96] resulted from The Surgeon General's opposition to the integration of Negro and white personnel in providing medical service for the Army—a position in line with the War Department's general policy on the use of Negro personnel.[97] On 24 March 1942 the 25th Station Hospital, a 250-bed unit, was organized at Fort Bragg (North Carolina). All of its members were Negroes except four officers—the commander and his immediate staff. The use of white officers to command Negro units was a common practice of the War Department and was not considered a violation of the policy of segregation. Its

[96] See above, pp. 110–12.

[97] John H. McMinn and Max Levin, Personnel (MS for companion vol. in Medical Dept. series), HD., and Ulysses Lee, The Employment of Negro Troops, a forthcoming volume in the series UNITED STATES ARMY IN WORLD WAR II.

TABLE 9—USE OF NONAFFILIATED STATION HOSPITAL UNITS ACTIVATED DURING 1941

Unit Desig-nation	Date of Activation	Embarked During 1941		Embarked January–July 1942		Embarked After 1 July 1942	
		Date	Destination	Date	Destination	Date	Destination
1st	10 Feb 41			30 Jan 42	Christmas Island		
5th	7 Jan 41			17 Feb 42	Australia		
7th	10 Feb 41					26 Sep 42	N. Ireland.
8th	10 Feb 41			17 Jan 42	Bora Bora		
9th	11 Feb 41			23 Jan 42	Australia		
10th	10 Feb 41			14 Jan 42	N. Ireland		
11th	25 Jan 41	5 Sep 41	Iceland				
12th	10 Feb 41			18 Feb 42	Australia		
22d	10 Feb 41			27 Feb 42	Hawaii		
26th	10 Feb 41			31 Jan 42	Canton Island		
47th	18 Jun 41			18 Feb 42	Australia		
109th	1 Jun 41			23 Jan 42	New Caledonia		
151st	1 Jun 41			30 Jun 42	England		
152d	1 Jun 41					5 Aug 42	England.
153d	1 Jun 41			18 Feb 42	Australia		
154th	1 Jun 41					10 Dec 42	Iraq.
155th	1 Jun 41			18 May 42	Australia		
156th	3 Jun 41			11 Mar 42	Hawaii		
159th	1 Jun 41			19 Mar 42	India		
160th	1 Jun 41					5 Aug 42	England.
165th	1 Jun 41			27 Feb 42	Hawaii		
166th	1 Jun 41			19 May 42	Australia		
167th	12 Jul 41	5 Sep 41	Iceland				
168th	12 Jul 41	5 Sep 41	Iceland				

Sources: Unit cards filed in Orgn and Directory Section, Oprs Br, AGO, and annual reports filed in HD.

advisability for hospital units was later questioned, and it was not followed in the case of other Negro hospital units activated during World War II. An advanced detachment of the 25th Station Hospital embarked in May 1942 for Liberia to support a force of construction engineers, personnel of the Air Transport Command and the Royal Air Force, natives employed by the Army at Roberts Field, and elements of a task force charged with protecting an airstrip and American rubber interests. After quarters were constructed overseas, the remainder of the unit, including its nurses, joined the advanced detachment on 10 March 1943. About the same time an all-Negro 150-bed unit, the 268th Station Hospital, was activated at Fort Huachuca (Arizona). After a period of training, it embarked for the Southwest Pacific theater in October 1943 and arrived in Australia in November.[98]

Establishing a Basis for Future Planning

Toward the end of 1942 the shift in emphasis from defensive measures to preparations for the offensive made it necessary to take stock of hospitalization already supplied in order to plan effectively for the future. Records of the number of hospital units shipped did not necessarily represent the number of beds available in the several theaters. In some instances, for reasons not often divulged to The Surgeon General, OPD diverted

[98] (1) An Rpt, 25th Sta Hosp, 1943, and Quarterly Hist Rpt, 268th Sta Hosp, 7 Jul 44. HD. (2) Diary, Col Stephen D. Berardinelli, 21 Jun 42 to 21 Dec 43. In his possession. (3) Interv, MD Historian with Col Berardinelli, formerly CO of 25th Sta Hosp, 24 Feb 50. HD: 000.71.

TABLE 10—USE OF NONAFFILIATED EVACUATION HOSPITAL UNITS ACTIVATED DURING 1940 AND 1941

Unit Designation	Date of Activation	Supplied Enlisted Personnel for Affiliated Units			Went to Theaters of Operations		Disbanded after Supplying Enlisted Personnel to Other Units (Date)
		Unit Designation	Date of Embarkation	Destination	Date of Embarkation	Destination	
1st	1 Aug 40				4 Mar 42	Australia	
3d	1 Aug 40	8th	2 Nov 42	N. Africa			24 Aug 42
4th	10 Feb 41	2d	4 Sep 42	N. Ireland			24 Aug 42
		48th	18 Jan 43	India			
6th	10 Feb 41	9th	26 Sep 42	England			24 Aug 42
10th	10 Feb 41				4 Mar 42	Australia	
11th	10 Feb 41				2 Nov 42	N. Africa [a]	
15th	1 Jun 41				7 Feb 43	N. Africa [a]	
19th	1 Jun 41	7th	7 Apr 42	Tongatabu			25 Aug 42
		12th	6 Jan 43	England			
23d	16 May 41	25th	19 Oct 42	New Zealand			18 Aug 42
		52d	23 Jan 42	New Caledonia			
36th	1 Jun 41	56th	16 Apr 43	N. Africa	19 Feb 44	New Guinea [a]	
37th	1 Jun 41	16th	14 Apr 43	N. Africa			13 Nov 42
41st	1 Jun 41				13 Nov 43	England [a]	
42d	1 Jun 41	27th	3 Apr 44	N. Africa			15 Oct 42
		77th	5 Aug 42	England			
43d	1 Jun 41	14th	10 Jul 43	India			15 Aug 42
53d	1 Jun 41	21st	29 Aug 43	Guadalcanal			17 Aug 42
		73d	20 Jan 43	India			
54th	2 Jun 41				31 Jul 43	Australia [a]	
68th	10 Feb 41	51st	3 Apr 44	N. Africa			23 Oct 42
		59th	12 Dec 42	N. Africa			

[a] Converted from 750- to 400-bed evacuation hospitals before being sent overseas.

Sources: Unit cards filed in Orgn and Directory Section, Oprs Br, AGO, and annual reports filed in HD.

units to different destinations from those for which they were originally earmarked. It sometimes happened that units arrived at overseas ports without equipment, which was shipped on other vessels, and therefore could not set up for actual operations. At other times assemblages were shipped as expansion units, for theaters to issue as needed to numbered hospitals that were already operating, to overseas hospitals that had operated during peacetime and were now being expanded, or to provisional hospitals that were being established with theater personnel. Furthermore, the U.S. Army was receiving hospitalization in some areas through reverse lend-lease. Thus The Surgeon General could not rely upon records of shipment of hospital units and assemblages for accurate information about beds available overseas. Nor could he depend upon statistical health reports (Medical Department Form No. 86ab). Designed to supply his Office regularly with information about admissions and dispositions of patients and about available and occupied beds in all Army hospitals, these reports often reached Washington only after considerable delay and differed in many instances from other available records.[89]

[89] Memo, SG for Oprs Div SOS, 31 Oct 42, sub: Bed Capacities for Fixed Hosps at Overseas Bases. SG: 632.2.

TABLE 11—USE OF NONAFFILIATED SURGICAL HOSPITAL UNITS ACTIVATED DURING 1940 AND 1941

Unit Designation	Date of Activation	Redesignation in U. S.		Date of Embarkation	Initial Destination	Redesignation Overseas	
		Unit	Date			Unit	Date
6th Surg Hosp	1 Aug 40	91st Evac (Mtz)	31 Aug 42	12 Dec 42	N. Africa		
7th Surg Hosp	1 Aug 40	92d Evac (Mtz)	25 Aug 42	28 Jun 43	Australia		
28th Surg Hosp	10 Feb 41			4 Mar 42	Australia	360th Sta Hosp	28 Oct 43
33d Surg Hosp	25 Jan 41			4 Mar 42	Australia	361st Sta Hosp	28 Oct 43
48th Surg Hosp	10 Feb 41			2 Aug 42	England	128th Evac (SM)	1 May 43
61st Surg Hosp	1 Jun 41	93d Evac (Mtz)	25 Aug 42	16 Apr 43	N. Africa		
63d Surg Hosp	1 Jun 41	94th Evac (Mtz)	25 Aug 42	28 Apr 43	N. Africa		
74th Surg Hosp	1 Jun 41	95th Evac (Mtz)	25 Aug 42	16 Apr 43	N. Africa		

Sources: Unit cards filed in Orgn and Directory Section, Oprs Br AGO, and annual reports filed in HD.

In July 1942, therefore, to get more accurate and more current information than he had, The Surgeon General called upon SOS headquarters for assistance.[100] Finding that neither SOS headquarters nor OPD had accurate records of the beds available in various theaters, the SOS Hospitalization and Evacuation Branch requested the latter, on 6 August 1942, to require all overseas commanders to submit a report on the capacities and numerical designations of their fixed hospitals.[101] This request was approved and, as the reports came in, the Surgeon General's Office, the SOS Hospitalization and Evacuation Branch, and OPD were able to get an accurate picture of hospitalization overseas at that time. It showed that the ratio of fixed beds to troop strength ranged from 2.09 percent in some areas to 24.1 percent in others.[102]

Even after reports of overseas bed capacities had been received and tabulated, several obstacles to planning for the future had to be removed. In the first place, The Surgeon General was uncertain about his authority to make recommendations concerning overseas hospitalization, in view of the hospitalization and evacuation policy which was published on 18 June 1942 making overseas commanders responsible for "the operation of all medical facilities under their control and *for future planning in connection therewith*" (italics added).[103] Despite this policy, SOS headquarters assured him that he could make recommendations about hospitalization and evacuation in theaters whenever appropriate. The Surgeon General also felt that he received insufficient information, both from higher authorities in the War Department and from surgeons in thea-

[100] (1) Memo, SG for Dir Oprs SOS, 11 Jul 42. SG: 632.2. (2) Memo, SG for Oprs Div SOS, 29 Jul 42, sub: Fixed Hosp Beds Overseas. HD: 632.-1 "Hosp Overseas, Bed Status."

[101] (1) Memos SPOPM 323.7 and SPOPH 632, CG SOS for ACofS OPD WDGS, 6 and 27 Aug 42, sub: Fixed Hosp Fac Available to Overseas Forces. HD: Wilson files, "Book I, 26 Mar 42–26 Sep 42." (2) 1st ind, CG SOS to SG, 14 Aug 42, on Memo, SG for Oprs Div SOS, 29 Jul 42, sub: Fixed Hosp Beds Overseas. HD: 632.-1, "Hosp Overseas, Bed Status."

[102] (1) Memo SPOPH 632(Hosp), CG SOS for SG, 20 Oct 42, sub: Bed Capacities of Fixed Hosps at Overseas Bases. HD: 632.-1 "Hosp Overseas, Bed Status." (2) Memo, SG for Oprs Div SOS, 31 Oct 42, same sub, with 1st ind SPOPH 632(10-31-42), CG SOS to SG, 16 Nov 42. Same file.

[103] Ltr AG 704 (6-17-42)MB-D-TS-M, TAG to CGs AGF, AAF, SOS, Theaters, etc., 18 Jun 42, sub: WD Hosp and Evac Policy. HD: 705.-1.

ters, to enable him to plan intelligently and effectively for overseas hospitalization. While much information he desired from higher authorities was classified for security reasons, the SOS Hospitalization and Evacuation Branch attempted to provide him with more information about operational plans than he had previously received.[104] Furthermore, in collaboration with the Surgeon General's Office that Branch took action which led to the establishment in January 1943 of a system of montly reports from overseas commands. Submitted first as sections of the Monthly Sanitary Reports and after July 1943 as Reports of Essential Technical Medical Data (ETMD's), these reports contained information about admission and evacuation rates, availability of hospital beds, suitability of hospital units and their equipment, and other factors of importance to The Surgeon General in planning theater medical services.[105] In addition, beginning with General Magee's trip to North Africa in the winter of 1942–43, representatives of the Surgeon General's Office made personal inspections of overseas areas in order to gain firsthand information about their medical services.[106]

Further obstacles to planning were lack of sufficient experience with battle casualties thus far in World War II to estimate accurately hospital admission rates and lack of an official evacuation policy—that is, a policy governing the selection of patients for evacuation to the United States in terms of the days of hospitalization which they were expected to require. In their absence The Surgeon General used for planning purposes the battle-casualty admission rates of World War I and assumed a policy of returning to the United States all patients who required 120 or more days of hospitalization. To establish a firmer basis for planning, he recommended in the spring of 1943 the establishment of an official evacuation policy but such action was not taken until later in the year.[107]

In providing hospitals for overseas service early in the war, the Medical Department discovered and attempted to correct shortcomings and errors in its prewar planning. It was discovered early that the activation and training of normal Army units was more valuable in meeting emergency hospital needs than the formation and organization of units affiliated with civilian hospitals and schools. Moreover, it soon appeared that units planned for theaters of operations were not suitable for all situations encountered in a modern global war and units of new types had to be de-

[104] (1) Memo SPMCP 704.-1, Act SG for Oprs Div SOS, 16 Nov 42, sub: Status of Hosp Overseas, with 1st ind SPOPH 701 (11-16-42), ACofS Oprs SOS to SG, 24 Nov 42. (2) Memo SPOPH 701 (11-16-42), CG SOS for ACofS OPD WDGS, 24 Nov 42, same sub. (3) Memo OPD 701 (11-24-42), ACofS OPD WDGS for CG SOS, 23 Jan 43, same sub. All in HD: 632.-1 "Hosp Overseas, Bed Status."

[105] (1) Rad CM-OUT 5938-5957, TAG to CGs Overseas Comds. SG: 370.2-1. (2) Memo SPOPH 440, CG SOS for TAG, 28 Dec 42, sub: ETMD from Overseas Forces, with Memo for Record. HD: Wilson files, "Book IV, 16 Mar 43-17 Jun 43." (3) Diary, SOS Hosp and Evac Br, 4 Dec 42. HD: Wilson files, "Diary." (4) Ltr AG 350.05 (12-28-42)OB-S-SPOPH-M, TAG to CGs Overseas Comds, 2 Jan 43, sub: ETMD from Overseas Forces. HD: Wilson files, "Experience in Med Matters from Overseas Forces." (5) Ltr AG 350.05 (28 Jun 43)OB-S-D-M, TAG to CGs Overseas Comds, 14 Jul 43, same sub. HD: 350.05 "Mil Info."

[106] Memo, SG for CG SOS, 12 Jan 43. HRS: Hq ASF, Gen [Wilhelm D.] Styer's files, "Med Dept."

[107] (1) Memo SPMCP 704.-1, Act SG for Oprs Div SOS, 16 Nov 42, sub: Status of Hosp Overseas, with 1 incl. HD: 632.-1 "Hosp Overseas, Bed Status." (2) Memo, Dir Control Div ASF for CG ASF, 2 Apr 43, sub: Situation with Respect to Army Hosp. SG: 322.15. (3) Memo, SG for CG ASF, 15 Apr 43, sub: Evac Policy for Overseas Theaters. SG: 705.-1. (4) See below, pp. 215-16.

veloped—field hospitals, motorized evacuation hospitals, and portable surgical hospitals. The size and weight of equipment of all hospital units had to be reduced and new methods of packing had to be developed in order to increase the mobility and transportability of hospitals. Shortages of Medical Corps officers appeared and required reductions in the number authorized by tables of organization developed during the emergency period. Shortages of equipment continued to plague the Medical Department and partially accounted for The Surgeon General's insistence upon withholding its issuance until hospital units were assigned to missions involving the care of patients. In this connection, The Surgeon General also resisted demands of higher authorities to plan for the use of numbered hospitals in the zone of interior medical service. Meanwhile other units were being activated and trained, and toward the end of General Magee's administration measures were taken to find out what hospital facilities theaters actually had and to place planning for future needs on a sounder basis.

PART THREE

HOSPITALIZATION IN THE LATER WAR YEARS MID–1943 TO 1946

Introduction

By the middle of 1943 the peak of the preparation phase of the war had been reached, and the United States and its Allies were ready to assume the offensive against the Axis powers. From then until the spring of 1945 troops moved steadily overseas, the number in the United States dropping from 5,355,683 to 2,753,455 and the number overseas growing from 1,637,419 to 5,403,931. In the fall of 1943, one body of American troops landed in Italy, carrying the offensive from North Africa to the European continent; others, by their attacks upon islands in the Gilbert and Marshall groups in the Pacific, began a two-pronged drive toward Japan. By the middle of the following year the Allies mounted their main attack against Germany, landing on the coast of France on 6 June 1944. Soon afterward the Central Pacific advance reached the Marianas and Southwest Pacific forces returned to the Philippines. Despite a German counteroffensive in December 1944, Allied forces moved inexorably toward victory in Europe and on 7 May 1945 Nazi Germany surrendered. Meanwhile, American troops in the Pacific pushed closer to the main Japanese islands, completing the reconquest of the Philippines and gaining control of islands in the Ryukyus chain. Then, on 10 August 1945, the Japanese Government sued for peace. Immediately afterward the Army's strength began to decline. By the beginning of 1946 the number of troops overseas dropped to 1,573,620 and of those in the United States to 1,895,652.[1]

Combat developments inevitably influenced the provision of hospitalization. With the movement of troops overseas the need for beds in station hospitals in the United States declined rapidly. On the other hand requirements for beds in hospitals of all types in theaters as well as in hospitals caring for overseas evacuees in this country mounted. The number of casualties and of soldiers with serious illnesses grew with the widening scope and increasing intensity of combat and the exposure of larger groups to disease hazards in various parts of the world. Estimating the number of beds that would be needed under such circumstances proved to be considerably more difficult than calculating the number needed for an Army in training. Moreover, to meet requirements for hospitalization, whatever they might be, the Medical Department had only limited means. New construction had been curtailed as the peak of the training phase had been reached; demands of overseas theaters for troops for combat operations and of the home front for civilian employees to produce war materials reduced the manpower pool, both military and civilian, upon which the Medical Department could draw; and in the fall of 1943 the number of doctors allowed the Army was limited to 45,000. These limitations meant that emphasis had to be placed upon more effective use of the means

[1] (1) Strength of the Army, STM-30, 1 Mar 47. (2) *Biennial Report . . . Chief of Staff, 1943-45*, pp. 1-87.

available. Instead of building new hospital plants, for example, the Medical Department had to expand and improve those already built or use vacated station hospitals and troop housing. Changes had to be made in the hospital system to avoid waste of personnel and equipment. Policies for hospitalization had to be modified in order to hold bed requirements to the lowest practical number. And the organization and administrative procedures of hospitals had to be standardized and simplified to permit relatively smaller and more heterogeneous staffs to operate them.

The task of using limited means effectively and of planning their allocation among major commands in the United States and among theaters in all parts of the world fell to Surgeon General Kirk when he succeeded General Magee in June 1943. General Kirk maintained continuity in the program of hospitalization, preserving many established policies and furthering developments already begun, but he also evolved new policies to meet changing situations and established new methods of operation. Meanwhile, he expanded and strengthened his own office and sought changes in the existing War Department organization to facilitate discharge of his responsibility for the health and medical care of the Army.

CHAPTER IX

Further Changes in Organization and Responsibilities for Hospitalization

Relationship of The Surgeon General With Other War Department Agencies

With the emergence of problems created by a shift from the defensive to the offensive phase of the war, changes occurred in the organization for hospitalization. One of the most fundamental was implicit in a gradual change in the relationship of The Surgeon General with ASF headquarters and the General Staff. Although The Surgeon General remained under the jurisdiction of ASF headquarters until after the end of the war, there was a growing trend in 1944 and 1945 toward his restoration to a position of direct contact with the General Staff. This trend resulted from efforts made by General Kirk to regain authority for his office commensurate with its responsibilities and from gradual resumption by the General Staff of some of the functions assumed earlier by the Army Service Forces.[1]

In the last half of 1943 the authority and responsibility of OPD for logistic matters as well as the strategic direction of theater forces were confirmed and strengthened. G–1 became concerned about allocation of personnel for medical service throughout the world, and G–4 devoted growing attention to bed requirements and the hospital system in general. In addition, two Special Staff units, the War Department Manpower Board and the Inspector General's Office, took a hand in such matters.

As this happened ASF headquarters lost some of its former authority and tended to become in some matters merely a formal channel of communication. Finally, early in 1945 this trend culminated in a War Department circular which, while not removing him from ASF jurisdiction, affirmed The Surgeon General's position as the chief medical officer of the Army and officially authorized him to deal directly with the Chief of Staff and

[1] For full information on this development see John D. Millett, *The Organization and Role of the Army Service Forces* (Washington, 1954), Chs. IX and X; and Ray S. Cline, *Washington Command Post: The Operations Division* (Washington, 1951), Ch. XIV; both in UNITED STATES ARMY IN WORLD WAR II.

the General Staff, without interference by ASF headquarters, on matters affecting the health of the Army.[2] In approving the publication of this circular the Secretary of War announced that it should be further interpreted as also giving The Surgeon General direct access to the Secretary himself.[3]

A change in the organization of ASF headquarters reflected both its decrease of authority in phases of hospitalization in which the General Staff took a more active interest as well as a gradual return to the Surgeon General's Office of certain functions connected with hospitalization and evacuation. In April 1943 the ASF Hospitalization and Evacuation Branch, whose head after February 1943 was Col. Robert C. McDonald, was reduced to a section of the Zone of Interior Branch of the Planning Division. In the following November the statement of this section's functions was revised to eliminate wording that could be interpreted as giving it operational responsibilities for any aspect of hospitalization. Meanwhile, Medical Department officers who had been assigned there in 1942 were transferred to other posts, two of them to the Surgeon General's Office. In February 1944 the entire section was abolished and its remaining functions were transferred to other units of the ASF Planning Division.[4] This Division, along with others such as the Mobilization and Control Divisions, continued to exercise considerable authority over hospitals at ASF installations and over ASF hospital units being prepared for overseas service.[5]

Another aspect of General Kirk's drive to regain authority with which to discharge responsibilities of his office was his effort to increase control by the Medical Department in general and by his Office in particular over medical installations, including hospitals, in service commands. Soon after he took office, General Kirk tried to have service command surgeons recognized as staff officers of service commanders rather than as chiefs of medical branches under the intermediate control of supply divisions. His efforts were not at first successful, but toward the end of 1943 General Somervell directed service command headquarters to conform as closely as practical to ASF headquarters. In most service commands the surgeon was then elevated, as were other technical service heads in the service commands, to a position as staff officer directly under the service commander himself.[6] After that, the Surgeon General's Office began to achieve closer co-ordination with service command surgeons and, through them, to exercise closer supervision over hospitalization.

Early in 1944 comparative studies of matters affecting the operation and administration of hospitals, such as the amount of personnel assigned to them, the efficiency with which they treated and disposed of patients, and the number of beds which they set up for use, were made by the Surgeon General's Office, and letters calling attention to the implications of these studies were sent to service command surgeons monthly.[7] Also, in 1944

[2] (1) WD Cir 120, 18 Apr 45. (2) Millett, *op. cit.*, pp. 298–310.

[3] Memo, SecWar for [CofSA], 6 Apr 45. HRS: G–1 file, 020 "SGO (10 Feb 45) 20 Apr 45."

[4] History of Planning Div, ASF, vol. I, pp. 33, 40–45, 61, 67, 78, 79, 80, 81. HRS. Officers transferred from ASF headquarters to SGO were Lt. Col. John C. Fitzpatrick and Maj. Henry McC. Greenleaf.

[5] (1) ASF Manual M 301, ASF Orgn, 15 Aug 44.

[6] Edward J. Morgan and Donald O. Wagner, The Organization of the Medical Department in the Zone of the Interior (1946), HD., pp. 97–99.

[7] Such letters are filed in SG: 323.7–5 for each service command.

the Surgeon General's Office adopted the "flying circus" method of inspection for hospitals. Representatives of such segments of the Office as the Professional Consultants Divisions, the Nursing Division, the Supply Service, the Personnel Service, and the Construction Branch, under the leadership of the chief of the Hospital Division and accompanied by service command surgeons or their representatives, flew from one hospital to another making thorough inspections of their operations. Such inspections achieved closer co-ordination between offices of The Surgeon General and service command surgeons and reduced confusion in the field which had formerly resulted from successive inspections by separate individuals and from the receipt of instructions from different staff officers.[8]

Only minor changes were made in the division of responsibility for numbered hospital units between the Ground and Service Forces. Upon recommendation of AGF headquarters and the Surgeon General's Office, responsibility for portable surgical hospitals was lodged with the Ground Forces in the winter of 1943–44.[9] In the middle of the next year the Ground Surgeon concurred in a recommendation of the Surgeon General's Office for transfer of responsibility for convalescent hospitals (units designed for the care of short-term patients in combat zones) from the Service to the Ground Forces.[10] Whereas both the Surgeon General's Office and ASF headquarters joined with the General Staff and the Ground Forces in establishing a general basis for the allotment of mobile hospital units to theaters, AGF headquarters was primarily responsible for the more detailed preparation of mobile hospitalization for separate theaters. Planning for fixed hospitalization in theaters for troops of all major commands—Air, Ground, and Service Forces—continued to be, but not without opposition by the Air Forces, a responsibility of the Surgeon General's Office and ASF headquarters.[11]

Uncertainty about the extent of the Air Forces' authority over hospitalization continued. Surgeon General Kirk believed that all hospitals in the United States should be combined into one system under his supervision,[12] but the Air Surgeon renewed his efforts to establish a separate and complete hospital system for the Air Forces. Activities in this connection caused a major change in the zone of interior hospital system.[13] Attempts to establish separate AAF hospitals in theaters of operations, though less successful, exemplified the Air Surgeon's drive for a completely separate medical service.

[8] Tab F, sub: Dev of a New Syst of Hosp Insp, to Memo, Dir Hosp Div SGO and Resources Anal Div SGO for Dir HD SGO thru Chief Oprs Serv SGO, 18 Jun 45, sub: Add Mat for An Rpt for FY 1945. HD: 319.1-2. Examples of reports of flying circus inspections are found in SG: 333.1 for each service command.

[9] (1) Memo for Record, by [Col] R. B. S[kinner], 26 Aug 43. Ground Med files: Transfer Binder Journal, 1943. (2) 6th ind SPMCP 322.15-17 (Cp Mackall)C, Chief Oprs Serv SGO to SG, 11 Nov 43, on Ltr, CG Airborne Comd AGF to CG AGF, 4 Sep 43, sub: Ptbl Surg Hosp. AGF: 321 No 5. (3) Memo 353-GNGPS (4 Sep 43), CofS AGF for CofSA attn ACofS G-3 WDGS, 29 Nov 43, sub: Ptbl Surg Hosp. AGF: 321 No 5. (4) Memo, ACofS G-3 WDGS to CG ASF, 1 Dec 43, sub: Ptbl Surg Hosp. AGF: 321 No 5.

[10] (1) Memo SPMOO 400.34 (24 Jul 44), CG ASF for CG AGF thru SG, 25 Jul 44, sub: Present Status of Certain MAC Offs with Conv Hosps, with inds and incls. (2) DF 320.3 (24 Feb 44), Dep ACofS G-3 WDGS to CG ASF, 22 Jul 44, same sub. Both in SG: 320.3-1.

[11] Interv, MD Historian with Col Arthur B. Welsh, 27 Dec 50. HD: 000.71.

[12] Rpt, SGs Conf with Chiefs Med Br SvCs, 14–17 Jun 43, p. 7. HD: 337.

[13] See below, pp. 182–85.

Efforts of the Air Surgeon To Get Separate Hospitals for Theater Air Commands

Under the War Department reorganization and policies established early in 1942, theater air commands, unlike ground commands, had no authority or control over hospital units used in support of troops in combat zones. Like ground forces, on the other hand, they were dependent upon service forces hospitals for the care of personnel in communications zones. In some theaters local air and theater surgeons arranged for the attachment, but not the assignment, of a limited number of either mobile or fixed hospitals to theater air commands,[14] but the Air Surgeon considered this arrangement unsatisfactory. He wanted theater air commands to have complete control of their own hospitals. The reasons he most often gave for this position were the loss of control by air commands of personnel sent to service forces hospitals, the loss of man-days caused by transferring patients to service forces hospitals and awaiting their return to duty through the replacement system, the lowered morale of air forces personnel which resulted from their temporary absence from air commands, and the need of air forces men for professional care that was "directed from an aero-medical viewpoint."[15] The Surgeon General, on the other hand, believed that supplying fixed hospitals to overseas areas on a theater basis, rather than on a major command basis, achieved a more effective use of available resources.

In the fall of 1943 the Air Surgeon attempted to get numbered hospital units included in the War Department troop basis as AAF units. Success would have meant that such units would be activated and trained by the Air Forces and would be sent to theaters as air units for use by air commanders and not by theater or communications zone commanders. This attempt failed because of lack of support by the Air Staff and opposition of the Surgeon General's Office and ASF headquarters.[16] To secure data for use in winning greater support from the Air Staff and in countering ASF arguments, the Air Surgeon in March 1944 sent to surgeons of all theater air commands a questionnaire about the desirability of separate hospitals for air forces personnel.[17]

Meanwhile there arose the question of the assignment to air commands of hospitals located in Newfoundland at bases transferred in the fall of 1943 from the Newfoundland Base Command to the Air Transport Command. After several months of negotiations, AAF headquarters, ASF headquarters, the Surgeon Gen-

[14] (1) Air Evaluation Board, SWPA, The Medical Support of Air Warfare in the South and Southwest Pacific, 7 December 1941–15 August 1945, pp. 431ff. HD. (2) Ltr, Surg 9th AF to Air Surg, 20 Aug 44. HD: TAS, "9th AF (Col Kendricks)."

[15] Study, unsigned, n d [1944], sub: Study of Overseas Hosp. HD: TAS, "Hosp for AAF Units Overseas." Also see Ltrs from Air Surg, cited below.

[16] (1) Memo, Air Surg for C of Air Staff, 29 Nov 43. (2) Comment 2, Col H. C. Chenault, MC, Air Surg Off to AC of Air Staff, Personnel, 6 Dec 43, on above. (3) Comment 1, Col H. C. Chenault, MC to AC of Air Staff OC & R, 13 Dec 43, sub: Air Base Hosps for Overseas Air Bases in 1944 AAF Trp Basis, on unknown basic memo. (4) Memo, unsigned [CG AAF] for CofSA, n d, sub: Hosp at AF Bases and Stas Outside Continental Limits of US. (5) Memo, CG AAF for CG ASF, 16 Feb 44, sub: Med Care of AAF Pers, with incl. All in HD: TAS, "Hosp for AAF Units Overseas." A full discussion of the Air Surgeon's attempts to get separate hospitals for theater air commands is in Hubert A. Coleman, Organization and Administration, AAF Medical Services in the Zone of the Interior (1948), pp. 409–32. HD.

[17] Study, unsigned, n d [1944], sub: Study of Overseas Hosp. HD: TAS, "Hosp for AAF Units Overseas."

eral's Office, and the General Staff agreed that the numbered hospitals at such bases would be returned to the United States and that the North Atlantic Wing of the Air Transport Command would operate dispensaries in their place. While such installations were in reality small hospitals, use of the term "dispensaries" kept nominally intact the War Department policy of having service forces provide fixed hospitalization for all forces in theaters of operations.[18]

Before this decision had been reached the President received complaints about the hospitalization of air troops in the United Kingdom, and in March 1944 he sent a committee composed of Surgeon General Kirk, Air Surgeon Grant, and Dr. Edward A. Strecker, a prominent civilian physician, to investigate the hospital situation there. They found insufficient cause for complaints and in April the President approved their recommendation that no change be made in the hospital system in the European Theater.[19]

Planning for the B–29 very-long-range-bomber program in April 1944 presented a favorable opportunity for pressing for separate air forces hospitals in the Pacific. When an OPD representative stated that ASF hospital units were not available for assignment to the Central Pacific area for the XXI Bomber Command, AAF headquarters offered to furnish them. OPD was on the verge of authorizing it to do so when the Surgeon General's Office proposed instead the transfer of certain hospital units from the less active South Pacific to the Central Pacific.[20]

The Air Surgeon then urged the Air Staff to take such "drastic" action that the Army Chief of Staff would be forced to make a decision as to whether or not theater air forces could have separate hospitals.[21] To support his position the Air Surgeon used replies which he had received from his March questionnaire. While they did not show a unanimous desire among air command surgeons for separate hospitals, they gave the Air Surgeon substantiating data for his position. The Air Staff remained nonetheless unconvinced of the wisdom or desirability of pressing for separate air forces hospitals generally. Instead, the Air Staff directed the Air Surgeon to prepare a study showing the need of the XX Bomber command, at that time located in India, for separate hospitals. Because he found it hard to divorce a desire for separate hospitals in all theaters from the question of separate hospitals for the XX Bomber Command, the Air Surgeon had difficulty preparing a study which the Air Staff would approve. He finally succeeded, only to be turned down by the commanding general of the Air Forces, who knew, according to officers in

[18] (1) Diary, Hosp Div SGO, 4 Apr 44. HD: 024.7–3. (2) 1st ind, SG to ACofS OPD WDGS, thru CG ASF, 5 Sep 44, on DF OPD 320.2 (30 Aug 44), ACofS OPD WDGS to CG ASF, 30 Aug 44, sub: Designation of Certain AAF Sta Hosps. SG: 322 "Hosp Misc 1944."

[19] (1) Memo, F. D. R[oosevelt] for Gen Marshall, 26 Feb 44. (2) Memo WDCSA 632 (28 Feb 44), CofSA for The President, 29 Feb 44. (3) Memo, Air Surg, and Dr. Edward A. Strecker for CofSA thru Dep Theater Comdr ETOUSA, 20 Mar 44. (4) Ltr, SecWar to The President, 29 Mar 44. (5) Memo, Sec WDGS for CG ASF, CG AAF, SG, and Air Surg, 10 Apr 44. All in AG: CofS files 632, 1944–46.

[20] (1) Comment 1, Air Surg to AC of Air Staff OC & R, 5 May 44, sub: Med Serv for XXI Bomber Comd. HD: TAS, "Hosp for AAF Units Overseas." (2) Memo, Dep Dir MOOD SGO for Record, 15 May 44. HD: MOOD "Pacific." (3) Memo OPD 320.3 PTO (17 May 44), ACofS OPD WDGS for CG ASF and CG AAF, 17 May 44, sub: Air Base Hosps in Support of VLR, with Memo for Record. HD: TAS, "Hosp for AAF Units Overseas."

[21] Memo, Air Surg for C of Air Staff, 26 Jun 44, sub: AAF Med Serv and Hosp Overseas. HD: TAS, "Hosp for AAF Units Overseas."

AAF headquarters, that the Army Chief of Staff opposed "duplicate medical services." [22] Thus, overseas air forces never received official authority to establish separate hospitals. In some theaters they set up hospitals under the guise of dispensaries, while in others they operated hospitals that were loaned to them by theater commanders.[23]

Expanding and Strengthening the Surgeon General's Office

Correlative to General Kirk's attempts to gain greater authority and higher status for The Surgeon General was the expansion and strengthening of his own Office.[24]

In July 1943 The Surgeon General combined his Hospitalization and Evacuation Division with his Hospital Construction Division to form a single unit: the Hospital Administration Division. Proposed by ASF headquarters as a means of simplifying the organization of the Surgeon General's Office,[25] this step concentrated related functions—hospital construction, hospital administration, and evacuation—under one officer, who was subordinate in turn to the new chief of the Operations Service, Col. (later Brig. Gen.) Raymond W. Bliss. The new Division, whose director from August 1943 to August 1945 was Col. Albert H. Schwichtenberg, had four branches. The Policies Branch, under Lt. Col. Basil C. MacLean until he was succeeded by Lt. Col. James T. McGibony in the fall of 1944, was responsible for establishing and publishing policies on hospital administration. The Evacuation Branch was in charge of the bed-credit system in general hospitals. The Construction Branch, whose new chief after 5 October 1943 was Lt. Col. (later Col.) Achilles L. Tynes, was responsible for co-ordinating the work of the Surgeon General's Office with the Engineers in the construction and maintenance of hospital plants. The fourth branch, the Liaison Branch, was new and was established to meet needs that had developed in the course of the war. It was charged with maintaining liaison with the Transportation Corps in the movement of patients, with The Provost Marshal General in the hospitalization of prisoners of war, and with the Women's Army Corps in the hospitalization and employment of Wacs.[26]

During the winter of 1943–44 a major expansion and reorganization occurred. Personnel limitations and prospective combat-casualty loads complicated problems of planning and providing hospitalization for the Army. Furthermore, there was some belief in both ASF headquarters and the Surgeon General's Office that the latter should be more active than in the past in planning hospitalization and in

[22] (1) Comments 1 to 12, on Memo, Air Surg for C of Air Staff, 26 Jun 44, sub: AAF Med Serv and Hosp Overseas. (2) Memo, unsigned [CG AAF] for CofSA, 23 Jul 44, sub: Twentieth AF Responsibilities. (3) Comments 13 to 16, on Memo, unsigned [CG AAF] for CofSA, n d, sub: XX Bomber Comd. All in HD: TAS, "Hosp for AAF Units Overseas."

[23] This statement is based upon numerous letters between Col. Walter S. Jensen, MC, Chief Surgeon of Hq. AAF, Pacific Ocean Area, and Maj. Gen. David N. W. Grant, USA, Air Surgeon. HD: TAS, "20th AAF/POA (Col Jensen)."

[24] Although reorganizations that were made were general and affected many units of his Office, only those concerned with hospitalization and evacuation will be considered here. For a discussion of the general reorganization, see Blanche B. Armfield, Organization and Administration (MS for companion vol. in Medical Dept. series), HD.

[25] Memo, SG for CG ASF, 18 Jun 43, sub: Orgn of SGO, with 1st ind, CG ASF to SG, 1 Jul 43, and 2d ind, SG to CG ASF, 7 Jul 43. SG: 024.-1.

[26] Morgan and Wagner, *op. cit.*, pp. 28–33. Information about personnel assignments was taken from SG office orders and personnel records on file in SGO.

supervising hospital operations.[27] Perhaps with tongue in cheek, the director of The Surgeon General's Control Division proposed in September 1943 that this should be considered a "new activity." [28] At any rate, early the next year the Surgeon General's Office began to negotiate with ASF headquarters for the transfer of personnel to establish a "Facilities and Personnel Utilization Branch" in the Hospital Administration Division. Organized by Dr. Eli Ginzberg, an economist and statistician on loan from the ASF Control Division, this Branch was charged in February 1944 with making comprehensive hospitalization plans, including the calculation of bed and personnel requirements, the utilization of available buildings and personnel, and the modification of the hospital system to achieve greater efficiency and economy in operations.[29] Soon afterward, in an attempt to achieve greater co-ordination among operational segments of his Office, The Surgeon General reorganized his entire Operations Service.[30] The revamped Service had two deputy chiefs. One was responsible, among other things, for the provision of hospitals for theaters of operations, while the other dealt with hospitalization and evacuation in the zone of interior.

Under the Deputy Chief for Hospitals and Domestic Operations were a Hospital Division and four liaison units. Three of the latter had previously existed as sections of the Liaison Branch of the Hospital Administration Division: the Prisoner-of-War Liaison Unit, the Women's Medical Unit, and the Transportation Liaison Unit. The fourth, the Army Air Forces Liaison Unit, was mainly a paper unit, for it was headed by the Hospital Division director who was already charged with maintaining liaison with the Air Surgeon's Office. Like the Hospital Administration Division which it succeeded, the Hospital Division had four branches. The Evacuation and Construction Branches continued without change; the Policies Branch was renamed the Administration Branch; and there was the newly created Facilities Utilization Branch.[31]

These changes were more apparent than real because Colonel Schwichtenberg, who was already serving as chief of the Hospital Division, continued in that post and became also the Deputy Chief for Hospitals and Domestic Operations. Thus, chiefs of the branches of the Hospital Division and heads of the liaison units continued under his supervision in much the same relationship as before. The changes were significant, however, in that (1) the person responsible for hospital activities was given higher status than formerly, (2) the new branch of the Hospital Division, the Facilities Utilization Branch, was charged with making comprehensive plans for hospitalization in the United States and with arranging for the execution of those plans with other interested units in the Surgeon General's Office, and (3) the amount of personnel available for work on hospital plans and operations was increased until there were twenty-three officers and thirty-six civilians un-

[27] (1) Memo, Dir Control Div SGO for [Maj] Gen [Norman T.] Kirk, 13 Jan 44, sub: Proposal for Overall Plan for Most Effective Util of Off Almt, Civ Pers, and Space in the SGO and for Modifications in Present Orgn. SG: 320.3 GG. (2) Tab A, sub: Estab of a Statistical Management Unit in the Oprs Serv, to Memo cited n. 8.

[28] Memo, Dir Control Div SGO for Chief Liaison Br Oprs Serv SGO, 30 Sep 43. Off file, Gen Bliss' Off SGO, "Util of MCs in ZI" (19) # 1.

[29] Diary, Hosp Admin Div SGO, 3 and 8 Jan 44; and Diary, Fac Util Br (later Resources Anal Div) SGO, [7 Feb 44]. HD: 024.7-3.

[30] Morgan and Wagner, *op. cit.*, pp. 44-51.

[31] *Ibid.*

der the supervision of the Deputy Chief for Hospitals and Domestic Operations in July 1944.[32]

The Office of the Deputy Chief for Plans and Operations replaced the old Plans Division, which had been headed since July 1943 by Col. Arthur B. Welsh. In this Office were three divisions: the Mobilization and Overseas Operations Division, the Technical Division, and the Special Planning Division.

The Mobilization and Overseas Operations Division, developed from a branch of the same name in the former Plans Division, had three branches. Its Theater Branch maintained current information on the status of Medical Department units in each overseas theater; made studies of bed requirements of the several theaters; formulated plans for the employment of Medical Department units, personnel, and equipment in each theater; and prepared recommendations to higher commands on changes in the status or organization of medical services overseas. In this work it maintained close liaison with the ASF Planning Division. The Troop Units Branch planned and recommended the types and numbers of ASF medical units required under current authorizations for each theater; planned the activation, reorganization, shipment, disbandment and inactivation of such units; and maintained liaison with the ASF Mobilization Division. The Inspection Branch, formerly a branch of the Plans Division, continued to receive and review reports from theaters of operations, such as the reports of essential technical medical data (ETMD's); maintained records of trips of inspection made by representatives of the Surgeon General's Office; and interviewed and circulated reports of interviews with medical personnel returned from overseas areas.

The Technical Division included among its many duties the preparation and revision of tables of organization and equipment, Medical Department equipment lists, and tables of allowances.

The Special Planning Division was responsible for plans for the demobilization of the Medical Department and for the medical care of civilians in occupied countries.[33]

A separate unit of the Operations Service, the Strategic and Logistic Planning Unit, was responsible for determining "the adequacy of all phases of Medical Department operations, and plans therefor, to the extent necessary to insure timely placing of sufficient personnel, equipment and supplies to meet all authorized requirements," [34] from March to November 1944. On the latter date it was absorbed by the Mobilization and Overseas Operations Division.[35]

This multiplicity of offices might give an erroneous impression of division of responsibility were it not pointed out that one man, Colonel Welsh, served at the same time as Deputy Chief of the entire Operations Service, Deputy Chief for Plans and Operations, and Director of the Mobilization and Overseas Operations Division.[36] *(Chart 7.)*

Further changes, representing perhaps a logical extension of those already made, occurred during the remainder of the war.

[32] An Rpt, FY 1944, Hosp and Dom Oprs SGO. HD.

[33] (1) Morgan and Wagner, *op. cit.*, pp. 44–51. (2) An Rpts, MOOD SGO, FY 1944 and 1945. (3) An Rpt, Spec Planning Div SGO, FY 1944. (4) An Rpt, Tec Div SGO, FY 1945. All in HD.

[34] Memo, Dir Strategic and Logistic Planning Unit SGO for Chief Oprs Serv SGO, 6 Jun 44, sub: Rpt of Accomplishments of the SGO. HD: 319.1–2 (MOOD Oprs Serv SGO).

[35] An Rpt, MOOD SGO, FY 1945. HD.

[36] Orgn Directory, SGO, 20 Mar 44. HD: 461.

Chart 7—Organization of the SGO for Hospitalization and Evacuation, 1943–45

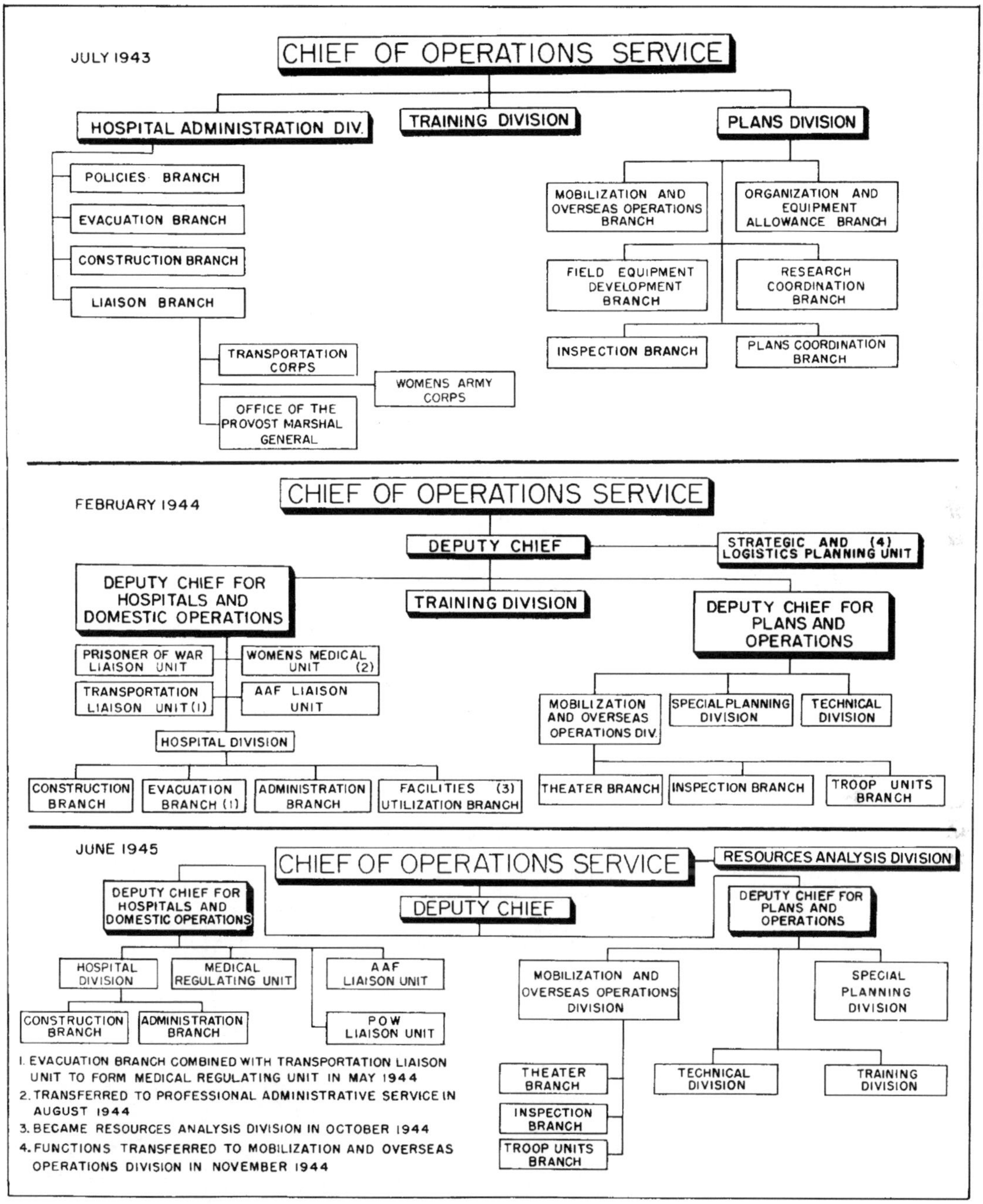

In May 1944 the Evacuation Branch was removed from the Hospital Division and was merged with the Transportation Liaison Unit to form a Medical Regulating Unit under Lt. Col. John C. Fitzpatrick.[37] This step combined under one head the control of the use of beds in general hospitals and the movement of patients to those beds. In August 1944 the Women's Medical Liaison Unit, whose function was more advisory than operational, was transferred from the office of the Deputy Chief for Hospitals and Domestic Operations to the new Professional Administrative Service. In October 1944 the Facilities Utilization Branch was removed from the Hospital Division and given higher status and responsibility, as the Resources Analysis Division, under the direct supervision of the chief of the Operations Service. Its head was Doctor Ginzberg, who by this time had been formally transferred from ASF headquarters to the Surgeon General's Office.[38] Continuing the trend of centralizing operational activities and separating administrative from advisory functions, responsibility for the operation of the reconditioning program was transferred in April 1945 to the Hospital Division, leaving the Reconditioning Consultants Division free to concentrate in an advisory capacity on matters of policy.[39]

Other units in the Surgeon General's Office continued to contribute, in varying degrees, to hospital operations. Among them, the Personnel and Supply Services were perhaps the most important. As increasing attention was given to management techniques, the Control Division entered the hospital operations field and, in co-operation with the Hospital Division, attempted to standardize and simplify hospital administrative procedures.[40]

---

[37] Memo for Record, by Col Tracy S. Voorhees, Dir Control Div SGO, 3 May 44, sub: The MRO Set-up. SG: 024.-1.

[38] An Rpt, Resources Anal Div SGO, FY 1945. HD.

[39] (1) Morgan and Wagner, *op. cit.*, pp. 49, 50, and 69.

[40] See below, pp. 261-65.

CHAPTER X

Adjustments and Changes in the Zone of Interior Hospital System

As the tempo and extent of the war increased, changes and adjustments were made in the hospital system. Among the more important reasons for them were the necessity of using limited personnel resources—particularly doctors—more effectively than formerly; the continuing efforts of the Air Surgeon to gain greater control over hospitalization of Air Forces men; the necessity of caring for large numbers of prisoners of war; and the growing number of patients requiring specialized treatment and care. In the fall of 1943 several groups attempted to solve the problem of limited personnel resources. Among them were the "Kenner Board," a group of officers appointed by The Surgeon General and headed by Brig. Gen. Albert W. Kenner to study Medical Department personnel utilization; the Hospital and Control Divisions of the Surgeon General's Office; the ASF Control Division; and the Inspector General's Office. These groups agreed that certain steps were desirable: reduction in size and number of station hospitals; merger of neighboring hospitals to eliminate overlapping and duplication; and removal of convalescent patients from the wards of general hospitals. They disagreed on the question of how to operate two sets of hospitals (those of the Army Air Forces and those of the rest of the Army) with a minimum of duplication of facilities and waste of personnel. Subsequently their opinions were reflected in changes made in the hospital system.[1]

Closure of Surplus Station Hospital Facilities

The first adjustment needed was the closure of station hospital plants, or parts of them, to keep step with the shrinkage in military population as troops moved over-

[1] (1) Mins of Mtgs and Rpt of Bd of Off to Study the Util of MC Offs, 17 Sep 43–6 Nov 43. HD: 334 "Kenner Bd." (2) Memo, Dr. Eli Ginzberg, Control Div ASF for Chief Oprs Serv SGO thru Dir Control Div ASF, 30 Nov 43, sub: Surv of Gen Hosps. SG: 333.1-1. (3) Memo, Lt Col Basil C. MacLean, Hosp Admin Div SGO for Gen [Raymond W.] Bliss thru Col [Albert H.] Schwichtenberg, 6 Nov 43, sub: Observations Based on Recent Visits . . . to 9 Gen Hosps. Off file, Gen Bliss' Off SGO, "Util of MCs in ZI" (19)#1. (4) Notes on Visit to McCloskey, O'Reilly, and Percy Jones Gen Hosps, 11 Dec 43, by Col Tracy S. Voorhees, Control Div SGO. SG: 333.1-1. (5) Memo, WDCSA 333 (4 Nov 43), DepCofSA for IG,4 Nov 43, sub: Util of Med Off Pers in ZI Instls. AG: 320.2 (18 Apr 44) (1).

seas. When this was done doctors no longer needed to care for troops in training could be released for assignment either to hospitals scheduled for overseas service or to general hospitals in this country. In the fall of 1943 both the Surgeon General's and the Air Surgeon's Offices made surveys to this end.[2] By the close of the year "considerable reductions" had been made in the sizes of AAF hospitals, and the Surgeon General's Office was planning a general procedure for adjusting capacities of all station hospitals to the troop populations which they served.[3] To avoid overcrowding in hospital plants that were by then larger than needed, The Surgeon General's Hospital Administration Division proposed a resumption of the practice of placing beds in wards only and of allotting to each bed 100 square feet of floor space, a practice which had been abandoned earlier when the need for beds was greater. This Division also recommended that local commanders be held responsible for reducing the sizes of station hospitals to authorized capacities.[4]

ASF headquarters and the General Staff approved these proposals and published regulations to effect them early in 1944.[5] Concurrently The Surgeon General's Facilities Utilization Branch began to urge service command surgeons to increase efforts to shrink station hospitals under their supervision.[6] To judge the progress made, The Surgeon General changed the way in which station hospital beds were reported in the summer of 1944. Until that time hospitals reported "constructed capacities"—that is, the number of beds which plants were constructed to hold—and hence reports showed neither the number of beds actually in use nor the number currently authorized. Under the new system they reported "authorized beds"—that is, beds for which were allotted supplies and personnel. The first such reports revealed that considerable progress had been made in the contraction of station hospitals.[7] On 26 May 1944 the reported capacity (constructed capacity) of all AAF and ASF station hospitals had been about 259,000, or 6.2 percent of the zone of interior troop strength. By 7 July 1944 the "authorized capacity" of station hospitals was reported to be about 134,000 (3.3 percent of the troop strength at that time) and of station and regional hospitals together about 198,000 (4.9 percent).[8]

Establishment of Regional Hospitals

Closure of surplus AAF and ASF station hospitals did not eliminate the problem of operating dual sets of hospitals (for the Air Forces and for the rest of the Army) without duplication of plants and

[2] (1) Ltr, Asst to Chief Med Br S&S Div Hq 9th SvC to COs ASF Hosps 9th SvC, 26 Oct 43, sub: Util of Hosp Fac. SG: 632.-1. (2) Ltr, SG to CG 2d SvC attn SvC Surg. 23 Dec 43, sub: Anal of Data Obtained in Recent Questionnaire of SG on Req Hosp. SG: 705.-1 (2d SvC)AA. (3) Tabs C and D of Memo, CG AAF (Air Surg) for CofSA attn G-4, 7 Oct 44, sub: Reduction of ZI Hosps. HRS: G-4 file, "Hosp and Evac Policy."

[3] Ltr, SG to Budget Off for WD, 27 Dec 43, sub: Sta Hosp Beds in ZI Instls. SG: 632.-2.

[4] (1) Diary, Hosp Admin Div SGO, 4 Jan 44. HD: 024.7-3. (2) Ltr, SG to Budget Off for WD, 27 Dec 43, sub: Sta Hosp Beds in ZI Instls. SG: 632.-2.

[5] (1) WD Cir 43, 1 Feb 44.*(2) AR 40-1080, C 2, 9 Jun 44. (3) ASF Cir 196, 27 Jun 44.

[6] Ltr, CG ASF by SG (Oprs Serv Hosp Div, Fac Util Br) to CGs SvCs attn SvC Surg, 28 Apr 44, sub: Redesignation of Sta Hosp Bed Capacities. HD: Resources Anal Div file, "Hosp."

[7] Form SG-396, Weekly Health Report, was revised 1 May 1944. The revised version was first used in Report 27, vol. IV, for the week ending 7 July 1944. Weekly Rpts, AML.

[8] (1) Weekly Health Rpts, vol. IV, No 21, and No 27. AML. (2) ASF Monthly Progress Rpt, Sec 7, *Health*, 31 Jul 44, p. 34, compared bed capacities of ASF sta hosps as of 26 May 44 and 30 Jun 44.

waste of personnel, and attempts to solve it led to a major change in the hospital system early in 1944. Although prohibited from operating general hospitals and caring for overseas patients, the Air Forces, it will be recalled, had built up station hospitals to the point where many were staffed and equipped to give general-hospital-type care, and the Air Surgeon opposed transferring Air Forces patients to general hospitals, operated by the Service Forces, when there were AAF station hospitals capable of treating and caring for them. On the other hand, Surgeon General Kirk opposed separate Air Forces station hospitals.[9] If they were to continue, he contended, their staffs should be reduced in quantity and quality to the level required to care for only minor ills and injuries, and patients from the Air Forces as well as from the rest of the Army who required treatment for serious ills and injuries should be concentrated, along with specialists to treat them, in general hospitals. In the fall of 1943 he attempted to achieve this goal (1) by requesting the General Staff either to permit him to reassign doctors from AAF hospitals as he saw fit or to direct the Air Forces to release specialists for duty with the Service Forces[10] and (2) by proposing a revision of the policy governing transfer of patients to general hospitals. ASF headquarters approved the latter suggestion and a revised policy was published in November 1943. In addition to establishing criteria for the selection of cases for transfer to general hospitals, this policy clearly limited station hospitals to such operations as appendectomies, herniotomies, and the treatment of simple fractures of the extremities.[11] The inference was that specialists were not needed in station hospitals.

Almost immediately the Air Forces protested that such restrictions would reduce their hospitals to dispensaries and would waste the skills and abilities of their staffs.[12] Despite The Surgeon General's insistence that, on the contrary, Medical Corps officers would be used more effectively if specialists and patients requiring specialized care were concentrated rather than scattered,[13] the Deputy Chief of Staff of the Army directed a compromise between the positions of the Air Surgeon and The Surgeon General. The Air Forces were to release some medical officers for ASF assignments but the policy on the transfer of patients to general hospitals was to be revised to permit AAF station hospitals to perform any operations, however complicated, for which they had adequate staffs.[14]

Early in 1944 The Inspector General reopened the question of the manning and use of AAF station hospitals. Reporting on a survey made by General Snyder, he

[9] Statement of Maj Gen Norman T. Kirk, Rpt, SGs Conf with Chiefs Med Br SvCs, 14–17 Jun 43, pp. 7–8. HD: 337.

[10] (1) Memo, SG for CofSA thru CG ASF, 13 Sep 43, with 1st ind, CG ASF to CofSA, 13 Sep 43. HRS: Hq ASF Gen Styer's files, "Med Dept." (2) Memo SPGAP 320.2 (8 Nov 43), Dir MPD ASF for ACofS G–1 WDGS, 8 Nov 43, sub: Critical Shortage of Med Specialists in ASF. SG: 322.051–1.

[11] (1) Ltr SPMCR 300.5–5, SG to AG, 10 Nov 43, sub: Policy Regarding Trf of Pnts to Named Gen Hosps. AG: 704.11 (10 Nov 43) (1). (2) WD Cir 304, 22 Nov 43.

[12] Memo, CG AAF for ACofS G–1 WDGS, 2 Dec 43, sub: Med Serv. AG: 704.00 (2 Dec 43).

[13] (1) Memo SPMC 701.–1, SG for Dir MPD ASF, 9 Dec 43, sub: Med Serv–AF. (2) T/S SPGAM 705 (Gen) (3 Dec 43)–31, CG ASF to ACofS G–1 WDGS, 13 Dec 43, same sub. (3) Ltr SPMCM 322.051–1, SG to CG ASF, 15 Dec 43, sub: MC Offs for Asgmt to ASF T/O Units. All in AG: 704.11 (2 Dec 43).

[14] (1) Memo WDCSA 705 (24 Dec 43) DepCofSA for ACofS G–1 WDGS, 24 Dec 43, sub: Sec 2, WD Cir 304, 22 Nov 43. AG: 704.11 (2 Dec 43). (2) WD Cir 12, 10 Jan 44.

recommended on 13 January 1944 that AAF station hospitals that were staffed and equipped to serve as general hospitals should be used in that capacity for patients not only from the Air Forces but from the Service and Ground Forces as well. The Deputy Chief of Staff accordingly directed the commanding generals of the Air and Service Forces to prepare a combined plan for hospitalization "on a regional and military population basis, irrespective of command or service jurisdictional boundaries." [15]

To comply with this directive and still maintain the status quo, The Surgeon General drew up a plan based upon the Secretary of War's policy of permitting only the Service Forces to operate general hospitals and of assigning all overseas evacuees, with few exceptions, to their care. He proposed that general hospitals should be of two types, those staffed for specialized treatment and those staffed for "all work," and that station hospitals of both the Air and Service Forces should be staffed according to manning tables applicable to both alike.[16] The Air Surgeon, on the other hand, attempted to use this opportunity to get authority to operate hospitals equal in all respects to those of the Service Forces. He proposed that hospitals be designated as specialized hospitals, regional hospitals, and station hospitals; and that they be staffed on the basis of their workloads and functions instead of by manning tables.[17] Since none were to be called general hospitals, none would be restricted by the Secretary of War's policy and hospitals of all three types could presumably be operated by both the Air and Service Forces.

When representatives of the Air Surgeon and The Surgeon General could not agree upon a plan to submit to the Deputy Chief of Staff, the Air Forces designated certain of their installations as "regional hospitals" and called attention to this development as their way of complying with the directive.[18] Subsequently, the entire problem of agreement upon a joint plan was referred to the Chiefs of Staff of the Air and Service Forces for solution.[19]

The outcome was a major change in the hospital system. Agreed upon by the AAF and ASF Chiefs of Staff, approved by the Deputy Chief of Staff of the Army, and authorized in April 1944, it represented a compromise between the proposals of The Surgeon General and the Air Surgeon. To the familiar station and general hospitals were now added the regional hospital, an entirely new species, and the convalescent hospital, an outgrowth of the convalescent centers and annexes already in use on a small scale. The Service Forces alone were to continue to operate general hospitals, but both the Air and Service Forces were to operate station, regional, and convales-

[15] (1) Ltr IG 333.-Med Pers, IG to DepCofSA, 13 Jan 44, sub: Util of Med Off Pers in ZI Instls. (2) Memo, DepCofSA for CGs ASF and AAF, 26 Jan 44, same sub. Both in Off file, Gen Bliss' Off SGO, "Util of MCs in ZI" (20) #2.

[16] Memo, SG for CG ASF, 29 Feb 44, sub: Util of Med Off Pers in ZI Instls, in Rpt to CG ASF from SG, Plan for Util of Med Off Pers in ZI, 29 Feb 44. HD: 322.051-1.

[17] (1) Memo, Hq AAF for SG, 26 Feb 44, sub: Proposed Plan, SGO, for the Util of MC Offs in ZI. Off file, Gen Bliss' Off SGO, "Util of MCs in ZI" (19) #1. (2) Draft Memo, CGs AAF and ASF for DepCofSA, [Feb 44], sub: Util of Med Off Pers in ZI Instls, prepared by Hq AAF. HD: Resources Anal Div files, "Hosp."

[18] (1) A History of Medical Administration and Practice in the Fourth Air Force (1945), vol. I, pp. 43-44. HD: TAS. (2) An Rpt, 1944, AAF Regional Hosp Maxwell Fld. HD. (3) Draft Memo, CGs AAF and ASF for DepCofSA, [Feb 44], sub: Util of Med Off Pers in ZI Instls, prepared by Hq AAF. HD: Resources Anal Div files, "Hosp."

[19] History of Control Division, ASF, 1942-45, App, p. 246. HD.

cent hospitals. Regional hospitals were to be staffed not only to care for patients requiring merely the treatment usually given in station hospitals but also to serve as general hospitals for zone of interior patients. General hospitals were to have the most highly specialized staffs and to them were to be transferred all patients evacuated from theaters of operations, except those needing only convalescent care. General hospitals were also to accept patients from the zone of interior who needed specialized treatment not given in regional hospitals. Hospitals of all four types were to serve troops on an area basis, irrespective of the command to which the troops or the hospital belonged, and a hospital was to transfer patients to another having better qualified personnel only if patients needed treatment which the transferring hospital was not staffed to give.[20] Thus, while the Service Forces retained the right to operate all general hospitals and in them to care for all theater of operations evacuees who needed further hospital treatment, the Air Forces gained the right to operate regional hospitals which were, in effect, general hospitals for zone of interior patients.

Although this change in the hospital system did not achieve integration of Air and Service Forces hospitalization, it did produce certain advantages. In June the War Department designated as regional hospitals thirty AAF and thirty ASF station hospitals agreed upon between The Surgeon General and the Air Surgeon.[21] Soon afterward both The Surgeon General and the Air Surgeon issued directives covering the transfer of patients from station to regional hospitals.[22] For several months ASF station hospitals had difficulty in adjusting to the idea of transferring complicated cases to regional instead of general hospitals, and there was little joint use of hospitals by the Air and Service Forces;[23] but by the latter part of 1944 The Inspector General reported that the establishment of regional hospitals had eliminated much duplication.[24] During 1945, when the patient load became heavy because of the influx of patients from theaters of operations, the care of the more serious and complicated cases from the zone of interior in regional hospitals permitted general hospitals to devote themselves almost entirely to the treatment of overseas evacuees.[25]

The question of whether regional hospitals could take over still more of the general hospital load—and perhaps become general hospitals themselves—came up early in 1945. When The Surgeon General asked for about 70,000 more beds in gen-

[20] WD Cir 140, 11 Apr 44.

[21] Memo, CG ASF for DepCofSA, 31 May 44, sub: Designation of Regional Hosps and Conv Hosps. AG: 705 (3 Apr 44)(1) "Util of Med Off Pers in ZI Instls." (2) WD Cir 228, 8 Jun 44. The number of regional hospitals was adjusted later as the need arose. For example, see WD Cirs 352, 30 Aug 44, and 115, 11 Apr 45.

[22] (1) Ltr, SG to CGs SvCs attn SvC Surg, 6 Jul 44, sub: Bed Credits in Regional and Gen Hosps, Tab G to IG Rpt, 28 Dec 44. (2) Ltr, CG AAF (Air Surg) to CG Tng Comd AAF, 2 Sep 44, sub: Bed Credits. (3) AAF Reg 25–17, 6 Jun 44, sub: AAF Hosp and Evac in Continental US. All in HRS: WDCSA 632 (25 Sep 44), "Hosp in ZI."

[23] (1) Ltr, CG ASF (Dep SG) to CG 9th SvC, 21 Sep 44, sub: Specialized Hosp. SG: 323.3 (9th SvC)AA. Similar letters found under same file number for different service commands. (2) Memo, 1st Lt Robert J. Myers, AUS, Med Stat Div SGO for Capt Edward A. Lew, 18 Sep 44, sub: Distr of Pnts in Regional Hosps as of 25 Aug 44. SG: 632.2.

[24] Memo, Act IG for DepCofSA, 28 Dec 44, sub: Hosp Fac in ZI. HRS: WDCSA 632 (25 Sep 44) Case No 28, "Hosp Fac in ZI."

[25] (1) Tab B of Memo, Dir Hosp Div and Dir Resources Anal Div SGO for Dir HD SGO thru Chief Oprs Serv SGO, 18 Jun 45, sub: Add Mat for An Rpt for FY 1945. HD: 319.1–2. (2) Interv, MD Historian with Lt Col James T. McGibony, MC, formerly Chief Hosp Div SGO, 20 Feb 50. HD: 000.71.

eral and convalescent hospitals to handle the growing influx of patients from overseas, G–4 directed the Air Forces to investigate the possibility of caring for overseas patients in AAF regional hospitals.[26] Taking the position that maximum use had to be made of all available beds in order to justify requests for additional beds in general and convalescent hospitals, G–4 later directed that overseas casualties should be placed in 4,000 beds in AAF regional hospitals which the Air Surgeon offered for that purpose. G–4 stated that this was an emergency measure and did not alter current policies (presumably the policy established by the Secretary of War in 1943 that all overseas patients, with minor exceptions, should be treated in general hospitals).[27] The Air Surgeon, who formerly had attempted to get separate general hospitals for the Air Forces and wanted to care for overseas casualties in AAF hospitals, urged immediate compliance with G–4's directive.[28]

The Surgeon General opposed this move. Having previously estimated that there were 12,000 vacant beds in AAF and ASF regional hospitals, he agreed that regional hospitals could be used for the purpose proposed but held that there were certain objections to doing so and that the expedient should be resorted to only in an emergency which, he contended, had not yet arisen.[29] ASF headquarters supported The Surgeon General and appealed G–4's directive to the Deputy Chief of Staff. The latter referred the question for investigation on 19 March 1945 to The Inspector General, who recommended two months later (14 May) that vacant beds in both ASF and AAF regional hospitals should be used in the manner proposed by G–4. G–4 then sought the Secretary of War's approval of a directive making this recommendation effective. On 20 June the Secretary met with G–4 and The Surgeon General, whose opinions on The Inspector General's report he had already received. By that time "events had overtaken this disagreement," G–4 reported, for the war in Europe had ended, and "there was no longer a necessity" of using regional hospital beds to take the load off the general hospital system. The Surgeon General concurred with this statement and the original demand was accordingly dropped.[30]

This development did not alter the fact that occupancy of general hospital beds at the end of June—despite provision of addi-

[26] Memo WDGDS 7486, ACofS G–4 WDGS for CG AAF, 11 Jan 45, sub: Care of Add Pnts at AAF Regional Hosps. HRS: G–4 file, "Hosp and Evac Policy."

[27] (1) Memo, CG AAF (Air Surg) for ACofS G–4 WDGS, 13 Feb 45, sub: Care of Overseas Casualties in AAF Regional Hosps. HRS: G–4 file, "Hosp and Evac Policy." (2) Memo WDGDS 9049, Dep ACofS G–4 for CG AAF and ASF, 27 Feb 45, same sub. HRS: G–4 file, "Hosp, vol. II." (3) Memo, Lt Col C. A. Dixon, G–4 for ACofS G–4 WDGS, 3 Mar 45, sub: Conf on Use of AAF Regional Hosp Beds. Same file.

[28] Memo, Air Surg for ACofS G–4 WDGS, 22 Mar 45, sub: Progress Rpt on Care of Overseas Casualties in AAF Regional Hosps. HD: TAS 210.721b, "Care of Overseas Casualties in AAF Hosps." Other memorandums on this subject are in the same file.

[29] T/S, Act SG to ACofS G–4 WDGS thru CG ASF, 22 Feb 45, sub: Care of Overseas Casualties in AAF Regional Hosps. HRS: G–4 file, "Hosp, vol. II."

[30] (1) 1st ind SPOPG (27 Feb 45), CG ASF to DepCofSA, 5 Mar 45, on Memo WDGS 9049, Dep ACofS G–4 WDGS for CGs ASF and AAF, 27 Feb 45, sub: Care of Overseas Casualties in AAF Regional Hosps. HRS: Hq ASF Planning Div file, 700 "Hosp and Evac." (2) Memo, DepCofSA for IG, 19 Mar 45, sub: ZI Hosp. HRS: Hq ASF Lt Gen Lutes' files, "Hosp and Evac, Jun 43–Dec 46." (3) Memo WDSIG 333.9–Hosp Fac (2), IG for DepCofSA, 14 May 45, sub: Rpt of Surv of ZI Hosps. SG: 333 WDCSA 632 (14 May 45). (4) Memo, Chief Planning Br G–4 for ACofS G–4 WDGS, 21 Jun 45, sub: Conf with SecWar on Rpt of Surv of ZI Hosps, with incl, Memo, Col Kyle (aide to SecWar) for SecWar [31 May 45], sub: ZI Hosps. HRS: G–4 file, "Hosp, vol. IV."

tional beds in the first half of 1945, placing large numbers of general hospital patients on leave and furlough for 90 days, and adoption of measures to speed the disposition of patients—ran above what was normally considered the saturation point (80 percent of capacity) while the occupancy of regional hospital beds was considerably lower.[31] Whether this situation was preferable to redistributing the patient load depended on the cogency of arguments against the suitability of regional hospitals for handling overseas patients. Several were of doubtful weight, such as that the use of these hospitals would "not have facilitated" observance of the War Department's policy of hospitalizing patients near their homes. On this point the Inspector General's Office and indeed The Surgeon General's own Resources Analysis Division estimated that 15 to 20 percent of the beds available in regional hospitals were located in areas where population was dense but general hospital beds few in number. To the argument that existing space in general hospitals (that is, on 5 March 1945) was still adequate, the reply might have been that it was being kept so partly by establishing additional beds in general hospitals which The Surgeon General had requested. It was also argued that filling the beds of regional hospitals with long-term patients would use up excess capacity needed to provide extra hospitalization for troops that would be returned from Europe for redeployment to the Pacific. To this the Inspector General's Office replied that the need in the latter case would arise only after the peak load had been passed. Nor did the Inspector General's Office agree with The Surgeon General's contention that difficulties would result from mixing overseas patients with those from the zone of interior in regional hospitals. Greater importance may or may not be attached to The Surgeon General's argument that the administrative difficulties of adding a large number of hospitals to those already treating overseas patients would have outweighed the gain of 12,000 beds. But it could not be denied, of course, that "diversion of patients from the general hospital system would prevent control of treatment by the agency now charged with their care."[32]

This last argument perhaps held the key to the entire matter. After the establishment of regional hospitals to serve in effect as general hospitals for zone of interior patients, the chief remaining distinction between hospital systems of the Air and Service Forces was that ASF general hospitals, but no AAF hospitals at all, were authorized to care for patients returning from overseas areas for further medical

---

[31] See below, pp. 210–12. Normally a hospital was considered full when 80 percent of its beds were occupied, because some of its beds were always required for dispersion. In August 1944 the Facilities Utilization Branch, SGO, proposed reducing the "dispersion factor" in estimating requirements from 20 to 15 percent because of a "liberal furlough policy." (Memo, Eli Ginzberg for SG, 18 Aug 44. HD: Resources Anal Div file, "Hosp.") In estimating requirements in January 1945 no beds for dispersion were included "on the assumption that furloughs will provide the necessary number of empty beds." (Memo, Asst SG for Act Dir Plans and Oprs ASF, 8 Jan 45, sub: Gen Hosp Program, ZI. SG: 323.3.)

[32] (1) 1st ind SPOPG (27 Feb 45), CG ASF to DepCofSA, 5 Mar 45, on Memo WDGDS 9049, Dep ACofS G–4 WDGS for CGs ASF and AAF, 27 Feb 45, sub: Care of Overseas Casualties in AAF Regional Hosps. HRS: Hq ASF Planning Div file, 700 "Hosp and Evac." (2) T/S, Act SG to Dep ACofS G–4 WDGS thru CG ASF, 22 Feb 45, same sub. HRS: G–4 file, "Hosp, vol. II." (3) Memo WDSIG 333.9–Hosp Fac (2), IG for DepCofSA, 14 May 45, sub: Rpt of Surv of ZI Hosps. SG: 333 WDCSA 632 (14 May 45). (4) Memo, Dir Resources Anal Div SGO for Chief Oprs Serv SGO, 20 Jan 45, sub: Sta and Regional Hosp Backup for Gen Hosp Syst. SG: 632.2.

and surgical treatment. To have placed some of them in AAF regional hospitals would have narrowed if not eliminated that distinction. An officer who participated in these transactions afterward interpreted the controversy in these terms—the desire of the Air Surgeon to eliminate that distinction and the determination of The Surgeon General to maintain it.[33] This view seems plausible when the previous efforts of the Air Surgeon to secure a hospital system equal to that of the Service Forces are considered. It may also derive color from the fact that The Surgeon General, in tracing for the benefit of the Secretary of War the events leading up to the controversy, started with a reference to the Air Surgeon's attempt to secure general hospitals for AAF casualties in 1943.[34] Further evidence to support such an interpretation is the accusation by the Air Surgeon and members of his staff that The Surgeon General was using delaying tactics. They charged that while he agreed to employ regional hospital beds for overseas casualties in an emergency he deliberately spun out negotiations in an effort to avoid taking that step at all.[35] In any event, the distinction between general and regional hospitals remained, and it continued to be the official policy of the Army to treat overseas evacuees in general hospitals only.

Development of Convalescent Hospitals

Convalescent hospitals were first authorized as types of Army hospitals in the zone of interior in April 1944, but their origin lay in the early war years.[36] Under authority granted by the Secretary of War in July 1943, the Air Forces announced the establishment of eight convalescent centers in September 1943. They were to operate in conjunction with station hospitals and were to rehabilitate AAF patients who had been treated in other hospitals or who had been evacuated from theaters of operations solely because of operational fatigue.[37] In June 1943 the Service Forces began to establish convalescent annexes in hospital barracks, leased schools and inns, or vacated Army housing. Operated as parts of general hospitals, such annexes normally housed convalescent patients only from the hospitals to which they belonged, but one of them—the convalescent annex of England General Hospital, set up in leased hotels with a capacity for 2,600 patients—served as a convalescent center for patients from other general hospitals as well.[38] Partly because of difficulties in finding suitable housing for annexes, the program was slow in getting under way and convalescent patients accounted for approximately 75 percent of the patient load of general hospitals in the fall of 1943. Groups studying the hospital system at that time agreed that convalescent patients should be removed from the wards

---

[33] Interv, MD Historian with Col John C. Fitzpatrick, MC, formerly MRO, SGO, 18 Apr 50. HD: 000.71.

[34] Memo, Chief Planning Br G–4 for ACofS G–4 WDGS, 21 Jun 45, sub: Conf with SecWar on Rpt of Surv of ZI Hosps. HRS: G–4 file, "Hosp, vol. IV."

[35] (1) Record of Tel Conv between [Maj] Gen [D. N. W.] Grant and [Brig] Gen Raymond W. Bliss, 7 Mar 45. HD: TAS 210.721b "Care of Overseas Casualties in AAF Hosps." (2) Memo, [Lt Col Alonzo A. Towner, MC] for Gen Grant, n d. Same file.

[36] See above, pp. 117–20.

[37] AAF Memo 20–12, 18 Sep 43. HD: AAF Memo 5–20 series.

[38] (1) 1st ind SPRMC 322 (18 Jun 43), CG ASF to SG, 22 Jun 43, on unknown basic ltr. SG: 632.–1. (2) Res Adopted by Fed Bd of Hosp, incl to Memo SPRMC 632 (19 Oct 43), CG ASF for CofEngrs, 27 Oct 43, sub: Auth for Estab of Conv Retraining Units at Gen Hosps. CE: 683 Pt I. (3) Ltr, SG to CG ASF, 30 Oct 43, sub: Program for Providing Conv Fac. SG: 632.-1. (4) An Rpt, 1944, Surg 2d SvC. HD.

of general hospitals to permit fuller use of the latter's highly specialized staffs.[39]

During 1944 the convalescent hospital program received impetus from several sources. Early that year, after his Office had estimated the patient load for 1944, The Surgeon General requested that additional beds be provided in convalescent "facilities," rather than in general hospitals, to save personnel and to permit the reconditioning of patients for return to duty in a nonhospital atmosphere. In March ASF headquarters approved this proposal, and during subsequent months service commands, acting under ASF authority, established convalescent centers in vacated barracks at Daytona Beach (Florida), Camp Lockett (California), Camp Carson (Colorado), Camp Atterbury (Indiana), Fort Sam Houston (Texas), Fort Custer (Michigan), and Fort Devens (Massachusetts).[40]

Meanwhile, a War Department circular authorized convalescent hospitals, as distinct from convalescent centers, annexes, and facilities. Accordingly, in June 1944 the War Department designated as convalescent hospitals two ASF and five AAF convalescent centers which The Surgeon General and the Air Surgeon selected for that purpose. Two months later, thirteen additional ASF convalescent centers were designated as hospitals, and subsequently other changes were made in the number in operation.[41] These hospitals remained in an experimental stage for the rest of 1944. Those of ASF served as places for housing and feeding ambulatory patients and for preparing them through physical and military training for return to duty. Changes in barracks provided for such hospitals were held to a minimum. They therefore lacked classrooms, shops, and gymnasiums that were later—in 1945—considered essential. In addition, the scope of activities of convalescent hospitals was not clearly defined; their organization was not precisely outlined by higher authorities; and they had little personnel and equipment of their own.[42]

An exception to this general situation was the Old Farms Convalescent Hospital, in Avon, Conn. Established in May 1944 as a result of The Surgeon General's and the President's interest in the rehabilitation of blinded war casualties, this hospital soon afterward received personnel and equipment for a social-adjustment training program which continued throughout the war.[43]

In the fall and winter of 1944 several events brought the convalescent hospital program to full fruition. During a movement of higher authorities to reduce the numbers of beds in the United States, G–4 took up the matter of convalescent hospitals and in November, as a part of a compromise solution of the bed requirement problem, authorized 40,000 beds in AAF

[39] (1) Memo, unsigned and unaddressed, 23 Aug 43, sub: Status of Program for Estab of Conv Retraining Units. SG: 632.-1. (2) Memo, Dir Hosp Admin Div SGO for Chief Oprs Serv SGO, 4 Dec 43, sub: Rpt of Trip to . . . Gen Hosps. SG: 333.1-1.

[40] (1) See below, pp. 201–02. (2) Memo, SG for CG ASF, 10 Mar 44, sub: Conv Fac. Off file, Gen Bliss' Off SGO, "Med Clarification of Disposition Policy." (3) ASF Cir 93, 4 Apr 44. (4) An Rpts, 1944, Surg 1st, 4th, 5th, 6th, and 7th SvCs; and An Rpts, 1944, Brooke Gen and Conv Hosps and Mitchell Conv Hosp. HD.

[41] WD Cirs 140, 11 Apr 44; 228, 7 Jun 44; and 352, 30 Aug 44.

[42] (1) Memo, SG for Dir Pers ASF, 22 Jul 44, sub: Estab of Conv Hosps. HD: 322 "Estab of Conv Hosps." (2) Memo, Eli Ginzberg for Pres WDMB, 23 Aug 44. HRS: ASF Planning Div file, 700 "ZI Hosp." (3) ASF Monthly Progress Rpt, Sec 7, *Health,* 31 May 44. (4) An Rpts, 1944, Surg 2d, 4th, 5th, and 7th SvCs; An Rpt, 1944, Mitchell Conv Hosp; An Rpts, 1945, Brooke and Wakeman Hosp Ctrs. HD.

[43] (1) History, Old Farms Convalescent Hospital [1947]. HD: 319.1-2. (2) SG Ltr 162, 11 Sep 43.

and ASF convalescent hospitals.[44] This established a basis for the procurement of personnel and equipment for such installations. A few weeks later, on 4 December 1944, the President directed the Secretary of War to permit no overseas casualty to be discharged from the service until he had received "the maximum benefits of hospitalization and convalescent facilities," including "physical and psychological rehabilitation, vocational guidance, prevocational training and resocialization." [45] Such unlimited support from the Commander in Chief helped the Medical Department to get necessary means for an elaborate convalescent program, which The Surgeon General's Reconditioning Consultants Division announced in December 1944.[46]

During the first half of 1945, ASF convalescent hospitals were supplied with personnel and equipment of their own; the barracks in which they were located were remodeled; shops, classrooms, gymnasiums and recreational facilities were provided; and elaborate programs consisting of technical and prevocational training, general education, vocational counseling, occupational therapy, recreation, athletics, and entertainment were set up.[47] Thus, toward the end of the war, emphasis in the convalescent program shifted from the preparation of patients for return to duty to their preparation for return to civilian life.

The operation of convalescent hospitals was a major factor in enabling the Medical Department to care for the peak load of patients in the summer of 1945. It contributed to maximum use of specialists in general hospitals. Furthermore, convalescent hospitals provided a better psychological environment for the care of many patients, especially those suffering from neuropsychiatric disorders, than did general hospitals.[48] Their value in the treatment of medical and minor surgical cases, however, was questioned in the middle of 1945,[49] and general hospitals gradually adopted a practice of discharging patients of those types directly to civilian life.

Merger of Adjacent Hospitals

Besides suggesting the removal of convalescent patients from general hospitals, groups studying the hospital system in the fall of 1943 proposed the merger of adjacent hospitals into single installations. The establishment of regional hospitals accomplished this in part, for in some cases nearby station hospitals were either wholly or partially merged with regional hospitals.[50] In the same period the Ninth Service Command consolidated the Vancouver Barracks Station Hospital with Barnes General Hospital, which was located on the same post.[51] The next April The Sur-

[44] Memo, ACofS G-4 WDGS for CGs ASF and AAF, 17 Nov 44, sub: ZI Hosps. SG: 322 "Hosp Misc."

[45] Ltr, Franklin D. Roosevelt to SecWar, 4 Dec 44. HRS: ASF Control Div file, 705 "Cut-back in Gen and Conv Fac."

[46] (1) ASF Cir 419, 22 Dec 44, sub: Conv Hosp Revised Program. (2) TM 8-290, Educ Reconditioning, Dec 44. (3) TM 8-291, Occupational Therapy, Dec 44. (4) TM 8-292, Physical Reconditioning, Dec 44.

[47] (1) An Rpt, FY 1945, SG. HD. (2) Richard L. Loughlin, [History of] Reconditioning [in the U. S. Army in World War II], (1946), HD. (3) Memo WDSIG 333.9 Hosp Fac (2), IG for DepCofSA, 14 May 45, sub: Rpt of Surv of ZI Hosps. SG: 333 WDCSA 632 (14 May 45). (4) An Rpts of Conv Hosps for 1945. HD. (5) Memo, Lt Col Gerard R. Gessner for Chief Hosp Div SGO, 4 Jun 45. HD: 333.1-1.

[48] An Rpt, FY 1945, SG; and An Rpt, FY 1945, Hosp and Dom Oprs. SGO. HD.

[49] Memo, Dir Resources Anal Div SGO for Chief Oprs Serv SGO, 7 Jun 45, sub: Criteria for Reduction in Hosp Fac. SG: 323.3 "Hosp."

[50] Memo, IG for DepCofSA, 28 Dec 44, sub: Hosp Fac in ZI. HRS: WDCSA 632 (25 Sep 44).

[51] 1st ind, CG 9th SvC to CG ASF attn SG, 22 Sep 43, on Ltr, SG to CG 9th SvC, 24 Aug 43, sub: Combination of Sta Hosp with Gen Hosp. SG: 323.7-5 (Barnes GH)K.

geon General's Facilities Utilization Branch made a study of other sets of general and station hospitals located on the same Army posts, comparing personnel required to operate them as separate installations with that needed for their operation as consolidated hospitals. It appeared that fewer Medical Corps officers, particularly specialists, and fewer nurses would be needed if station hospitals were merged with near-by general hospitals.[52] The Surgeon General's Office anticipated more efficient operation from the supervision of the activities of two installations by one rather than two commanding officers. Moreover, the commaders of general hospitals were subject to less control by post commanders than were those of station hospitals—an advantage from The Surgeon General's viewpoint. The mergers were not expected to increase the number of general hospital beds immediately, because general hospitals thus enlarged would still have to care for troops stationed on their posts. Later as troops moved overseas, beds formerly used for station hospital patients could be transferred to general hospital use.[53] Accordingly, five station hospitals were consolidated with five general hospitals in the summer of 1944, as follows: Fort Devens Station Hospital with Lovell General Hospital, Fort Dix Station Hospital with Tilton General Hospital, Fort Bliss Station Hospital with William Beaumont General Hospital, Fort Benjamin Harrison Station Hospital with Billings General Hospital, and Dante Hospital in San Francisco with Letterman General Hospital.[54]

Attempts To Limit the Use of General Hospitals as Debarkation Hospitals

Another change in the hospital system occurred when The Surgeon General modified the existing practice of using general hospitals located near ports as receiving and evacuation hospitals. Throughout the later war years Halloran, Stark, and Letterman General Hospitals continued to serve as debarkation hospitals, the latter two being devoted almost exclusively to that function as the evacuation load grew heavier. At various times during 1944 and 1945 other general hospitals—Lovell, Barnes, McGuire, Birmingham, LaGarde, Madigan, and Mason—served also in that way.[55] General hospitals accepted their roles as receiving and evacuation, or debarkation hospitals reluctantly because the processing of patients in transit did not require the fullest use of specialized equipment and staffs and because hospitals engaged in that function had alternating periods of activity and idleness, depending upon the arrival of ships with patients.[56] Several officers in the Surgeon General's Office were also dissatisfied with the practice of having

[52] Memo, Chief Fac Util Br SGO for Chief Oprs Serv SGO, 24 Apr 44, sub: Pers Study of Five Contiguous Sets of Sta and Gen Hosps. HD: Resources Anal Div file, "Hosp."

[53] (1) Ltr, SG to Fed Bd Hosp, 27 Jun 44, sub: Combination of Named Gen Hosp and Adj Sta Hosp. SG: 323.7-5. (2) Draft Ltr, SecWar (prepared by SGO) to Fed Bd Hosp, 12 Jul 44. SG: 322 "Hosp." (3) Interv, MD Historian with Maj Gen Norman T. Kirk, 20 Nov 51. HD: 314 (Correspondence on MS)V.

[54] Diary, Hosp Cons Br SGO, 15 and 20 Jul 44. HD: 024.7-3.

[55] (1) Weekly Health Rpts, vol. IV, No 1, 7 Jan 44; No 24, 16 Jun 44; No 32, 11 Aug 44; No 34, 25 Aug 44; and No 40, 6 Oct 44. AML. (2) An Rpt, FY 1945, Hosp and Dom Oprs, SGO. HD. (3) Memo, Dir Resources Anal Div SGO for Dir HD SGO, 25 Sep 45, sub: Operational Problems and Accomplishments in Med Serv, World War II. HD: 319 "Hosp." (4) Memo, SG for WDMB, 4 Oct 44, sub: Debarkation Hosps. SG: 322 "Hosp."

[56] (1) Memo, CO Halloran Gen Hosp for CG 2d SvC attn Surg, 21 Feb 44, sub: Increased Bed Capacity. SG: 632.2 (Halloran GH)K. (2) Diary, Hosp Admin Div SGO, 11 Jan 44. HD: 024.7-3. (3) S/S, SG to CG ASF, 25 Nov 44, sub: 300-Bed Expansion by Conversion, McGuire Gen Hosp, with inds. SG: 632.-1 (McGuire GH)K.

general hospitals perform dual functions. The Medical Regulating Officer, for example, thought that this practice interfered with efficient operation of the evacuation system, and others agreed with hospital commanders that it was wasteful of both personnel and equipment.[57] When changes in the hospital system were being considered early in 1944. The Surgeon General proposed establishment of a new type of hospital, to be known as a receiving and evacuation hospital and to be manned and equipped to perform only the processing of patients in transit.[58] This proposal was not accepted, and the circular outlining the revised hospital system in April 1944 provided for the continued use of existing types of hospitals—station, general, or regional—for debarkation purposes.[59] After that, in the summer of 1944, Stark, Letterman, and Halloran separated general hospital functions from debarkation work, becoming to that extent two hospitals in one.[60]

As the need for beds in both general and debarkation hospitals increased, The Surgeon General attempted to keep to a minimum the use of general hospitals for debarkation processing. In the summer of 1944 he secured approval of ASF headquaters to use the Camp Edwards Station Hospital, instead of Lovell General Hospital, as a debarkation hospital for the port of Boston. This action, he explained, would make available more general hospital beds in New England, a heavily populated section with only two general hospitals. It would also help to economize in the use of Medical Corps officers, since debarkation hospitals required less elaborate staffs than general hospitals.[61] In the winter of 1944, as he planned to meet higher bed requirements which his Office had estimated for 1945, The Surgeon General proposed to use other station hospitals—those located at staging areas and operated by the Chief of Transportation—to free some general hospitals of debarkation work and to provide additional debarkation beds that would be needed for the anticipated load of casualties.[62] A survey made by the Inspector General's Office had already shown that staging area hospitals were being used only slightly, since few troops were being moved overseas.[63] The Chief of Transportation agreed to convert hospitals in the staging areas of the ports of Boston (Camp Myles Standish), New York (Camp Kilmer and Camp Shanks), and Hampton Roads (Camp Patrick Henry) into debarkation hospitals.[64] This action made it

[57] (1) Memo, Lt Col John C. Fitzpatrick, MRO, for Col A. H. Schwichtenberg, Hosp Div SGO, 23 May 44. TC: 370.05. (2) Memo, Same for Chief Oprs Serv SGO, 1 Sep 44, sub: Rpt of Visit to San Francisco. HD: 705 (MRO, Fitzpatrick Stayback). (3) Memo, Lt Col Basil C. MacLean for Brig Gen R. W. Bliss, Chief Oprs Serv SGO thru Col A. H. Schwichtenberg, Dir Hosp Admin Div, 2 Feb 44, sub: The More Efficient Util of Army Hosp Fac. Off file, Gen Bliss' Off SGO, "Util of Army Hosp Fac."

[58] Classification of Med Instls, Tab B to SGs Plan for the Util of Med Off Pers in ZI, 29 Feb 44. HD: 322.051-1.

[59] WD Cir 140, 11 Apr 44.

[60] An Rpts, 1944, Stark, Halloran, and Letterman Gen Hosps. HD.

[61] (1) Memo, Dep SG for CG ASF, 1 Jun 44, sub: Util of Comd Fac: Designation of Cp Edwards a Gen Hosp. Off file, Gen Bliss' Off SGO, "Util of Army Hosp Fac." (2) Ltr, CG 1st SvC to CG ASF attn SG, 7 Jun 44, sub: Instls for Debarkation Hosp. SG: 322.15-1. (3) An Rpt, 1944, Cp Edwards Sta Hosp. HD.

[62] Memo, SG for Act Dir Plans and Oprs ASF, 8 Jan 45, sub: Gen Hosp Program, ZI. SG: 323.3.

[63] Memo, Act IG for DepCofSA, 28 Dec 44, sub: Hosp Fac in ZI. HRS: OCS 632 (25 Sep 44) Case No 28, "Hosp Fac in ZI."

[64] (1) 1st ind SPTOM 632, CofT to SG, 17 Jan 45, on Memo, SG for Med Liaison Off, OCofT, 9 Jan 45. SG: 632. (2) Diary, Lt Col H. A. Huncilman, Planning Div ASF, 25, 27, and 29 Jan 45. HRS: Hq ASF Planning Div file, 700 "ZI Hosps." (3) Diary, Hosp Div SGO, 31 Jan 45. HD: 024.7-3.

TABLE 12—ASF DEBARKATION HOSPITALS

Port and Hospital	October 1944			March 1945			June 1945			August 1945		
	Total Beds	Dbktn Beds	Gen Hosp Beds	Total Beds	Dbktn Beds	Gen Hosp Beds	Total Beds	Dbktn Beds	Gen Hosp Beds	Total Beds	Dbktn Beds	Gen Hosp Beds
Boston												
Edwards	2,128	2,128	0	[a] 3,200	800	2,400	2,950	900	2,050	([b])	......	......
Boston POE	......	......	......	1,700	1,700	0	1,700	1,700	0	......	......	......
New York												
Halloran	4,134	2,799	1,335	5,350	2,700	2,650	5,350	2,700	2,650	5,350	2,700	2,650
Kilmer	......	......	......	2,000	2,000	0	2,000	2,000	0	2,000	2,000	0
Shanks	......	......	......	2,300	2,300	0	2,300	2,300	0	......	......	......
Mason	......	......	......	3,032	1,000	2,032	2,532	500	2,032	3,032	500	2,532
Hampton Roads												
McGuire	1,777	1,577	200	......	......	......	......	......	......	......	......	......
Patrick Henry	......	......	......	1,100	1,100	0	1,100	1,100	0	......	......	......
Charleston												
Stark	2,400	2,162	238	2,400	2,125	275	2,400	2,125	275	2,400	2,125	275
New Orleans												
LaGarde	926	150	776	1,176	0	1,176	1,300	0	1,300	......	......	......
Los Angeles												
Birmingham	1,727	717	1,010	1,777	800	977	......	......	......	......	......	......
Camp Haan	......	......	......	......	......	......	800	800	0	800	800	0
San Francisco												
Letterman	2,338	2,000	338	3,500	3,140	360	3,500	3,140	360	3,500	3,140	360
Seattle												
Madigan	3,880	500	3,380	4,300	1,000	3,300	4,300	1,000	3,300	4,380	1,000	3,380
Total	19,310	12,033	7,277	31,835	18,665	13,170	30,232	18,265	11,967	21,462	12,265	9,197
All Sta Hosps Used for Debarkation purposes	2,128	2,128	0	7,100	7,100	0	7,900	7,900	0	2,800	2,800	0
All Gen Hosps Used for Debarkation purposes	17,182	9,905	7,277	24,735	11,565	13,170	22,332	10,365	11,967	18,662	9,465	9,197

[a] Camp Edwards Station Hospital was designated a General Hospital in February 1945.
[b] In this table no figures are listed for beds in hospitals at the times when those hospitals were not being used for debarkation purposes.

Sources: (1) Memo SPMCH, SG for WDMB, 4 Oct 44, sub: Debarkation Hosp. SG: 322 Hosp. (2) Weekly Hosp Rpts, vol. II, No. 13, 30 Mar 45; No. 25, 22 Jun 45; and No. 35, 31 Aug 45.

unnecessary to devote more space in Halloran General Hospital to debarkation work and made it possible to free all of McGuire General Hospital and the Camp Edwards Station Hospital, which was converted into a general hospital, for specialized medical and surgical treatment. *(Table 12)* Later in 1945 the Camp Haan Regional Hospital took over from Birmingham General Hospital the processing of patients debarked at Los Angeles.[65] Thus, the Surgeon General's Office tried gradually to limit the practice of using general hospital facilities for debarkation work.

As the evacuation of patients by air increased during 1944 and 1945 the Air Forces selected certain station and regional hospitals located near important landing fields to receive and process patients

[65] (1) Memo, Dir Resources Anal Div SGO for Maj [James J.] Souder, 22 Mar 45, sub: Debarkation Beds. HD: Resources Anal Div file, "Hosp." (2) Diary, Hosp Div SGO, 7 and 11 Apr 45. HD: 024.7-3. (3) Memo, CG ASF for CofEngrs, 11 Apr 45, sub: Pnt Unloading Fac, Cp Haan Hosp. SG: 322 "Hosp."

brought to them. By October 1944 beds were set aside in eleven AAF hospitals for this purpose.[66] Six were used for debarking patients in emergencies only. The other five, located at Mitchel Field (New York), Coral Gables (Florida), Hamilton Field (California), Great Falls (Montana), and Portland (Oregon), were devoted almost exclusively to processing patients evacuated by air.[67] In the late spring of 1945 the Air Forces, with the concurrence of The Surgeon General, planned to establish a new type of zone of interior installation, called a holding facility, at the Fairfield-Suisun Field (California). It was designed to perform only one function—the processing of patients who were in transit to other hospitals for definitive treatment.[68] Although the war ended before it was constructed, its approval represented a further development in the movement toward the use of less elaborate facilities than general hospitals for debarkation purposes.

Extension of the Practice of Establishing Specialized Centers

Extension and further development of the practice of establishing centers for specialized treatment in general hospitals constituted another adjustment in the hospital system during the later war years. Until the middle of 1944 specialty centers in general hospitals took up only a small proportion of their total beds and were established piecemeal to meet needs as they arose, without regard to eventual requirements for beds for specialized treatment. This situation came about because an army in training needed less specialized care than one in combat, because it was difficult to predict types and amount of specialized treatment that would be needed, and because hospitals themselves opened successively rather than all together. By the time of the invasion of Europe, the peak patient load had been estimated and the last of the general hospitals, with the exception of four temporary ones authorized in 1945, were about to begin operation. Enough experience in hospital admissions had accumulated to permit a breakdown of the anticipated patient load in terms of types of wounds, diseases, and injuries. Furthermore, an increasing shortage of specialists made their concentration for maximum use more imperative than ever. Thus, whatever the need for a thoroughgoing program earlier, it became more important and easier to formulate one by the middle of 1944. Therefore, in the summer of that year The Surgeon General's Facilities Utilization Branch collaborated with his professional consultants in a study of the need for specialized centers and in the preparation of a comprehensive plan to meet it.[69]

The general features of this plan, announced in a War Department circular in August 1944, remained unchanged through the remainder of the war. Related

[66] AAF Debarkation Hosp, incl to Memo, SG for WDMB, 4 Oct 44, sub: Debarkation Hosp. SG: 322 "Hosp."

[67] Memo, Act IG for DepCofSA, 28 Dec 44, sub; Hosp Fac in ZI. HRS: OCS 632 (25 Sep 44) Case No 28, "Hosp Fac in ZI."

[68] (1) S/S, CG AAF to ACofS G-4 WDGS, CofSA, and SecWar, 27 Apr 45, sub: Debarkation Hosp, Fairfield-Suisun Army Air Fld. (2) DF WDGDS 12801, ACofS G-4 WDGS to CofSA, 10 May 45, same sub. (3) Ltr, SecWar to Brig Gen Frank T. Hines, Chairman Fed Bd Hosp, 15 May 45. All in HRS: OCS 632.

[69] (1) Ltr, SG to CG 4th SvC attn SvC Surg, 14 Jun 44, sub: Specialized Gen Hosp. SG: 323.7-5 (4th SvC)AA. Similar letters were sent to the rest of the service commands. (2) Plan for Specialized Hosp, by [Dr.] Eli Ginzberg, Spec Asst to Dir Hosp Div SGO, 27 Jul 44. HD: Resources Anal Div file, "Hosp." (3) ASF Monthly Progress Rpt, Sec 7, *Health*, 31 Jul 44, pp. 29-31.

specialties were grouped in the same hospital to improve the quality of professional care. For example, neurosurgical and neurologic centers were established together, and centers for general medicine were set up in hospitals specializing in the treatment of arthritis, tuberculosis, and rheumatic fever. Attempts were made to locate specialty centers in relation to population density, to permit compliance as far as possible with the policy of hospitalizing patients near their homes. Success in such attempts was limited by at least two factors: (1) there were proportionately fewer general hospitals in densely populated areas such as the Northeast than there were in the South and Southwest, where they had been located initially to serve large concentrations of troops in training, and (2) it was either possible or desirable to establish only a limited number of centers—in some instances as few as two—in certain specialties such as tuberculosis, arthritis, and treatment of the blind.

The size of centers increased as the patient load grew. Although professional consultants of the Surgeon General's Office believed that they should be kept reasonably small, the Facilities Utilization Branch considered it more economical of personnel, particularly specialists, to limit the number but increase the size of centers. In the fall of 1944, for example, amputation centers were increased from 500 to 750 beds each and neurosurgical centers from 250 to 500. Subsequently, to care for the peak patient load, capacities were further increased, some centers having 2,000 or more beds.

Centers for additional specialties were established to meet new needs and achieve fuller use of specialists of all kinds. For example, patients suffering from tropical diseases and trench foot became so numerous as to warrant the designation of centers for the treatment of those conditions, and a shortage of internists prompted the establishment of general medicine as a specialty. General and orthopedic surgery also became specialties as the field of surgery was narrowed by the establishment of centers for various surgical specialties. As a result, the major portion of beds in general hospitals was gradually given over to specialized treatment, and general hospitals became in effect specialized hospitals. By the time the peak patient load was reached in June 1945, there were 234 centers for 21 specialties with a total of 132,178 beds in 65 general hospitals in the United States.[70]

General Hospitals for Prisoners of War

A further change in the hospital system resulted from the capture by American forces of large numbers of prisoners of war. For German and Italian prisoners who became sick or were injured while in internment camps in this country, the system of hospitalization formerly established was changed only slightly during the latter half of the war. Such prisoners continued to be treated in station hospitals located either in internment camps or on near-by Army posts and, when they needed a higher type of care, in general

[70] (1) See last note above. (2) WD Cir 347, 25 Aug 44. (3) ASF Cir 284, 30 Aug 44. (4) Ltr SPMCH 323.3 (7th SvC)AA, SG to CG 7th SvC attn Surg, 10 Aug 44, sub: Specialized Gen Hosps. HD: Resources Anal Div file, "Hosp." (5) Tab B to Memo, Dir Hosp Div and Dir Resources Anal Div for Dir HD SGO, 18 Jun 45, sub: Add Mat for An Rpt for FY 1945. HD: 319.1–2. (6) Table entitled "Authorized Patient Capacities in General Hospitals by Specialty as of 30 June 1945," prepared by Resources Analysis Division, 30 June 1945. Off file, Resources Analysis Div, SGO.

hospitals operated for U. S. Army patients. All Japanese prisoners were concentrated, since they were few in number, in the station hospital at Camp McCoy, Wis.[71]

In the second half of 1943 the offices of The Surgeon General and The Provost Marshal General collaborated in establishing procedures for the reception, examination, and transportation of a new category of prisoners—those evacuated as patients from theaters of operations.[72] Early the next year they restated these procedures and designated five general hospitals located near ports to receive and sort such patients and to transfer them to other hospitals for further treatment. At the same time, they specified certain general hospitals for the care of tuberculous, insane, blind, and deaf prisoners; and, in order to simplify the observance of security and administrative regulations, they adopted a practice of concentrating all prisoners who needed general-hospital-type care—those evacuated as patients from theaters of operations as well as those transferred from internment camps—in one general hospital if possible, and in not more than three in any instance, in each service command.[73] These steps did not solve all problems. Some general hospitals continued to be inadequately prepared to carry out security measures; and even though prisoners were concentrated more than formerly, they were still scattered among hospitals in nine service commands. Such dispersal made difficult the work of a commission charged with determining the eligibility of some prisoners for repatriation as well as that of a group responsible for certifying others for "protected status" as medical personnel, under the terms of the Geneva Convention.[74]

In anticipation of an influx of prisoner-of-war patients after the invasion of Europe and in the hope of solving some of the administrative problems caused by the existing system of hospitalization, The Surgeon General's liaison officer with The Provost Marshal General proposed in July 1944 that at least one general hospital be devoted exclusively to German prisoners of war. It could be used to sort incoming patients, to treat those needing general-hospital-type care, to process those eligible for repatriation, and to hold others awaiting certification as protected personnel.[75] His superior, the Deputy Chief for Hospitals and Domestic Operations, adopted this idea and announced on 21 July 1944 that The Surgeon General was designating Glennan General Hospital as a German prisoner-of-war general hospital.[76]

Two months later The Surgeon General asked for an entire Army post for use as a second hospital of this type. Because of

[71] (1) WD Cirs 235, 12 Jun 44, and 347, 25 Aug 44. (2) PW Cirs 18, 29 Mar 44; 20, 7 Apr 44; and 38, 15 Jul 44. Off file, PW Off, OPMG. (3) TWX, PMG to CG each SvC, 4 Jan 45, in An Rpt, FY 1945, PW Liaison Unit SGO. HD. (4) Diary, Hosp Div SGO, 7 Oct 44. HD: 024.7-3. (5) Hosp, Evac, and Disposition of PW Pnts in US, by Lt Col James T. McGibony, MC. HD: 383.6.

[72] WD Cir 214, 15 Sep 43.

[73] PW Cir 11, 8 Feb 44. Off file, PW Off, OPMG.

[74] (1) Memo SPMGA 383.6 (59), Maj Rene H. Juchli for Act Dir PW Div OPMG, 23 Feb 44, sub: Rpt of Second Repatriation of German PW. (2) Memo SPMGA 383.6 (59), same for Asst PMG, 10 Apr 44, sub: Immed Designation of Cp for Reception of Protected Pers and Repatriable PW. (3) Ltr, same to PMG, 13 May 44, sub: Rpt of Third Repatriation Move, German PW. (4) Ltr, same to Dir Hosp Admin Div SGO, 13 Aug 44, sub: Rpt of Handling PW as Observed at NYPE and Halloran Gen Hosp. All in HD: 319.1-2.

[75] Memo, Chief PW Liaison Unit SGO for SG attn Col A. H. Schwichtenberg, 17 Jul 44, sub: Reception, Hosp, Treatment, and Disposition of Pnts among PW and Protected Pers. HD: 319.1-2.

[76] Memo, Dep Chief for Hosp and Dom Oprs SGO for PMG, 21 Jul 44, sub: Hosp Fac for PW. HD: Resources Anal Div file, "Hosp."

pressure at this time to reduce the number of beds in hospitals in the United States, ASF headquarters suggested the use of vacant beds in existing hospitals instead. The Surgeon General objected to this proposal, averring that all existing general hospital beds—according to his estimates—would be needed by the end of the year for American patients, that the treatment of prisoner-of-war patients who needed general-hospital-type care in station hospitals would violate the terms of the Geneva Convention, and that the dispersion of prisoner-patients among many regional and station hospitals was wasteful of both medical and police personnel. Early in October, therefore, ASF headquarters and G–4 approved the designation of the station hospital at Camp Forrest (Tennessee) as Prisoner of War General Hospital No. 2.[77] The establishment of a third prisoner-of-war general hospital was made unnecessary by a change in policy. At the end of October 1944 the Chief of Staff directed the European theater not to transfer prisoner-of-war patients to the United States except rabid Nazis and those desired for questioning for intelligence purposes.[78] After V-E Day, the repatriation of prisoners made it possible to return Glennan General Hospital to the treatment of Americans in June 1945, to discontinue the general hospital at Camp Forrest in December 1945, and to close that camp itself in April 1946.[79]

The operation of two general hospitals devoted exclusively to the care of prisoner-of-war patients simplified administrative and security problems and ultimately saved American medical personnel. Prisoner-patients arriving at ports in this country were transferred to either Glennan or Camp Forrest. There they were sorted into three groups. Those who were convalescent were transferred to convalescent annexes; those requiring care for only minor ills or injuries were sent to near-by prisoner-of-war station hospitals; and those requiring more specialized treatment were kept at one of the prisoner-of-war general hospitals. In addition, prisoners who were eligible for repatriation or for certification as protected personnel were held in special facilities at these hospitals. After their eligibility had been verified, the former were returned to Germany and the latter were assigned to the staffs of prisoner-of-war hospitals to care for their compatriots.[80] For a time, prisoner-of-war general hospitals had duplicate staffs of American and German personnel. In January 1945 the chief of The Surgeon General's Prisoner of War Liaison Unit reported that the German staffs of such hospitals were requesting repatriation because they were given little opportunity to do actual medical and surgical work. He recommended the removal of all American medical personnel except the minimum required for key supervisory positions. The next month the Surgeon General's Office issued directives

[77] (1) Memo, SG for CG ASF, 13 Sep 44, sub: Add Hosp Fac for PW Pnts. SG: 383.6. (2) Memo, SG for CofS ASF, 4 Oct 44, sub: Hosp Fac for German PW Pnts. SG: 322 "Hosp." (3) Diary, Hosp Div SGO, 6 Oct 44. HD: 024.7–3.

[78] (1) Rad CM–OUT–53129, Marshall to Eisenhower, 27 Oct 44. SG: 383.6. (2) Memo SPMOC 383.6 (30 Oct 44), CG ASF for SG, n d, sub: Hosp Fac for German PW Pnts. Same file.

[79] (1) Diary, Hosp Admin Br Hosp Div SGO, 8 May 45. HD: 024.7–3. (2) Diary, PW Liaison Unit SGO, 24 May 45. Same file. (3) Hosp, Evac, and Disposition of PW Pnts in the US, by Col McGibony, MC. HD: 383.6.

[80] (1) Diary, Hosp Div SGO, 7 Oct 44. HD: 024.7–3. (2) Memo, Chief Med Liaison Br for Asst PMG, 27 Jan 45, sub: Study of Enemy Repatriation. HD: 319.1–2. (3) Ltr, Chief PW Med Liaison Unit SGO to SG and PMG, 7 Apr 45, sub: Rpt of Visit to PW Gen Hosp No 2, Cp Forrest, Tenn. Same file.

to require compliance with this recommendation.[81]

Establishment of Hospital Centers

A final change in the hospital system was the establishment of hospital centers. During 1944 convalescent hospitals were opened in several instances on the same posts as general hospitals. With the expansions of 1945 these hospitals grew beyond all previous expectations. For example, by April 1945 the Percy Jones General and Convalescent Hospitals, with their annexes, had a strength, including both patients and operating personnel, of more than 16,500. This was greater than that of an infantry division. These installations occupied not only the Percy Jones General Hospital building, located in Battle Creek, Mich., but also almost all of Fort Custer, which was situated near by. In most instances such installations operated under separate commanders. Each had its own administrative organization for activities such as receiving and disposing of patients; feeding, clothing, and paying both patients and operating personnel; and handling mail, personnel records, and legal problems. Each exercised administrative control over its own patients, requiring the transfer of records and a change of command every time a patient was transferred from one to the other.[82]

Early in 1945, the chief of the Surgeon General's Operations Service decided that combination of such installations under a hospital center commander would simplify the administration of supply and service activities and would permit the transfer of patients between adjacent general and convalescent hospitals without red tape. This had proved to be true when hospital centers were established overseas. Meanwhile, the Percy Jones General Hospital had already begun to centralize under a single head each activity common to both hospitals. Therefore the Operations Service sent representatives to observe its organization and operations, and to discuss with its commander plans for establishing hospital centers. These representatives found merit in such centralization, and the SurgeonGeneral's Office decided to apply it to other installations.[83]

In establishing hospital centers the Medical Department encountered several difficulties. There was opposition in the General Staff, because G–3 feared that additional personnel would be requested to man hospital center headquarters.[84] The Surgeon General's Office believed that the integration of activities common to both general and convalescent hospitals under a single command would actually save personnel and therefore agreed to a condition imposed by the General Staff in approving hospital centers. Personnel for center headquarters would be a part of, and not an addition to, that already provided for general and convalescent hospitals.[85] On 11 April 1945 the War Depart-

[81] (1) Memo SPMGO(4)383.6, Chief Med Liaison Br SGO for Dep Chief Hosp and Dom Oprs SGO, 8 Jan 45, sub: Util of Enemy Protected Pers. HD: 319.1–2. (2) Rad, Lull (SGO) to CGs 4th, 7th, 8th, and 9th SvCs, 5 Feb 45. HD: 319.1–2. (3) An Rpt, FY 1945, Hosp and Dom Oprs SGO. HD.

[82] An Rpts, 1945, Percy Jones, Wakeman, and Cps Butner and Carson Conv Ctrs. HD.

[83] Interv, MD Historian with Col McGibony, MC, 20 Feb 50. HD: 000.71.

[84] Diary, Hosp Div SGO, 31 Mar and 2 Apr 45. HD: 024.7–3.

[85] (1) WD AGO Form No 026, Request and Justification for Publication, prepared by SGO, 24 Feb 45, sub: Hosp Ctr (ZI). (2) Memo SPMCH 300.5 (WD Cir), SG for TAG thru CG ASF, 6 Mar 45, sub: Proposed Amendment to WD Cir 140, 1944. (3) Memo, SG for ACofS G–4 WDGS, 31 Mar 45, same sub. (4) DF WDGDS 11065, ACofS G–4 WDGS to TAG, 2 Apr 45, same sub. All in AG: 705 (4–3–44) (1). (5) WD Cir 105, 4 Apr 45.

ment announced that nine hospital centers, each composed of a general and a convalescent hospital, would be established at Camp Pickett, Va.; Camp Butner, N. C.; Camp Edwards, Mass.; Camp Carson, Colo.; Camp Atterbury, Ind.; Fort Custer, Mich.; Fort Sam Houston, Tex.; Fort Lewis, Wash.; and Camp Forrest, Tenn.[86] Local commanders then ran into problems in consolidating and reorganizing general and convalescent hospitals into hospital centers. Lacking authoritative standard guides, center commanders proceeded according to their own ideas or the demands of the local situation to set up organizations, establish administrative procedures, and work out relationships with subordinate components, on the one hand, and with post headquarters, on the other.[87]

Despite these difficulties the establishment and operation of hospital centers proved advantageous. The administration of supply and service activities by center headquarters freed hospital commanders of administrative detail, saved personnel, and avoided duplication of effort in those fields. Centralization also made it easy to shift personnel between hospitals as it was needed. Finally, the operation of a single registrar's office for both general and convalescent hospitals made it possible to move patients from one to the other by simple inter-ward transfers, rather than by the complicated procedures required when they were moved between separate installations.[88]

The establishment of hospital centers represented the last of a succession of adjustments in the hospital system during the war. While most of them were prompted primarily by the necessity of using limited resources effectively, other considerations entered in. For example regional hospitals developed partially from attempts of the Air Forces to establish a completely separate medical service while convalescent hospitals received an additional impetus from a belief that convalescent patients could best be restored to physical condition for full duty or prepared for return to civilian life in an installation with a nonhospital atmosphere. Some of the changes made in the latter part of the war, such as specialization in general hospitals, had their origins earlier and were designed to improve the quality of hospital care. Others, such as the merger of adjacent station and general hospitals and the establishment of hospital centers, were expected to improve administration. Since most of the changes were the result of wartime demands, when peace came the need for them no longer existed and the hospital system in the United States reverted to its prewar form.

[86] WD Cir 115, 11 Apr 45.

[87] (1) An Rpt, FY 1945, Percy Jones Hosp Ctr; and An Rpt, FY 1945, Hosp and Dom Oprs SGO. HD. (2) Edward J. Morgan and Donald O. Wagner, The Organization of the Medical Department in the Zone of the Interior (1946), pp. 162–64. HD.

[88] An Rpts, 1945, Percy Jones, Wakeman, and Cps Carson and Butner Hosp Ctrs; and An Rpt, FY 1945, Hosp and Dom Oprs SGO. HD.

CHAPTER XI

Bed Requirements in the Zone of Interior

While most changes in the hospital system, discussed in the foregoing chapter, were expected to conserve medical resources, especially physicians, they obviously were not expected to reduce the total number of beds that would be needed. In some instances, such changes actually tended to increase bed requirements, for policies making it impossible to place patients of a particular type in any available vacant bed occasionally required the provision of more beds than otherwise needed. Under current policies, for example, vacant beds in regional hospitals could not be used for overseas patients to reduce the number of additional beds required in general hospitals. Also, vacant beds in station hospitals could not be used for prisoner-of-war patients requiring general-hospital-type care to avoid the establishment of special prisoner-of-war general hospitals. Furthermore, the practice of providing different types of hospitals for different types of patients complicated the calculation of requirements, since beds needed for different groups had to be estimated separately. Another factor which increased the difficulty of estimating bed requirements was the transition from the defensive to the offensive phase of the war. Because of uncertainty about the tempo and scope of combat operations and about the kind of warfare to be encountered it was always more difficult to predict numbers of combat casualties than numbers of patients resulting from the normal incidence of diseases and accidental injuries. Nevertheless, estimates had to be made and it was important to make them as accurate as possible. Failure to have enough beds at any particular moment would not only subject The Surgeon General and the Army to severe criticism but would also jeopardize the treatment of American casualties. To have more beds than were needed would waste personnel and might mean, in the face of the ceiling imposed upon Medical Corps officers, inadequate manning of the hospitals provided. The Surgeon General's Office, ASF headquarters, the General Staff, and other agencies of the Government participated in determining bed requirements, and differences of opinion that arose among them illustrated the complexity of the process.

Despite the restrictive personnel situation in the fall of 1943, The Surgeon General's Hospital Division continued to consider the problem of meeting bed requirements primarily in terms of construction. Following the former practice of figuring bed requirements on the basis of World War I experience, it estimated that the number of required station hospital beds would decrease from about 256,000 in December 1943 to about 80,000 in December 1945, but that the number of beds needed in general hospitals would increase from about 98,500 to over 122,000 in the same period.[1] To meet the anticipated need for general hospital beds, The Surgeon General in September 1943 requested ASF headquarters to earmark and retain funds that had been appropriated but not used for the construction of approximately fifteen additional general hospitals. The latter refused, insisting that any additional general hospital beds that would be needed could be established without further construction in station hospital buildings that would become surplus as troops moved overseas.[2]

First Attempt To Base Requirements on an Estimate of the Patient Load

Late in 1943 the prospect of the invasion of Europe, along with limited amounts of available personnel, and uncertainty about the patient load, necessitated a more realistic appraisal of requirements and resources than any formerly made. The Surgeon General borrowed personnel from ASF headquarters, it will be recalled, to establish a special group in his Office for this purpose. In the winter of 1943–44 this group, later known as the Facilities Utilization Branch, attempted to predict the size of the patient load throughout the world during 1944.[3] It admitted that it was "up against the difficulty of working with figures that had little firmness," [4] and its calculations rested upon a series of estimates: the number of troops to be engaged in combat; the rate at which troops in theaters would suffer wounds, accidental injuries, and diseases; and the proportion of patients in theaters that would be evacuated to the United States.

Some of the estimates were based on current World War II information while others rested primarily upon World War I experience. Projected troop strengths for theaters were known, but the proportion of troops to be engaged in combat had to be estimated. Records were available to show the rate at which disease and nonbattle injuries occurred, but information about World War II battle-injury rates was meager. To estimate these rates the experience of the Meuse-Argonne fighting in World War I was combined with that of the Tunisian campaign (1943), Tarawa operation (1943), and the German campaign in Russia (1941). Information about the German campaign, incidentally, was found in a study prepared by the Office of Strategic Services. The proportion of overseas patients who would be evacuated to the United States was estimated on the basis of World War I experience, "reinforced by the derived estimate of the German experience in the Russian campaign." This estimate—30 percent of estimated battle casualties and 3 percent of estimated disease and nonbattle-injury cases—differed only slightly from figures for World War I. These estimates were used to calculate the number of patients who would need beds in theaters of operations as well as the number who would be evacuated to the United States. To arrive at the number of patients from the zone of interior who

[1] (1) Memo, SG (Hosp Cons Br) for CofEngrs, 24 Aug 43, sub: Review of Est for FY 1944. SG: 632.–2. (2) Ltr, SG (Hosp Cons Br) to CofEngrs, 18 Nov 43, sub: MD Cons Reqmts for FY 1945. SG: 632.–1. (3) 1st ind, SG (Hosp Cons Br) to CofEngrs, 24 Jan 44, on Ltr, CofEngrs to SG, 18 Jan 44, sub: Engr . . . Estimates, FY 1945. SG: 632.–1.

[2] Ltr, SG to CG ASF, 2 Sep 43, sub: Retention of Appropriated Funds for Gen Hosp Cons, with 1st ind, Reqmts Div ASF to SG, 19 Sep 43. SG: 632.–1.

[3] (1) An Rpt, FY 1944, Dep Chief Hosp and Dom Oprs SGO. HD. (2) Tab A, sub: Estab of a Statistical Management Unit in the Oprs Serv, to Memo, Dir Hosp Div SGO and Dir Resources Anal Div SGO for Dir HD SGO, 18 Jun 45, sub: Add Mat for An Rpt for FY 1945. HD: 319.1–2. (3) Ltr, [Dr.] Eli Ginzberg to Col Calvin H. Goddard, 2 Jan 52. HD: 314 (Correspondence on MS)V.

[4] Hosp and Evac: A Re-estimate of the Pnt Load and Fac, Feb 44, Introduction, p. 1. HD: 705.–1.

would need beds in general hospitals, recent experience in transfers from station hospitals (0.5 percent of the troop population) was applied to the projected strength for 1944.

From the calculations and interpretations of this study the Surgeon General's Office estimated that 140,000 beds would be required during 1944 to accommodate patients evacuated from theaters of operations and transferred from zone of interior hospitals. Such patients would normally have been provided for in general hospitals, but on this occasion The Surgeon General did not ask for an increase in general hospital beds to 140,000 or even to the 115,000 which, according to his previous calculations on the old percentage basis, would be needed by the end of 1944. Instead, in view of the limited number of physicians available and the fact that about 75 percent of the patients in general hospitals were convalescent, he accepted the existing authorization of 100,000 general hospital beds and proposed in February 1944 that an additional 40,000 beds be provided in convalescent "facilities." Such facilities could be operated either as annexes of general hospitals or as separate installations and would require lower ratios of personnel (especially physicians) to patients than did general hospitals.[5]

Suspecting that The Surgeon General's figures were too high, ASF headquarters made a thoroughgoing study of its own. Its Planning Division conferred with representatives of the Surgeon General's Office, the Office of the Chief of Transportation, and other interested staff divisions of ASF headquarters. It also communicated with the chief surgeons of the European and North African theaters. Different agencies, using battle-casualty admission rates that varied widely, arrived nonetheless at similar estimates of the patient load, particularly for the first ninety days of operations on the European continent.[6] In March 1944, therefore, ASF headquarters for the most part approved The Surgeon General's recommendation. It authorized the conversion of vacant barracks to provide 25,000 beds for convalescent patients and agreed to earmark space for 25,000 more if needed.[7] The Surgeon General then began to establish convalescent facilities thus authorized but ASF headquarters apparently did not seek approval of the General Staff (G-4) for the expansion. As a result the Medical Department failed to get adequate personnel and equipment for the facilities that were established until the approval of G-4 was finally obtained in the fall of 1944.

Movement To Reduce the Number of Hospital Beds in the United States

During the spring and summer of 1944 other problems, such as changes in the hospital system and the provision of medical support for theaters of operations,[8] demanded more attention than zone of

[5] The above two paragraphs are based on the following: (1) Hosp and Evac: A Re-estimate of the Pnt Load and Fac, Feb 44. HD: 705.-1. (2) Memo, SG for Dir Plans and Oprs ASF, 22 Feb 44, sub: Hosp and Evac. HRS: Hq ASF Planning Div Program Br file, "Hosp and Evac, vol. 3." (3) Ltr, Eli Ginzberg to Col Calvin H. Goddard, 2 Jan 52, HD: 314 (Correspondence on MS)V.

[6] (1) Memo, Dir Plans and Oprs ASF for Dir Planning Div ASF, 28 Feb 44, sub: Hosp and Evac. HRS: Hq ASF Gen Lutes' files, "Hosp and Evac, 1943-46." (2) Memo, Dir Planning Div ASF for Dir Plans and Oprs ASF, 1 Mar 44, sub: Hosp and Evac. HRS: Hq ASF Planning Div Program Br file, "Hosp and Evac, vol. 3." (3) Memo, Dir Planning Div ASF for Chief ZI Br Planning Div ASF, 2 Mar 44, same sub. Same file. (4) Hosp and Evac: An Anal, Mar 44. HRS: Hq ASF Planning Div Program Br file.

[7] Memo, CofS ASF for Dir Plans and Oprs ASF, 28 Mar 44, sub: Conf on Hosp and Evac. HRS: ASF Planning Div Program Br file, "Hosp and Evac, vol. 3."

[8] See above, pp. 181-99, and below, pp. 214-37.

interior bed requirements, but gradually a tendency developed among many agencies to question the need for all of the beds previously authorized. By the fall of 1944 this tendency developed into a general movement to reduce their number.

The demand to reduce the number of beds in zone of interior hospitals arose at first from observation of the low rate of occupancy. Statistics published by the Surgeon General's Office showed that only about half of the beds in all hospitals in the United States were used during most of 1944.[9] *(Chart 8.)* Furthermore, optimism about an early end of the war made it seem unlikely to officers in ASF headquarters and the General Staff that the occupancy rate would increase appreciably.[10] Meanwhile various expedients were being used to supply theaters with their quotas of beds, among them the shipment of hospital units without full complements of professional personnel.[11] The Deputy Chief of Staff expressed the opinion that this practice would be unnecessary if medical personnel and facilities were properly used. He therefore directed The Inspector General in September 1944 to investigate duplication of hospitalization in the United States.[12] By that time ASF headquarters, the War Department Manpower Board, and divisions of the General Staff had already begun to make their own estimates of bed requirements in the zone of interior.

A reduction in the authorized ratio of station hospital beds had been made several days before the Deputy Chief of Staff criticized the use of medical resources. As early as May 1944, in the course of discussions with the General Staff about nurse requirements, The Surgeon General's Facilities Utilization Branch had informally proposed a reduction from 4 to 3.6 percent of troop strength.[13] The General Staff accepted this suggestion immediately, but it was not until 20 September 1944 that a new ratio of 3.5 percent—formally proposed by The Surgeon General in August—was established by War Department directive.[14] The same directive, however, authorized for the first time a ratio for regional hospital beds: 0.5 percent of troop strength. Formerly used to estimate the number of beds in general hospitals needed to care for zone of interior patients transferred from station hospitals, this figure was adopted because such patients were eventually to be transferred to regional instead of general hospitals. Since no corresponding reduction was made in the number of beds authorized for general hospitals it is difficult to see that the reduction in the station hospital bed ratio meant any reduction in the total number of beds authorized. In any event, this action must have seemed to authorities higher than The Surgeon General as only a step in the right direction.

The ASF Director of Plans and Operations proposed a reduction in the number

[9] (1) Weekly Health Rpts, vol. IV, Nos 1–39, 1944. AML. (2) ASF Monthly Progress Rpts, Sec 7, *Health*, Mar–Aug 44.

[10] (1) Remarks by Col Albert H. Schwichtenberg, MC, in Notes on Conf of AAF Comd Surgs, Off of Air Surg, 16–20 Apr 45. SG: 337. (2) Interv, MD Historian with Lt Col James T. McGibony, MC, 20 Feb 50. HD: 000.71.

[11] See below, pp. 218–28.

[12] (1) Mins, Mtg of Gen Council, 25 Sep 44. HRS: AGO Reference Collection. (2) Memo WDCSA 632 (25 Sep 44), DepCofSA for IG, 25 Sep 44, sub: Hosp Fac in ZI. HRS: WDCSA 632 (25 Sep 44), Case 28, "Hosp Fac in ZI."

[13] Memo SPMCH 211 Nurses, Eli Ginzberg for Maj Armour, G–3 WDGS, 25 May 44, sub: Almt of Nurses. HRS: G–3 files, 210–219 incl, "vol. II."

[14] (1) DF, Dep ACofS G–3 WDGS to WDMB, G–1 and G–4, 10 Jun 44, sub: Almt of Nurses. HRS: G–3 files, 210–219 incl, "vol. II." (2) Memo, SG (init E. G[inzberg]) for ACofS G–3 and G–4 WDGS thru CG ASF, 29 Aug 44. SG: 632.2. (3) Memo WDGCT 211 (26 May 44), Dep ACofS G–3 WDGS for CG ASF, 18 Sep 44, sub: Almt of Nurses. Same file. (4) AR 40–1080, C 3, 20 Sep 44.

CHART 8—HOSPITAL BEDS AUTHORIZED AND OCCUPIED BY TYPE OF HOSPITAL IN CONTINENTAL UNITED STATES 1943 AND 1944

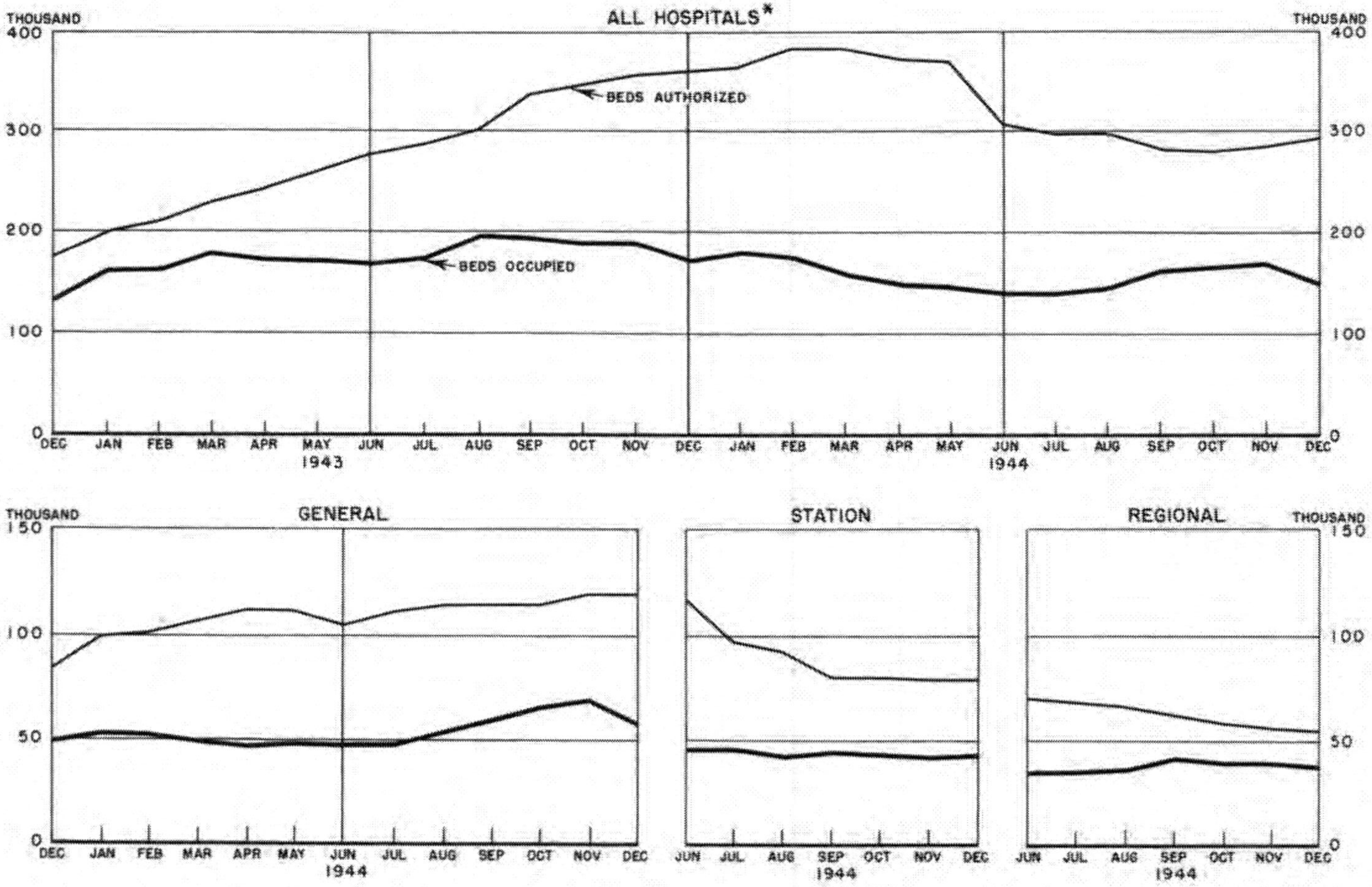

*Excludes dispensaries, convalescent facilities (but includes convalescent hospitals after establishment in June 1944), venereal disease facilities, college training units, and nonfixed hospitals at maneuver areas.

Source: Weekly Health Reports, ASF, Med Statistics Div, SGO.

of beds in all hospitals on 4 September 1944. Pointing to the low occupancy rate, to the expectation that regional hospitals would relieve general hospitals of zone of interior patients, and to the fact that battle casualties and their evacuation from overseas had been less than estimated, he called upon The Surgeon General to analyze the entire hospital program with a view to reducing the number of beds in station and regional hospitals by 25 percent and in general hospitals to 80,000.[15] To effect this reduction would have meant closing from twelve to twenty general hospitals—a proposal made verbally by the War Department Manpower Board during the same month.[16]

The Surgeon General agreed that too many station hospital beds had been provided, but he pointed out that he had already begun to reduce their number. In opposing other reductions he emphasized future possibilities. He called attention to the tendency of sick rates and hospital occupancy to be higher in winter than in summer, to the likelihood of heavier battle casualties, to the prolongation of the war beyond what had been expected, to the expectation that patients from overseas would need longer periods of hospitalization in the United States than anticipated, and to the prospect that more beds would be needed in all types of zone of interior hospitals when the war in Europe ended and redeployment to the Pacific began. He also pointed out that the transfer of patients from Europe and North Africa had hardly begun because of the European theater's opposition to evacuating patients in troop transports and North Africa's lack of adequate shipping.[17] The bed surplus, in short, was only temporary and earlier estimates would prove correct. These arguments failed to change the opinion of the ASF Director of Plans and Operations, but on 25 September 1944 his proposal to require The Surgeon General to make the desired reductions was quashed by General Somervell, who considered it unwise to order such cuts in the face of The Surgeon General's opposition.[18]

Two days before, on 23 September 1944, G–4 directed both AAF and ASF headquarters to reduce the beds in station and regional hospitals to the number authorized by the new ratios (3.5 and 0.5 percent of troop strength respectively) and to plan a further reduction of 25 percent in each—the same cut proposed earlier by ASF headquarters.[19] Later G–4 apparently directed ASF headquarters to plan reductions in the number of general hospital beds also.[20] The Air Surgeon and The Surgeon General readily agreed to reduce beds to current authorizations, but they objected to a further lowering of the bed ratio. Such action, they said, would allow no vacant beds for dispersion or epidemics. It would limit beds in station hospitals to 2.6 percent and in regional hospitals to

[15] Memo SPOPP 632 (23 Aug 44), CG ASF (Dir Plans and Oprs) for SG, 4 Sep 44, sub: ZI Hosp Program. HRS: ASF Planning Div file, 700 "ZI Hosp."

[16] (1) Remarks by Col Schwichtenberg, MC, in Notes on Conf of AAF Comd Surgs, Off of Air Surg, 16–20 Apr 45. SG: 337. (2) Transcription of written answers by Maj Gen Norman T. Kirk, USA, Ret, to questions in Ltr of 10 Nov 50, from Editor, Hist Med Dept in World War II. HD: 314 (Correspondence on MS)I.

[17] Memo, SG (init E. G[inzberg]) for CG ASF, 15 Sep 44, sub: ZI Hosp Program. HRS: Hq ASF Planning Div file, 700 "ZI Hosp."

[18] (1) Memo, Dir Plans and Oprs ASF for CG ASF, 23 Sep 44, sub: ZI Hosp Program, with incl. HRS: ASF Planning Div file, 700 "ZI Hosp." (2) MRS, [Gen] Somervell to [Maj Gen Wilhelm D.] Styer, 25 Sep 44, atchd to Memo just cited. Same file.

[19] Memo WDGDS 3221, ACofS G–4 WDGS for CGs AAF, AGF, ASF, 23 Sep 44, sub: Reduction of ZI Hosp. SG: 322 "Hosp Misc."

[20] S/S WDGDS 4166, ACofS G–4 WDGS to DepCofSA, 20 Oct 44, sub: ZI Hosp Reqmts. HRS: G–4 files, "Hosp and Evac Policy."

0.4 percent of troop strength, while beds actually occupied in station hospitals ranged from 2.5 to 2.7 percent of troop strength.[21] While this argument was in progress the question of general-hospital bed requirements was being discussed among G–4, The Surgeon General, and the War Department Manpower Board.

In these discussions the Manpower Board raised two new issues: the propriety of lumping together the capacities of all types of hospitals when considering present and future needs and of counting beds in convalescent facilities as part of these resources. The Manpower Board followed both practices. It considered all beds in convalescent facilities as hospital beds and added to them the beds in station, regional, and general hospitals to arrive at a total number of beds already established. Comparing the number of patients in all hospitals with this total, the Board concluded that a surplus of 78,000 beds existed in the United States.[22] The Surgeon General contended that beds in convalescent facilities should not be considered as hospital beds, since the Board had until then refused to allocate personnel for them. He insisted, moreover, that beds in hospitals of different types were not interchangeable. For example, under existing policies vacant beds in station and regional hospitals could not be used for overseas evacuees. Nor were all beds in general hospitals available for the treatment of such patients. Some were used for prisoners of war, non-Army patients, and Army patients from surrounding areas who needed only minor care and treatment, while others had to be set aside to receive evacuees in transit from ports to hospitals of definitive treatment. He argued, therefore, that the Manpower Board's conclusion about a surplus of hospital beds was invalid.[23]

The final decision which the General Staff made in the face of conflicting arguments proved to be a compromise. After further study by G–4 of the beds required in all types of hospitals, the Staff agreed in November 1944 to authorize 40,000 convalescent beds—10,500 of them in AAF hospitals. This was substantially the number recommended by The Surgeon General and the Air Surgeon and already set up in convalescent hospitals. The Manpower Board now reluctantly agreed to provide staffs for them. Moreover, the Staff required no cut in the existing number of beds in general hospitals or in the ratio authorized for regional hospitals. On the other hand it directed a cut in the ratio of station hospital beds, but only from 3.5 to 3 percent of troop strength instead of to the 2.6 percent first suggested.[24] The Air Surgeon apparently considered this

[21] (1) Memo, CG AAF for CofSA attn G–4, 30 Sep 44, sub: Reduction of ZI Hosp. HRS: G–4 files, "Hosp and Evac Policy." (2) Memo, CG AAF (Air Surg) for CofSA attn G–4 Div, 7 Oct 44, same sub. Same file. (3) T/S SPMC 322 Hosp, SG to Dir Plans and Oprs ASF, 30 Sep 44, same sub. HRS: Hq ASF Planning Div file, 700 "ZI Hosp." (4) Memo, SG (init E. G[inzberg]) for Dir Plans and Oprs ASF, 25 Oct 44, same sub. SG: 632.2. (5) Memo SPOPP 700, CG ASF for ACofS G–4 WDGS, 30 Oct 44, same sub. AG: 323.3 (4 Sep 44)(1).

[22] Memo WDSMB 323.3 (Hosp), Pres WDMB for CofSA, 16 Oct 44, sub: ZI Hosp Reqmts. HRS: G–4 files, "Hosp and Evac Policy."

[23] (1) Memo, Eli Ginzberg, Spec Asst, Dir Hosp Div SGO for Pres WDMB, 23 Aug 44. (2) Memo, SG for CG ASF, 15 Sep 44, sub: ZI Hosp Program. (3) Inf Memo, Dir Resources Anal Div SGO for Lt Col Huncilman (ASF), 26 Dec 44, sub: Background for Staffing Conv Hosps. All in HRS: Hq ASF Planning Div file, 700 "ZI Hosp."

[24] (1) S/S WDGDS 4166, ACofS G–4 WDGS to Dep CofSA, 20 Oct 44, sub: ZI Hosp Reqmts. (2) S/S WDGDS 4956, same to same, 8 Nov 44, same sub. (3) Memo, CG AAF (Air Surg) for ACofS G–4 WDGS, 31 Oct 44, sub: AAF Conv Hosps. (4) Memo, Dep SG (init A. H. S[chwichtenberg] and E. G[inzberg]) for ACofS G–4 WDGS, 2 Nov 44, sub: Reqmts for ASF Conv Fac. (5) S/S WDSMB 323.3 (Hosp), Pres WDMB to CofSA, 13 Nov 44, sub: ZI Hosps. All in HRS: G–4 files, "Hosp and Evac Policy."

compromise satisfactory, but The Surgeon General's representatives insisted that no reduction at all should be made.[25] In announcing the Staff's decision on 17 November 1944, G-4 directed both AAF and ASF headquarters to study the hospital situation further in the light of actual experience and to submit by 15 January 1945 any recommendations which they might have on changes in requirements.[26]

Changes in the Manner of Reporting Beds

The movement to reduce the number of hospital beds caused a change in the method of reporting them. ASF headquarters decided that "unrefined data" on hospitalization, published by the Surgeon General's Office in Weekly Health Reports and in ASF Monthly Progress Reports, gave erroneous impressions and made it difficult to arrive at sound conclusions about the adequacy of hospital facilities.[27] Earlier the Surgeon General's Office had warned that a distinction needed to be made between the total number of beds in general hospitals and the smaller number available for "true general-hospital cases." To obtain the latter figure one must subtract from the total the number of beds necessarily vacant because of the practice of distributing patients into wards according to disease, sex, and rank, as well as those set aside for other purposes—such as the care of station-hospital-type patients, civilians, veterans, and Navy personnel, and the debarkation processing of patients arriving from theaters of operations.[28] This implied that to get a true picture of hospitalization not only the capacity of hospitals by type but their capacity to handle particular types of patients should be known, and that the number of beds set aside for special purposes and lost through dispersion should be taken into account.

The Surgeon General's regular reports began to take notice of this latter factor in statistics for the end of September 1944. Previously he had reported the number of beds authorized (which was reasonably close to the number normally available) and the number occupied. Now he added a figure for "effective beds" in general hospitals. It was obtained by subtracting an allowance for dispersion and for "debarkation beds" from the number of authorized beds. The following month he presented similar figures for regional and station hospitals, and at the same time gave the percentage of effective beds occupied in each class of hospital. This percentage, for all general hospitals, was 76.5; the percentage of authorized beds that were occupied (a figure previously given but now dropped) would have been 58.1. The next month, instead of reporting simply beds occupied, The Surgeon General showed "patients remaining," a figure which included not only the number of patients occupying beds but also the number temporarily absent on sick leave, on furlough, and without leave. The ratio of "patients remaining" to "effective beds" was given. In the case of general hospitals, taken collectively, this ratio amounted to

[25] (1) Memo, CG AAF (Air Surg) for CofSA attn G-4, 7 Oct 44, sub: Reduction of ZI Hosps. HRS: G-4 files, "Hosp and Evac Policy." (2) Diary, Plans and Policy Sec, ASF Planning Div, 31 Oct 44. HRS: Hq ASF Planning Div file, 700 "ZI Hosp." (3) Memo, Dir Hosp Div (init E. G[inzberg]) for Col [William B.] Higgins, G-4, 31 Oct 44, sub: Sta and Reg Hosp Bed Reqmts. SG: 632.2.

[26] Memo WDGDS 5391, ACofS G-4 WDGS for CGs AAF and ASF, 17 Nov 44, sub: ZI Hosps. SG: 322 "Hosp Misc."

[27] (1) Memo SPOPP 705, CG ASF for SG, 20 Nov 44, sub: Data on Status of Hosp Beds and Pers, ZI. AG: 323.3 (4 Sep 44) (1). (2) Memo, Maj Gen W. D. Styer for Gen Lutes, 9 Nov 44. HRS: Hq ASF Planning Div file, 700 "ZI Hosp."

[28] Memo, Eli Ginzberg, Spec Asst, Dir Hosp Div SGO for Pres WDMB, 23 Aug 44. HRS: Hq ASF Planning Div file, 700 "ZI Hosp."

91.3 percent. The ratio of beds occupied to "effective beds" would have been 73.9 percent; of beds occupied to beds authorized, 56.4 percent.[29] Thus, although there was little change in actual occupancy, the new system of reporting makes it appear that hospitals were being more fully utilized than formerly.

By this time (November 1944) a series of conferences on bed reporting had already started under the auspices of ASF headquarters,[30] and in February 1945 conclusions were reached regarding the other factor considered necessary to a true presentation of the hospital situation. In that month the Surgeon General's Office and the ASF Planning Division agreed upon a system of reporting beds, patients, and operating personnel in terms of types of care or types of beds, regardless of their location in particular types of hospitals.[31] Four months later the ASF Monthly Progress Report carried such information. It showed that although there were 213,-373 beds in general and convalescent hospitals, only 180,760 were used as general and convalescent hospital beds.[32]

Meeting Increased Requirements for the Peak Patient Load

Meanwhile the tide had long since turned in the drive to reduce hospital bed capacity. Not long after G-4's compromise decision of 17 November 1944, The Surgeon General's Resources Analysis Division made a new study of bed requirements that showed a need for more beds in general and convalescent hospitals than G-4 had authorized. There were several reasons for this study: completion by the Medical Regulating Officer of new estimates of patients to be evacuated from theaters during 1945, the prospect that redeployment would interfere with the use of station hospital buildings for any possible overflow from general hospitals, and G-4's directive that further recommendations about bed requirements be submitted by 15 January 1945.[33]

In this study the Resources Analysis Division concentrated upon general and convalescent hospitals rather than upon station and regional hospitals, for there was little possibility either that G-4 would raise the bed ratio for the last two or that the Surgeon General's Office would recommend reducing it. In estimating requirements for beds in general and convalescent hospitals, the Division calculated the numbers of beds that would be needed for three groups of patients: debarkees, zone of interior and non-Army patients, and overseas patients. The minimum number of debarkation beds needed, it was assumed, was one half the anticipated monthly evacuee load, or approximately 17,500. Experience showed that 33,000 beds in general hospitals were used by zone of interior and non-Army patients

[29] ASF Monthly Progress Rpts, Sec 7, *Health*, 30 Sep, 31 Oct, and 30 Nov 44.

[30] (1) Memo SPOPP 720 (9 Nov 44), Dir Plans and Oprs ASF for CofS ASF, 30 Nov 44, sub: Status of Hosp Beds and Med Pers, ZI. AG: 323.3 (4 Sep 44)(1). (2) Diary, ASF Planning Div (Lt Col H. A. Huncilman), 28 Nov 44. HRS: Hq ASF Planning Div file, 700 "ZI Hosp." (3) Memo SPOPP 700, Dir Planning Div for Gen Wood, 26 Dec 44, sub: ZI Hosps. HRS: Hq ASF Planning Div file, "Hosp and Evac." (4) Memo, Maj W. H. Hastings (ASF) for Lt Col H. A. Huncilman, 25 Jan 45, sub: Hosp Occupancy Data for Monthly Progress Rpt. HRS: Hq ASF Planning Div file, 700 "ZI Hosp."

[31] ASF Cir 68, 26 Feb 45.

[32] ASF Monthly Progress Rpt, Sec 7, *Health*, 30 Jun 45.

[33] (1) Interv, MD Historian with Col John C. Fitzpatrick, MC, formerly MRO, SGO, 18 Apr 50. HD: 000.71. (2) Memo, Eli Ginzberg for the Record, 28 Nov 44. HD: 560.-2 (Hosp Ships). (3) Memo for Record on Memo, CG ASF for SG, 13 Dec 44, sub: Gen Hosp Program, ZI. HRS: Hq ASF Planning Div file, "Hosp and Evac." Documents dealing with conflicting claims to the use of station hospitals are in HRS: G-4 file, 602.3. (4) Memo SPOPP 322, CG ASF for SG, 7 Dec 44, sub: ZI Hosps. SG: 322 "Hosp Misc."

despite the policy of transferring complicated cases from station to regional, instead of general, hospitals. Beds for overseas evacuees receiving definitive treatment were computed on the basis of the number to be brought in each month, as forecast in the study made by the Medical Regulating Officer, and on the average length of time they were expected to stay in hospitals. From these calculations, it appeared that patients in general and convalescent hospitals would reach a peak number of 198,000 in August 1945. If 17,500 beds were set aside for debarkation processing, a total of about 215,000 beds would then be needed. Additional beds for dispersion were not included in this number because it was anticipated that the patient load would ordinarily be lower than the estimated peak and that many patients would leave beds vacant when they went on leaves and furloughs.[34]

This study led The Surgeon General on 8 January 1945 to ask for 70,000 additional general and convalescent hospital beds. He proposed that 49,500 of them should be in general hospitals and that they should be provided as follows: 10,000 by converting the convalescent annexes of general hospitals into wards; 17,500 by using hospital barracks for patients instead of enlisted men of the medical detachment, for whom other housing would be provided; 8,000 by placing ambulatory patients of general hospitals in post barracks; 9,000 by converting four station hospitals into temporary general hospitals; and 5,000 by using beds in staging area hospitals for debarkation purposes, thus freeing an equal number of beds in general hospitals for patients needing prolonged care. The Surgeon General suggested that about 20,500 additional beds in convalescent hospitals could be provided by using vacant barracks located near by. In this connection it should be noted that he followed a policy of expanding existing hospitals rather than establishing new ones because smaller ratios of personnel to patients were required for large than for small installations and scarce specialists were used more advantageously by concentrating rather than dispersing them.[35]

A combination of circumstances intervened in December 1944 and January 1945 to cause the General Staff to consider favorably this request. In mid-December the Battle of the Bulge put to flight all thoughts of an early end to the war in Europe. About the same time, approval by the Joint Chiefs of Staff of the Medical Regulating Officer's estimates of evacuees to be received during 1945 made it appear that the number of patients in zone of interior hospitals would increase. In addition, a directive from the Chief of Staff on 3 December 1944 requiring the European theater to use transports for evacuation assured the early return to the United States of many patients from that area.[36] Of perhaps more importance, the Secretary of War wrote to the Chief of Staff early in January: "If we later prove to

[34] (1) Memo SPMCH 322 (Hosp-Cp Edwards)C, SG for CG ASF, 21 Nov 44, sub: Use of Cp Edwards as a Debarkation Hosp. HRS: G-4 file, 602.3. (2) Memo, Asst SG for Act Dir Plans and Oprs ASF, 8 Jan 45, sub: Gen Hosp Program, ZI with tabs and incls. HRS: Hq ASF Planning Div file, "Hosp and Evac." (3) Diary, Resources Anal Div, SGO, 19, 20, 22, and 23 Dec 44. HD: 024.7-3.

[35] (1) Memo, Asst SG for Act Dir Plans and Oprs ASF, 8 Jan 45, sub: Gen Hosp Program, ZI, with Tabs A-J. HRS: Hq ASF Planning Div file, "Hosp and Evac." (2) Memo, SG for CG ASF, 4 Jan 45, sub: Gen and Conv Hosps. Same file. (3) Memo, SG for Col Prichard, 22 Feb 45, sub: Background Info Covering the Gen Hosp Expansion Program. SG: 632.

[36] (1) Interv, MD Historian with Lt Col J[ames] T. McGibony, MC, 20 Feb 50. HD: 000.71. (2) JCS Document 1199, 16 Dec 44. SG: 560.2. (3) Rad CM-OUT-72113 (3 Dec 44), CofSA to CG Hq ComZ ETO and CG UK Base Sec, 3 Dec 44. SG: 560.2.

have erred [in forecasting requirements] I want to make sure that we have erred on the side of too much." [37] Finally, The Surgeon General's Resources Analysis Division seems to have established better relations than formerly with the War Department Manpower Board and a new Deputy Chief of Staff of the Army, perhaps inclined to be more favorable to The Surgeon General's position than his predecessor, had taken office in October 1944.[38] During the early part of January 1945, Surgeon General Kirk vigorously pushed his program for additional beds in personal conferences with the commanding general of the Service Forces, members of the General Staff, the Deputy Chief of Staff, the Chief of Staff, and perhaps also the Secretary of War. On 20 January 1945 it was approved.[39]

In succeeding months G–4 and The Surgeon General differed about the number of additional beds actually required. G–4 suggested, it will be recalled, that the number might be reduced by placing overseas patients in vacant beds in AAF regional hospitals. The Air Forces offered beds for that purpose and emphasized, along with G–4, the desirability of using them to reduce the number of additional beds required in other hospitals. When The Surgeon General and ASF headquarters argued that no emergency existed to require such use of regional hospitals, G–4 asked ASF headquarters on 3 April 1945 for a justification of the number of beds authorized in January.[40]

Meanwhile the Surgeon General's Office had reappraised its former estimate of requirements. Beginning in December 1944 the number of evacuees arriving in the United States from all theaters increased each month until in March 1945 it surpassed by about 12,000 the monthly average on which planning at the end of December had been based.[41] This trend indicated that the peak load in general and convalescent hospitals would occur in June, two months earlier than previously expected, and that it would be higher by 46,000 patients than the 198,000 estimated in December 1944. Accordingly, in the latter part of March 1945 the Surgeon General's Office asked ASF

[37] Memo, SecWar for CofS, n d, included as Tab B to Memo, WDCSA 700 (13 Jan 45), Asst DepCofSA for ACofS G–1, G–2, G–3, G–4, and OPD WDGS and for CGs ASF, AGF, and AAF, 13 Jan 45, sub: Med Mission Reappraised. HRS: G–4 file, "Hosp, vol. II."

[38] Weekly Diary, Resources Anal Div SGO, 13 Jan 45. HD: 024.7–3. Lt. Gen. Joseph T. McNarney was succeeded by Lt. Gen. Thomas T. Handy as Deputy Chief of Staff, United States Army, in October 1944. Info supplied by OCS files.

[39] General Kirk had a conference with the Chief of Staff on 26 December 1944, with the commanding general, ASF, on 5 and 8 January 1945, and with members of the General Staff and the Deputy Chief of Staff on 18 January 1945. (1) Memo WDCSA 632 (26 Dec 44), Gen George C. Marshall for Gen Thomas T. Handy, 26 Dec 44. HRS: OCS 632. (2) Notes for Gen Kirk on Conf with Gen Marshall, Summary, 25 Dec 44. HD: Resources Anal Div file, "Hosp." (3) MRS SPGAA 705 (4 Jan 45), MPD ASF for Dir Plans and Oprs ASF, 11 Jan 45, sub: Gen and Conv Hosps. HRS: Hq ASF Planning Div files, "Hosp and Evac." (4) Weekly Diary, Resources Anal Div, SGO, 13 Jan 45. HD: 024.7–3. (5) Memo, Lt Col Huncilman, ASF for the Record, 19 Jan 45. HRS: Hq ASF Planning Div files, "Hosp and Evac." (6) DF WDGDS 7623, SecWar (G–4) to CG ASF, 20 Jan 45, sub: Gen Hosp Program, ZI. HD: Resources Anal Div file, "Hosp."

[40] (1) See above, pp. 185–86. (2) DF WDGDS 11208, ACofS G–4 WDGS to CG ASF, 3 Apr 45, sub: Gen Hosp Program for ZI. HRS: Hq ASF Planning Div file, 700 "Hosp."

[41] The increase by month from November 1944 through March 1945 was as follows:

Year and Month	*Total Patients Returned to U.S.*
November 1944	19,700
December 1944	32,511
January 1945	33,382
February 1945	38,251
March 1945	44,845

These figures are from statistics compiled by the Medical Regulating Officer on the basis of monthly reports by port surgeons and the Air Transport Division. History . . . Medical Regulating Service. . . .

TABLE 13—HOSPITALIZATION DATA AS OF 29 JUNE 1945

Type of Hospital	Number of Authorized Beds	Number of Patients: Total	Occupying Beds: Army	Occupying Beds: Non-Army	Army—Absent on leave, furlough, or for other reasons	Patients Reported per 100 Beds	Percent Beds Occupied
General [a]	152, 971	186, 916	118, 717	5, 811	62, 388	122	81.4
Convalescent (AAF and ASF) [b]	59, 978	58, 345	41, 752	4	16, 589	97	69.6
AAF Convalescent	11, 600	6, 240	5, 534	0	706	54	47.7
ASF Convalescent	48, 378	52, 105	36, 218	4	15, 883	108	74.8
Regional (AAF and ASF)	50, 078	38, 045	33, 842	2, 944	1, 259	76	73.4
AAF Regional	19, 960	14, 554	13, 172	936	446	73	70.6
ASF Regional	30, 118	23, 491	20, 670	2, 008	813	78	75.2
Station (AAF and ASF)	51, 561	34, 980	28, 305	6, 338	337	68	67.1
AAF Station	21, 306	11, 728	10, 045	1, 577	106	55	54.5
ASF Station	30, 255	23, 252	18, 260	4, 761	231	77	76.0
General and Convalescent	212, 949	245, 261	160, 469	5, 815	78, 977	115	78.0
General, Convalescent and Regional	263, 027	283, 306	194, 311	8, 759	80, 236	107	77.2
All Hospitals	314, 588	318, 286	222, 616	15, 097	80, 573	101	75.5

[a] General hospitals—only general hospitals proper.
[b] Convalescent hospitals—included both separate convalescent hospitals and those operated in connection with general hospitals.
Source: Weekly Hospitalization Report, vol. II, No. 26. AML.

headquarters for 9,000 additional debarkation beds and for 25,000 additional convalescent beds.[42] Perhaps in recognition of the inconsistency of requesting additional beds at a time when they were arguing that no emergency existed to require the use of vacant beds in regional hospitals for overseas patients, representatives of the Surgeon General's Office and ASF headquarters agreed in conference on 5 April 1945 not to pass this request on to G–4. Instead, they would care for the higher number of patients in beds already authorized by placing more patients on leave and furlough, by speeding the disposition of cases being treated, and by limiting general and convalescent hospitals more strictly to overseas patients. ASF headquarters agreed to some additional construction to increase the capacity of existing debarkation facilities and justified the beds authorized in January by explaining to G–4 the upward trend in patient evacuation.[43]

The peak patient load in the zone of interior occurred at the end of June 1945, approximately two months after V–E Day.[44] An analysis of hospital-occupancy figures at that time shows that all beds in general, convalescent, and regional hospitals were needed and that even more might have been required if many patients had not been placed on leave or furlough. For example, the patient census of general, convalescent, and regional hos-

[42] (1) Memo, SG for Dir Plans and Oprs ASF, 19 Mar 45, sub: Temp Debarkation Reqmts. SG: 632.2. (2) Memo, SG for CG ASF, 23 Mar 45, sub: Gen Hosp Program, ZI. SG: 322 "Hosp."

[43] (1) Memo, SG for CG ASF, 6 Apr 45, sub: Gen Hosp Program, ZI, with 1st ind. SG: 322 "Hosp." (2) 1st ind, CG ASF to ACofS G–4 WDGS, 9 Apr 45, on DF WDGDS 11208, ACofS G–4 WDGS to CG ASF, 3 Apr 45, same sub. HRS: Hq ASF Planning Div file, 700 "ZI Hosp."

[44] This statement is based upon figures in Weekly Hospitalization Reports that include both Army and non-Army patients as of midnight of Friday of each week. *Statistical Review, World War II: A Summary of ASF Activities*, prepared by the Statistics Branch, Control Division, ASF, lists the average number of Army patients each month and shows the peak load occurring during July.

CHART 9—HOSPITAL BEDS AUTHORIZED AND OCCUPIED, AND PATIENTS REPORTED IN ALL HOSPITALS IN THE CONTINENTAL UNITED STATES: JUNE 1944–DECEMBER 1946

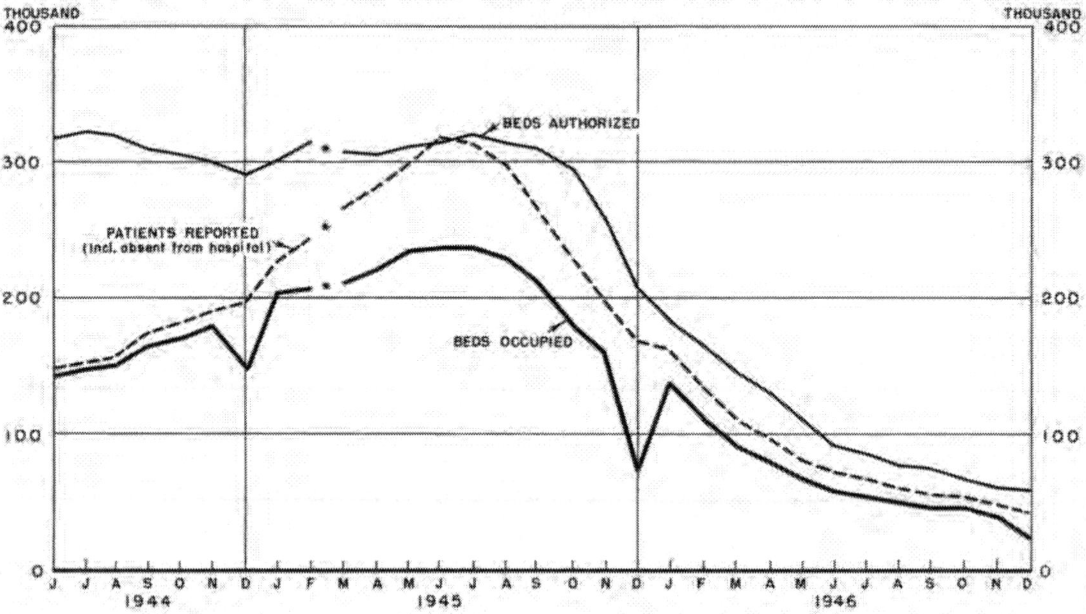

*Excludes debarkation beds and patients after February 1945.

Source: Weekly Health Reports, ASF, Med Statistics Div, SGO.

pitals was 283,306, while the number of beds in those hospitals was only 263,027. Of these beds, 203,070 were occupied. The rest of the patients—80,236—were absent from hospitals on leave or furlough. Not all hospitals were equally used, and the patient load was unevenly distributed. General hospitals were filled beyond the saturation point, normally considered to be 80 percent of their total bed capacities, and had more than 62,000 patients on leave. Regional hospitals, on the other hand, were only 73.4-percent occupied, and had few patients on leave. This suggests either that beds in these hospitals might have been reduced in number or that some might have been used for overseas patients to relieve general hospitals of part of their heavy load. In general, ASF hospitals showed higher occupancy ratios than did those of the Air Forces. This raises the question of whether the number of beds in the latter might have been reduced or vacant beds in them used for more non-AAF personnel. The low occupancy of both AAF and ASF station hospital beds indicates that the Staff had been justified in reducing their ratio to 3 percent and in suggesting even further reductions.

A more even distribution of patients and a fuller utilization of all hospitals would have been achieved, perhaps, by modifications of existing hospitalization policies but this was precluded chiefly by the separation of zone of interior hospitals into AAF and ASF hospitals and by the struggle for power between The Surgeon General and the Air Surgeon. *(Table 13, Charts 9, 10)*

CHART 10—HOSPITAL BEDS AUTHORIZED AND OCCUPIED, AND PATIENTS REPORTED BY CONVALESCENT, REGIONAL, GENERAL, AND STATION HOSPITALS IN CONTINENTAL UNITED STATES: JUNE 1944–DECEMBER 1946

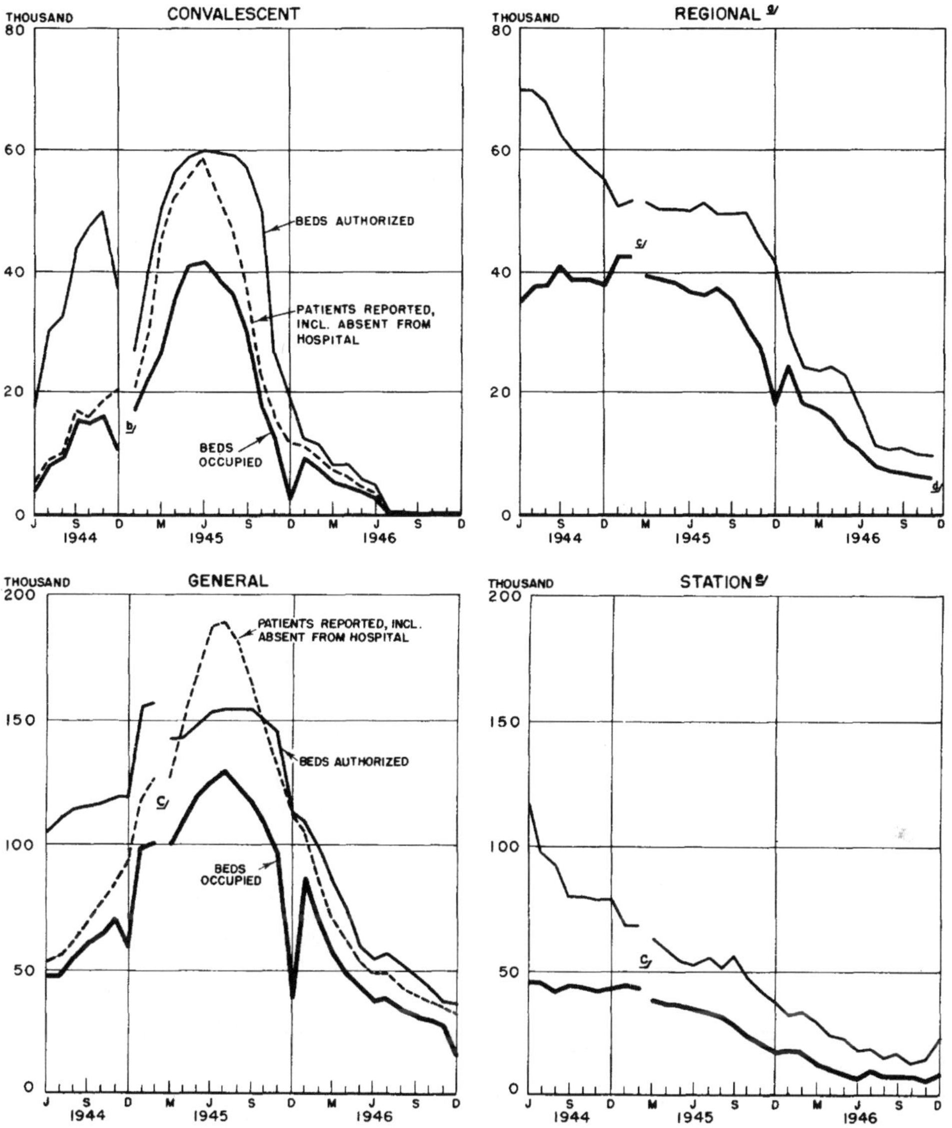

[a] Patients reported by regional hospitals, not shown, varied from 1,500 to 2,500 more than beds occupied.

[b] Includes convalescent facilities, but excludes convalescent annexes at general hospitals after December 1944.

[c] Excludes debarkation beds after February 1945.

[d] All regional hospitals became station hospitals in December 1946.

[e] Patients reported by station hospitals, not shown, usually ranged between 1,300 and 2,500 more than beds occupied. This applies to the period Dec 1944 to Sept 1945, the war months for which figures are available.

Source: Weekly Health Reports, ASF, Med Statistics Div, SGO.

CHAPTER XII

Estimating and Meeting Requirements of Theaters for Hospital Beds

Although estimates of beds required for theaters were generally made separately from those for the zone of interior, developments attending the estimation of requirements for both areas were in some respects similar. Such similarities occurred despite the fact that co-ordination between interested divisions of the Surgeon General's Office was incomplete.

Until the late summer of 1943 the Plans Division of the Surgeon General's Office continued to plan hospitalization for active overseas theaters on the basis of a 10- to 15-percent ratio of fixed beds to troop strength.[1] One reason for this high ratio was that the director of the Division, aware of public criticism which the Medical Department would incur if it ever failed to have enough beds, desired to have a sufficient number to meet promptly a greatly accelerated build-up of troops overseas and still have enough left to constitute a safety factor.[2] Another reason of equal cogency was that sufficient information about various factors that affected bed requirements during World War II was not yet available to justify the establishment of lower ratios than those derived from World War I experience.

Factors Influencing Bed Requirements

Among the factors that influenced bed requirements were: (1) overseas troop strengths, both actual and projected; (2) disease and nonbattle-injury hospital-admission rates; (3) battle-casualty hospital-admission rates; (4) the average length of time patients stayed in hospitals; and (5) evacuation policies. While troop strengths and admission rates for disease and nonbattle-injury cases could be determined with reasonable accuracy, admission rates for battle casualties could be estimated only roughly and were therefore uncertain at best. The average length of time that patients stayed in hospitals depended upon some factors that were uncontrollable, such as the severity of wounds and the seriousness of illnesses, and upon others, such as evacuation poli-

[1] For example, see Ltr, SG to CG ASF, 13 Jul 43, sub: Trp Basis for Pacific Area. SG: 320.2.

[2] Interv, MD Historian with Col Arthur B. Welsh, MC, 27 Dec 50. HD: 000.71. According to Colonel Welsh the safety factor was an undeployed reserve within the United States for use in case the enemy employed atomic, chemical, or biological weapons effectively.

cies, that could be determined by the War Department.

Evacuation policies governed the numbers and types of patients to be transferred from theaters to the zone of interior and were expressed in terms of days. For example, a theater which evacuated all patients requiring 120 or more days of hospitalization was said to have a "120-day policy." Under such a policy a theater would retain for treatment in its own hospitals all patients who, it was expected, could be returned to duty within 120 days and would evacuate the balance, not at the end of the 120-day period, but as soon as they were able to travel and conveyances were available. Under a 120-day policy the average length of stay of patients in theater hospitals was shorter than under a 180-day policy and more patients were evacuated to the zone of interior. It was estimated, for example, that 30 percent of all battle-casualty patients were returned to the United States under the former, while only 20 percent were returned under the latter. Thus the evacuation policy affected the number of hospital beds required in theaters. It also affected the number needed in the United States to hospitalize evacuees, the amount of transportation required for patients, and the number of replacements needed by theaters. From a theater commander's viewpoint, the ideal arrangement was to hospitalize in theaters those patients who could be returned to duty within a "reasonable" period of time, thus reducing the number of replacements needed, and to evacuate the rest as soon as possible, thus reducing the number of hospital units and the amount of equipment shipped into and used in the theater. The Surgeon General believed that a 120-day policy more nearly approached the ideal than did any other.[3]

Establishment of Official Evacuation Policies

Although the Surgeon General's Office and ASF headquarters had tried to get official evacuation policies established in the spring of 1943, final action was delayed until August. Being of vital concern to theaters, evacuation policies were normally established by the War Department only after consultation with theater headquarters, and several months were required to get comments on a proposal of The Surgeon General in May 1943 that a 120-day policy be officially adopted.[4] These replies revealed that all theaters except the European and Asiatic (China-Burma-India) agreed upon the desirability of that policy. Having enough beds to operate under a 180-day policy, both the European and Asiatic theaters preferred the latter. It permitted them to return to duty a greater proportion of experienced personnel. It also enabled them to save shipping required both to evacuate patients to the United States and to return replacements to theaters. In addition, the European theater favored a 180-day policy because it lacked hospital ships for evacuation and its chief surgeon opposed returning patients to the United States in transports. Although the South Pacific, Southwest Pacific, and North African theaters preferred a 120-day policy, they requested permission to continue operations under a 90-day policy because of short-

[3] (1) ASF Monthly Progress Rpt, Sec 7, *Health*, 31 Dec 44, pp. 29–34. HD. (2) Memo SPOPP 370.05, Dir Planning Div ASF for Dir Plans and Oprs ASF, 24 Jan 45, sub: Review of "Elements of an Evac Policy." HRS: ASF Hq Planning Div File, 370.05 "Hosp and Evac."

[4] WD Memo W40–12–43, Evac Policy for Overseas Comds, 8 May 43. HD: Wilson files, 008 "Policy re Evac for Overseas." See p. 165.

ages of beds. After analysis of these replies, the War Department announced on 28 August 1943 that it was establishing a 180-day policy for the European and Asiatic theaters and a 120-day policy for all others to become effective as soon as required hospital and transportation facilities were available.[5]

Establishment of Bed Ratios for Theaters of Operations

A few days before theater evacuation policies were announced, official bed ratios had been authorized for theaters for the first time in World War II. Early in August 1943, when the Surgeon General's Office and the General Staff were concerned about means of meeting the needs of the Army with the number of physicians authorized, The Inspector General reported that members of his staff, including General Snyder, had found in a survey of North African operations that battle-casualty rates had been lower than anticipated and that hospitalization requirements had been met during the first two campaigns with less than half the number of beds originally considered essential.[6] In view of this report the Deputy Chief of Staff of the Army directed OPD to survey bed requirements of all theaters "in the light of experience to date." Meanwhile, OPD was to limit the total number of beds shipped overseas, whether in fixed or mobile hospitals, to 8 percent of theater troop strengths.[7]

In the study that followed, both OPD and the Surgeon General's Office agreed that fixed and mobile beds should be estimated and authorized separately because they served different purposes. Designed to support divisions in combat, mobile hospitals cared for patients requiring only short-duration treatment before return to duty and prepared others for evacuation to the rear. Thus sufficient numbers of fixed hospital beds were needed in the rear to take over patients whom mobile hospitals could not return to duty. Both offices agreed also that theaters should be supplied with "50-percent expansion equipment"—that is, with enough equipment to permit each fixed hospital to expand its bed capacity for short periods of time by 50 percent, without any increase in its authorized personnel. This would provide a safety factor for emergencies. Both offices further agreed that combat operations up to that time furnished an insufficient basis for estimating future rates of battle-casualty admissions, but they differed as to how this should affect the establishment of fixed-bed ratios. A computation by the Surgeon General's Office of beds needed in each theater for disease and nonbattle-injury cases, based on experience between the last of 1941 and the early part of 1943, did not alter its opinion that the 10- to 15-percent ratio should still be adhered to. It therefore recommended that this ratio be officially authorized. Believing that fewer beds would suffice, OPD used The Surgeon General's rates for disease and nonbattle injuries along with limited information available about World War II battle-casualty rates to develop

[5] WD Memo W40–19–43, Policy on Evac of S&W from Overseas Comds, 28 Aug 43. HD: Wilson files, 008 "Policy re Evac from Overseas Comds." Replies of theaters to the War Department memorandum of 8 May 43 are found in SG: 705.–1.

[6] (1) Memo, IG for DepCofSA, 10 Aug 43, sub: Ests of Battle Casualties as Affecting Repls and Plans for Evac and Hosp. HRS: OPD, 700 "ETO." (2) Memo, IG for DepCofSA, 10 Aug 43, sub: Surv of the Orgn and Opr of the MD Fac in NATOUSA and Sicily. Same file.

[7] Memo WDCSA 333 (10 Aug 43), DepCofSA for ACofS OPD WDGS, 13 Aug 43, sub: Surv of the Orgn and Opr of the MD. HRS: OPD, 700 "ETO."

other ratios of fixed beds that ranged from a low of 4 percent for one theater to a high of 10 percent for others. Abandoning its former position because of the limited number of physicians now available, the Surgeon General's Office concurred in recommending these ratios.

As a result, on 24 August 1943, the Deputy Chief of Staff approved the proposal to authorize fixed and mobile beds separately, agreed to supply all theaters with 50-percent expansion equipment, and authorized ratios of fixed beds as follows: 8 percent for the European and Asiatic (China-Burma-India) theaters, 10 percent for the South and Southwest Pacific theaters, 6.6 percent for the North African theater, 6 percent for the Middle East-Central-African theater, and 4 percent for the American (the Western Hemisphere, exclusive of the United States) theater.[8] A short time later a ratio of 7 percent was established for the Central Pacific,[9] and the 8 percent ratio for the Asiatic theater, which at first applied only to American troop strength, was revised in February 1944 to provide 8 percent each for the American forces and the Chinese Army in India.[10] In establishing such ratios the Deputy Chief of Staff announced that he was not thereby authorizing additions to the troop basis. It remained to be seen whether quotas of beds authorized for various theaters could be met with units already included in the troop basis.

Mobile bed requirements were agreed upon in a conference which OPD held with representatives of G-3, G-4, ASF headquarters, the Ground Surgeon, and The Surgeon General, and were approved on 23 August 1943 by the Deputy Chief of Staff. For planning purposes, beds were authorized in evacuation hospitals for 3 percent, and in convalescent hospitals for 1 percent, of the troops in combat zones. Although there was misunderstanding about what this meant in terms of units, it was generally considered that one 400-bed evacuation hospital would be supplied for every division (except airborne divisions, which were not authorized evacuation hospitals) and for each group of army or corps troops equivalent in number to a division; that one 3,000-bed convalescent hospital would be supplied for each group of nine divisions; and that three portable surgical hospitals would be supplied, whenever theaters used them, for each division. If 750-bed evacuation hospitals were used, they were to be supplied in numbers sufficient to give a quantity of beds equal to that authorized in 400-bed hospitals. It was expected that portable surgical hospitals would be used only in the Pacific and Asiatic theaters and that convalescent hospitals would be used as mobile units chiefly in the European and North African theaters.[11] In addition, spe-

[8] (1) Memo, SG for ACofS OPD WDGS, 17 Aug 43, sub: Fixed Hosp, Overseas. SG: 701.-1. (2) Memo, Act ACofS OPD for DepCofSA, 20 Aug 43, sub: Surv of Orgn and Opr of the MD, with notation: "Approved as amended," by order of SecWar, by Col W. A. Schulgren, Asst Sec WDGS, 24 Aug 43. HRS: OPD, 700 "ETO."

[9] This ratio was established before April 1944. See Memo, CG ASF for CofSA thru ACofS G-4 WDGS, 10 Apr 44, sub: Overseas Hosp. HRS: ASF Planning Div Program Br file, "Hosp, Apr 44."

[10] (1) Memo OPD 632 (19 Sep 43), ACofS OPD WDGS for DepCofSA, 24 Sep 43, sub: Hosp—Asiatic Theater. HRS: WDCSA 632. (2) DF OPD 632 (22 Oct 43), ACofS OPD WDGS to TAG, 1 Feb 44, sub: Hosp in the Asiatic Theater (Beds). HRS: G-4 file, "Hosp and Evac Policy."

[11] (1) Memo, [Col] R[obert] B. S[kinner] for Record, 26 Aug 43. Ground Med files: Chronological file (Col Skinner). (2) Memo, Act ACofS OPD WDGS for DepCofSA, 28 Aug 43, sub: Surv of the Orgn and Opr of the MD. HRS: OPD, 700 "ETO." (3) Memo, Col A[rthur] B. Welsh for Record, 7 Sep 43. SG: 632.-2.

cial provision had to be made for the hospitalization of Chinese troops in the Asiatic theater. For the Chinese Army in India (which had an authorized strength of 57,000) beds were authorized in evacuation hospitals on a 2-percent ratio; and for the Chinese Army in China, beds were authorized in portable surgical hospitals at the rate of one such unit for each of twenty-seven divisions.[12]

Ratios of mobile beds authorized at this time remained unchanged during the war; [13] but some theaters never received full quotas and therefore had to improvise mobile hospitals, while others found it desirable to use, in addition to authorized mobile hospital units, some fixed hospital units (field hospitals) as mobile hospitals.[14]

Efforts to Provide Theaters With Authorized Quotas of Beds

After bed ratios and evacuation policies were established, adjustments had to be made in hospital facilities in each theater. Some, notably the South Pacific, Central Pacific, and European theaters, had less than their authorized quotas of mobile beds. Others, the Southwest Pacific, Asiatic, and North African, had more.[15] A few areas, for example Alaska and the Middle East, had more fixed beds than authorized, while others—the European, North African, Pacific and Asiatic theaters—had fewer.[16] Theaters that had too many mobile and too few fixed beds were permitted either to convert excess mobile hospital units into fixed hospital units, as was done in the Southwest Pacific area,[17] or to use mobile units as fixed units, without conversion or reorganization, as was done in the Asiatic and North African theaters.[18]

When these changes did not erase deficits of fixed beds, other methods of increasing capacities were employed. The most obvious was to send additional hospital units to theaters. Between September and December 1943, 24 general hospital units, 10 field hospital units, and 39 station hospital units were shipped from the United States,[19] but they were insufficient to supply all theaters with authorized bed capacities.

Another method was to enlarge hospitals already in theaters by increasing capacities authorized various units by tables of organization and equipment. This was economical of personnel. In the fall of 1943 a 750-bed station hospital, for example, required 40 officers (of whom 24 were Medical Corps officers), 75 nurses, and 392 enlisted men, while three 250-bed

[12] (1) Memo OPD 632 (19 Sep 43), ACofS OPD WDGS for DepCofSA, 24 Sep 43, sub: Hosp—Asiatic Theater. HRS: WDGSA 632. (2) DF OPD 632 (22 Oct 43), ACofS OPD WDGS to TAG, 1 Feb 44, sub: Hosp in the Asiatic Theater (Beds). HRS: G-4 file, "Hosp and Evac Policy."

[13] Memo SPMDA 322.05, SG for SecWar, 10 Jan 45, sub: The Med Mission Reappraised. HRS: G-4 file, "Hosp and Evac, vol. II."

[14] These developments will be discussed fully in a volume planned for this series on hospitalization and evacuation in theaters of operations.

[15] Table Showing Mobile Hosp Units in Theaters, Tab X to Memo, Act ACofS OPD WDGS for DepCofSA, 28 Aug 43, sub: Surv of Orgn and Opr of the MD. HRS: OPD, 700 "ETO."

[16] See *Chart 11*.

[17] (1) Memo OPD 320.2 (5 Oct 43), ACofS OPD WDGS for CG ASF, 9 Oct 43, sub: Evac Policy for Overseas Comds (Hosp Units). SG: 320.2. (2) Ltr AG 322 (14 Oct 43) OB-I-SPMOU-M, TAG to Comdr-In-Chief SWPA, 18 Oct 43, sub: Reorgn and Redesignation of Certain Hosp Units, SWPA. SG: 320.3-1.

[18] (1) DF OPD 632 (22 Oct 43), ACofS OPD WDGS to TAG, 1 Feb 44, sub: Hosp—Asiatic Theater (Beds). HRS: G-4 file, "Hosp and Evac Policy." (2) Rpt, Asst Comdt MFSS, Carlisle Bks to SG, 29 Nov 43, sub: Visit to ETO and NATO, 1 Sep-24 Oct 43. SG: 333.1.

[19] An Rpt, MOOD SGO, FY 1944. HD.

station hospitals required 63 officers (of whom 39 were Medical Corps officers), 90 nurses, and 450 enlisted men.[20] For this reason the Surgeon General's Office had proposed as early as the summer of 1943 that from 66⅔ to 80 percent of all fixed beds should be in general hospitals (1,000-bed capacity) and the remainder in smaller units.[21] In the fall of 1943 the Central Pacific theater enlarged the table-of-organization capacities of some of its hospitals in order to provide additional fixed beds with a minimum of additional personnel,[22] and in December 1943 The Surgeon General asked other theaters to do likewise.[23]

A third method of increasing numbers of fixed beds was to expand hospitals beyond table-of-organization capacities—that is, to have a 1,000-bed general hospital, for example, set up beds and temporarily care for more than 1,000 patients without any increase in personnel. Anticipated in the provision that theaters be authorized 50-percent expansion equipment, this method was used in many instances, particularly in the Southwest Pacific and North African theaters, in the fall and winter of 1943.[24]

If bed capacities were not increased sufficiently by these means, theaters were permitted temporary "reductions" in official evacuation policies to enable them to transfer more patients to the United States. The South Pacific theater, for example, operated under a 60-day evacuation policy until January 1944 and changed to a 90-day policy in February, while the North African theater followed a 90-day policy until May 1944.[25]

Although some theaters objected to using the expedients discussed above,[26] all succeeded in meeting hospitalization needs during the winter of 1943-44. While none having a deficit of fixed beds in the fall of 1943 reached its authorized quota by the end of the year, only one—the North African theater—had more patients than it did table-of-organization beds.[27]

While efforts were being made to supply theaters with authorized quotas of fixed beds, the Surgeon General's Plans Division was looking toward the future. As theaters built up troop strengths and planned combat operations, they called upon the War Department for specific types and numbers of units to meet anticipated needs. The OPD and G-3 Divisions of the General Staff, attempting to meet theater requests if possible, periodically issued a "Six Months Forecast"—a document showing units needed and the time

[20] See T/O 8-560, Sta Hosp, 22 Jul 42 with C 1, 5 Sep 42, and C 2, 18 Sep 42.

[21] (1) Draft Rad, CG ASF to CGs NATO, SWPA, USAF CBI, SPA, and ETO, 21 Jun 43. HD: Wilson files, "Day File, Jun 43." (2) Memo for Record on Draft Memo, Asst to CofS ASF for ACofS OPD WDGS, 23 Jun 43, sub: Proposed Rad for Certain Overseas Theaters Concerning Fixed Hosp Policy. Same file. It is not readily apparent how such a percentage could be applied generally, unless the essential difference between functions of general and station hospitals were to be ignored.

[22] Ltr AG 322 (24 Sep 43)OB-I-SPMOU-M, TAG to CG USAFCPA, SG, and Chiefs of Tec Servs, 28 Sep 43, sub: Reorgn of Sta and Gen Hosps in CPA. SG: 320.3-1.

[23] (1) Diary, MOOB SGO, 4-10 Dec 43. HD: 024.7-5, "MOOB Diary." (2) Rad CM-OUT-8738 (23 Dec 43), CG ASF to theater commanders. SG: 322.15-1.

[24] (1) Notes atchd to Memo, Col William L. Wilson, MC for Chief Control Div [SGO], 1 Nov 43, sub: Visit to SWPA. SG: 333.1-1 (Aust)F. (2) Rad CM-IN-9494 (15 Jan 44), Algiers to AGWAR, 14 Jan 44. SG: 322.15-1.

[25] (1) Rad CM-IN-18720 (25 May 44), CG NATO to WD, 24 May 44. HRS: G-4 file, "Hosp and Evac Policy." (2) Rad CM-OUT-42858 (28 May 44), WD to CG NATO, 27 May 44. Same file.

[26] Theater objections will be discussed in a volume planned for this series on hospitalization and evacuation in theaters of operations.

[27] See *Chart 11*.

Chart 11—Fixed Hospital Bed Capacity, and Occupancy in Overseas Theaters: March 1943–December 1945

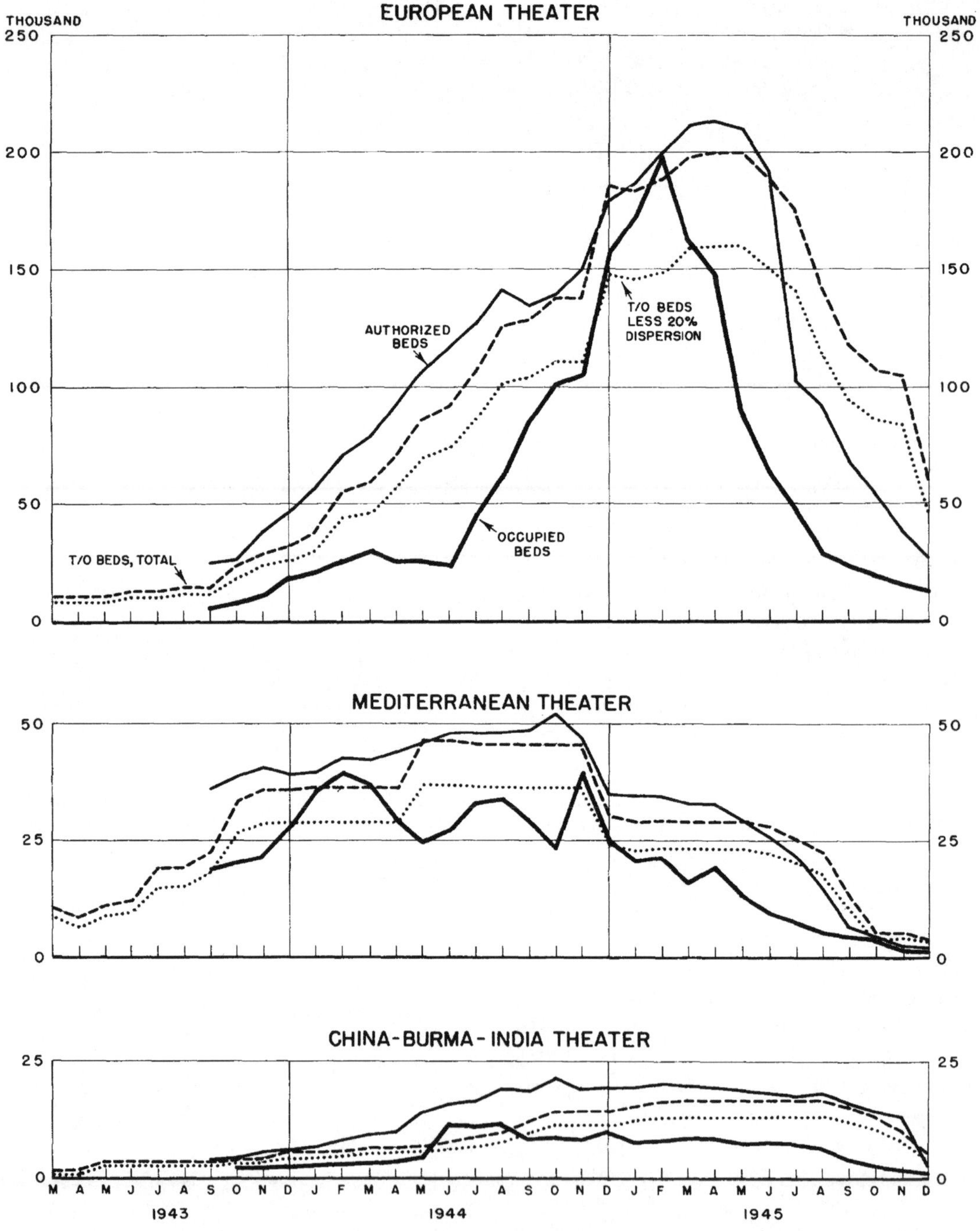

Chart 11—Fixed Hospital Bed Capacity, and Occupancy in Overseas Theaters: March 1943–December 1945—Continued

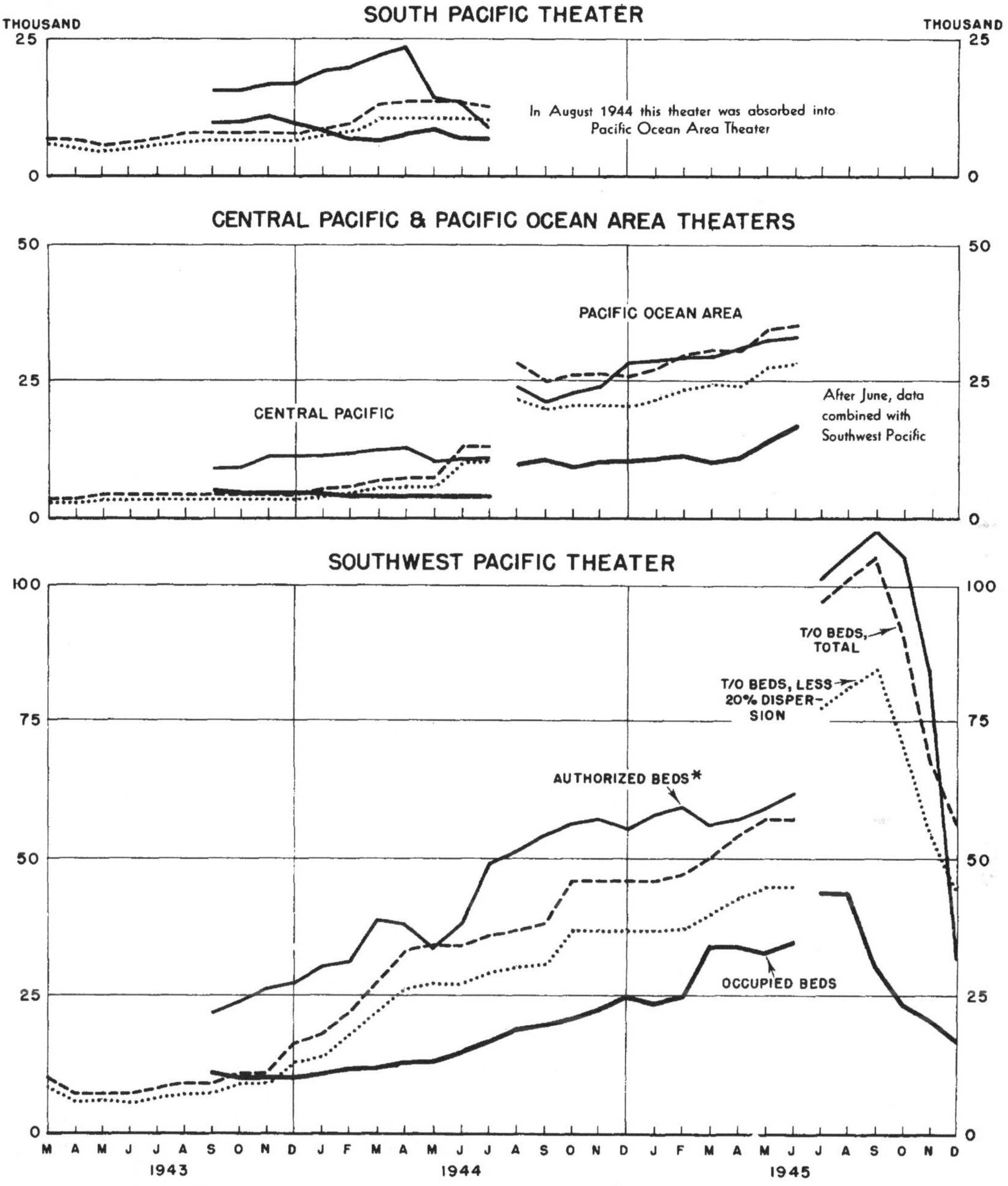

* Based on War Department determined percentage of troop strength.

Source: Hospitalization Overseas—Authorized Fixed Beds. HD: 024, Mob. and Overseas Oper. Div., Oper. Serv., SGO.

of their shipment.[28] Hospital units listed in the "Forecast" did not always exist in this country, and it was sometimes necessary to make adjustments among units already activated. The Surgeon General's Plans Division proposed such action. For example, in November 1943 the Mobilization and Overseas Operations Branch made a study of units required by the eighth revision of the "Forecast" and found that more station hospital units of 750-, 250-, 200-, 150-, 100-, and 25-bed capacities had been activated than were needed but that fewer general and field hospital units had been activated than were required. The Surgeon General's Office then recommended the inactivation and reorganization of certain station hospital units in order to supply personnel for the required number of general and field hospitals.[29] ASF headquarters approved this recommendation and orders were issued to make it effective. At successive times later, as for example in September 1944, the Surgeon General's Office suggested similar action to insure the availability of units in the types and sizes desired by theaters.[30]

In addition to recommending adjustments among types of hospital units being prepared for overseas service, the Surgeon General's Office took other actions in the fall of 1943 to meet future needs. After the Deputy Chief of Staff authorized 50-percent expansion equipment for fixed hospitals in theaters, the Mobilization and Overseas Operations Branch co-operated with the Supply Service of the Surgeon General's Office in securing authority to procure the equipment thus authorized.[31] In addition, the troop basis of 1944 was reviewed and G–3 agreed to increase the number of fixed hospital units included in it to provide 20,000 additional beds. Even so, the troop basis did not list enough units to supply all theaters with quotas authorized by the Deputy Chief of Staff in August 1943.[32] Finally, and not of least importance, under a system of telegraphic reporting initiated in July 1943, the Surgeon General's Office began to receive from theaters fuller, more accurate, and more current data on which to base studies of admission rates.[33]

Problems encountered in the fall and winter of 1943 in providing theaters with authorized quotas of fixed beds were merely a preview of 1944. The increasing scope and intensity of combat operations created more pressing needs for hospitalization and at the same time, by using up more personnel in the form of replacements, accentuated the shortage of men for assignment to hospital units. From the early part of 1944 this shortage was so great that it became one of the controlling factors in planning overseas hospitalization. Early in February 1944 the Surgeon General's Office warned ASF headquar-

[28] An example of this document, Twentieth Revision of the Six Months Forecast, Units and Availability, Data as of 20 Oct 44, Based on OPD Reqmts 5 Oct 44, G–3 Div WDGS is on file HD: 370.5.

[29] (1) An Rpt, MOOD SGO, FY 1944. HD. (2) Diary, MOOB, 27 Nov–3 Dec 43. HD: 024.7–5, "MOOB Diary." (3) Ltr, SG to CG ASF, 5 Nov 43, sub: Activations, Reorgns and Inactivations of Non-Div Med Units. SG: 322.3–1.

[30] Ltr, SG to CG ASF, 8 Sep 44, sub: Reorgn of Med Units. SG: 320.3–1.

[31] (1) Memo, SG for ACofS OPD WDGS, thru CG ASF, 9 Dec 43, sub: Recommended Changes in Victory Program Trp Basis, Revision of 22 Nov 43, with ind. SG: 322.15–1. (2) Memo, Act Chief Sup Serv SGO for SG, 28 Dec 43, sub: Fixed Beds Overseas in Army Sup Program. SG: 632.–2. (3) Memo, Dep Chief Oprs Serv SGO for SG, 30 Dec 43. SG: 632.–2.

[32] Memo for Record on DF, ACofS G–3 WDGS to ACofS OPD WDGS, 26 Jan 44. HRS: G–3 file, 700–800.

[33] Memo WDGDS 6442, Act ACofS G–4 WDGS for CG ASF, 7 Sep 43, sub: Hosp in Overseas Theaters, with 1st ind, SG to ACofS G–4 WDGS, 17 Sep 43. SG: 701.–1.

ters that it would be impossible to meet theater requirements unless enlisted men were supplied in sufficient numbers to activate and train the units authorized.[34] Soon afterward ASF headquarters informed G-3 that the Service Forces had 72,813 fewer men than were needed to activate units according to schedule and that 27,160 men were needed for Medical Department units alone.[35] Urgent requests from ASF headquarters for more men were of little avail, and during the first four months of 1944 only 12 general, 1 station, and 11 field hospital units were activated. In May the Medical Department received its first substantial allotment of personnel for numbered hospitals during 1944 and activated that month 11 general and 3 field hospital units. Then, during subsequent months, as a result of the policy of releasing from zone of interior installations men who were qualified for overseas service, additional men became available, and during the five months beginning with June and ending with October 98 general, 8 station, and 43 field hospital units were activated.[36] Thus few hospital units were activated during 1944 until the latter half of the year.

The Medical Department also had difficulty in procuring enough Medical Corps officers to man the units activated. As early as February 1944 the director of the Surgeon General's Military Personnel Division stated that there would not be enough Medical Corps specialists to staff hospitals being sent overseas and that some units would have to be shipped without specialists.[37] A month later the Surgeon General's Office reported to ASF headquarters that physicians to staff forty general hospital units then in training could not be procured until June and that full officer strength for nine of the general hospitals activated in March would not be available until August.[38]

Use of Negro Hospital Units

The use of Negro personnel—doctors, nurses, and enlisted men—to help relieve the general personnel shortage and meet theater needs for hospital units was complicated by existing policies and practices and by the attitude of theater commanders and surgeons.[39] Following a practice adopted early in the war—the organization of all-Negro units to provide opportunities for the use of Negro doctors and nurses—the War Department activated a third Negro hospital unit—the 335th Station Hospital—in August 1943. Meanwhile the 268th Station Hospital unit, which had been activated five months earlier, completed its training and in October 1943 embarked for the Southwest Pacific.[40]

[34] (1) Ltr, SG to CG ASF, 15 Feb 44, sub: Projection of Non-Div Med Units. SG: 322.3-1. (2) An Rpt, MOOD SGO, FY 1944. HD.

[35] (1) Memo, CG ASF for ACofS G-3 WDGS thru ACofS OPD WDGS, 18 Mar 44, sub: Projection of Non-Div Med Units, with incls. HRS: Hq ASF, Lt Gen LeR. Lutes' file, "Hosp and Evac, Jun 43 thru Dec 46." (2) Memo, CG ASF for ACofS G-3 WDGS, 26 Mar 44, sub: Med Units. Same file.

[36] An Rpt, MOOD SGO, FY 1944. HD.

[37] Memo, Dir Mil Pers SGO for Chief Oprs Serv SGO, 12 Feb 44, sub: Staffing of Gen Hosp Destined for Shipment to ETO. SG: 320.3-1.

[38] Memo, Dir Mob Div ASF for Dir Plans and Oprs ASF, 25 Mar 44, sub: Status of Med Units. HRS: Hq ASF, Lt Gen LeR. Lutes' file, "Hosp and Evac, Jun 43 thru Dec 46."

[39] These questions will be discussed fully in John H. McMinn and Max Levin, Personnel (MS for companion vol. in Medical Dept. series), HD. Also see Ulysses Lee, The Employment of Negro Troops, forthcoming volume in UNITED STATES ARMY IN WORLD WAR II.

[40] (1) An Rpt, 335th Sta Hosp, 1944. HD. (2) Quarterly Rpt, 268th Sta Hosp, Jul 44. HD.

With the need to use Negro personnel increasing as difficulties in meeting theater requirements mounted, the War Department in January 1944 requested all theaters to state whether or not they would use all-Negro hospital units. Most replied negatively. Fearing loss of the services of the 335th Station Hospital unit, The Surgeon General in May 1944 appealed to ASF headquarters for "efforts [to] be made to obtain an appropriate assignment" for it.[41] The same month he appealed personally to the chief surgeon of the European theater to use Negro nurses in at least one hospital.[42] The chief surgeon agreed, and in July 1944 sixty-three Negro nurses, among whom were some who had formerly served with the 25th Station Hospital in Africa and had been returned to the United States at the end of 1943, arrived in the European theater. After a period of training they were assigned in September to replace white nurses in the 168th Station Hospital.[43]

Meanwhile an assignment for the 335th Station Hospital had been found. In June 1944 the chief surgeon of the China-Burma-India theater made a trip to Washington to explain in person his desperate need for additional hospital units. Among the means of meeting the need, in view of the general shortage of units for shipment overseas, the low priority of the China-Burma-India theater, and the demands of other theaters, the use of the 335th Station Hospital was proposed. The theater surgeon agreed to accept this unit with an overstrength of sufficient size to permit the organization of an additional hospital in the theater.[44] As a result the 335th Station Hospital embarked in August 1944 and was stationed on the Stillwell Road after its arrival in Asia. According to plan, it was reorganized in December 1944 and its capacity was reduced from 150 to 100 beds. The personnel thus made surplus, along with that carried as overstrength, was used to form another 100-bed all-Negro hospital unit—the 383d Station Hospital. Both units continued to serve together as one hospital until the 383d was sent to the Philippines in August 1945.[45]

Thus, although Negroes served in the Medical Department overseas in organic medical units of divisions and in such other units as sanitary companies, the use of Negro professional personnel in hospital units was limited to the 25th Station Hospital (a Negro unit with four white officers in command and supervisory positions), the 268th, 335th, and 383d Station Hospitals (all-Negro units), and the 168th Station Hospital (a white unit with Negro nurses).

Estimating Requirements for Major Combat Operations

Before the full impact of personnel shortages was felt, the Surgeon General's Office began early in 1944 to estimate hospitalization and evacuation requirements for full-scale combat operations. In November and December 1943 the Com-

[41] Memo, SG for Dir Planning Div ASF, 17 May 44, sub: Overseas Employment of 335th Sta Hosp (Colored). AG: 370.05 (335th Sta Hosp)1944–I.

[42] Ltr, SG to Chief Surg, ETOUSA, 16 May 44. HD: ETO file, "Kirk-Hawley Corresp."

[43] An Rpt, 168th Sta Hosp, 1944. HD.

[44] (1) Memo for Record, 30 Jun 44, sub: Hosp in CBI, by Chief Theater Br MOOD SGO. HD: 024 "MOOD (CBI)." (2) Ltr, Col Robert P. Williams, Theater Surg USAF in CBI to Col George E. Armstrong, Dep Theater Surg USAF in CBI, 30 Jun 44. Same file. (3) Interv, MD Historian with Brig Gen Robert P. Williams, 13 and 15 Feb 50. HD: 000.71.

[45] (1) An Rpt, 335th Sta Hosp, 1944. HD. (2) Final Rpt, 383d Sta Hosp, Jul 45. HD. (3) AG Unit Card, 383d Sta Hosp. Orgn and Directory Sec, Oprs Br, Admin Servs Div, AGO.

bined Chiefs of Staff met with President Roosevelt and Prime Minister Churchill at the SEXTANT conference in Cairo and then with the President, the Prime Minister, and Marshal Stalin at Teheran.[46] The decision of these conferences to mount both OVERLORD (the invasion of Europe from England) and ANVIL (the invasion of Southern France from bases in the Mediterranean) during May 1944 focused attention on the European and North African theaters,[47] and twice during the winter of 1943-44 the Surgeon General's Office made studies of their need for hospital beds. On the basis of the first, made by the Mobilization and Overseas Operations Branch,[48] The Surgeon General recommended to ASF headquarters that North Africa be supplied with additional hospital units and with additional personnel for existing units to raise its bed capacity to its authorized quota, and to G-4 that the current bed ratios of both the European and North African theaters be raised.[49] Both recommendations were disapproved. OPD was handling requests from North Africa for additional personnel and hospital units. Because of the shortage of personnel in the United States, it proposed that the North African theater increase is fixed-bed capacity by using personnel already in the theater to expand existing hospitals.[50] G-4 disapproved raising current bed ratios because it believed hospital units supplied under them would provide sufficient beds for the early phases of operations on the European continent. If additional beds should then be needed, they could be sent later. Meanwhile, both theaters could use expansion equipment to increase capacities of existing hospitals for emergencies, and the European theater, if it should have a shortage of beds, could reduce its evacuation policy from 180 to 120 days and thus send a larger proportion of patients to the United States.[51]

The Surgeon General "strongly urged" that the decision not to send additional personnel and units to North Africa be reconsidered. He concurred in the decision not to raise bed ratios, but recommended that it be considered temporary, pending accumulation of more definite information about needs. Furthermore, he warned that evacuation facilities (ships and planes) would have to be adequate to remove patients from theaters if they were not given additional beds.[52] Meanwhile, his office had begun another study of the needs of overseas theaters.

The second study, made by the Facilities Utilization Branch of the Hospital Administration Division in connection with its attempt to estimate the number of beds that would be needed in the United States, covered estimated requirements of

[46] *Biennial Report . . . Chief of Staff, 1943-45*, p. 27.

[47] Memo SPOPP 337, Dir Plans and Oprs ASF for Dir Sup and Mat ASF; Chiefs of TC *et al.*, 15 Dec 43, sub: Sextant Decisions. HRS: Hq ASF Planning Div Program Br file, "Gen, vol. 2, 17 Jul 44." The invasions actually occurred later than planned.

[48] (1) Diary, MOOB SGO, 11-17 Dec 43. HD: 024.7-5, "MOOB Diary." (2) DF WDGDS 9381, ACofS G-4 WDGS to ACofS OPD WDGS and CG ASF, 11 Jan 44, sub: Fixed Bed Hosps, NATO and ETO. HRS: G-4 file, "Hosp and Evac Policy."

[49] Memo, SG for Dir Planning Div ASF, 17 Jan 44, sub: Serv Units for NA Forces. HRS: Hq ASF Planning Div Program Br file, "Hosp and Evac, vol. 3."

[50] Rad CM-OUT-8230 (21 Jan 44), ACofS OPD WDGS to CG NATO, 20 Jan 44. SG: 322.15-1.

[51] DF WDGDS 9381, ACofS G-4 WDGS to ACofS OPD WDGS and CG ASF, 11 Jan 44, sub: Fixed Bed Hosps, NATO and ETO. HRS: G-4 file, "Hosp and Evac Policy."

[52] (1) Memo, SG for CG ASF, 17 Feb 44, sub: Serv Units for NA forces. HRS: Hq ASF Planning Div Program Br file, "Hosp and Evac, vol. 3." (2) T/S, SG to ACofS G-4 WDGS thru CG ASF Planning Div, 9 Feb 44, sub: Fixed Bed Hosps, NATO and ETO. SG: 632.2.

all theaters as well as of the United States for hospitalization and evacuation facilities. Among the general conclusions drawn from this study were the following: under existing plans there would be a shortage of beds in both the European and North African theaters after the mounting of OVERLORD and ANVIL; the number of patients that would be brought back to the United States each month would rise to 40,000, of whom 60 to 70 percent would be in the "helpless" category; there would be a shortage of space on transports and hospital ships for evacuation from the European and North African theaters; using only the evacuation facilities planned, not more than 20 percent of all patients would be returned on hospital ships; and air evacuation offered little promise of supplementing ships in view of past accomplishments.[53] Ultimately action was taken upon each of these problems, but only those pertaining to theater hospitalization will be discussed at this point.

Decisions concerning overseas hospitalization were made at a conference on 28 March 1944. At that time General Somervell directed (1) that the number of beds supplied to Europe and North Africa under existing ratios should be increased, (2) that the General Staff should be requested to raise the authorized ratio for North Africa from 6.6 to 8.5 percent, and (3) that bed requirements for all theaters should be reviewed.[54] Plans to supply additional beds to Europe and North Africa were colored by the shortage of personnel and of trained hospital units in the United States. To furnish the European theater with a total of ninety-one general hospitals by the end of July, some had to be shipped before completion of training.[55] The shortage of fixed beds in North Africa was alleviated, as OPD had suggested earlier, by expanding table-of-organization capacities of existing hospitals with personnel available in the theater. With War Department approval, that theater inactivated six 250-bed station hospitals and with personnel formerly assigned to them expanded twelve 1,000-bed general hospitals to 1,500-bed capacities and five to 2,000-bed capacities. This increased the fixed-bed capacity by 9,500 beds and brought the ratio of available beds to troops up to 6.4 percent.[56]

The question of raising the ratio for North Africa became involved in a general review of bed requirements for all theaters because the General Staff refused to consider the former before completion of the latter.[57] Prepared by the ASF Planning Division and the Strategic Logistics Planning Unit of the Surgeon General's

[53] (1) Hosp and Evac: A Re-estimate of the Pnt Load and Facilities. Feb 44. HD: 705.-1. (2) Memo, SG for CG ASF, 22 Feb 44, sub: Hosp and Evac. HRS: Hq ASF Planning Div Program Br file, "Hosp and Evac, vol. 3."

[54] (1) Memo, CG ASF for Dir Planning Div ASF, 28 Mar 44, sub: Hosp. HRS: Hq ASF Planning Div Program Br file, "Hosp and Evac, vol. 3." (2) Memo, CG ASF for Dir Plans and Oprs ASF, 28 Mar 44, sub: Conf on Hosp and Evac. Same file.

[55] Memo, Chief Program Br Planning Div ASF for Col Bogart, ASF, 4 Apr 44, sub: ETO Hosp. HRS: Hq ASF Planning Div Program Br file, "Hosp and Evac, vol. 3."

[56] (1) Rad CM-IN-16542 (23 Mar 44), CG USAF NATO to WD, 23 Mar 44, sub: Expansion of Hosp. SG: 322.15-1. (2) Rad CM-OUT-20160 (7 Apr 44), War (OPD) to CG USAF NATO, 7 Apr 44. Same file. (3) Memo SPOPI 632, Dir Plans and Oprs ASF for ACofS G-3 WDGS, 29 Mar 44, sub: Expansion of Gen Hosps in NATO. HRS: Hq ASF Planning Div Program Br file, "Hosp and Evac, vol. 3."

[57] (1) Memo, CG ASF for CofSA, 30 Mar 44, sub: Deficiency of Fixed Hosp Units in NATO. HRS: Hq ASF Planning Div Program Br file, "Hosp and Evac, Apr 44." (2) Memo WDGSA/371 NATO (31 Mar 44), CofSA for CG ASF thru ACofS OPD WDGS, 4 Apr 44, sub: Deficiency of Fixed Hosp Units in NATO. HRS: Hq ASF Planning Div Program Br file, "Hosp and Evac, vol. 3."

Office, the general review was presented to the General Staff on 10 April 1944.[58] It was based upon recommendations of theaters, the average occupancy of beds in theaters during the previous six months, and the number of hospital units included in the troop basis. It represented an attempt to balance bed requirements against the number of hospital units already authorized.

Most of its proposals were accepted by G–4: that the bed ratio of the Southwest Pacific should be reduced from 10 to 8 percent, and of the Central Pacific from 7 to 5 percent, and that ratios for the European, Middle East, and American theaters should remain unchanged. G–4 rejected the proposal to raise the North African bed ratio above 6.6 percent, stating that the theater had gotten along satisfactorily on it and that the invasion of Southern France was uncertain. North Africa's later request (in May 1944) to change its evacuation policy from 90 to 120 days indicates that this decision was justified. G–4 also believed that the South Pacific ratio should be reduced from 10 to 6 percent (since the theater itself had recommended only 5 percent) instead of to 7 percent as ASF headquarters and the Surgeon General's Office proposed. While the two latter authorities recommended that the China-Burma-India ratio be reduced from 8 to 7 percent, G–4 thought that beds for the Chinese Army in India should remain at 8 percent and that the ratio for American troops only should be reduced to 7 percent.

The Deputy Chief of Staff approved G–4's findings. This meant that 351,528 of the 370,500 beds in units in the troop basis would be distributed among theaters, but that the remainder (18,972 beds) would be held in the United States as an undeployed reserve to meet unforeseen contingencies.[59]

Movement To Reduce Authorized Bed Ratios

Continuing Difficulty in Providing Authorized Quotas of Beds

Although beds authorized for theaters in the spring of 1944 did not exceed the number in hospital units in the troop basis, personnel shortages made it difficult to supply theaters with authorized quotas. A method formerly used—expansion of the table-of-organization capacities of the hospitals already in theaters—was applied again, particularly in the Southwest Pacific, where the closure of small hospitals released enough officers to expand capacities of larger hospitals by 7,250 beds and to permit the assignment elsewhere of 259 Medical Corps officers.[60] Occasionally, reductions in bed ratios and in troop

[58] (1) Memo, Dep Dir Plans and Oprs ASF for CG ASF, 4 Apr 44, sub: Overseas Hosp. HRS: Hq ASF Planning Div Program Br file, "Hosp and Evac, vol. 3." (2) Memo, Dir Strategic Logistics Planning Unit SGO for Chief Oprs Serv SGO, 6 Jun 44, sub: Rpt of Accomplishments of SGO. HD: 319.1–2 (MOOD Oprs Serv SGO).

[59] (1) Memo, CG ASF for CofSA thru ACofS G–4 WDGS, 10 Apr 44, sub: Overseas Hosp, with Tabs A–F. HRS: Hq ASF Planning Div Program Br file, "Hosp and Evac, Apr 44." (2) Memo WDGS 13077, ACofS G–4 WDGS for CG ASF, 27 Apr 44, sub: Overseas Hosp. HRS: Hq ASF Planning Div Program Br file, "Staybacks, 14 Apr–8 Aug 44." (3) Memo, Dep Dir Plans and Oprs ASF for SG, 29 Apr 44, sub: Overseas Hosp. Same file. (4) Rad CM–OUT–42858 (28 Mar 44), Marshall to CG USAF NATO, 27 May 44. HRS: G–4 file, "Hosp and Evac Policy."

[60] (1) Memo for Record, by Lt Col Lamar C. Bevil, SGO, 4 Jul 44, sub: Conf with Surg SOS SWPA. SG: MOOD "Pacific." (2) Memo, Dep Chief Oprs Serv SGO for SG, 5 Sep 44, sub: Anal of CM–IN–2287 (3 Sep 44) for SWPA. Same file. (3) An Rpt, MOOD SGO, FY 1945. HD.

strengths of one theater released hospital units for transfer elsewhere. In the summer of 1944, for example, units no longer needed in the South Pacific area were transferred to the China-Burma-India, Central Pacific, and Southwest Pacific theaters.[61] Moreover, changes in the zone of interior hospital system were expected not only to use personnel more efficiently at home but also to release some physicians for assignment to units earmarked for theaters. In addition, ratios of doctors, nurses, and enlisted men to beds were decreased in numbered hospital units as well as in zone of interior hospitals.[62] Furthermore, hospitals were "short-shipped" to the European theater—that is, before completion of training and without balanced or full staffs of physicians. In such cases, the theater was expected to complete the training of units and to supply missing specialists and other Medical Corps officers. Such personnel was believed to be available from several sources: from affiliated hospital units overstaffed with specialists and already in the theater, from hospital units in the theater that were being reorganized under revised tables of organization; and from infantry regiments where Medical Administrative Corps officers were replacing Medical Corps officers as battalion surgeons' assistants.[63] Finally, it was recognized that authorized bed quotas of theaters in some instances could not be met even by expedients just discussed, and that a theater would then have "to take care of its own requirements."[64]

Review of Requirements of European Theater

As difficulties were encountered in the summer and early fall of 1944 in meeting authorized fixed-bed quotas, The Surgeon General's Mobilization and Overseas Operations Division began to review the needs of theaters to see if estimates had been too high and if authorized bed ratios might therefore be lowered. As early as July 1944 there were "preliminary indications" that ratios authorized for both the European and the Southwest Pacific theaters could be lowered,[65] but a directive of the Deputy Chief of Staff that requirements of the European theater be reviewed 30 days after the initial landing in France (or the mounting of OVERLORD)

[61] (1) Rad WARX 62981, Marshall to Comdr-in-Chief SWPA; CG USAF CPA; CG USAF SPA; CG USAF CBI, 10 Jul 44, sub: Movement of Ptbl Surg Hosp in Pacific. (2) Rad WARX 72125, Marshall to CG USAF CBI, 26 Jul 44, sub: Departure of 18th and 142d Gen Hosps from SPA. (3) Rad CM-IN-25976, CG USAF SPA to WD and CG USAF CPA, 31 Jul 44. All in SG: 322 "Hosp Misc 1944."

[62] See below, pp. 181–99, 248–50.

[63] (1) Mins, Mtg of Staff Conf ASF, 13 Jul 44, incl 4 to Memo SPOPP 320.2, Act Dir Plans and Oprs ASF for Act CofS ASF, 21 Jul 44, sub: Status of Hosp units. HRS: Hq ASF Planning Div Program Br file, "Hosp and Evac, vol. 3." (2) Rad CM-OUT-34789 (10 May 44), Marshall (OPD) to Eisenhower, 10 May 44. SG: 320.3. (3) Rad CM-IN-11147 (15 May 44), CG USF ETO to WD, 15 May 44. Same file. (4) Memo, Dep SG for CG ASF, 27 Jul 44. HD: MOOD "ETO." (5) Rad CM-OUT-77546 (8 Aug 44), Marshall to Eisenhower, 8 Aug 44. Same file. (6) Rad CM-IN-2778 (30 Aug 44), Eisenhower to WD, 29 Aug 44. Same file. (7) Memo, SG for ACofS OPD WDGS thru CG ASF, 31 Aug 44, sub: Hosp in ETO. Same file. (8) Memo. SG for CG ASF, 5 Oct 44. SG: 322 "Hosp Misc 1944."

[64] (1) Memo with Memo for Record, Dir Plans and Oprs ASF for Joint Logistics Plans Cmtee, 6 May 44, sub: Med Reqmts—Twentieth AF. HRS: Hq ASF Planning Div file, "Hosp and Evac." (2) Memo, Lt Col Lamar C. Bevil for Col Arthur B. Welsh, 18 Aug 44, sub: Est of Med Situation in CBI. HD: MOOD "CBI." (3) Draft rad, ACofS OPD WDGS to CG USAF NATO, 12 Jul 44, with Memo for Record. HRS: OPD, 632 "Security Sec I."

[65] Memo, Act Dir Plans and Oprs ASF for Act CofS ASF, 25 Jul 44, sub: Hosp Reqmts, ETO. HRS: Hq ASF Planning Div Program Br file, "Staybacks, 15 Apr 44–8 Aug 44."

focused attention upon that theater.[66]

During July 1944 the Surgeon General's Office analyzed reports of hospital admissions for the first 32 days of operations in France and computed actual hospital admission rates for that period. This analysis showed that the average battle-casualty rate had been lower than anticipated—51 per 1,000 per month instead of 60—although during one week it had been as high as 89 per 1,000. Other studies showed that the average length of time that patients stayed in hospitals in the North African theater between the fall of 1942 and the middle of 1944 was 23.7 days. This was shorter than the average in Europe during World War I—27.29 days. If admission rates in the future should approximate those of the 32-day period of operations in France and if the average number of days patients stayed in hospitals should be as low as in the North African theater, the European theater would need fewer beds than at first anticipated. The Surgeon General's Office computed the number that would be required under a variety of combinations of admission rates, lengths of stay, and evacuation policies, and then calculated bed ratios that might be required under different sets of circumstances. It appeared that, under a 180-day evacuation policy, the highest ratio that would be needed under the most unfavorable circumstances was 12.05 percent and the lowest, under more favorable circumstances, was 5.46. Under a 120-day policy, the highest would be 8.06 and the lowest, 3.90 percent. It was thought that such ratios would provide sufficient beds not only for all patients hospitalized by the Army, including civilians and prisoners of war, but also for their dispersion in wards. The Surgeon General therefore considered it safe to reduce the bed ratio of the European theater from 8 to 7 percent if at the same time the evacuation policy should be reduced from 180 to 120 days.[67]

ASF headquarters arrived at the same conclusion after taking into consideration certain additional facts. General and convalescent hospitals in the United States had about half of their beds empty during the first half of 1944.[68] At the same time, the European theater was not sending to the United States as many patients as it could on returning troop transports.[69] Presumably a reduction in the evacuation policy would require the theater to return a great number of patients to the zone of interior and would therefore result in fuller use of available evacuation space on transports and of hospital beds in the United States. It would also make possible a reduction in the bed ratio of the European theater and, consequently, in the number of hospital units that would have to be sent there. In view of these considerations, ASF headquarters recommended on 11 August 1944 that the authorized bed ratio for the European theater be reduced from 8 to 7 percent and that its evacuation policy be lowered from 180 to 120 days.[70] The Deputy Chief of Staff ap-

[66] Memo with Memo for Record SPOPP 337, Plans and Oprs ASF for ACofS OPD WDGS, 1 Jul 44, sub: Fixed Hosp Data, with incls. HRS: Hq ASF Planning Div, "Hosp and Evac."

[67] (1) Ltr, SG to CG ASF, 1 Aug 44, sub: Overseas Hosp, with 2 incls. HRS: Hq ASF Planning Div Program Br file, "Hosp and Evac." (2) An Rpt, MOOD SGO, FY 1945. HD.

[68] See above, pp. 202–07.

[69] Memo, SG for ACofS OPD WDGS thru CG ASF, 31 Aug 44, sub: Hosp in ETO. HD: 705 (MRO Fitzpatrick Staybacks, 1 May 44–29 Oct 44).

[70] 3d ind SPOPP 370.05 (8 Aug 44), Plans and Oprs ASF to ACofS G–4 WDGS, 11 Aug 44, with Memo for Record, on Ltr, SG to CG ASF, 1 Aug 44, sub: Overseas Hosp. HRS: Hq ASF Planning Div, "Hosp and Evac."

proved this recommendation and the War Department informed the theater of the changes on 5 October 1944.[71]

Shift of Attention to the Pacific

The review of fixed-bed requirements of the European theater had hardly been completed when the Chief of Staff of the Army Service Forces, returning from a visit to the Pacific, turned attention in that direction.[72] He reported that increased operations against islands nearer the Japanese homeland and the necessity of caring for civilians on such islands might require more hospitals than those already planned for the Pacific. ASF headquarters then directed The Surgeon General on 8 September 1944 to re-examine plans for hospitalization and evacuation in that area.[73]

In complying with this directive The Surgeon General's Mobilization and Overseas Operations Division computed bed ratios by a different method from that used for the European theater. From statistical reports it determined the actual ratio of occupied beds to troop strength during 1943 and 1944 and to this ratio it added estimated ratios of beds to troop strength to provide for casualties from increased combat operations, for dispersion within hospitals, for dispersion of hospitals within theaters (that is, to permit some beds to be vacant or unused either because hospitals were situated in places with little or no combat or because they were being moved from one place to another), for soldiers of Allied armies, for prisoners of war, and for patients evacuated from mobile hospitals to permit such units to move. For example, in the Southwest Pacific area the ratio of occupied beds had been 3.75 percent; to this ratio were added the following: 1.00 percent for increased operational requirements, .90 percent for hospital dispersion, .45 percent for theater dispersion, .45 percent for Allied soldiers and prisoners of war, and .45 percent for patients from mobile hospitals.[74] The sum of these ratios was 7.00 percent and was considered the ratio of fixed beds to troop strength that would be required for the Southwest Pacific area. Ratios for other areas of the Pacific were also computed according to this method and on 14 September 1944 The Surgeon General recommended a reduction in the ratio for the Southwest Pacific from 8 to 7 percent and an increase in that for the Pacific Ocean areas (a theater formed in August 1944 by the combination of the Central and South Pacific areas) from 6 percent in the South Pacific and 5 percent in the Central Pacific to 7 percent for the entire area. At the same time he recommended that the 120-day evacuation policy should remain in effect and that the Army Medical Department should continue free of responsibility for the care of civilians in occupied islands.[75]

---

[71] Memo AG 704 (30 Sep 44) OB–S–SPOPP, TAG for CG ETO, 5 Oct 44, sub: Hosp and Evac Policy for the ETO. HD: MOOD "ETO."

[72] Memo, CofS ASF for SG, 27 Aug 44. HRS: Hq ASF Planning Div, "Hosp and Evac."

[73] Memo SPOPP 632.2, CG ASF for SG, 8 Sep 44, sub: Hosp and Evac, POA and SWPA. HRS: Hq ASF Planning Div, "Hosp and Evac."

[74] The reason for adding in the ratio of beds to troop strength to provide beds for patients evacuated from mobile hospital units to permit them to move is not clear. Actually, one of the chief functions of fixed hospitals was to receive patients evacuated from mobile hospitals to insure mobility. This had been pointed out by the Surgeon General's Office in August 1943, and as a result the General Staff had agreed that fixed- and mobile-bed requirements would be computed separately.

[75] 1st ind, SG to Dir Plans and Oprs ASF, 14 Sep 44, on Memo SPOPP 632.2, Dir Plans and Oprs ASF for SG, 8 Sep 44, sub: Hosp and Evac, POA and SWPA. HRS: Hq ASF Planning Div, "Hosp and Evac."

ASF headquarters approved these recommendations, with minor modifications, but the General Staff took no final action upon them because a new study of hospital bed requirements for all theaters soon superseded the study of requirements for the Pacific.[76]

The Manpower Board Estimates Requirements

The drive of the War Department Manpower Board to save personnel by reducing the number of hospitals in the Army—a drive which threatened the closure of some hospitals in the United States in the fall of 1944—extended to overseas areas also.[77] The method which the Board used to compute theater bed requirements differed from The Surgeon General's. The Board proposed that the average noneffective rate (that is, the number of persons per 1,000 per day unfit for duty because of sickness or other disability) be converted into a ratio for authorizing fixed beds. Thus the number of authorized fixed beds would equal but not exceed the number of noneffectives. The Board contended that this method would provide sufficient hospitalization for all theaters, since beds were not actually needed for all noneffectives (some being treated in quarters) and since all hospitals could expand authorized capacities by 50 percent. If any theater should by chance accumulate more patients than beds, the Board stated, it could transfer greater numbers of patients to the United States, because in the Board's opinion evacuation facilities and zone of interior hospital capacities already exceeded requirements. Arriving on the basis of statistics published by the Surgeon General's Office at an average noneffective rate of 50, the Board concluded that not more than 250,000 beds were needed for the 5,000,000 troops in all theaters of operations. It therefore advocated deleting from the troop basis fixed hospital units containing 120,000 beds in excess of this number.[78]

On the basis of this study, G–3 recommended on 29 September 1944 that all inactive general, station, and field hospital units (having authorized capacities totaling 44,000 beds) should be deleted from the troop basis; that no further fixed hospital units be sent to theaters of operations; that the active units in training in the United States, with a total authorized capacity of 20,000 beds, be kept in this country in the strategic reserve; and that the bed requirements of all theaters be restudied by 1 November 1944.[79]

Although OPD believed that these recommendations were "premature,"[80] G–4 directed ASF headquarters on 11 October 1944 to make an immediate review of fixed-bed requirements of all theaters on the basis of "the latest and most complete current experience data available to The Surgeon General" and warned that it was "particularly desired that no attempt be made in this study to arbitrarily justify

[76] (1) Memo with Memo for Record SPOPP 370.05, CG ASF for ACofS OPD WDGS, 16 Sep 44, sub: Hosp and Evac, POA and SWPA. HRS: Hq ASF Planning Div, "Hosp and Evac." (2) Memo WDGDS 3710, ACofS G–4 WDGS for DepCofSA, 5 Oct 44, sub: Hosps for SWPA and POA. HRS: OPD, 632 "Security Sec I."

[77] See above, pp. 203–05.

[78] Memo WDSMB 323.3 (Hosp) (25 Sep 44), WDMB for ACofS G–3 WDGS, 25 Sep 44, sub: Fixed Hosp Reqmts for Overseas Theaters. HRS: G–4 file, "Hosp and Evac Policy."

[79] Memo WDGCT 705.1 (29 Sep 44), ACofS G–3 WDGS for CofSA, 29 Sep 44, sub: Fixed Bed Reqmts. HRS; G–4 file, "Hosp and Evac Policy."

[80] DF, Act ACofS OPD WDGS to ACofS G–4 WDGS, 7 Oct 44, sub: Fixed Bed Reqmts, with Memo for Record. HRS: OPD, 632 "Security Sec I."

present figures on fixed bed hospitalization for theaters."[81]

General Review of Bed Requirements

The study which the Surgeon General's Office prepared in compliance with the G–4 directive was impressive. It included estimates of requirements of all theaters arrived at by two methods—the "admission rate" method used earlier for the European theater and the "beds occupied" method used earlier for the Pacific. Each was supposed to serve as a check on the other. All estimates were based upon certain principles or assumptions which the Mobilization and Overseas Operations Division considered important. First, hospitals could operate with 50 percent more patients than authorized beds for only short emergency periods and hence expansion capacities could not be considered available for normal needs. Second, beds for dispersion would be needed within hospitals and within theaters. Vacant beds in contagious wards could not be used for surgical patients, for example, and some hospitals would always be only partially filled because the shifting fortunes of war temporarily left them on quiet fronts. Finally, though evacuation policies might be changed in emergencies to permit theaters to transfer larger proportions of patients to the United States, the maintenance of policies already established was desirable.

As much as possible this study was based upon World War II statistics, but in some instances rates and ratios still had to be estimated without the benefit of such data. For estimates by the "admission rate" method the Mobilization and Overseas Operations Division used actual admission rates for disease and nonbattle-injury patients for the period from July 1943 to June 1944 for most theaters. In some instances, these rates had to be adjusted. For example, the daily admission rate (the number of patients admitted to hospitals per 1,000 men per day) for disease and nonbattle injuries for the Pacific Ocean area had been 1.7, but in anticipation of higher disease incidence in future operations nearer Japan an admission rate of 2 was used. While the length of stay in hospitals—also used in this method—differed from one theater and from one time to another, ranging from 18 to 21 days, the actual average length of stay in hospitals in all theaters during World War II was used. In estimates of requirements by the "beds occupied" method the ratio of occupied beds to theater troop strength during 1943 and 1944 was considered as a base to which were added ratios of beds for patients resulting from increased operations; those needed for transient, Navy, Allied, and prisoner-of-war patients; and those required for dispersion. The ratio of occupied beds was actual, based on statistical reports, but the other ratios were estimated.

Different ratios of beds for the same theater resulted from the use of the two methods of estimating requirements. For the European theater under a 120-day evacuation policy, for example, a ratio of 7.73 percent was needed according to estimates made by the "admission rate" method and of 7 percent according to the "beds occupied" method. Lower ratios of beds would be needed with 90-, 60-, or 30-day evacuation policies. Because zone of interior hospitalization and evacuation

[81] DF WDGDS 3918, ACofS G–4 WDGS to CG ASF, 11 Oct 44, sub: Fixed Bed Reqmts for Overseas Theaters, with 1 incl. HRS: Hq ASF Planning Div, "Hosp and Evac." Also, SG: 632.2 "Bed Reqmts."

facilities had been planned on the basis of a 120-day evacuation policy and because such a policy seemed more economical of personnel and shipping than lower ones, The Surgeon General recommended that the 120-day policy be continued and that estimated ratios of beds required under it be approved. Those ratios were the same as the ones already authorized for all theaters except the American, China-Burma-India, Southwest Pacific, and Central Pacific. For the first three of these, The Surgeon General proposed reductions in ratios from 4, 7, and 8 percent to 3, 6, and 7 percent respectively. For the last, he proposed an increase from 5 to 6 percent. In addition, he recommended that beds be provided in hospital units in the strategic reserve for 4 percent of the troops in that reserve. He proposed further that theaters be asked what evacuation policies and bed ratios they wanted and that, until their answers were received, no reduction should be made in the number of units in the troop basis, no personnel should be diverted from training for those units, and hospital units should continue to be shipped overseas as planned. ASF headquarters approved this study and its recommendations.[82]

Faced with varying estimates of bed requirements made by the War Department Manpower Board and G–3 on the one hand and by the Surgeon General's Office and ASF headquarters on the other, G–4 had the problem of considering both and of arriving at recommendations that could be presented to the Deputy Chief of Staff for approval. As a result of conferences with representatives of The Surgeon General and G–3,[83] and of analyses of the different studies, G–4 arrived at a compromise which favored The Surgeon General and on 2 November 1944 sent the following recommendations to the Deputy Chief of Staff: (1) that the bed ratios recommended by The Surgeon General be approved, with minor exceptions; (2) that the evacuation policies already authorized remain in effect; (3) that the shipment of hospital units to the European theater be slowed down in order to permit them to be better staffed and trained and to see if they were actually needed; and (4) that the four general hospital units and the four field hospital units that were in the troop basis but were not scheduled by OPD for shipment to any theater be deleted. On 22 November 1944, the Deputy Chief of Staff approved G–4's recommendations. The bed ratios thus authorized were as follows: for the European and Southwest Pacific theaters, 7 percent; for the Mediterranean theater (formerly North African), 6.6 percent; for the Pacific Ocean areas (formerly the Central and South Pacific), 6 percent; for the Middle Eastern theater, 6 percent; for the China and India-Burma theaters, 6 percent for all American troops and for 102,000 Chinese troops in India; and for the American theater, 3 percent.[84]

---

[82] (1) 1st ind, SG to CG ASF, 18 Oct 44, with Tabs A through D, on Memo SPOPP 370.05, CG ASF for SG, 13 Oct 44, sub: Fixed Bed Reqmts for Overseas Theaters, with 1 incl. (2) 1st ind SPOPP 705, CG ASF to ACofS G–4 WDGS, 24 Oct 44, with Memo for Record, on DF WDGDS 3918, ACofS G–4 WDGS to CG ASF, 11 Oct 44, sub: Fixed Bed Reqmts for Overseas Theaters. Both in HRS: Hq ASF Planning div file, "Hosp and Evac."

[83] DF WDGDS 4602, Act ACofS G–4 WDGS to ACofS G–3 WDGS, 1 Nov 44, sub: Fixed Bed Reqmts, with Memo for Record. HRS: G–4 file, "Hosp and Evac Policy."

[84] (1) Memo WDGDS 4434, Act ACofS G–4 WDGS for DepCofSA, 2 Nov 44, sub: Fixed Hosp Bed Allowances for Overseas Theaters, with Tab A. HRS: Hq ASF Planning Div, "Hosp and Evac." (2) Memo WDGDS 4477, ACofS G–4 WDGS for CG ASF, 22 Nov 44, sub as above. Same file.

This re-examination of the needs of theaters for fixed beds achieved in part the desired end—saving of personnel through a reduction in the number of hospital units the Army would have. While it was being made, the General Staff deleted six general hospital units from the troop basis. Afterward it deleted four more general and four field hospitals.[85] These were units which OPD had not scheduled for shipment but which the Surgeon General's Office wished to hold in the United States as an undeployed reserve. The shipment of hospital units to the European theater was also slowed down. With the concurrence of that theater, the General Staff planned to send 11 general hospital units to Europe during the last two months of 1944, instead of 30 that were scheduled, and to send the remaining 19 early in 1945.[86] Although these actions may have helped the Medical Department, they did not solve all problems caused by personnel shortages and it was still necessary to ship hospital units with less than full complements of personnel. For example, eleven of the general hospitals sent to Europe during the winter of 1944–45 had no nurses assigned to them upon departure from the United States.[87]

Experiences of theaters in hospitalization from November 1944 to May 1945 showed that enough fixed beds were supplied to meet actual requirements. During this period only two theaters, the Southwest Pacific and the Asiatic, failed to receive enough beds to fill authorized quotas. The others had numbers that either exceeded quotas consistently or reached them and then wavered slightly above or below. Even during periods when theaters had fewer beds than authorized, they also had fewer patients than the number of fixed beds present, with one exception—the European theater. *(See Chart 11.)* In the winter of 1944–45, its patient load increased rapidly and by January and February 1945 the number of patients occupying fixed beds was greater than the number of normal beds present in the theater.[88] For a short time, then, attention was centered upon this problem. *(Table 14.)*

The Problem of the European Theater in the Winter of 1944–45

The situation in which there were more patients than normal fixed beds in the European theater arose from a variety of causes. During November and December 1944 hospital admissions increased rapidly. In addition, stoppage by the War Department in the fall of 1944 of the transfer (with few exceptions) of prisoner-of-war patients to the United States resulted in the accumulation of 14,000 German patients in theater hospitals by the end of December. Furthermore, failure of the European theater to follow evacuation policies set by the War Department (because of a shortage of hospital ships and the chief surgeon's opposition to the use of transports for evacuation) created a backlog of Army patients awaiting

[85] (1) Memo SPMDA 322.05, SG for SecWar, 10 Jan 45, sub: Med Mission Reappraised. HRS: G-4 file, "Hosp, vol. II." (2) Memo for Record on Memo, CG ASF (SG) for CofSA, 17 Dec 44, sub: Adequacy of Hosp and Evac, ETO. HRS: Hq ASF Planning Div file, "Hosp and Evac."

[86] (1) Memo WDGDS 4434, Act ACofS G-4 WDGS for DepCofSA, 2 Nov 44, sub: Fixed Hosp Bed Allowances for Overseas Theaters. HRS: Hq ASF Planning Div file, "Hosp and Evac." (2) MRS, Col Durward G. Hall (SGO) to Gen [George F.] Lull then Col A[rthur] B. Welsh then Col Carl [C.] Sox, 14 Nov (1944?). SG: 322 "Hosp Misc."

[87] Memo, Chief Atlantic Sec Theater Br MOOD SGO for Record, 8 Mar 45, sub: Substitution of Enlisted Technicians for Nurses in ETO Hosps. HD: MOOD "ETO."

[88] An Rpt, SG, FY 1945, pp. 53–54. HD.

TABLE 14—EVACUATION POLICIES AND AUTHORIZED BED RATIOS, MAJOR THEATERS OF OPERATIONS

Year and Month	Europe			North Africa (Mediterranean)			Pacific							Asiatic			
							South Pacific			Central Pacific		Southwest Pacific		China-Burma-India			
	Evacuation Policy		Fixed-Bed Ratio	Evacuation Policy		Fixed-Bed Ratio	Evacuation Policy		Fixed-Bed Ratio	Evacuation Policy	Fixed-Bed Ratio	Evacuation Policy	Fixed-Bed Ratio	Evacuation Policy		Fixed-Bed Ratio	
1943	*Official*	*De Facto*[a]		*Official*	*De Facto*[a]		*Official*	*De Facto*[a]									
August	180	180+	8%	120	90	6.6%	120	60	10%	120	7%	120	10%	180		8% US Army	
September																	
October																	
November																	
December																	
1944																	
January																	
February								90								8% US Army & 8% CAI[b]	
March																	
April									6%		5%		8%			7% US Army & 8% CAI[b]	
May																	
June					120												
July							Pacific Ocean Area							China		India-Burma	
August							Evacuation Policy		Fixed-Bed Ratio					Evacuation Policy	Fixed-Bed Ratio	Evacuation Policy	Fixed-Bed Ratio
September																	
October	120	180	7%														
November							120		6%			120	7%	180	6%	180	6% US Army & 6% CAI[b]
December																	
1945																	
January		120															
February		90															
March		60															
April	60		7%	60	60	6.6%	AFPAC										
May							Evacuation Policy			Fixed-Bed Ratio							
June																	
July																	
August	120	90	4%	120	90	4%	60			6%				Evacuate all Patients by 1 March 1946 Regardless of Evacuation Policy			
September		120			120												
October																	
November																	
December							120			4%				↓	4%	↓	4%

[a] Dates of change are approximate.
[b] Chinese Army in India.

Source: Documents cited in footnotes to relevant portions of Chapters XII and XVIII

transfer to the zone of interior. Meanwhile, the theater actually had fewer fixed beds than it was credited with, because many of its field hospitals (normally counted as fixed hospitals) were being used as forward-area surgical hospitals and evacuation holding units.[89] Informed of this situation early in December 1944,[90] the General Staff, ASF headquarters, and the Surgeon General's Office turned their attention to a solution of some of the theater's problems.

Difficulties of the War Department in meeting authorized quotas of fixed beds for all theaters precluded shipment to Europe of more hospitals than already scheduled. Therefore, G–4 decided that the European theater would have to care for prisoner-of-war patients in hospitals that were manned primarily by captured German medical personnel. On 28 December 1944 the War Department informed the theater of this decision,[91] and by February 1945 it had in operation or in the process of organization prisoner-of-war hospitals containing 13,000 beds.[92]

Failure of the theater to use vacant evacuation space on troop transports threatened not only to continue to contribute to a shortage of beds in Europe and insufficient use of those in the United States but also to create a serious evacuation problem. If patients were not evacuated as they accumulated it would be difficult to get them out of the theater after the defeat of Germany, because transports would then be diverted to the Pacific and hospital ships would be unable to move the patient load as rapidly as desirable. On 3 December 1944, therefore, the Chief of Staff of the Army ordered the commanding general of the European theater to use all evacuation space on transports, even if it required the theater to lower its evacuation policy to 90 days or less.[93] As a result, the theater evacuated patients under a 120-day policy in January, a 90-day policy in February, and a 60-day policy in March and April.[94] By thus transferring a larger proportion of its patient load to the zone of interior, the European theater reduced its requirements for additional beds and contributed at the same time to the more effective use of beds in general hospitals in the United States.

To enable the theater to establish as many fixed beds as it was credited with having, The Surgeon General proposed that it be authorized additional fixed beds to replace those in field hospitals being used as mobile units.[95] The General Staff approved this proposal, and on 25 December 1944 the War Department authorized both the European and Mediterranean theaters to subtract from fixed-bed totals the beds in field hospitals being used as mobile units and to replace them by expanding table-of-organization capacities of station and general hospitals already present.[96] Later, ASF headquarters pro-

[89] (1) An Rpt, MOOD SGO, FY 1945. HD. (2) Interv MD Historian with [Maj] Gen [Paul R.] Hawley, 18 Apr 50. HD: 000.71.

[90] Ltr SHAEF 704–3 Med, SHAEF to CofSA thru ACofS G–4 WDGS, 4 Dec 44. SG: 632.2.

[91] Rad, ACofS OPD WDGS to CG ComZ ETO and CG USAF MTO, 28 Dec 44. HRS: Hq ASF Planning Div, "Hosp and Evac."

[92] An Rpt, MOOD SGO, FY 1945. HD.

[93] (1) Memo, Col William B. Higgins (G–4) for ACofS G–4 WDGS, 4 Dec 44, sub: Evac from ETO. HRS: G–4 file, "Hosp and Evac Policy." (2) Rad CM–OUT–72113 (3 Dec 44), CofSA to CG ComZ ETO and CG UK Base Sec, 3 Dec 44. SG: 560.2.

[94] Administrative and Logistical History of the Medical Service, Communication Zone-ETO, Ch 13, "Evacuation," pp. 32–34. HD.

[95] Memo, SG for CG ASF, 13 Dec 44. HRS: Hq ASF Somervell file, "SG 1944."

[96] Rad OPD 632 (26 Dec 44), ACofS OPD WDGS to CG ComZ ETO and CG USAF MTO, 26 Dec 44, sub: Hosp. HRS: Hq ASF Planning Div, "Hosp and Evac."

posed that other theaters be given similar authority.[97]

In addition to the measures just discussed, at the suggestion of the Chief of Staff G–4 sent to Europe one of its representatives, Col. (later Brig. Gen.) Crawford F. Sams, a Medical Corps officer, to discuss with the chief surgeon of the theater and the chief medical officer of SHAEF the most effective use of the beds present.[98] The situation in Europe was thereby so alleviated that by March it was possible to divert to the Pacific six of the general hospitals scheduled earlier for shipment to Europe.[99]

Meeting the needs of theaters for hospitalization in the latter part of the war was characterized by efforts to estimate requirements as realistically as possible and by the necessity of using a variety of expedients to provide quotas of beds actually authorized. Establishment in the second half of 1943 of official evacuation policies and bed ratios for various theaters placed planning on a sounder basis than formerly. The first ratios established were based only partially upon World War II experience; but as statistics of casualty and disease incidence accumulated they were studied repeatedly to determine whether or not ratios could be lowered. Though a reduction was at times possible, shortages of personnel continued to require some theaters to meet their quotas partially by expanding the table-of-organization capacities of some units, using the emergency expansion of others, and employing units shipped from the zone of interior incompletely trained and staffed. Toward the end of 1944 it was necessary to force the European theater to observe War Department policies on evacuation in order to relieve the load on theater hospitals by transferring part of it to the United States. That theater also had to use other expedients, such as the employment of captured enemy personnel in the the treatment of prisoners of war, in order to have sufficient fixed beds for American Army patients.

[97] Memo SPOPP 705, Act Dir Plans and Oprs ASF for ACofS OPD WDGS, 5 Jan 43, sub: Adequacy of Hosp in TofOpns—Deletion of Fld Hosps from Auth Fixed Beds, with Memo for Record. HRS: Hq ASF Planning Div, "Hosp and Evac."

[98] (1) Memo, G. C. M[arshall] (CofSA) for [Lt] Gen [Thomas T.] Handy, 26 Dec 44. WDCSA: 632 A 414. (2) Interv, MD Historian with Brig Gen Crawford F. Sams, 18 Jan 50. HD: 000.71.

[99] (1) Memo, Act CofS ASF for Dir Plans and Oprs ASF, 24 Mar 45, sub: Hosps in ETO. HRS: Hq ASF Control Div files, 323.3 "Hosps." (2) An Rpt, MOOD SGO, FY 1945. (3) Memo, Chief Planning Br G–4 WDGS for ACofS G–4 WDGS, 3 Apr 45, sub: Diversion of Hosps. HRS: G–4 files, "Hosp, vol. III."

CHAPTER XIII

Changes in Policies and Procedures Affecting the Occupancy of Hospital Beds in the Zone of Interior

An important feature of attempts to meet hospital requirements with limited resources was an extension of the practice begun on a small scale during the early war years of keeping patients who did not actually need hospital care from occupying beds. This could be done by limiting admissions and shortening length of stay.

Problem of Limiting Hospital Admissions

More was done to shorten periods of patient-stay than to limit admissions. Two factors worked against the latter: (1) the Medical Department's practice of admitting patients to hospitals before performing complete diagnostic procedures and (2) policies of the General Staff governing discharges from the Army. Normally, zone of interior patients were sent to hospitals after only preliminary examinations by dispensary physicians and were then given more thorough examinations by hospital staffs. Early in the war, it will be recalled, some hospitals had established diagnostic clinics for the examination of patients before their admission to wards. This practice did not become general, and hospitals continued to admit patients first and to perform diagnostic procedures afterward.[1] Some policies of the General Staff tended to increase rather than to limit hospital admissions. In July 1943, for example, the Staff issued a directive, against The Surgeon General's advice, to discharge from the Army men who did not meet minimum physical standards. This flooded hospitals with patients whose disabilities had to be observed and evaluated before they could be given disability discharges.[2] Toward the end of 1943, when a manpower short-

[1] See above, p. 121. Annual reports of hospitals are silent, with few exceptions, on the establishment of diagnostic clinics. See also *Federal Medical Services—A Report with Recommendations,* prepared for the Commission on Organization of the Executive Branch of the Government [Hoover Commission] by the Committee on Federal Medical Services (Washington, 1949), pp. 20–21.

[2] (1) WD Cir 161, 14 Jul 43. (2) An Rpt, 1943, Ft Bragg Sta Hosp. HD. (3) William C. Menninger, *Psychiatry in a Troubled World* (New York, 1948), pp. 551–52.

age developed, the Staff directed that men who could serve usefully in military assignments, despite minor ailments, should be kept in the Army.[3] While this reduced the disability-discharge load, it increased the number of men who returned to hospitals repeatedly with the same complaints and led to a tug of war between line officers and the Medical Department over whether those who were not physically disabled but were noneffective should be given medical or administrative discharges.[4] The Staff finally attempted to solve this problem by making it easier in the latter half of 1944 for line officers to grant administrative discharges and by authorizing in the spring of 1945 the discharge at separation centers of all combat-wounded enlisted men in the limited service category.[5] To some extent these actions relieved hospitals of the care of men who did not need actual treatment at a time when these installations were reaching their peak load.[6]

Measures to Shorten the Length of Patient-Stay

Shortening the time spent by patients in hospitals was another way of limiting occupancy of beds to patients actually needing hospital care. Controlling the length of stay in an effort to limit the occupancy of beds to patients actually needing hospital care was a complicated and difficult process, for many factors affected it, some tending to increase and others to shorten it. Among them—aside from the seriousness of patients' wounds, injuries, and illnesses—were the speed with which patients were transferred to proper types of medical installations, the degree of recovery they were expected to achieve while in Army hospitals, the efficiency with which hospitals completed diagnoses and treatments, and the administrative problems that were encountered in disposing of patients after completion of treatment. Beginning in the fall of 1943 the Surgeon General's Office devoted more attention than formerly to these factors in particular and to the length of stay in general.

The attention given to the general problem is illustrated by studies made in the Surgeon General's Office and letters sent to service commands. During 1944 and 1945 the Facilities Utilization Branch and its successor, the Resources Analysis Division, made monthly studies of the length of time different hospitals kept patients before disposing of them. In the absence of more reliable data, the Branch measured the average duration of patient-stay by means of an "activity index." This index was the ratio of total patient days to the sum of hospital admissions and dispositions. Over a long period of time a number twice the size of the activity index was considered a close approximation of the number of days that the average patient spent in a given hospital.[7] A low activity

[3] WD Cir 293, 11 Nov 43.

[4] (1) An Rpt, 1943 and 44, Ft Bragg Sta Hosp. HD. (2) An Rpt, 1944, Surg 7th SvC. HD. (3) Memo, SG for CG ASF, 1 Sep 44, sub: Disposition of Inapt and Inadaptable. SG: 300.3. (4) Memo, Dep SG for ACofS G-1 WDGS, 26 Sep 44, sub: WD Cir 370 (1944) II-EM. SG: 300.-5. (5) Memo, SG for CG ASF, 23 Mar 45, sub: Gen Hosp Program, ZI. SG: 322 "Hosp."

[5] (1) WD Cir 370, 12 Sep 44. (2) AR 615-368 and AR 615-369, 20 Jul 44. (3) WD Cir 71, 6 Mar 45.

[6] (1) Memo, Dir NP Consultants Div SGO for Dir Resources Anal Div SGO, 27 Nov 44, sub: Discharge of EM. SG: 220.811-1. (2) An Rpt, 1944, Surg 7th SvC. HD. (3) An Rpts, 1945, Baxter Gen Hosp and Ft Bragg Sta Hosp. HD.

[7] Draft article for ASF Monthly Progress Rpt, Sec 7, *Health*, entitled "The Disposition of Patients in Hospitals of Selected Size Groups [31 May 44]." HD: Resources Anal Div file, "Hosp."

index was therefore an indication that a hospital was treating and disposing of patients promptly. Monthly announcements of hospitals' activity indices kept before service command surgeons the importance of avoiding unnecessarily long patient-stays.[8] This indirect pressure upon hospitals seemed insufficient after the patient load began to increase rapidly in the spring of 1945. In March, therefore, The Surgeon General urged general and convalescent hospital commanders, as well as service command surgeons, to accelerate dispositions.[9] The following month he established tentative monthly quotas for the disposition of patients from convalescent hospitals.[10] Meanwhile, during the preceding year and a half, attention had been given to various individual factors which influenced the length of patient-stay.

One of these was the transfer of patients between hospitals. Failure to transfer patients promptly from station hospitals to better staffed and better equipped hospitals, after it had been determined that they needed a higher type of care than that afforded in station hospitals, retarded their recovery. On the other hand, unnecessary transfers of patients between hospitals of different types consumed the time of hospitals involved, put an extra load on overburdened transportation facilities, and increased the time patients stayed on hospital rolls by causing repetitive physical examinations and more administrative paper work. Several steps were therefore taken to regulate the transfer of patients. In the fall of 1943 the Deputy Chief of Staff ruled that zone of interior patients need not be transferred from station to general hospitals merely because their injuries or illnesses were of particular types, provided station hospitals were equipped and staffed to give them the care and treatment they needed.[11] In the spring of 1944, when regional hospitals were authorized, a policy was established under which patients were to be transferred "without any more delay than is compatible with sound professional judgment" to the "nearest adequate medical installations," regardless of their type—whether regional, convalescent, or general hospitals—and regardless of the command under which they operated.[12] To implement this policy, both the Air Surgeon and The Surgeon General applied to regional hospitals the bed credit system which had been developed earlier to facilitate the transfer of patients from station to general hospitals.[13] Soon afterward The Surgeon General established the Medical Regulating Unit (mentioned elsewhere) to control the transfer to general hospitals of patients debarked at ports in the United States. This office, in turn, devised an elaborate system by which general and convalescent hospitals reported vacant beds and debarkation hospitals reported patients received, indicating by code their sex, rank, home address, and disability.[14] Theoretically this system assured the transfer of patients directly to hospitals staffed

[8] These letters are found in SG: 323.7-5 (each service command).

[9] Ltr, CG ASF (SG) to CGs all SvCs attn SvC Surg, and to COs all Gen and Conv Hosps, 24 Mar 45, sub: Furlough and Disposition Policy. Off file, Gen Bliss' Off SGO, "Med Clarification of Disposition Policy."

[10] Ltr, SG to CO Ft Story Conv Hosp, 12 Apr 45. Off file, Gen Bliss' Off SGO, "Med Clarification of Disposition Policy."

[11] See above, p. 183.

[12] WD Cir 140, 11 Apr 44.

[13] (1) See above, pp. 35, 184–85. (2) The Planning and Oprs of ZI Hosps, Tab B to Memo, Dir Hosp Div and Dir Resources Anal Div SGO thru Chief of Oprs Serv SGO for Dir HD SGO, 18 Jun 45, sub: Add Mat for An Rpt for FY 1945. HD: 319.1-2.

[14] See below, pp. 346–49.

and equipped to care for their particular ills and injuries but it was not completely successful.

A study by the Resources Analysis Division early in 1945 showed that forty-five out of fifty-nine general hospitals were receiving patients who should have been sent to other medical installations. "Beyond a doubt," a report on the study continued, "there are a large number of overseas patients being transferred from the debarkation hospitals to the general hospitals who need little or no further surgical or medical treatment and could equally as well be cared for in convalescent hospitals. These cases consume a large amount of time in the general hospitals in examination and working up plus all the administration detail and the time involved in disposition." [15]

Another factor which affected the length of stay in Army hospitals was the degree of recovery which patients were expected to attain before being discharged. Those returned to duty were expected to be able to do an effective day's work as soon as they rejoined their outfits. To shorten the convalescent phase of hospitalization, The Surgeon General emphasized during 1944 the reconditioning program initiated the year before. Although no statistical studies were made of the effect of this program on the average period of hospitalization, many hospital commanders believed that it was shortened.[16] Patients who could not be reclaimed for military service could be transferred to Veterans Administration hospitals if they needed further care. In the early part of the war, it had been Surgeon General Magee's policy to transfer such patients as soon as the Medical Department determined that they could not be restored to duty, thus shortening the time they stayed in Army hospitals.[17] During 1943 public pressure upon the Army to keep patients for final treatment, along with the inability of Veterans Administration hospitals to accommodate large numbers of them [18] caused a change in policy that tended to lengthen the period of patient-stay. In December 1943 Army hospitals began to keep all patients whose disabilities were incurred in line of duty, except those who were tuberculous or psychotic, until their definitive treatment had been completed.[19] As seriously wounded casualties began to fill hospital beds during 1944, this policy had to be clarified for it was difficult to know when the definitive treatment of those with chronic disabilities was completed. In the fall of that year it was announced that such patients would be kept in Army hospitals until they had reached the "maximum degree of recovery." [20] In the following December, the President confirmed this policy and broadened its application to include patients whose disabilities had not been incurred in line of duty.[21] Hospital commanders interpreted this directive "very broadly," and by March 1945, as

[15] Memo, J. S. Murtaugh [Resources Anal Div, SGO] for Dr [Eli] Ginzberg, 16 Mar 45, sub: Summary of Replies to the Furlough and Disposition Study. Off file, Resources Anal Div, SGO.

[16] Richard L. Loughlin, [History of] Reconditioning [in the U.S. Army in World War II], (1946), pp. 198–208. HD.

[17] (1) See above, pp. 129–30. (2) AR 615–360, C4, 16 Apr 43.

[18] Ltr, Dep SG to Mr Donald C. Urquhart, Veterans of Foreign Wars of US, 24 Mar 44. SG: 220.-811-1.

[19] (1) WD AGO Form 026, prepared by Col William B. Foster, MC, SGO, 15 Nov 43, sub: Request and Justification for Publication. AG: 220.8 (2 Jun 42) (2) Sec 2. (2) AR 615–360, C 16, 15 Dec 43.

[20] (1) WD Cir 423, 27 Oct 44. (2) ASF Cir 374, 13 Nov 44.

[21] Ltr, Franklin D. Roosevelt to SecWar, 4 Dec 44. HRS: Hq ASF Control Div, 705 "Cutback in Gen and Conv Fac."

the patient-load neared its peak, The Surgeon General concluded that they were holding patients longer than necessary.[22] Two months later his Office attempted to define more precisely the term "maximum degree of recovery." This term, it was explained, referred to the point in a patient's treatment when progress appeared to have leveled off and no further substantial improvement could be anticipated. Patients reaching that point, even though they had not made full compensatory adjustment to disabilities, were not to be kept longer in Army hospitals.[23]

A third factor affecting the length of time patients stayed in hospitals was the efficiency with which hospital staffs made diagnoses and initiated treatment. In the fall of 1943 representatives of the Surgeon General's Office and the ASF Control Division complained that hospitals were delaying diagnoses and treatment by having unnecessary laboratory work performed for each patient.[24] At that time The Surgeon General urged hospitals to insist upon its elimination. A few months later he suggested that service command surgeons require hospitals to keep ward charts showing the duration of patient-stay, as a reminder that unnecessary procedures should be avoided and requisite medical treatment given promptly. Some, and perhaps all, service commands accepted this suggestion.[25]

A fourth factor affecting length of stay was the administrative work involved in disposition of patients, either by return to duty or by separation from the service. Their return to units or organizations from which they entered hospitals created no problem, but the reassignment of others who were physically unqualified for duty with their former units or whose units had gone overseas was fraught with delays. Reassignment was primarily an Army personnel procedure over which the Medical Department had no control. It was complicated by the fact that patients belonged to different major commands (Ground, Service, and Air Forces), were qualified for different types of duty (limited or full duty), came from different areas (theaters of operations or the zone of interior), and were of separate ranks (commissioned or enlisted). Because of these complications, directives governing the reassignment of men and women who had been hospitalized were numerous, frequently changed, often obscure in meaning, and sometimes in conflict with one another. Attempts were made to correct this situation, but the general problem so far as it pertained to Ground and Service Forces personnel remained unsolved throughout the war.[26] The Air Forces, on the other hand, adopted a system of assignment in the fall of 1944 that was simple and effective. AAF headquarters placed liaison officers in some AAF regional hospitals and, with the concurrence of ASF headquarters, in each general and ASF regional hospital.

[22] Memo, SG for CG ASF, 23 Mar 45, sub: Gen Hosp Program, ZI. SG: 322 "Hosp."

[23] Ltr, SG to CGs all SvCs attn COs Hosp Ctrs, Gen Hosps, and Conv Hosps, 28 May 45, sub: Med Clarification of Disposition Policy. HD.

[24] (1) Rpt of SGs Pers Bd, 3 Nov 43. HD. (2) Memo, Dr Eli Ginzberg, ASF Control Div for Chief Oprs Serv SGO thru Dir Control Div ASF, 30 Nov 43, sub: Surv of Gen Hosps. SG: 333.1-1.

[25] (1) SG Ltr 193, 30 Nov 43. (2) Ltr, SG (init A. H. S[chwichtenberg]) to Surg 2d SvC, 8 Feb 44, sub: Prompt Prof and Admin Practice in Army Hosps. SG: 705 (2d SvC)AA. Similar letters were sent to other service command surgeons. (3) Ltr, CG 5th SvC (Asst SvC Surg) to SG, 30 Mar 44, sub: Prompt Prof and Admin Practice in Army Hosps. SG: 705 (5th SvC)AA. (4) An Rpt, 1944, 2d SvC Surg. HD.

[26] (1) Mins, SvC Conf, Ft Leonard Wood, Mo, 27–29 Jul 44, p. 17. HD. (2) Memo, SG for CG ASF, 14 Mar 45, sub: Improvement in Hosp Admin Procedures. SG: 300.7. (3) History of Control Division, ASF, 1942–45, App, p. 199.

These officers acted as representatives of the commanding general, Army Air Forces, reassigning both commissioned and enlisted personnel of the Air Forces. Subsequently it was reported that they returned flying officers to duty in the Fourth Air Force in 10 percent of the time formerly required.[27]

Aside from the necessity of securing reassignments, there was another cause for delay in returning patients to duty: the administrative procedure for the physical reclassification of officers. In July 1943 the General Staff directed that officers found by hospital disposition boards to be permanently incapacitated for full military service should appear before Army retiring boards instead of being returned to duty in limited service assignments.[28] This meant that such an officer had to be kept in a hospital while its commander forwarded recommendations of his disposition board to service command headquarters; the service commander issued orders for the appearance of the officer before a retiring board; the board assembled and considered the case, and sent its findings to Washington for review by The Surgeon General, The Adjutant General, and the Secretary of War's Separation Board; and The Adjutant General issued orders for the officer's disposition. In the fall of 1944 the Surgeon General's Office, ASF headquarters, and the Adjutant General's Office attempted to find a way to avoid keeping such officers in hospitals after their treatment had been completed. The Adjutant General proposed returning them to their previous stations or to replacement pools after appearance before retiring boards, to await there the decision of agencies in Washington.[29] The ASF proposal, which went further than this, was approved by the General Staff. On 14 October 1944 a War Department circular authorized hospital and station commanders to return to duty officers recommended for limited service by disposition boards, without referring them, except in a few cases, to retiring boards.[30] This change in procedure reduced the length of stay in hospitals of officers in this category to such an extent that it saved, according to the estimate of ASF headquarters, 1,000 hospital beds annually.[31]

Improvements in Disability Discharge and Retirement Procedures

Officers and men whose physical disabilities prohibited return to duty were either retired or discharged from the service. Since both retirement and discharge for disability were personnel as well as medical administrative procedures, they involved agencies other than the Medical Department. Their simplification was therefore a complicated process and some-

---

[27] (1) A History of Medical Administration and Practice in the Fourth Air Force (1945), vol. I, pp. 79–81. HD: TAS. (2) Ltr, CG AAF to CG ASF, 25 Aug 44, sub: Disposition of AAF Pnts in Gen Hosps and Certain ASF Hosps. AG: 705(25 Aug 44)(1). (3) ASF Cir 296, 9 Sep 44. (4) AAF Ltr 25–1, 21 Sep 44, sub: AAF Liaison with Hosp. SG: 211 (Surg, Flight). (5) An Rpts, 1944, Fitzsimons, Thayer, and O'Reilly Gen Hosps. HD.

[28] Rad, ACofS G–1 WDGS to SvC Comdrs, Retiring Bds, and all Named Gen Hosps, 10 Jul 43. SG: 334.6–1 Retiring Bds.

[29] Draft of WD Cir, incl to T/S APGO–S 210.85 (6 Sep 44), TAG to SG, 8 Sep 44, sub: Disposition of Offs Appearing before Retirement Bds, with 1st ind, SG to TAG, 24 Oct 44. SG: 300.5 (WD Cir).

[30] (1) Memo, CG ASF for ACofS G–1 WDGS, 25 Sep 44, sub: Physical Reclassification of Offs. AG: 210.85 (25 Sep 44)(2). (2) DF WDGAP 210.01, ACofS G–1 WDGS to TAG, 7 Oct 44, same sub. Same file. (3) WD Cir 403, 14 Oct 44.

[31] Rpt, Economies Effected through Procedures Studies Made by or jointly with Control Div ASF, 13 Apr 45. HRS: Hq ASF Control Div file, "Est Admin Savings Resulting from Procedural Revisions."

times slow, but for the Medical Department it was important because any delay in either procedure wasted beds by lengthening the stay of patients in hospitals.

Despite earlier attempts to remove causes for delays, the disability discharge procedure took more time than was considered necessary and in the fall of 1943[32] both the Surgeon General's Office and ASF headquarters began studies to simplify and standardize it. Because its Control Division was engaged in a more general study of Army administrative procedures, ASF headquarters directed The Surgeon General to discontinue his study. The ASF Control Division proceeded thereafter, with assistance from the Surgeon General's Office, to develop and test a revised procedure for disability discharges.[33] In March 1944 this procedure was published in a tentative manual and each service command was directed to install it in one general and one station hospital for further testing. Reports from such tests were favorable, and on 24 July 1944 ASF directed all of its hospitals to begin using the new procedure. Six months later a War Department manual made it official for use in hospitals of the Air Forces as well as of the Service Forces.[34]

The new procedure for disability discharges covered actions taken within hospitals themselves, since measures adopted earlier had reduced administrative actions required by headquarters other than hospitals.[35] This goal was more completely achieved during 1944 when additional post commanders delegated to hospital commanders their functions relative to disability discharges, and the War Department delegated to commanders of regional and convalescent hospitals, as it had earlier to those of general hospitals, authority to grant discharges without reference to higher headquarters.[36] Under the new procedure, administrative actions within hospitals were simplified and speeded up. Hospital commanders were permitted to request records of former physical examinations and medical treatments from the Adjutant General's Office and from other hospitals as soon as ward officers made a diagnosis indicating eventual disability discharge, rather than after completion of treatment. This move was expected to eliminate delays in the consideration of cases by CDD (Certificate of Disability for Discharge) boards. To reduce the work of these boards and of all officers who participated in the procedure, paper work required for disability discharges was simplified. Separate forms and letters previ-

[32] (1) Memo, Dr Eli Ginzberg, Control Div ASF for Chief Oprs Serv SGO thru Dir Control Div ASF, 30 Nov 43, sub: Surv of Gen Hosps. SG: 333.1-1. (2) Notes on Visit to McCloskey, O'Reilly, and Percy Jones Gen Hosps, 11 Dec 43, by Col Tracy S. Voorhees, Control Div SGO. Same file.

[33] (1) Memo, SG (Control Div) for Dir Control Div ASF, 29 Oct 43, sub: Delays in Discharging Pnts from Hosps. (2) Memo, SG (Control Div) for CG Army Med Ctr, 29 Oct 43, sub: Delays in CDD Procedure. (3) Memo, CG ASF (Control Div) for SG attn Dir Control Div, 5 Nov 43, sub: Delays in Discharging Pnts from Hosps. (4) Memo, Act Dir Control Div SGO for Brig Gen Edward S. Greenbaum, Off of UnderSecWar, 16 Feb 44, sub: Improvements in CDD Procedures. All in SG: 220.811-1. (5) An Rpt, FY 1944, Control Div SGO. HD.

[34] (1) History of Control Division, ASF, 1942-1945, App, pp. 345-46. HD. (2) Memo, CG ASF for CG 1st SvC, 17 Mar 44, sub: Estab of Pilot Instl Covering Discharges and Release from AD. SG: 220.811-1. Similar letters were sent to each service command. (3) Draft of Tentative Procedures—Discharge and Release from AD, Hq ASF, 5 Mar 44. AG: 220.8. (4) ASF Cir 217, 13 Jul 44. (5) TM 12-235, Enl Pers—Discharge and Release from AD (Other than at Separation Ctrs), 1 Jan 45.

[35] See above, pp. 124-30.

[36] (1) AR 615-360, C 19, 17 Mar 44. (2) An Rpts, 1944, Fts Jackson, Bragg, and Cp Shelby Regional Hosps. HD. (3) WD Memo 615-44, 17 Aug 44, sub: Discharge Auth. (4) AR 615-360, 20 Jul 44, and C 1, 1 Feb 45.

ously used were eliminated or consolidated, and copies of different forms and the number of signatures required on them were limited. All forms were set up according to standard typewriter spacing to facilitate preparation and, in some instances, rubber stamp entries were authorized.[37] To insure speedy, well co-ordinated action by all hospital officers concerned with discharges, a time schedule was established. It listed the actions taken by each officer on the days following the admission of patients to hospitals, the day before the CDD board meeting, the day of the meeting, and the three following days. Finally, the manual on the discharge procedure showed graphically each step in a disability discharge.

Except in procuring adequate supplies of new forms, hospitals encountered little difficulty in installing the new procedure. Their reaction was almost immediately favorable. For example, by the end of 1944 one of them reported that disability discharges were "no longer a matter of concern." [38] The Surgeon General's Office likewise was pleased with the new procedure and with the saving in hospital beds which it produced.[39] According to an estimate of the ASF Control Division in April 1945, this saving amounted to an average of seventeen days for each disability discharge and to a total of 6,205,000 hospital bed-days (the equivalent of seventeen 1,000-bed hospitals) annually.[40]

As in the case of disability discharges for enlisted men, several agencies became concerned in the fall of 1943 about the time used in retiring officers for disability. Among them were the Adjutant General's Office, the Surgeon General's Office, and ASF headquarters.[41] During the next two years they worked together to speed the retirement process and thereby to shorten the period of hospitalization of officers disabled for military duty. One method was to shorten the time that elapsed between completion of an officer's treatment and his appearance before a retiring board. In the middle of 1943 the procedure for getting an officer before a retiring board was complicated. After completion of treatment, his case was reviewed by a hospital disposition board. If the board recommended retirement, its recommendation was sent to higher headquarters, such as that of a service command, for review. If that headquarters approved the recommendation, it ordered the officer to go before a retiring board. At that point, the hospital requested his personnel records from the Adjutant General's Office. After they arrived, the retiring board could consider the officer's case. In the fall and winter of 1943 steps were taken to get records

[37] (1) TM 12-235, Enl Pers—Discharge and Release from AD (Other than at Separation Ctrs), 1 Jan 45. (2) History of Control Division, ASF, 1942-45, pp. 183-86, and App, pp. 345-46. HD.

[38] An Rpt, 1944, O'Reilly Gen Hosp. HD. Letters from hospitals reporting on the new procedure, dated May-June 1944, are filed in HRS: Hq ASF Control Div file, "Disability Discharge Corresp." See also: An Rpts, 1944, Fts Jackson and Bragg Regional Hosps and Ashford Gen Hosp. HD.

[39] An Rpt, FY 1944, Control Div SGO, and An Rpt, FY 1945, Hosp and Dom Oprs SGO. HD.

[40] Rpt, Economies Effected through Procedures Studies Made by or jointly with Control Div ASF, 13 Apr 45. HRS: Hq ASF Control Div file, "Est Admin Savings Resulting from Procedural Revisions."

[41] (1) T/S, Dir Control Div AGO to Chief Insp and Investigation Br AGO, 28 Aug 43, sub: Retirement Procedures Affecting Offs. AG: 210.85 (12-17-42)(1). (2) Memo, SG for Gen Malin Craig, Pres Army Retiring Bd, 30 Aug 43. SG: 334.6-1. (3) Memo, Dir Control Div SGO for Brig Gen Charles C. Hillman, SGO, 8 Sep 43, sub: Retiring Bd Procedures. Same file. (4) Memo, Lt Col Basil C. MacLean, SGO for Gen [Raymond W.] Bliss thru Col A. H. Schwichtenberg, 6 Nov 43, sub: Observations Based on Recent Visits to Gen Hosps. Off files, Gen Bliss' Off SGO, "Util of MCs in ZI" (19) # 1.

from the Adjutant General's Office at an earlier point in the proceedings. In September, on The Surgeon General's recommendation, the General Staff authorized hospitals to request records of officers as soon as disposition boards recommended their appearance before retiring boards.[42] Later, on recommendation of the ASF Control Division, the Staff permitted hospitals to request these records as soon as it became obvious that officers would be considered for retirement, even though their cases had not been reviewed by disposition boards.[43] In the latter half of 1944 another cause for delay was eliminated when the Staff authorized hospital commanders to order officers to appear before retiring boards without reference to higher headquarters.[44]

Another method of speeding the retirement of officers was to prevent the development of backlogs of work for retiring boards. This could be done, in part at least, by increasing the number of such boards. Until the middle of 1943 retiring boards were few in number and could be appointed only by the Secretary of War.[45] In June of that year the Secretary delegated appointment authority to commanding generals of service commands and directed them to establish retiring boards at all general hospitals. Four months later the commanding general of the Air Forces, receiving similar authority, was directed to set up a retiring board at each AAF convalescent center.[46] In the middle of 1944 the right to have retiring boards was extended to all convalescent and regional hospitals.[47] Later, in October 1944, the number of cases referred to such boards was limited when, in connection with the movement to shorten the period of hospitalization of officers being physically reclassified for limited duty only, retiring boards were relieved of the consideration of such cases.[48]

An additional way of speeding officer retirements was to reduce the paper work of retiring boards. In the latter part of 1944 the ASF Control Division developed a standard form for such boards to use in reporting their proceedings.[49] Following the success of the new manual on disability-discharge procedures, the same Division developed and published in 1945 a technical manual on the retirement and reclassification of officers.[50] This manual, like that on the disability-discharge procedure, gave detailed instructions in diagrammatic and other explanatory forms on the completion of all administrative actions in the retirement process and established a time schedule to be followed by officers concerned. As a result, according to ASF headquarters, the period of hospitalization of officers awaiting disabil-

[42] (1) Memo SPMCH 300.3–1, Exec Off SGO for Publication Div AGO thru Procedure Br SGO, 7 Aug 43, sub: Proposed Change in AR 605–250. AG: 210.-85 (12–17–42)(1). (2) AR 605–250, C 1, 17 Sep 43.

[43] (1) Memo, Dir Control Div ASF for TAG, 18 Dec 43, sub: Request for Publication. AG: 210.85 (12–17–42)(1). (2) AR 605–250, C 5, 6 Jan 44.

[44] (1) T/S, Chief Insp and Investigation Br AGO to Dir Control Div AGO, 26 Jul 44, sub: Reasgmt of Pers Returned to Duty from Hosp. AG: 705 (5 Jul 44). (2) WD Cir 403, 14 Oct 44.

[45] AR 605–250, 1 Jun 43 and 28 Mar 44.

[46] WD Memo W605–28–43, 17 Jun 43, and WD Memo W605–41–43, 19 Oct 43, sub: Delegation of Auth to Appoint Retiring Bds. SG: 334.6–1.

[47] (1) AR 605–250, C 1, 22 Jun 44. (2) Mins, SvC Conf, Ft Leonard Wood, Mo, 27–29 Jul 44. HD.

[48] See above, p. 243.

[49] Memo, CG ASF (Dir Control Div ASF) for SG, 9 Oct 44, sub: Form for the Proceedings of Army Retiring Bds. SG: 315 "Gen."

[50] (1) Draft of Proposed WD Technical Manual, TM 12–245, Physical Reclassification and Retirement of Offs, 1 Jun 45. Off file, Physical Standards Div, SGO. (2) Tentative WD Technical Manual, TM 12–245, Physical Reclassification, Retirement, and Retirement Benefits for Offs, 1 Oct 45. Same file.

ity retirements was reduced enough to save 4,700 beds annually.[51]

The simplification and standardization of procedures for disability discharges and retirements were the culmination of efforts begun early in the war to limit the occupancy of hospital beds to persons actually needing them. Earlier measures to reform these procedures affected actions taken outside hospitals but were a necessary foundation for the later ones which were mainly intended to improve action within the hospitals themselves. Other efforts to restrict patients in hospitals to those needing medical and surgical treatment were less successful. Little if anything was done to screen patients by physical examination before admission to hospitals. The reassignment of those returning to duty continued to cause difficulty and delays in disposition. And the policy of giving all patients "maximum hospitalization," whether their disabilities had been incurred in line of duty or not, tended to lengthen the average period of hospitalization and hence to increase the occupancy of beds by men who could be of no further service to the Army.

[51] History of Control Division, ASF, 1942–45, App. pp. 481–83. HD.

CHAPTER XIV

Changes in Size and Make-Up of Staffs of Zone of Interior Hospitals

Changes in policies and procedures affecting the occupancy of beds resulted in part from limitations upon the amount of personnel available for the hospitals. One such limitation was a definite requirement that hospitals get along on proportionately smaller staffs than accustomed to. Although the Manpower Board and ASF headquarters were chiefly responsible for this development, the Surgeon General's Office participated indirectly. Established in March 1943 to advise the Chief of Staff on personnel matters,[1] the Manpower Board analyzed the functions of hospitals in the United States, as it did those of other installations, and developed "yardsticks" by which to measure their personnel requirements.[2] Using these yardsticks, the Board estimated the total amount of military and civilian personnel which ASF installations needed, and the General Staff normally accepted the Board's estimates in making personnel authorizations. ASF headquarters then subdivided its quota among service commands. Service commanders in turn authorized personnel for subordinate installations which then took similar action.[3] Under this system, despite its nominally advisory capacity the Manpower Board exercised a rigid control over the personnel which the Service Forces received, and subordinate commands might or might not authorize as much for hospitals as the Manpower Board's yardsticks showed they needed.[4] To provide a guide for subordinate commands in manning hospitals, and perhaps to influence service commanders in making authorizations, the Surgeon General's Office developed manning tables for general, regional, and station hospitals of various sizes and obtained sanction for them in a War Department circular issued in the spring of 1944.[5] They agreed gener-

[1] (1) Memo W600-27-43, 11 Mar 43, sub: WD Manpower Bd. (2) Ltr, CofSA to CG SOS, 12 Mar 43, same sub. Both in SG: 322.7-1 (Bds, etc.).

[2] (1) WDMB Yardstick No 7 for Measuring Pers Reqmts of Named Gen Hosps. SG: 323.7-5. (2) Rpt, SGO Bd of Offs on the Util of MC Offs, 19 Oct 43. Off file, Gen Bliss' Off SGO, "Util of MCs in ZI" (19) #1.

[3] (1) History of Control Division, ASF, 1942-45, pp. 31-33. HD. (2) ASF Cir 39, 11 Jun 43. (3) 1st ind, CG ASF to SG, n d, on Memo SPMDC 320.2 (2d SvC)AA, SG for CG ASF, 10 Apr 45, sub: Strength Auth, MD. HRS: ASF SPGA 320.2 "Med."

[4] For example, see Diary, Hosp Div SGO, 28 Sep 44 and 16 Mar 45. HD: 024.7-5.

[5] (1) Memo, Gilbert W. Beebe, Control Div SGO for Col Tracy S. Voorhees, Control Div SGO, 31 Oct 43. SG: 632.-2. (2) Memo SPMCH 300.5-5, SG for CofS ASF, 19 Apr 44, sub: Pers Strength Tables for Med Instls in ZI. AG: 320.3 (18 Apr 44)(1). (3) WD Cir 209, 26 May 44.

ally with the Manpower Board's yardsticks and with recommendations made by the Inspector General's Office. While they were not compulsory they served as guides supplied by the Medical Department for the reduction of hospital staffs.[6]

General Nature of Changes

The general reduction made in hospital staffs can be illustrated by changes in the ratio of employees to beds. In July 1943 the average number of employees (military and civilian) per 100 beds in general hospitals was 94. At that time 58.6 percent of all beds in general hospitals were occupied. Therefore the number of employees per 100 occupied beds was 160. By July 1944 the average number of employees per 100 beds in all general hospitals had dropped to 68.6. At that time, however, only 42 percent of the beds were occupied, and therefore the number of employees per 100 occupied beds was 160—the same as a year before. About a year later (June 1945), when 81.4 percent of all general hospital beds were occupied and the number of patients on the rolls of general hospitals (those absent from hospitals on leave or furlough as well as those occupying beds) was 122 percent of their bed capacities, the average number of employees per 100 beds was 71.1, but the average per 100 occupied beds was only 87. Thus, by the middle of 1945 the staffs of Army general hospitals in the United States had been reduced to the point where they had roughly only about half as many people to care for patients as in former years.[7]

Another general change in hospital staffs during the latter half of the war was the widespread substitution of civilians, Wacs, and limited service personnel for the enlisted men, officers, and nurses who were taken out of zone of interior hospitals for overseas assignments. This change resulted from a War Department policy governing the use of personnel by the Service Forces, reiterated by ASF headquarters in June 1943. In general, men qualified for overseas service were to be released as rapidly as possible from assignment to all zone of interior installations. In replacing them commanders were not to assign men to positions that could be filled by women; they were not to assign military persons, male or female, to those that could be filled by civilians; and they were not to assign officers to duties that could be performed by enlisted persons or civilians.[8] Compliance with this policy had two effects upon hospital staffs. In the first place, as officers, nurses, and men were withdrawn from hospitals for overseas service, hospital staffs were subject to a continuous personnel turnover. For example, during 1944 Birmingham General Hospital gained 53 Medical Corps officers, but lost 33; it gained 177 nurses, but lost 89; and it gained 758 enlisted men, but lost 416.[9] Redeployment following V-E Day and demobilization following V-J

[6] (1) Memo, SG for DepCofSA thru CG ASF, 10 May 44, sub: Pers Strength Tables. . . . (2) Memo, WDMB for ACofS G-4 WDGS, 25 Apr 44, sub: Anal of Proposed Strength Tables. . . . Both in AG: 320.2 (18 Apr 44)(1).

[7] (1) Tables on basic data and ratios of gen hosps. Off file, Resources Anal Div, SGO. (2) Statistical Health Rpts. Off file, Med Statistics Div, SGO. In 1939 civilian hospitals in the United States had an average of 83 employees per 100 beds and 121 employees per 100 patients. See Warren P. Morrill, "Ratio of Personnel to Patients," *Hospitals* (The Journal of the American Hospital Association), XIV (1940), pp. 47-49.

[8] ASF Cir 39, 11 Jun 43.

[9] An Rpt, 1944, Birmingham Gen Hosp. See also An Rpts, 1944 and 45, Ashford, Wakeman, Baker, and Lovell Gen Hosps and Waltham, Ft Geo. G. Meade, Cps Bowie, Crowder, and Shelby Regional Hosps. HD.

Day gave impetus to this turnover. Secondly, as hospitals replaced persons qualified for overseas service with those in other categories, their staffs gradually became heterogeneous mixtures of doctors, administrative officers, Army nurses, civilian nurses, paid nurses' aides, voluntary nurses' aides, general and limited service men, Wacs, skilled and unskilled civilians, and prisoners of war. Some of the problems involved in the reduction, turnover, and replacement of personnel in particular categories will now be considered.

Wider Use of Administrative Officers

Medical Corps officers available for assignment to zone of interior hospitals were limited in number. According to manning tables, the proper ratio of physicians to beds ranged from 2.5 per 100 in a 1,000-bed general hospital to 2 per 100 in a 4,000-bed installation. During 1944 the actual average ratio for all general hospitals was approximately 2.6 per 100 beds. The next year, with the expansion of the hospital system, that ratio dropped to about 2.3 per 100 and remained there until November 1945.[10] Hospital commanders apparently accepted the fact that additional doctors were not available, for they complained about shortages during this period less than earlier. In a few instances hospital commanders and service command surgeons reported that the quality of professional care declined. In others they called attention to the need for more specialists, such as neuropsychiatrists, orthopedic surgeons, and neurosurgeons.[11] More frequently, they complained about constant changes in professional staffs and about the inferior quality of replacements received.[12] Despite these complaints, there seem to have been enough Medical Corps officers to care adequately for all patients provided they were relieved of administrative work and permitted to devote full time and attention to professional activities.[13]

The chief method of relieving physicians of administrative work was the more extensive use of Medical Administrative Corps officers. It will be recalled that substitution of these for Medical Corps officers in strictly administrative positions had begun during the early war years, but had not reached widespread proportions. In the fall of 1943 a strict limitation upon the number of Army physicians combined with an increasing supply of Medical Administrative Corps officers to suggest to both the Surgeon General's Office and the medical officer on The Inspector General's staff a wider use of administrative officers, not only in administrative work unconnected with medical practice but also in jobs having semiprofessional aspects.[14] In November 1943, therefore, The Surgeon General proposed that Medical Administrative Corps officers be used throughout the Army in many positions

[10] Tables on basic data and ratios in gen hosps. Off file, Resources Anal Div SGO.

[11] An Rpts, 1944, 2d, 4th, 7th, and 9th SvC Surgs; An Rpts, 1945, 5th and 7th SvC Surgs; An Rpt, 1944, Ashburn Gen Hosp. HD.

[12] (1) An Rpts, 1944, 4th and 5th SvC Surgs; An Rpt, 1944, Ft Benning Regional Hosp; An Rpts, 1945, 1st, 4th, 5th, and 9th SvC Surgs; An Rpts, 1945, Beaumont Gen Hosp, Ft Bragg and Cp Lee Regional Hosps. HD. (2) Mins, Conf of Hosp Comdrs, 7th SvC, 22 Aug 45. HD: 337.

[13] (1) Memo, Act IG for CG ASF, 7 Feb and 15 Mar 45, sub: Med Pers and Hosp Fac in ZI. IG: 333.9–Med Pers (2). (2) Memo WDSIG 333.9–Hosp Fac (2), Act IG for DepCofSA, 14 May 45, sub: Rpt of Surv of ZI Hosps. SG: 333 WDCSA 632 (14 May 45). (3) Mins, 6th Conf of SvC Comdrs, Edgewater Park, Miss, 1–3 Feb 45. HD: 337.

[14] (1) Mins, Mtg of Bd of Offs to Study Util of MC Offs, 17 Sep 43. (2) Ltr IG 333.0–Med Pers, IG to DepCofSA, 13 Jan 44, sub: Util of Med Off Pers in ZI Instls. Both in Off file, Gen Bliss' Off SGO, "Util of MCs in ZI" (19) #1 and (20) #2.

previously held by doctors, such as battalion surgeons' assistants in the field and registrars in hospitals.[15] The General Staff approved this proposal.[16] In May 1944 this policy was reflected in hospital manning tables prepared by the Surgeon General's Office.[17]

The demand for Medical Administrative Corps officers to fill positions assigned to them under the new policy created a temporary shortage in the latter part of 1944. Gradually, as the supply of such officers increased they took over all customary administrative positions in hospitals in the zone of interior, except those of executive officer and commanding officer, as well as new positions established to handle such additional wartime functions as legal assistance, personal affairs, vocational counseling, and reconditioning. In addition, during 1944 and 1945 some hospital commanders appointed Medical Administrative Corps officers as assistants to doctors to relieve them of duties not directly connected with the treatment of patients. In such positions, Medical Administrative Corps officers assumed responsibility for all property in hospital wards, for the cleanliness of wards, and for the discipline of patients; granted passes, leaves, and furloughs to patients; and in some instances assigned and supervised the work of enlisted and civilian ward employees. Thus, by the end of the war Medical Administrative Corps officers, whose use had been almost negligible in 1942, had become an important part of Army hospital staffs.[18]

Alleviation of the "Shortage" of Army Nurses

During 1944 and the early part of 1945 hospital commanders and service command surgeons complained loudly of an "acute shortage" of Army nurses; but by the middle of 1945, they reported, the shortage had been eliminated and there were plenty of nurses for the rest of the year.[19] During the first four months of 1944 (for which figures are available) the average number of beds per Army nurse in general hospitals ranged from 21.2 to 23.8, but the average number of patients per Army nurse was between 10.1 and 13.7. In June 1945, when the peak patient load was reached, the average number of beds per nurse in general hospitals was 13.7, but the average number of occupied beds per nurse (11.2) remained about the same as the year before.[20] If one considers the general situation, and that only in terms of the ratio of occupied beds to nurses, there seems to have been no more reason for complaint in 1944 than later when hospitals reported that the shortage had been eliminated. At any rate, the validity of complaints made in 1944 was openly questioned by the commander of the Fifth Service Command.[21]

[15] Memo SPMCT 353.-1, SG for CG ASF, 25 Nov 43, sub: Conservation of MC Offs. AG: 320.2(10-30-41)(2) T/Os.

[16] DF WDGCT 322(25 Nov 43), ACofS G-3 WDGS to TAG, 1 Mar 44, sub: Conservation of MC Offs. AG: 320.3(10-30-41)(2) T/Os.

[17] WD Cir 209, 26 May 44.

[18] An Rpts, 1944, 5th and 9th SvC Surgs; An Rpts, 1944, Baker, Beaumont, Birmingham, O'Reilly, and Wakeman Gen Hosps and Cps Barkeley, Shelby and Ft McClellan Regional Hosps; An Rpt, 1945, 5th SvC Surg; An Rpts, 1945, Birmingham, Crile, and Lovell Gen Hosps. HD.

[19] An Rpts, 1944, 2d, 3d, 4th, 5th, and 9th SvC Surgs; An Rpts, 1945, 2d, 5th, 7th, and 9th SvC Surgs; An Rpts, 1944 and 45, Ashford, Fitzsimons, Baker, Halloran, O'Reilly, Baxter, Beaumont, Lovell, Birmingham, and Wakeman Gen Hosps and Waltham, Cps Barkeley, Crowder, and Shelby, and Ft McClellan Regional Hosps. HD.

[20] Tables on basic data and ratios of gen hosps. Off file, Resources Anal Div SGO. See Charts 8, 9, and 10, and Table 13.

[21] Mins, 6th Conf of SvC Comdrs, Edgewater Park, Miss, 1-3 Feb 45, pp. 202-03. HD: 337.

Hospital commanders may have been complaining about a potential rather than an actual shortage of nurses, but whether potential or actual there were reasons for their belief that it was serious. In the first place, the authorized ratio of nurses to beds during 1944 was lower than that to which hospitals had been accustomed. Early that year the Deputy Chief of Staff of the Army ordered it reduced from one for every ten beds to one for every fifteen.[22] Next, the number of nurses actually assigned to hospitals during 1944 was often lower than the number authorized[23] and there was thus a shortage of nurses to fill authorized quotas. If hospitals had been called upon to operate at full capacity at that time, they might have encountered serious difficulties. Furthermore, at the time when hospitals were required to adjust to lower ratios of nurses, their enlisted staffs were reduced also and some of their trained technicians were withdrawn for overseas service.[24] This situation perhaps contributed to a feeling on the part of nurses themselves that they were shorthanded and overworked, a feeling possibly heightened by the fact that nurses had to devote attention to new activities, such as the educational and physical reconditioning programs, that were being introduced during 1944.[25] Finally, the continuous turnover of personnel interfered with the achievement of stable, well-organized staffs to operate hospital wards. Whatever the reason, there was a widespread belief in Army hospitals during 1944 and the early part of 1945 that there was an "acute shortage" of nurses; and the Medical Department, from the Surgeon General's Office down, tried to alleviate that condition.[26]

A number of measures were adopted to insure an adequate nursing service for the Army's patients. Some, such as the elimination of inessential nursing records and the concentration of patients requiring continuous nursing care in as few wards as possible, were administrative.[27] Others, such as the employment of civilian registered nurses and senior student nurses, were designed to supplement the professional nursing service.[28] By April 1945 there were in general hospitals more than 2,000 cadet nurses and more than 1,000 civilian nurses.[29] A measure that was pro-

[22] (1) DF WDGAP 320.21, ACofS G–1 WDGS to CG ASF and SG, 8 Jan 44, sub: Nurse Pers Reqmts. HD: 211. (2) Memo, SG for DepCofSA thru CG ASF, 10 May 44, sub: Pers Strength Tables for Med Instls in ZI. AG: 320.2(18 Apr 44)(1). (3) WD Cir 209, 26 May 44.

[23] For example, see Conf, Post Surgs and COs of Gen Hosps, 2d SvC, 19–20 Jun 44. HD: 337.

[24] See below, pp. 253–56.

[25] An Rpts, 1944 and 45, Birmingham, Lovell, Wakeman, and Baker Gen Hosps. HD.

[26] Florence A. Blanchfield and Mary W. Standlee, Organized Nursing and the Army in Three Wars (1950) (cited hereafter as Blanchfield and Standlee, Organized Nursing) gives a full discussion of the nursing "shortage" in the winter of 1944–45. In general, the authors indicate that the Medical Department's estimate of nurse requirements was unrealistically high. In an interview on 20 November 1951 General Kirk stated that the Medical Department was "always short" of nurses until a draft was proposed in the winter of 1944–45. (HD: 314 Correspondence on MS) V. The question of whether or not there was a shortage of nurses in zone of interior hospitals was only part of a larger question of a shortage of nurses for use in theaters of operations as well as in the zone of interior. This question will be discussed more fully in John H. McMinn and Max Levin, Personnel (MS for companion vol. in Medical Dept. series). HD.

[27] (1) Mins, Conf of Post Surgs and COs of Gen Hosps, 2d SvC, 19–20 Jun 44, p. 128. HD: 337. (2) Mins, 6th Conf of SvC Comdrs, Edgewater Park, Miss, 1–3 Feb 45, pp. 191–93. Same file. (3) An Rpt, 1944, O'Reilly Gen Hosp. HD.

[28] An Rpts, 1944, 2d, 3d, 4th, 5th, and 9th SvC Surgs; An Rpts, 1944, Fitzsimons, Halloran, O'Reilly, Birmingham, and Baxter Gen Hosps, and Waltham, Cps Shelby and Crowder Regional Hosps. HD.

[29] Tables on basic data and ratios of gen hosps. Off file, Resources Anal Div SGO.

posed, but not adopted, was a draft of nurses.[30] Still another measure was the increased employment of ancillary personnel to relieve nurses of nonprofessional duties in the care of patients. During 1944 and 1945 hospitals hired civilian nurses' aides and ward orderlies, sought the services of volunteer Red Cross nurses' aides, and used both enlisted men and Wacs, as they were available, to assist nurses in the care of patients.[31]

Greater Use of Limited Service Men

Along with measures affecting the allotment of officers and nurses to hospitals, there were changes in the type of enlisted men employed during 1944 and 1945.[32] The existing policy of reassigning general service men from zone of interior installations to overseas units was made stricter and applied more widely during 1944 than before. In January ASF headquarters began a drive to have all general service men, except those who were more than thirty-five years old, those who had already served overseas, those who had had less than one year of Army service, and those who were considered to be in certain "key" categories, released from its installations by June; later, October.[33] This drive threatened to strip hospitals of even their trained technicians. In order to prevent this, the Surgeon General's Office got the Military Personnel Division of ASF headquarters to consider such men as dental laboratory technicians, meat and dairy inspectors, pharmacists, X-ray technicians, reconditioning instructors, medical technicians, surgical technicians, and laboratory technicians as being in "key" categories.[34] In July 1944 ASF headquarters announced that even "key" technicians, if physically qualified for overseas service, would be taken out of zone of interior installations as soon as replacements were available.[35] Service commands interpreted these directives differently, and some pulled "key" men out of hospitals without thought of the availability of properly trained replacements.[36] To recover for the Medical Department some of the technicians improperly transferred as well as those misassigned initially to the Ground Forces, the Surgeon General's Office succeeded in getting orders published during 1944 and 1945 requiring their retransfer to Medical Department units and installations. These actions saved enough technicians, so the Enlisted Personnel Branch of the Surgeon General's Office reported at the end of 1944, to man all hospitals properly,[37] but not all

[30] Blanchfield and Standlee, Organized Nursing, pp. 551–95.

[31] An Rpts, 1944 and 45, 2d, 3d, and 9th SvC Surgs; An Rpts, 1944, Deshon, Halloran, O'Reilly, Baker, Fitzsimons, Baxter, Wakeman, Birmingham, and Lovell Gen Hosps. HD.

[32] For example, see An Rpts, 1944 and 45, Fts Bragg and Knox, Cps Barkeley and Lee Regional Hosps, and Baxter, Beaumont, Halloran, Schick, and Wakeman Gen Hosps. HD. See also McMinn and Levin, *op. cit.*

[33] (1) ASF Cir 26, 24 Jan 44. (2) Quarterly Rpt, 3d Qtr 1944, Enl Pers Br, Mil Pers Div SGO. HD.

[34] (1) ASF Cir 193, 26 Jun 44. (2) WD Memo W615-44, 29 May 44, sub: Critically Needed Specialists. HD. (3) Quarterly Rpt, 3d Qtr 1944, Enl Pers Br Mil Pers Div SGO. HD. (4) Mins, Conf of Post Surgs and COs of Gen Hosps, 2d SvC, 19–20 Jun 44, p. 194. HD: 337.

[35] ASF Cir 239, 29 Jul 44.

[36] (1) Ltr, Capt Luther F. Dunlop, QMC, Hosp Div SGO to HD SGO, 4 Jul 44, sub: Summary of Civ Situation in Sta and Gen Hosps during the Past Few Months. HD: 230.-1 "Civ Pers (Gen)." (2) Quarterly Rpt, 4th Qtr 1944, Enl Pers Br Mil Pers Div SGO. HD. (3) An Rpts, Ft Bragg Regional Hosp and Beaumont Gen Hosp. HD.

[37] Quarterly Rpt, 3d and 4th Qtr 1944 and 2d Qtr 1945, Enl Pers Br Mil Pers Div SGO, and An Rpts, 1944, Baxter and Schick Gen Hosps. HD.

commanders were satisfied with saving technicians. Some complained loudly about the loss of certain clerical employees, such as those occupying the position of sergeant major, whom they considered also as "key" persons.[38]

One reason that hospital commanders complained about the loss of general service men was that they encountered personnel-management problems in using civilians, Wacs, and limited service men to replace them.[39] As a rule, limited service men assigned to hospitals came either from nonmedical units in the United States or from organizations overseas. Many were not trained for work in hospitals and had to be oriented and trained on the job, even in clerical positions. Some felt that they had already contributed their share toward winning the war and wished to be discharged from the Army. Others were psychoneurotic and their job-assignments had to be made with caution. Still others had mental limitations which made it difficult for them to absorb job-training. Many were physically handicapped and could not do heavy work. These restrictions on the use of limited service men complicated the problem of staffing hospitals.[40] Furthermore, the assignment of such men to hospitals often created morale problems. Under the ASF personnel-control system, each hospital was authorized a specific number of noncommissioned officers. So long as it had that number it could make no promotions.[41] Many limited service men assigned to hospitals held noncommissioned-officer grades which they had earned in nonmedical units. They were usually not qualified, either by experience or by training, to hold such grades in hospitals. When required to do work which they considered beneath the dignity of their grades, they became resentful. Moreover, their mere presence prevented the promotion of other men who, by reason of qualifications and jobs held, deserved to be noncommissioned officers. Lack of opportunities for promotion lowered the morale of these men.[42]

Hospital commanders were powerless to correct this situation, and the Surgeon General's Office tackled it. Hoping to solve the dual problem of having men with proper job qualifications assigned as replacements and of promoting men who deserved noncommissioned-officer grades, that Office in 1944 prepared tables of organization for zone of interior hospitals, showing job specifications and corresponding grades.[43] These tables were not published in 1944. In January 1945, after the problem of grades for enlisted men was made more acute by the proposal to assign WAC companies to hospitals,[44] Surgeon General Kirk appealed to the Secre-

[38] For example, see remarks of hospital commanders in the following: (1) Mins, Conf of Post Surgs and COs of Gen Hosps, 2d SvC, 19–20 Jun 44, pp. 204 and 209. HD: 337. (2) An Rpt, 1944, Ashford Gen Hosp. HD.

[39] In the middle of 1943 the Army abolished the term "limited service" but continued to classify men as qualified or not qualified for overseas service. Unofficially men not qualified for overseas service continued to be called limited service men.

[40] An Rpts, 1944, 2d, 4th, 5th, 7th, and 9th SvC Surgs; An Rpts, 1944, Halloran, Beaumont, Wakeman, Baxter, Baker, Ashford, and Birmingham Gen Hosps and Cps Barkeley, Lee, and Ft Knox Regional Hosps. HD.

[41] ASF Cir 39, 11 Jun 43.

[42] (1) An Rpt, 1943, 2d SvC Surg; and An Rpts, 1944, Wakeman and Birmingham Gen Hosps. HD. (2) Mins, 6th Conf of SvC Comdrs, Edgewater Park, Miss, 1–3 Feb 45, p. 190. HD: 337.

[43] An Rpt, FY 1944, Enl Pers Br Mil Pers Div SGO. HD.

[44] See below, pp. 256–59.

tary of War to approve the table-of-organization method of manning hospitals in the zone of interior.[45] The Secretary approved this proposal in principle, and the Surgeon General's Office revised the tables it had prepared in 1944.[46] During the following six months, the latter attempted to have them published. For some reason, perhaps simply red tape, this was not done and the problem of job qualifications and grades remained unsolved in ASF hospitals.[47]

Replacement of Military by Civilian Employees

Although limited service men were authorized as replacements for men physically qualified for overseas service, chief emphasis of War Department policy regarding nonprofessional personnel was on the use of civilians to replace military employees, whether general service men, limited service men, or enlisted women. Beginning in 1943 civilians were used actually to replace enlisted men, rather than to supplement them. Under the ASF personnel-control system established in June of that year, hospitals had personnel ceilings which they could not exceed, and as they employed additional civilians they had to release proportionate numbers of enlisted men.[48] The War Department's goal during 1944 and 1945 was to replace military personnel with civilians up to about half the total force.[49] This goal—one to which Surgeon General Magee had objected vigorously in the fall of 1940 [50]—was approached, though not reached, during the later war years. In June 1944 ASF station and regional hospitals employed 33,023 enlisted men and women, but only 19,469 civilians, exclusive of registered nurses—a ratio of approximately 17 military to 10 civilian employees. During the following year civilians replaced enlisted persons at such a rate that in June 1945 such hospitals had 17,673 enlisted men and women and 11,703 civilians—approximately 10 civilians for every 15 enlisted men and women.[51] General hospitals used civilian employees in greater proportion. In March 1944 the ratio of enlisted to civilian workers in all general hospitals was about 10 to 10.5, for there were 28,060 enlisted men and women and 29,546 civilians employed in those installations. About a year later, when general hospitals employed 40,659 enlisted and 45,793 civilian workers, the ratio had changed to about 10 enlisted persons to 11 civilians.[52]

In replacing military with civilian employees, hospitals encountered difficulties,

[45] Memo SPMDA 322.05, SG for SecWar, 10 Jan 45, sub: Med Mission Reappraised. HRS: G-4 file, "Hosp, vol. II." It should be noted that this was a reversal of The Surgeon General's traditional opposition to staffing zone of interior hospitals according to tables of organization.

[46] (1) DF WDGAP 321 Med, ACofS G-1 WDGS for ACofS G-4 WDGS, 29 Jan 45, sub: Med Mission Reappraised. HRS: G-4 file, "Hosp, vol. II." (2) Diary, Hosp Div SGO, 31 Jan 45. HD: 024.7-3. (3) Quarterly Rpt, 1st Qtr 1945, Enl Pers Br Mil Pers Div SGO. HD. (4) Unsigned Memo for Record, 22 Feb 45. SG: 320.3 "(T/O) Jan-Mar 45."

[47] (1) Memo, Dir Resources Anal Div SGO for Gen Bliss, 20 Jun 45, sub: Pers Guides. HD: Resources Anal Div file, "Hosp." (2) 2d ind, Dep SG to CG ASF, 14 Jul 45, on basic not located. Same file.

[48] ASF Cir 39, 11 Jun 43.

[49] Mins, Conf of Post Surgs and COs of Gen Hosps, 2d SvC, 19-20 Jun 44, pp. 197, 207, and 208; and Mins, 6th Conf of SvC Comdrs, Edgewater Park, Miss, 1-3 Feb 45, pp. 193-94. HD: 337.

[50] See above, pp. 31-32.

[51] Tables on basic data and ratios for sta, regional, POW, and conv hosps. Off file, Resources Anal Div SGO.

[52] Tables on basic data and ratios for gen hosps. Off file, Resources Anal Div SGO.

as they had earlier.[53] They still had trouble recruiting civilians in sufficient numbers, maintaining stable civilian-personnel forces, and using women and elderly or partially disabled men. They had to hire civilians who were not qualified for jobs they were to hold, and train them afterward. For example, hospitals in the Fourth Service Command trained civilians as apprentice dietitians, dental assistants, dental mechanics, laboratory helpers, X-ray technicians, guards, firefighters, telephone operators, steamfitters, refrigeration and air-conditioning mechanics, laundry operators, ward attendants, mess attendants, orthopedic shoe mechanics, cooks, and meatcutters. Furthermore, particularly in wards, hospital commanders confronted the difficulty of replacing enlisted men who worked twelve hours a day with civilians who worked only eight. Hoping to solve this problem, The Surgeon General asked for replacements on a basis of three civilians for two enlisted men. Some service commands followed this practice, but the War Department Manpower Board disapproved it and recommended allotments of civilian replacements for enlisted men on a one-for-one basis.[54] Hospitals then used split shifts for civilian employees and made other changes in work schedules, in order to have sufficient numbers on duty during the hours when work was heavy. Other difficulties for hospital commanders resulted from their lack of control over civilians, who often failed to show up for work, refused to work on night shifts, and, because of civil service regulations, could not be moved from one job to another to meet emergency needs. In such instances it was necessary to assign enlisted personnel to fill the vacancies. Finally, hospitals began to employ a different type of civilian during the later war years—paid nurses' aides—who, although not numerous, often created morale problems among enlisted Wacs by their mere presence.[55]

Use of Wacs in Army Hospitals

Although the Medical Department had begun to use Wacs[56] in hospitals earlier, by the middle of 1943 their number was small in proportion to that of enlisted men and civilians. Apparently WAC headquarters could not supply more, for in January

---

[53] See above, pp. 33, 135. This paragraph is based in general upon the following: An Rpts, 1944, Surgs 4th, 5th, 7th, and 9th SvCs, and 1945, 2d and 5th SvCs; and An Rpts, 1944 and 45, Brooke, Halloran, O'Reilly, Ashford, Baker, Birmingham, Wakeman, Baxter, Beaumont, Ashburn, and Battey Gen Hosps and Regional Hosps, Cps Shelby, Polk, Lee and Crowder, Scott and Keesler Flds, and Fts Bragg, Knox, and Meade, all in HD; and Ltr, Capt Luther F. Dunlop, QMC, Hosp Div SGO to HD SGO, 4 Jul 44, sub: Summary of Civ Situation in Sta and Gen Hosps during Past Few Months, in HD: 230.-1 "Civ Pers (Gen)."

[54] (1) Memo, WDMB for ACofS G-3 WDGS, 25 Apr 44, sub: Anal of Proposed Strength Tables for Med Instls in ZI. (2) Memo, SG for DepCofSA thru CG ASF, 3 May 44, same sub. (3) Memo WDSMB 323.3 (Hosp), WDMB for CofSA, n d, sub: WD Cir 209, 1944. (4) Memo SPMDM 300.5, SG for ACofS G-1 WDGS, 17 Feb 45, same sub. (5) Memo WDGSA 200.3 (3 Mar 45), Asst DepCofSA for ACofS G-1 WDGS, 7 Mar 45, same sub. All in AG: 320.2 (18 Apr 44)(1). (6) WD Cir 87, 19 Mar 45. (7) Mins, Conf of Post Surgs and COs of Gen Hosps, 2d SvC, 19-20 Jun 44, p. 199. HD: 337.

[55] ASF Cir 226, 20 Jul 44. The best discussion available of the employment of civilian nurses' aides in Army hospitals is in Blanchfield and Standlee, Organized Nursing, pp. 487-89, 492-93, 568.

[56] The Women's Army Corps (WAC) was authorized by Congress to supersede the WAAC on 1 July 1943. For a general discussion of the use of Wacs by the Medical Department see McMinn and Levin, *op. cit.*, and Mattie E. Treadwell, *The Women's Army Corps* (Washington, 1954), Chap XIX, in UNITED STATES ARMY IN WORLD WAR II.

1944 The Surgeon General's Hospital Administration Division reported that many unfilled requisitions were on hand.[57] As the withdrawal of general service men from zone of interior hospitals and the lack of sufficient nurses to fill authorized quotas increased the need of hospitals for ancillary personnel, The Surgeon General approved the use of Wacs and of both voluntary and paid nurses' aides. During 1944 and 1945 special recruiting campaigns were conducted both by WAC headquarters for additional Wacs and by the Red Cross for civilian nurses' aides. By the spring of 1945 a surplus of Wacs had been recruited for the Medical Department.[58] In order to use all of them, and at the same time to offset the shorter hours which Wacs were by then authorized to work, The Surgeon General requested their allotment to replace enlisted men in a ratio of three Wacs for two men. The Staff refused this request, and some of the Wacs recruited for the Medical Department had to be transferred to other assignments.[59]

As hospitals began to use more Wacs, a controversy developed over policies governing their employment. Basically, it sprang from the question of whether Wacs were to be considered primarily as women or as enlisted personnel. The director of the Women's Army Corps placed more emphasis on their sex than on their enlisted status. Interested in their welfare and in the success of recruiting programs, she wanted Wacs to work shorter hours than was customary for enlisted men assigned to ward duties, to be used only as technicians and not as ward orderlies or kitchen workers, and to be given grades commensurate with technical duties performed.[60] Aware of difficulties which hospital commanders encountered in manning installations in compliance with War Department policies, The Surgeon General wished to give them as much flexibility as possible in the employment of military personnel. Therefore, he emphasized the enlisted status of Wacs and insisted that they should not be given preferential treatment, just because they were women, in jobs, work-hours, or grades.[61] This attitude, along with the kind of jobs to which some Wacs in hospitals were assigned, laid the Medical Department open to the accusation in the fall of 1944 that it sidestepped recruiting promises.[62]

In the winter of 1944–45 The Surgeon General almost lost out in the controversy over policies on Wac employment. In December 1944 G–1 ruled that Wacs should work the same hours as nurses

[57] (1) Tables on basic data and ratios of gen, regional, sta, and conv hosps. Off file, Resources Anal Div SGO. (2) Diary, Hosp Admin Div, 25 Jan 44. HD: 024.7–3.

[58] (1) Treadwell, *op. cit.*, Ch. XIX, gives from the WAC viewpoint a full discussion of both the recruiting of Wacs for, and their use by, the Medical Department. (2) Blanchfield and Standlee, Organized Nursing, pp. 489–93, have a discussion of the nurses' aide recruiting campaign.

[59] (1) Ltr, SG to CG ASF attn Dir Mil Pers Div, 23 May 45, sub: Asgmt of MD Enl Pers (WAC). SG: 322.5–1(WAC) 1945. (2) Ltr, SG to CG ASF attn Dir Mil Pers Div, 23 Jun 45, sub: Tng of Enl Pers (WAC). Same file. (3) Quarterly Rpts, 2d and 3d Qtrs (1 Jun and 1 Oct) 1945, Enl Pers Br Mil Pers Div SGO. HD.

[60] Ltr WDWAC 720 (29 Jun 44), Dir WAC to CG ASF, 29 Jun 44, sub: WAC Duties on KP Detail and Hosp Orderly Asgmt. AG: 220.3 "WAC(29 Jun 44) (2)."

[61] (1) T/S, SG to ACofS G–1 WDGS, 31 Oct 44, sub: WAC Pers Asgd to Hosp Duties. AG: 220.3 "WAC (29 Jun 44)(2)." (2) Memo, Dir Tng Div SGO for Chief Prof Admin Serv SGO, 22 Nov 44. HD: 353 "WAC Gen."

[62] (1) T/S SPGAM/322.5 WAC(6 Sep 44)–97, CG ASF to ACofS G–1 WDGS, 12 Sep 44, sub: WAC Duties on KP Detail and Hosp Orderly Asgmts. AG: 220.3 "WAC(29 Jun 44)(2)." (2) Blanchfield and Standlee, Organized Nursing, p. 494.

(normally less than those of enlisted men employed in wards).[63] The following month the Chief of Staff, in approving a recruiting program for Wacs for the Medical Department, directed that WAC table-of-organization or table-of-distribution companies should be organized for general hospitals. The table of distribution that was adopted listed only technical jobs, except for company administrative work, and contained no grades lower than that of technician fifth grade (the equivalent of corporal).[64] If the wishes of the WAC director had been followed, all of the Wacs already serving in hospitals under the bulk-allotment system would have been either assigned to these companies or transferred from hospitals. Either action would have deprived hospitals of the use of Wacs as ward orderlies, drivers, clerks, cooks, and bakers. The Surgeon General objected to such an arrangement and the General Staff then agreed that general hospitals might retain some Wacs, without assigning them to table-of-distribution companies, for use in nontechnical jobs.[65] After V-J Day WAC companies were disbanded and the Medical Department returned to the former system of employing enlisted women, along with enlisted men, as part of its bulk allotment of military personnel.

As hospital commanders employed greater numbers of Wacs, some reported that they could be used in all departments on almost every type of job, but others believed that Wacs could not replace enlisted men on a one-for-one basis in the wards and kitchens of hospitals, where the work was heavy and the hours long.[66] To keep enough men in such places for heavy work, the General Staff approved The Surgeon General's proposal that the number of enlisted women assigned to wards and diet kitchens should not exceed 40 percent of the total enlisted staff.[67]

While some hospital commanders resented limitations upon their authority to select the jobs and set the duty-hours of Wacs, the most common problem in employing them was one of morale. Nurses rarely thought of enlisted women in terms of the nursing service and objected to their assumption of many professional nursing duties.[68] Because of misleading recruiting publicity, Wacs came to expect more opportunities in the nursing care of patients than was warranted, and many were disillusioned and disappointed when they found their actual jobs less glamorous than had been depicted.[69] Enlisted men resented the preferential treatment which Wacs received in the matters of rank and working conditions. Wacs in turn resented

[63] DF WDGAP 220.3 WAC, ACofS G-1 WDGS to SG thru CG ASF, 26 Dec 44, sub: WAC Pers Asgd to Hosp Duties. AG: 220.3 "WAC (29 Jun)(2)."

[64] T/D 8-1037, WAC Hosp Co (ZI), 17 Feb 45. SG: 322.5-1 (WAC) 1945.

[65] (1) Mins, Mtg Held in Off of Dir WAC, 9 Mar 45. SG: 322.5-1 (WAC) 1945. (2) Memo, Act Chief Pers Serv SGO for SG, 14 Mar 45, sub: WAC Recruiting Program for T/D Co at Named Gen hosps. Same file. (3) Memo, Lt Col E. R. Whitehurst for Dir Tng Div SGO, 18 Jul 45. Same file. (4) Quarterly Rpt, 1st and 2d Qtrs, 1945, Enl Pers Br Mil Pers Div SGO. HD.

[66] (1) An Rpts, 1944 and 45, Lovell, Wakeman, Baker, Percy Jones, Baxter, Birmingham, Beaumont, Ashford, and Crile Gen Hosps, and Waltham, Ft. Knox, and Cps Polk and Barkeley Regional Hosps; and Quarterly Rpt. 3d Qtr (2 Oct 44) 1944, Enl Pers Br Mil Pers Div SGO. HD. (2) Weekly Summary of Daily Diaries, Hosp and Dom Oprs SGO, 14 Jul 45. HD: 024.7-3.

[67] (1) Memo SPMCQ 300.5(WD Cir), SG for Dir Publication Div AGO thru CG ASF and ACofS G-1 WDGS, 31 Jan 45, sub: Proposed WD Cir. . . . AG: 220.3 "WAC (29 Jun 44)(2)." (2) WD Cir 71, 6 Mar 45.

[68] Blanchfield and Standlee, Organized Nursing, pp. 487, 594.

[69] Treadwell, *op. cit.*, Ch. XIX, and Blanchfield and Standlee, Organized Nursing, p. 487.

preferential treatment accorded civilian nurses and nurses' aides.[70] Despite these difficulties, Wacs became valuable and integral parts of hospital staffs by the end of the war.[71]

Use of Prisoners of War in Army Hospitals

A final category of personnel which proved advantageous in the operation of hospitals in the United States was prisoners of war. Hospitals began to use them during 1944 and by the end of the year some general hospitals employed as many as two or three hundred each. They continued to be used until their repatriation in 1945. Normally, prisoners of war were not used in wards in the care of patients. The most common place for their employment was in kitchens and messes and on buildings and grounds. In some hospitals they served also in warehouses, motor pools, laundries, post exchanges, and orthopedic shops. Some prisoners had skilled trades and others were skilled technicians. Hospital commanders used them, when desirable, on jobs for which they had been trained. Generally, prisoners of war seem to have been an industrious, easily managed lot, who did their work efficiently and well so long as they were properly supervised.[72]

The record of the Medical Department's experience in manning hospitals leads to two conclusions. In the first place, during the earliest part of the war Army hospitals had larger staffs than they actually needed to maintain a satisfactory standard of care, for the Surgeon General's Office itself was agreeable to some reductions in 1944 when necessity required them. It is a moot point whether or not the reductions required by policies and practices of the War Department Manpower Board and ASF headquarters were too great. In the second place, experience showed that hospitals could be operated with a lower ratio of doctors and able-bodied enlisted men to total hospital staffs than had been thought possible. The Surgeon General's Office resisted the substitution of Medical Administrative Corps officers for doctors in administrative positions as well as the substitution of civilians, limited service enlisted men, and Wacs for able-bodied enlisted men; but when necessity or directives from higher authority compelled these steps to be taken experience proved that they were not disastrous.

This is not to say that the practice of reducing the staffs of hospitals and of substituting personnel of various kinds for able-bodied enlisted men had no adverse effect upon hospital operations. On the contrary, as shown above, changes in personnel created serious problems for hospital commanders. Furthermore, opinion differed about the effect of those changes upon the quality of professional care. Many hospital commanders reported that

[70] (1) Draft Ltr, SG to CG ASF, 23 Jul 45, sub: Discipline and Morale of ASF Trps. (2) Memo, Consultant Women's Health and Welfare Unit SGO for Chief Pers Serv SGO, 28 Jul 45, sub: Use of WAC in Army Med Instls. Both in SG: 322.5-1 (WAC).

[71] (1) Rpt, Subcmtee on Employment of Mil Med Resources to the Exec Sec, Cmtee on Med and Hosp Serv of the Armed Forces, 25 May 48, p. 542. HD. (2) Memo, Dep Dir Educ and Tng Div SGO for Spec Planning Div SGO, 17 Apr 46, sub: Wacs in Postwar Mil Estab. HD: 353 "WAC Gen."

[72] (1) An Rpts, 1944, Percy Jones, Ashford, Baker, Letterman, and Halloran Gen Hosps, and Cp Barkeley and Ft McClellan Regional Hosps; and An Rpts, 1945, Birmingham, Lovell, Baker, Baxter, and Ashford Gen Hosps and Waltham and Cp Shelby Regional Hosps. HD. (2) Mins, 6th Conf of SvC Comdrs, Edgewater Park, Miss, 1-3 Feb 45, p. 192. HD: 337.

they continued to maintain high standards; but some, as well as certain service command surgeons and indeed the chief of the Surgeon General's Hospital Division, believed that medical care suffered as a result of changes in both the quality and quantity of personnel assigned to hospital staffs.[73]

On the other hand, a group of nonmedical officers who investigated complaints of the hospital commander at Fort Jackson (South Carolina) during the spring of 1944 believed that many hospital commanders became "panicky" when faced with changes in their staffs and that most of their problems were capable of solution through "determined and efficient personnel management." [74] Certainly the problems of hospital commanders would have been fewer and the possibility of adverse effects upon professional care less if changes eventually made in hospital staffs, as well as measures to improve personnel management in hospitals, had been initiated early in the war by the Medical Department itself.

[73] (1) See above, pp. 249–59. (2) Interv, MD Historians with Brig Gen Albert H. Schwichtenberg, 29 Apr 52. HD: 000.71.

[74] Proceedings, Bd of Offs Held at Ft Jackson, SC, 1–4 May 44, Pursuant to Verbal Orders CG [ASF]. HRS: SPGA/320.2 Med.

CHAPTER XV

Improvements in the Internal Organization and Administration of Hospitals in the United States

In the latter half of the war, reductions in the staffs of hospitals and changes in their make-up made more imperative than formerly the improvement of hospital organization and administration. It will be recalled that the Wadhams Committee had recommended such action as early as November 1942 and as a result The Surgeon General had brought into his Office in the spring of 1943 an experienced hospital administrator, Lt. Col. Basil C. MacLean. In his opinion preliminary studies confirmed the need for improvement.[1] Moreover, as the Army's manpower shortage became serious in the fall of 1943, ASF headquarters began a general program for the more efficient use of personnel. Extending to all technical and supply services, including the Medical Department, it comprehended the standardization of organization, the elimination of nonessential activities and records, the simplification of work methods, and the improvement of administrative procedures.[2] As a part of this program and of efforts to shorten periods of patient-stay in hospitals, the ASF Control Division and the Surgeon General's Office began work in the fall of 1943 on the simplification and standardization of the disability-discharge procedure, already discussed. By the following January, General Somervell informed Surgeon General Kirk that he considered improvement of hospital administration one of the Medical Department's major problems. About a month later, at a service command conference in Dallas, Tex., he directed the chief of the Surgeon General's Operations Service, Brig. Gen. Raymond W. Bliss, to "undertake to be the lead-off man in a study of

[1] (1) Memo, Lt Col Basil C. MacLean, SGO, for Brig Gen Raymond W. Bliss thru Col A[lbert] H. Schwichtenberg, 6 Nov 43, sub: Observations Based on Recent Visits . . . to Nine Gen Hosps. Off files, Gen Bliss' Off SGO, "Util of MCs in ZI" (19) #1. (2) Memo, MacLean for Bliss thru Schwichtenberg, 2 Feb 44, sub: More Efficient Util of Army Hosp Fac. Off files, Gen Bliss' Off SGO, "Util of Army Hosp Fac."

[2] History of Control Division, ASF, 1942-45, pp. 31-55, 160-66, 182-83. HD.

the simplification of this Medical Department paper-work." [3]

Simplification of Administrative Procedures

A basis for the study directed by General Somervell was laid during the spring of 1944. Work on the disability-discharge procedure had already demonstrated the value of simplification and standardization and about a week before the Dallas conference the Surgeon General's Hospital Division had asked his Control Division to review hospital administrative procedures generally. The latter Division called for assistance upon the ASF Control Division, which had had experience and which had personnel qualified in such matters. In April 1944 these Divisions, assisted by service command control divisions, surveyed records and procedures used at Schick, O'Reilly, and Halloran General Hospitals and outlined a broad program for succeeding months. Studies were to be made to simplify hospital organization, hospital admissions, ward administration, fiscal procedures, mess management, hospital statistics, nursing administration procedures, personnel office procedures, information office procedures, and hospital dispositions. To prevent swamping hospitals with revised but imperfect procedures, the Hospital and Control Divisions of the Surgeon General's Office insisted that each revised procedure should be approved by professional consultants of that Office and tested in selected hospitals before general adoption. To avoid unnecessary delays in their use, procedures were to be studied separately and, when revised and tested, were to be issued as parts of a loose-leaf manual on hospital administration.[4]

Several difficulties were encountered in carrying out this program. Short of personnel because it had reduced its own staff as an example to others, the Surgeon General's Control Division had only one officer who could devote his full time to that work. The Division also lacked personnel qualified by training and experience to make procedural studies and to draft procedural manuals in the form desired by ASF headquarters. Furthermore, its director was absent on special overseas missions during much of 1944 and work on the program suffered from his absence. To overcome some of these difficulties, the Surgeon General's Office temporarily borrowed personnel from the ASF Control Division, from Army hospitals, and from other installations. Even so, the ASF Control Division considered progress on the program unsatisfactory and threatened, early in 1945, to take over its completion. The Surgeon General prevented such action, but friction between his Office and the ASF Control Division continued.[5] As a result of these difficulties, and of delays

[3] (1) Memo, Lt Gen Brehon B. Somervell, CG ASF for SG, 18 Jan 44. HRS: Hq ASF Somervell files, "SG 1944." (2) Mins, ASF Conf of CGs of SvCs, Dallas, Tex., 17–19 Feb 44. HD: 337.

[4] (1) Memo, Act Dir Control Div SGO for Dir Control Div ASF, 10 Feb 44, sub: Proposed Study of Admin Procedures and Records Used in Gen Hosps. SG: 323.7-5 (Gen Hosp). (2) Memo, Dep SG for CG ASF attn Dir Control Div ASF, 14 Mar 45, sub: Improvement of Hosp Admin Procedures. SG: 300.7. (3) History of Control Division, ASF, 1942–45, App, pp. 357–59. HD.

[5] (1) Memo, Maj J. B. Joynt, Control Div ASF for Col A. G. Erpf, Control Div ASF, 18 Dec 44, sub: Problems on Hosp Manual. (2) Memo, Col A. G. Erpf, Control Div ASF for Col O. A. Gottschalk, Control Div ASF, 18 Dec 44, sub: Control Div SGO. (3) Memo SPMCQ 300.7, Dep SG for CG ASF attn Dir Control Div ASF, 14 Mar 45, sub: Improvement in Hosp Admin Procedures. (4) Memo, Col A. G. Erpf for Col O. A. Gottschalk, 17 Mar 45. All in HRS: Hq ASF Control Div file, "SGO." (5) Memo, Act Dir Control Div ASF for Act CofS ASF, 5 Apr 45, sub:

inherent in testing revised procedures before adopting them for general use, only one chapter of the projected manual—that on hospital admissions—was published before the peak patient load was reached in the United States. Other revised procedures—those for linen control, disability discharges, and disability retirements—were published in separate manuals or circulars before that date.

The hospital admissions procedure can be used to illustrate both the manner in which new procedures were developed and the methods used to simplify hospital paper work. The Control Division of the Surgeon General's Office, in consultation with the Hospital Division, developed a tentative procedure for the admission of patients, and, along with it, the forms to be used. Before these forms were published, they were approved by the ASF Control Division, the Air Surgeon's Office, the Surgeon General's Control, Professional Services, Hospital, and Medical Statistics Divisions, and the Adjutant General's Methods Management Branch.[6] The new procedure was then given a preliminary trial in three hospitals—two of the Service Forces and one of the Air Forces.[7] After they had commented on its advantages and disadvantages, it was revised and published in a tentative manual of hospital procedures.[8] Soon afterward, the Surgeon General's Office called a conference in Washington to explain the new procedure to representatives of various hospitals.[9] Selected hospitals, serving as pilot installations, then began to use the procedure and to teach representatives from other hospitals how to employ it.[10] Finally, early in 1945, the new procedure was published in final form as a chapter of the new manual on hospital administration (TM 8-262), and by the middle of that year almost all hospitals with as many as ten admissions a day had begun to adopt it.[11]

While the revised procedure covered in somewhat greater detail than did the old one the various steps taken in the admission of patients, its greatest significance lay in changes in hospital admission records and their preparation. Two basic forms were prepared for the admission of patients to hospitals: the clinical record brief and the medical report card. In addition, other records such as deposit slips for patients' funds and locator cards for use by interested groups in hospitals were prepared to meet local needs only. Under

Status of Hosp Admin Procedures. SG: 323.3 (Hosp). (6) Memo, CG ASF for SG, 7 Apr 45, same sub. Same file. (7) Memo, SG for Act CofS ASF, 12 Apr 45, same sub. Same file. (8) Memo, Dir Control Div [SGO] for Dir HD [SGO], 23 Jun 45, sub: An Rpt of Control Div for FY 1945. HD: 319.1-2-(Control Div, SGO) FY 1945. The reason that Colonel MacLean took little or no part in the development of simplified administrative procedures, and left the Surgeon General's Office in the fall of 1944, is not clear to the writer.

[6] (1) Diary, Hosp Div SGO, 12 and 14 Jun 44. HD: 024.7-3. (2) Ltrs, SG to Chief Forms Design and Standardization Sec Methods Management Br Control Div ASF, 13 Jul 44, sub: Revision of MD Form 52 and Revision of WD MD Form 55A. SG: 315.

[7] (1) Memo, Capt H. S. Press, SGO for Mr W. A. Archibald, SGO, 30 Jun 44, sub: Progress of Hosp Procedures Simplification Project. SG: 323.7-5 (Gen Hosp).

[8] Manual of Hosp Procedures (Tentative), prepared by SGO Control Div, 1 Sep 44. HD.

[9] Ltr, CO Regional Hosp Cp Swift to CG 8th SvC attn SvC Surg, 1 Oct 44, sub: Rpt of Hosp Admin Procedure Conf Held in Washington, 25 Sep 44. SG: 337.-1.

[10] For example, see: An Rpts, 1944, Schick Gen Hosp, and Ft Jackson and Cp Swift Regional Hosps. HD.

[11] (1) Memo SPMCQ 300.7, SG for CG ASF, 14 Mar 45, sub: Improvement in Hosp Admission Procedures. HRS: Hq ASF Control Div file, "SGO." (2) An Rpt, FY 1945, Control Div SGO. HD. (3) TM 8-262, Admin of Fixed Hosps, ZI, Ch II, Hosp Admissions, 1 Feb 45.

the old procedure the two basic forms had to be typed in separate operations, for even though much information was common to them both, such as the patient's name, rank, serial number, organization, age, race, length of service, etc., those forms were blocked off differently. Other records had to be made up separately also, many by offices needing information found either on the clinical record brief or on the hospital's daily admission and disposition sheet. Under the revised procedure, all forms containing common information were blocked off alike and a mimeograph duplicator was used to transfer that information to as many copies as needed throughout the hospital. Thus one typing replaced fifteen or twenty under the old system. The chapter on the new admissions procedure illustrated each of these forms and gave detailed instructions for their preparation and distribution. In the opinion of the Surgeon General's Office, the new procedure speeded up the admission of patients, eliminated the duplication of records, supplied operating units of hospitals with information they had not formerly received, and saved in the hospitals where adopted a total of about 3,333 man-days of work per week.[12] Hospital commanders encountered only minor difficulties in installing the new procedure and, with few exceptions, considered it an improvement over the old one.[13]

As in the development of the admissions procedure which saved work for administrative officers, the Surgeon General's Office was equally interested in procedures that would relieve ward officers of administrative details in order to permit them to devote more time to professional work. One of the procedures developed during 1944, that for the control and distribution of hospital linens, was designed for this purpose. Developed in a manner similar to the hospital admissions procedure, the linen control procedure was published in December 1944 in an ASF circular rather than as a chapter of the hospital-administration manual.[14] Under the old procedure physicians were charged with the linen used in wards and clinics. In order to avoid being "caught short," they required ward personnel to count soiled linen as it left the ward and clean linen as it was returned. Furthermore, they required periodic inventories and some tended to hoard linen unnecessarily. Additional linen-counts were made at intermediate storage points and at hospital laundries. Under the new procedure each hospital had a linen officer who was responsible for all linen used. All counts of linen in wards and intermediate stations were eliminated; and linen officers, rather than ward officers, made periodic inventories. According to some hospitals, a disadvantage of this procedure was an excessive loss of linens. This was compensated for, in the opinion of the Surgeon General's Office and many hospital commanders, by the saving of about 1,250 man-days of work per month and

[12] (1) TM 8-262, Admin of Fixed Hosp, ZI, Ch II, Hosp Admissions, 1 Feb 45. (2) An Rpt, FY 1945, Control Div SGO; and An Rpt, FY 1945, Hosp and Dom Oprs SGO. HD.

[13] For example see: An Rpts, 1944, Baxter and Fitzsimons Gen Hosps; An Rpt, 1945, Birmingham Gen Hosp; An Rpts, 1944, Cps Crowder and Swift, and Ft Jackson Regional Hosps; An Rpts, 1945, Cp Wolters and Ft Bragg Regional Hosps. HD.

[14] (1) ASF Memo for Record, 11 Nov 44. AG: 427 (11 Nov 44) (2). (2) Ltr SPMCH 300.5 (ASF Cir), SG to AG, 30 Nov 44, sub: Proposed ASF Cir on Linen Control and Distribution Systems. Same file. (3) Rpt of Economies Effected through Procedures Studies Made by or jointly with Control Div ASF, 13 Apr 45. HRS: Hq ASF Control Div file, "Est Admin Savings Resulting from Procedural Revisions." (4) ASF Cir 395, 2 Dec 44.

the relief of doctors of administrative details. It was also reported that the new procedure decreased the hoarding of linen and speeded up its distribution to places where needed.[15]

The use of dictaphones in hospitals was not called for by manuals or circulars, but nevertheless constituted an important change in the method of preparing clinical records. Lack of enough medical stenographers in hospitals, as a result of the civilian labor shortage and of hospital personnel ceilings, made it necessary during 1943 for doctors themselves to prepare clinical records, sometimes in longhand. To relieve them of such a time-consuming process, hospitals began early in 1944 to acquire dictaphones. At convenient times doctors recorded on these machines consultation reports, progress notes, case histories, and final summaries. Clerks organized in central pools then transcribed the information recorded. This system of preparing clinical records permitted doctors to keep more complete and more legible records and to devote more attention to care of patients. It also contributed to the more efficient use of clerical personnel. Finally, by enabling doctors to keep clinical records up to date it helped to speed the disposition of patients and to shorten their period of hospitalization.[16]

The simplification of other administrative procedures was not completed before the peak patient load was reached, but work on the program continued during the winter of 1944 and the spring of 1945. Beginning in July 1945 chapters in the hospital-administration manual were published on the following subjects: Patients' Funds and Valuables (1 July 1945); Hospital Organization (1 July 1945); Ward Administration (1 October 1945 and 15 February 1946); Accounting Procedures for Hospital Funds (1 October 1945); Mess Administration (15 November 1945); Personnel Administration (28 December 1945 and 15 February 1946); Clinical Procedures (15 February 1946); and Supply Procedures (1 March 1946).[17]

Work-Measurement and Work-Simplification Programs

Delay in completing the manual on hospital administration did not interfere with the simplification of administrative procedures and work methods by hospitals themselves. As part of its program for efficient personnel utilization, early in 1943 ASF headquarters began to require subordinate installations to set up programs of "work simplification" and "work measurement." Work simplification was the process of reducing the jobs of individual workers, or the operations of groups of workers, to their simplest forms and eliminating from them all lost motion. Work measurement was the determination by various standards of the number of employees required for certain jobs or operations.[18] During 1944 and 1945 hos-

[15] (1) An Rpt, FY 1945, Hosp and Dom Oprs SGO; An Rpts, 1944, Lawson, Thayer, Oliver, and Ashburn Gen Hosps, and AAF Regional Hosp Keesler Fld; An Rpts, 1945, Birmingham and Lovell Gen Hosps, and Surg 7th SvC. HD. (2) Mins, Hosp Comdrs Conf, 7th SvC, 22 Aug 45. HD: 337.

[16] (1) Excerpts from rpts of various hosps on the use of dictaphones, Jun–Jul 44. SG: 413.51. (2) An Rpts, 1944, Ashburn, Deshon, Beaumont, Baxter, and Birmingham Gen Hosps, and Regional Hosps at Fts McClellan and Meade, Maxwell and Scott Flds, and Cps Shelby, Barkeley, Swift, and Crowder. HD.

[17] (1) TM 8–262, Admin of Fixed Hosps, ZI, dates listed. (2) An Rpt, FY 1945, Hosp and Dom Oprs SGO. HD.

[18] (1) History of Control Division, ASF, 1942–45, pp. 160–63; App, pp. 141–44 and 151–53. HD. (2) Memo, CG SOS for Dir Staff Divs, Cs of Sup and Admin Servs, CGs all SvCs, 1 Mar 43, sub: Work Simplification. SG: 024.–1.

pital control officers appointed as a result of ASF headquarters' emphasis upon management techniques (or administrative engineering) conducted work-measurement and work-simplification studies and proposed changes to save time and personnel in a multiplicity of functions and activities.[19] For example, a survey of ward attendants' duties at Walter Reed General Hospital in the spring of 1944 showed that attendants spent 20 percent of their time in off-the-ward errands. To correct that situation a delivery service staffed with twenty people was set up, and forty ward attendants were released.[20] Another hospital, Thayer General Hospital, made changes in its system of trash collection that saved 200 man-hours per month. At still another Ashford General Hospital, a reallocation of individual duties and a rearrangement of office and desk space in the registrar's office permitted the completion in 1944 of 4,911 more work-units in 9,600 fewer work-hours than in the year before. Seventeen work-measurement and work-simplification studies made at Newton D. Baker General Hospital during 1944 resulted in the saving of 2,844 man-hours per month. Other hospitals reported similar savings from local changes.[21] In this way, hospitals adjusted their operations to performance by reduced staffs and management control became an established function in all large Army hospitals.[22]

Additional Activities and Their Place in the Organizational Structure of Hospitals

In the latter half of the war new professional and administrative activities were added to Army hospitals. When convalescent reconditioning was established as an Army program, hospital commanders placed that activity in a variety of locations in their organizational structures; but by February 1944 the Surgeon General's Office concluded that reconditioning should be considered as a professional service on a par with medical and surgical services. The next month, with the approval of ASF headquarters, the chief of The Surgeon General's Reconditioning Division announced this decision as policy at a conference of reconditioning officers at Schick General Hospital.[23] Two other changes occurred in the professional services during 1943 and 1944. Gradually hospitals began to list nursing as a professional rather than an administrative service and to show neuropsychiatry as an independent service rather than as a section of the medical service.[24]

---

[19] In an interview on 20 November 1951 General Kirk stated that he thought too much emphasis had been placed upon the "workload business." In his opinion workload studies were expensive and "did not pay more than ten cents on the dollar." HD: 314 (Correspondence MS)V.

[20] Work Simplification Rpt, 8 Apr 44, sub: Delivery Serv, Walter Reed Gen Hosp. SG: 323.7-5(Walter Reed GH)K.

[21] An Rpts, 1944, Thayer, Ashford, Newton D. Baker, O'Reilly, Kennedy, Baxter, Schick, and Birmingham Gen Hosps; An Rpts, 1945, Crile and Battey Gen Hosps. HD.

[22] (1) Memo, Dir Control Div SGO for Dir HD SGO, 23 Jun 45, sub: An Rpt of Control Div for FY 1945. HD: 319.1-2 (Control Div, SGO) FY 1945. (2) SG Cir 119, 15 Sep 50, sub: Orgn of US Army Hosps Designated as Class II Instls or Activities, provided for a management office in each Army hospital designated as a Class II installation or activity (that is, general hospitals operating in 1950 under the direct control of SGO).

[23] (1) An Rpts, 1944, Baxter, Finney, Crile, Lawson, Vaughan, and Fletcher Gen Hosps. HD. (2) Ltr, Act SG to CG ASF, 15 Mar 44, sub: Orgn Chart, Reconditioning Program, with 1st ind, CG ASF to SG, 17 Mar 44. Off file, Physical Med Consultants Div SGO, "Reconditioning, Gen (Policy)." (3) An Rpt, Reconditioning Conf, Schick Gen Hosp, 21-22 Mar 44, p. 17. HD: 353.9 Schick Gen Hosp.

[24] See annual reports of hospitals on file in HD.

Additional administrative activities in hospitals came largely as a result of their introduction generally in ASF installations. Revision of the ASF organization manual in December 1943 caused addition of control officers to serve as staff advisers on administrative, procedural, and management problems.[25] About the same time authority was granted all ASF installations having a strength of 2,000 or more to appoint special services officers to conduct athletics and recreation programs and orientation officers (later called information and education officers) to conduct information and education programs.[26] In February 1944 ASF headquarters directed the establishment on each of its posts of a personal affairs division to assist soldiers in handling their personal affairs.[27] In the following December the War Department directed separation centers and many hospitals (those separating from the service one hundred or more persons monthly) to set up classification and counseling units to assist soldiers in planning their return to civilian life.[28] General hospitals with few exceptions and regional hospitals in some instances came within the purview of these directives and acted accordingly. These new activities—special services, information and education, personal affairs, and classification and counseling—were to be known later as "welfare services" or as "individual services."

Effect on Hospitals of the ASF Standard Plan for Post Organization

The general program of ASF headquarters to standardize organization throughout the Service Forces continued, as it had earlier, to influence the organization of general hospitals.[29] In December 1943 the standard plan for the organization of ASF posts was revised. At that time a control officer and a post inspector general were added to form, along with the existing public relations officer, the commanding officer's immediate staff. Furthermore, the seven functional divisions which previously comprised all post activities were replaced by seven administrative and seven technical staff units. To make this change, the erstwhile Administrative Division, a functional division which had included the adjutant, judge advocate, and fiscal officer, was abolished and its officials were listed among the seven administrative staff units. Certain technical services—quartermaster, ordnance, chemical warfare, signal, and transportation—were relieved from their former subordination to the Supply Division and were established as independent technical staff units. Medical and engineer activities, considered as functional divisions under the old plan, now became technical staff units. All welfare activities continued, under the new post plan, to be grouped under the Personnel Division.[30]

General hospitals attempted to adjust themselves to the new organizational plan for ASF posts as they had to its predecessor. In each hospital, professional services and some administrative units peculiar to hospitals, such as the registrar's office and the dietetics division, had to be added to the units included in the standard ASF plan. In the administrative field, hospitals made adjustments in various ways. Baxter

---

[25] For example, see An Rpts, 1944, Baxter, Woodrow Wilson, Schick, and Mayo Gen Hosp. HD.

[26] (1) ASF Cir 127, 20 Nov 43. (2) WD Cir 360, 5 Sep 44.

[27] ASF Cir 31, 7 Feb 44.

[28] WD Cir 486, 29 Dec 44.

[29] See above, p. 123.

[30] ASF Manual M 301, Pt IV, Rev 2, 15 Dec 43. Also see above, *Chart 13*.

General Hospital, for example, followed the ASF plan carefully, at least in its organization chart, and only added to the post organization a reconditioning division, a medical supply office, a medical detachment, and a professional division that included the professional services and such administrative units as the registrar's and dietitian's offices. Mayo General Hospital adhered less strictly to the ASF plan. Although it had most of the officers which that plan called for, it placed many who were supposed to be grouped under an intermediate supervisor, such as special services and personal affairs officers, in a direct relationship with the commanding officer.[31] *(Chart 12)* Hospitals that thus multiplied the number of officers reporting directly to the commander violated one of the ASF principles of organization, namely, that the number of such officers should be kept as small as possible.[32] Several hospitals on the other hand followed that principle (and incidentally a recommendation made by the Wadhams Committee in the fall of 1942) by combining their administrative services under a single director and their professional services under another.[33] In February 1945 the commanding officer of Darnall General Hospital suggested that this grouping of professional and administrative services under separate directors, who in turn were responsible to the commanding officer, might be followed with advantage by all other hospitals.[34]

Two other changes were considered desirable to make the ASF post organization applicable to all hosiptals. Officers in the Third Service Command headquarters and in the Surgeon General's Office, as well as some hospital commanders, believed that technical service officers with only minor functions in hospitals, such as those of the Chemical Warfare Service, Ordnance Department, and Transportation Corps, should be either eliminated or subordinated—as they had been under the previous ASF post organization—to a director of supply.[35] Conversely, because officers concerned with the individual welfare of soldiers (special services, personal affairs, information and education, and classification and counseling officers) assumed more importance in hospitals than in other installations, some hospital commanders and service command surgeons felt that they should be grouped together under a director of individual services rather than under the director of personnel.[36]

Emergence of Standard Plans for Hospitals

Early in May 1944 the Surgeon General's Office announced that it was planning to publish a standard plan for the organization of general hospitals, but its development was delayed because of shortage of personnel in the Control Divi-

[31] See annual reports of hospitals named. HD

[32] ASF Manual M 301, 15 Aug 44, Pt I, Sec 103.02, sub: Principles of Orgn.

[33] (1) An Rpts, 1944, Cp Barkeley and Scott Fld Regional Hosps. HD. (2) 1st ind, CO Staten Island Area Sta Hosp to CG 2d SvC attn SvC Surg, 3 Mar 45, on Ltr, CG 2d SvC (Surg) to CO Staten Island Area Sta Hosp, 24 Feb 45, sub: Orgn Chart. HD: 323 "Hosp Orgn."

[34] Ltr, CO Darnall Gen Hosp to CG 5th SvC attn SvC Surg, 22 Feb 45, sub: Standard Orgn Charts of Gen, Regional, and Sta Hosps, with incl. HD: 323 "Hosp Orgn."

[35] (1) Orgn Chart prepared by 3d SvC Hq, [1944]. HD: 323 "Hosp Orgn." (2) Interv, MD Historian with Dr. H. A. Press, formerly of SGO Control Div, 1944–45, 9 Oct 50. HD: 000.71. (3) An Rpts, 1944, Mayo, Valley Forge, Ashburn, and Baker Gen Hosp. HD.

[36] Ltrs from 4th and 5th SvC Surgs, and COs of Darnall, Nichols, O'Reilly, and Schick Gen Hosps. HD: 323 "Hosp Orgn."

CHART 12—ORGANIZATION OF MAYO GENERAL HOSPITAL, 1944

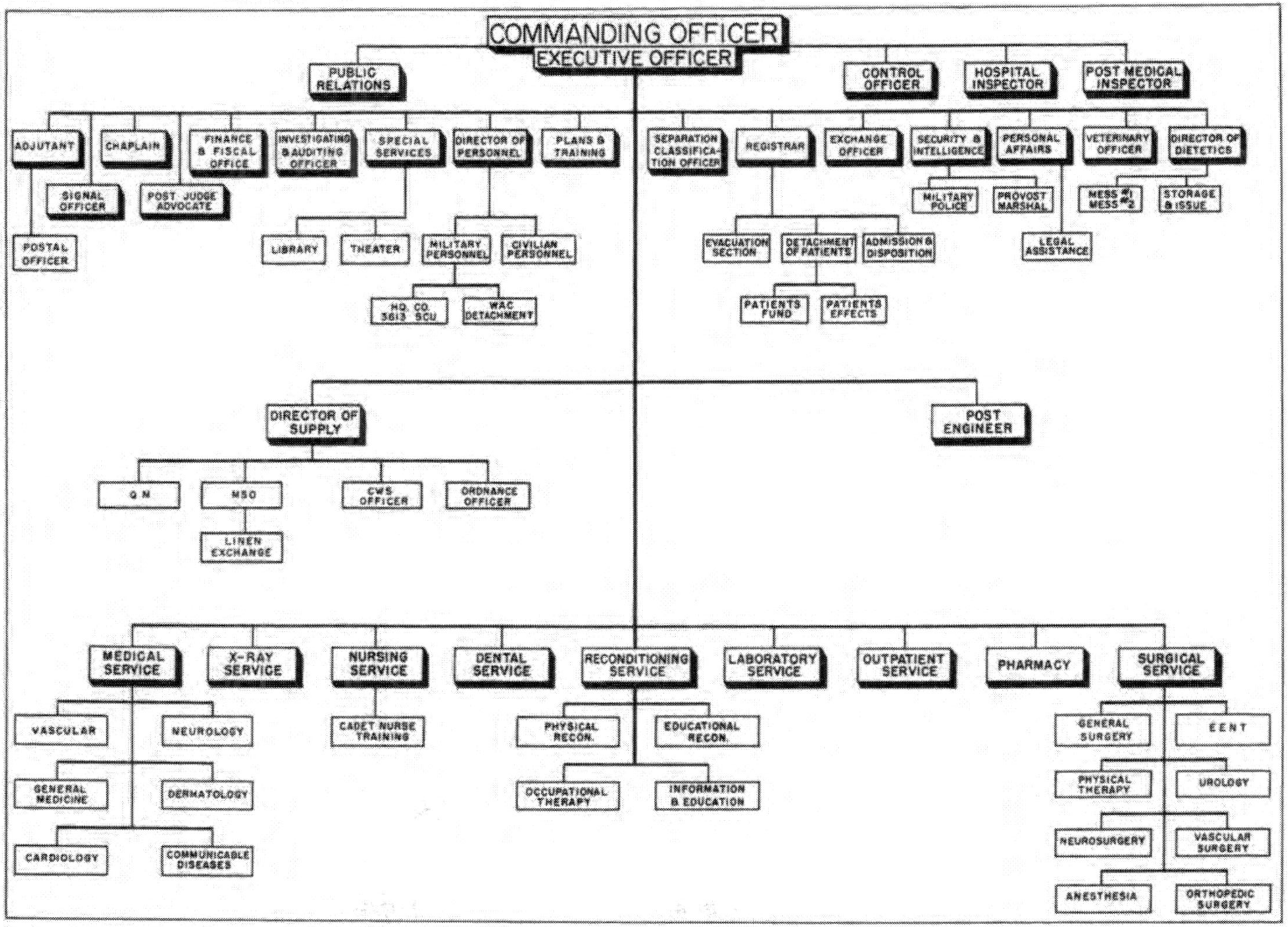

sion and priority given to procedures for disability discharges and hospital admissions.[37] Meanwhile, the surgeon of the Fourth Service Command worked out a standard plan for the organization of hospitals under his supervision.[38] Then, in June and July 1944 the surgeon and the control officer of the Third Service Command, with assistance from the Surgeon General's Office, developed a standard plan for hospitals in that Command. After it had been tested for about six months, The Surgeon General submitted it for comment in February 1945 to other service commands. On the basis of their suggestions, he made minor changes in the Third Service Command plan and adopted it as standard for general, regional, and station hospitals.[39] It was published in July 1945 as a chapter of the manual on hospital administration.[40] The Surgeon General's Office also worked during this period on the organization of convalescent hospitals and hospital centers. Tentative plans were published in 1944 and 1945. The final plan for convalescent hospitals was published in December 1945, but that for hospital centers remained unpublished because they began to close before it was completed.[41]

During the movement to standardize hospital organization, the merits of such a step were freely discussed. Hospital commanders generally and service command surgeons in some instances raised arguments against inflexible standardization. One feared that it would crystallize hospital organization, increasing efficiency in the operation of some installations but prohibiting imaginative and capable commanders from making valuable innovations in others.[42] Some felt that standardization would prevent hospital commanders from adjusting to local conditions. For example, hospitals giving little outpatient care might not need to establish separate outpatient services. Others believed that commanders needed freedom to fit their organizations to the personalities of officers assigned to them. An eye, ear, nose, and throat specialist of intense individualism and higher rank than a chief of surgical service, for instance, could hardly be successfully subordinated, in an EENT section, to the latter.[43] On the other hand, there was some feeling that men should be fitted to jobs, not jobs to men, and that the standardization of organization would help to solve problems raised by clashing personalities. The most telling arguments in favor of standardization were that it was the first step toward the simplification and standardization of administrative procedures, that it facilitated the measurement of work and of personnel require-

[37] (1) Rad, SG to CG 4th SvC attn SvC Surg, 3 Mar 44. SG: 323.7–5(4th SvC)AA. (2) Edward J. Morgan and Donald O. Wagner, The Organization of the Medical Department in the Zone of the Interior (1946), p. 145. HD. (3) Interv, MD Historian with Dr. Press, 9 Oct 50. HD: 000.71.

[38] (1) Rad, SG to CG 4th SvC attn SvC Surg, 3 Mar 44. SG: 323.7–5(4th CA)AA. (2) 1st ind, CG 4th SvC (Surg) to SG, 9 Mar 45, on Ltr SPMCH 323.3 (4th SvC)AA, SG to CG 4th SvC attn SvC Surg, 16 Feb 45, sub: Standard Orgn Charts of Gen, Regional, and Sta Hosps. HD: 323 "Hosp Orgn."

[39] (1) Ltr 323.3 (1st SvC)AA, SG to CG 1st SvC attn SvC Surg, 16 Feb 45, sub: Standard Orgn Charts of Gen, Regional, and Sta Hosps. Identical letters were sent to all service commands; these letters, with their replies, are on file in HD: 323 "Hosp Orgn." (2) Status of Procedures being Developed in SGO, [Apr 45]. HD.

[40] TM 8–262, Ch. I, Hosp Orgn, 1 Jul 45.

[41] (1) ASF Cirs 419, 22 Dec 44; 135, 16 Apr 45; and 445, 14 Dec 45. (2) Morgan and Wagner, *op. cit.*, p. 162.

[42] 1st ind, CG 7th SvC (Surg) to SG, 8 Mar 45, on Ltr 323.3 (7th SvC)AA, SG to CG 7th SvC attn SvC Surg, 16 Feb 45, sub: Standard Orgn Charts of Gen, Regional, and Sta Hosps. HD: 323 "Hosp Orgn."

[43] Letters from hospital commanders and service command surgeons expressing these opinions are on file, HD: 323 "Hosp Orgn."

ments, and that it promoted manpower economy.[44] At any rate, both the Surgeon General's Office and ASF headquarters were committed to standardization of hospital organization by the winter of 1944. That they did not insist on inflexibility was demonstrated by a proviso that hospital commanders might deviate from the standard plan if their respective service commanders approved.[45]

Details of the Medical Department's Standard Plans

The standard plan for the organization of general hospitals, published in July 1945, resembled the ASF plan for post organization and reflected the experience of hospitals in making adjustments to it. In both plans, the commander's immediate staff included public relations officers, control officers, and inspectors (called inspectors general on posts and medical inspectors in hospitals). General hospitals, according to the standard plan, were to have six of the seven administrative staff divisions of posts. The seventh, training, was to be subordinated to the personnel division. In addition, they were to have four administrative staff units not called for in the post organization plan. These were the station complement (medical detachment), the dietetics division, the veterinarian's office (for food inspection), and the registrar's office. The plan for hospitals had no technical staff divisions as such. Some, such as ordnance and chemical warfare, were eliminated completely; others, such as quartermaster and transportation, were subordinated to the supply division; and another, the engineer, was placed on the administrative staff. The welfare services, despite the wishes of hospital commanders, were left subordinated to the personnel division. The plan for hospital organization naturally included professional services. There were nine in general hospitals, including the reconditioning service, the neuropsychiatric service, and the nursing service. In this field hospital commanders were left with more latitude than in the administrative because, the manual stated, the professional services "function solely in a professional manner and are subject to constant variation by reason of changes in types of patients treated." The standard plan for regional and station hospitals resembled that for general hospitals. The chief differences were that administrative and technical units which existed as parts of post and general hospital organizations were eliminated and the neuropsychiatric service was subordinated, as a section, to the medical service.[46] *(Chart 13)*

Publication of the standard plan for the organization of general, regional, and station hospitals had little appreciable effect upon their organization.[47] The chief reason, perhaps, was that the plan itself reflected experiences of hospitals in conforming with ASF directives on organization.[48] Nevertheless it officially sanctioned their conformity and provided them with a detailed statement of the functions of all major units within hospitals. Undoubtedly its value would have been greater if pub-

[44] Ltr, SG to CG 1st SvC attn SvC Surg, 16 Feb 45, sub: Standard Orgn Charts of Gen, Regional, and Sta Hosps, with 1st ind and incl. HD: 323 "Hosp Orgn."

[45] TM 8-262, Ch. I, Sec I, 1 Jul 45.

[46] TM 8-262, Ch. I, 1 Jul 45.

[47] Morgan and Wagner, *op. cit.*, pp. 147-51, arrive at this conclusion after examining the data on organization given in the annual reports of 14 general and 19 regional hospitals for 1944 and 1945.

[48] Interv, MD Historian with Dr. Press, 9 Oct 50. HD: 000.71.

Chart 13—Comparison of Standard Plans for Organization of ASF Posts and ASF General Hospitals, 1945

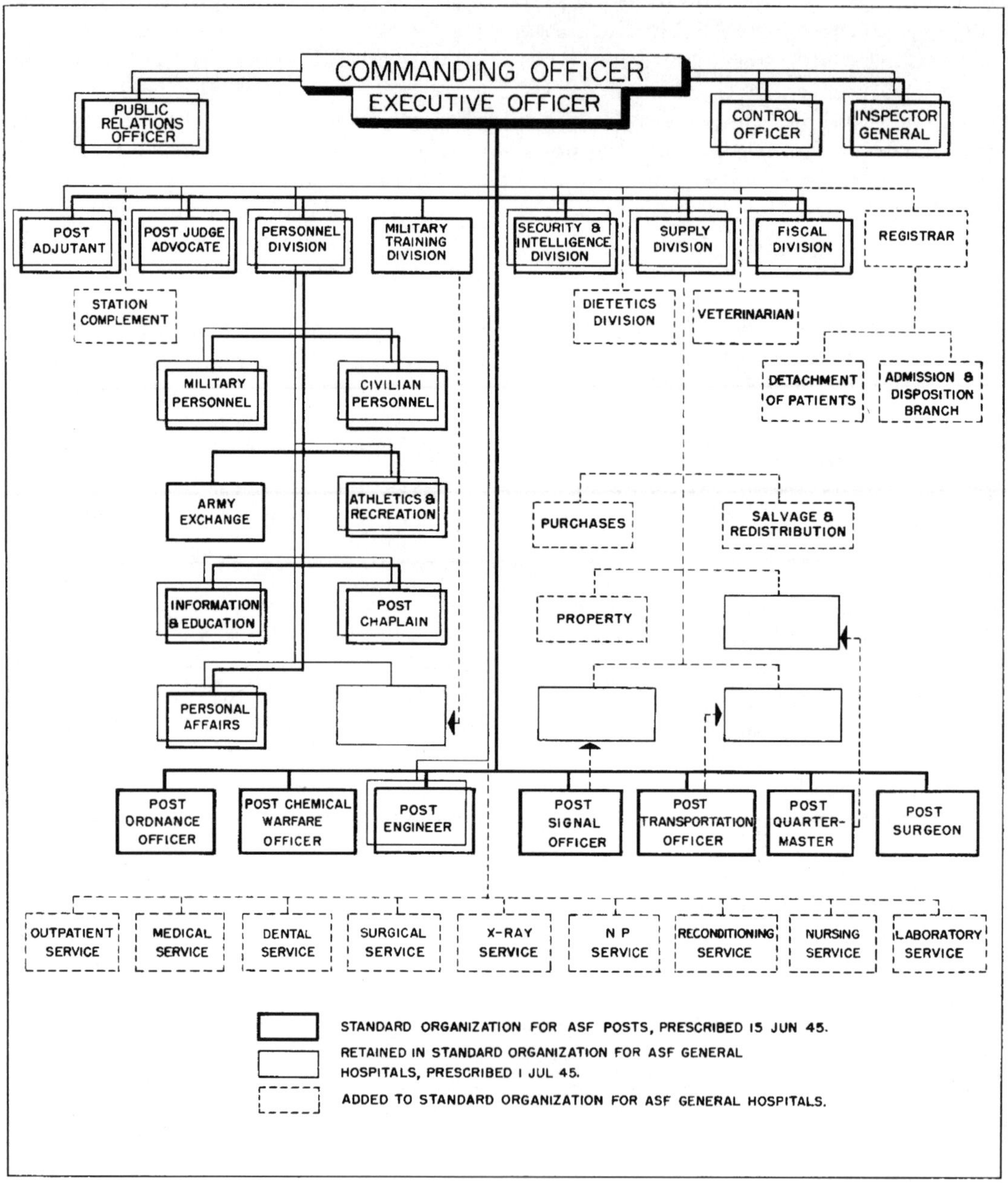

lished four years earlier, at a time when new hospitals were beginning to open with staccato rapidity.[49]

The development of standard organizational plans for convalescent hospitals and hospital centers came even later than for general hospitals and was therefore of less value. Having only limited amounts of personnel and no guides for organization, ASF convalescent hospitals were organized by their commanding officers to fit individual circumstances. Consequently they differed from one another in many respects. Convalescent hospitals that were separate installations attempted generally to organize administrative activities according to the standard ASF post plan.[50] Those that operated in conjunction with general hospitals depended upon the latter for some administrative services and organized for the rest as the personnel assigned to them permitted.[51] Gradually a common feature began to emerge. It was the establishment of a reconditioning section and the grouping of patients into companies, battalions, and/or regiments for administration and supervision.[52] In the winter of 1944, when additional emphasis was placed upon the convalescent program, the Surgeon General's Office developed and published a guide [53] which left the organization of administrative activities of convalescent hospitals almost entirely to the discretion of their commanders. The result was that, as they received more patients and operating personnel, some set up administrative offices that duplicated, or at least paralleled, those of the general hospitals located near by.[54] The guide showed in more detail the organization of convalescent activities. They were to be grouped in three divisions: a receiving division, an infirmary division, and a reconditioning division. The infirmary division was not to be established in convalescent hospitals located near general hospitals. The reconditioning division was to have a twofold function: it was to exercise command over patients who were to be organized in three battalions (neuropsychiatric, primary reconditioning, and advanced reconditioning), and it was to conduct the convalescent training program. This program was to include occupational therapy, physical reconditioning, educational reconditioning, and classification and counseling. The plan served as a guide to convalescent hospitals that remained separate installations during 1945, and it was used to some extent, particularly for the organization of convalescent activities, by those that became parts of hospital centers in the spring of that year. That hospitals considered it as a guide only is indicated by differences

[49] The plan of 1945 for general hospitals remained in force for five years. The Surgeon General's Office then published, on 15 September 1950, a new standard plan for their organization. It is of interest that this plan called for fewer major units within a hospital and charged two officers, the executive officer and the deputy commanding officer, with the co-ordination, if not the supervision, of the administrative and professional services respectively. SG Cir 119, 15 Sep 50, sub: Orgn of US Army Hosps Designated as Class II Instls or Activities.

[50] An Rpts, 1944, Mitchell Conv Hosp and Surg 4th SvC. HD.

[51] (1) An Rpts, 1944, Madigan and Percy Jones Gen and Conv Hosps. HD. (2) An Rpts, 1945, Brooke and Wakeman Hosp Ctrs, have reference to 1944 orgn. HD.

[52] An Rpts, 1944, Wakeman and Lovell Gen and Conv Hosps, and Cp Carson Conv Hosp. HD.

[53] ASF Cir 419, 22 Dec 44, Pt II, Conv Hosp—Revised Program.

[54] An Rpts, 1945, Percy Jones, Wakeman, and Cps Butner and Carson Hosp Ctrs. HD. These reports have discussions of organization of convalescent and general hospitals before they were combined to form centers.

CHART 14—STANDARD PLAN FOR ORGANIZATION OF ASF CONVALESCENT HOSPITALS, 1945

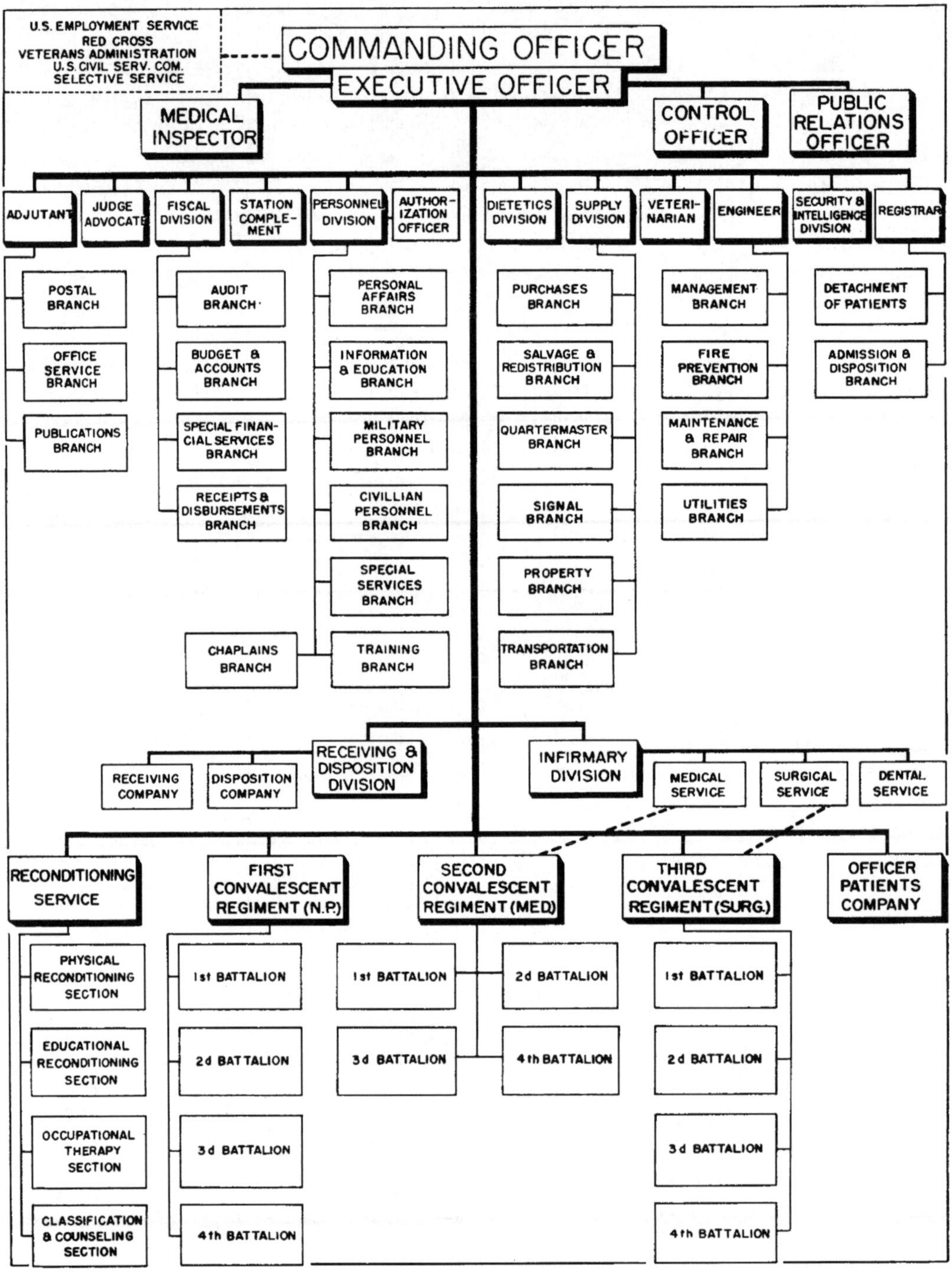

that continued to exist in the organization of different installations.[55]

At the end of 1945 a second plan for the organization of convalescent hospitals was developed by the Surgeon General's Office and published by ASF headquarters.[56] A combination of the old plan for convalescent hospitals and the new standard plan for general hospitals, it showed the administrative organization of convalescent hospitals in more detail than did the old one. The immediate staff of the commanding officer and the administrative staff units of convalescent hospitals were to be essentially the same as those prescribed for general hospitals. The convalescent services were to be similar to those called for by the 1944 guide for convalescent hospitals. The most important change was the separation of the reconditioning, or convalescent training, program from the administration of companies of patients. The chief of the reconditioning service was to have charge of the former, while the hospital commander was to supervise directly the commanders of the 1st convalescent regiment (neuropsychiatric), 2d convalescent regiment (medical), and 3d convalescent regiment (surgical). Publication of this plan after convalescent hospitals had already begun to close undoubtedly limited its effect upon the organization of such installations. *(Chart 14)*

The establishment of hospital centers in the spring of 1945 was expected to eliminate duplication of administrative activities involved in the operation at the same location of both convalescent and general hospitals. The Surgeon General's Office expected that administrative functions common to both would be centralized under center headquarters, but a guide for the organization of hospital centers published in April 1945 was sufficiently general to leave to local commanders the decision as to how much centralization there would be.[57] For that reason, and because of differences among hospital centers—some being located on posts with other activities and some constituting posts in themselves—centers varied in organization from one to another.[58] Two extremes were represented by the Percy Jones Hospital Center and the Wakeman Hospital Center. *(Chart 15)* The former, a post itself, had operating as well as supervisory functions, and administrative activities common to both the general and convalescent hospitals assigned to it were performed by center headquarters.[59] Wakeman, on the other hand, was located on a post with other Army activities that were nonmedical in character. Post headquarters furnished some administrative services for both the general and convalescent hospitals; each hospital performed the others itself; and center headquarters served in a supervisory, not an operational, capacity.[60]

In the hope of achieving a measure of uniformity in the organization of hospital centers, the Surgeon General's Office in July 1945 sent out the Percy Jones plan for comment by hospital center commanders

[55] (1) An Rpts, 1945, Welch and Cp Upton Conv Hosps. HD. (2) Orgn and Functional Charts, Percy Jones Hosp Ctr, 24 Apr 45; Orgn and Functional Charts, Brooke Hosp Ctr, 16 Aug 45; Orgn and Functions, Cp Edwards, Mass, Embracing the Post and the Hosp Ctr, 20 Aug 45; Orgn and Functional Manual, Cp Carson Hosp Ctr, 31 Jul 45. HD: 323 "Hosp Orgn."

[56] ASF Cir 445, 14 Dec 45, Pt II—Conv Hosp—Revised Program.

[57] (1) See above, pp. 198–99. (2) WD Cir 105, 4 Apr 45. (3) ASF Cir 135, 16 Apr 45.

[58] Morgan and Wagner, *op. cit.*, pp. 163–64.

[59] An Rpt, 1945, Percy Jones Hosp Ctr. HD.

[60] 2d ind, CO Wakeman Hosp Ctr to CG 5th SvC attn SvC Surg, 18 Jul 45, and 3d ind, Surg 5th SvC to SG, 9 Aug 45, on Ltr, SG to CG 5th SvC attn SvC Surg, 9 July 45, sub: Standard Orgn Charts for Hosps. SG: 323.3(5th SvC)AA.

CHART 15—ORGANIZATION OF PERCY JONES HOSPITAL CENTER, 1945

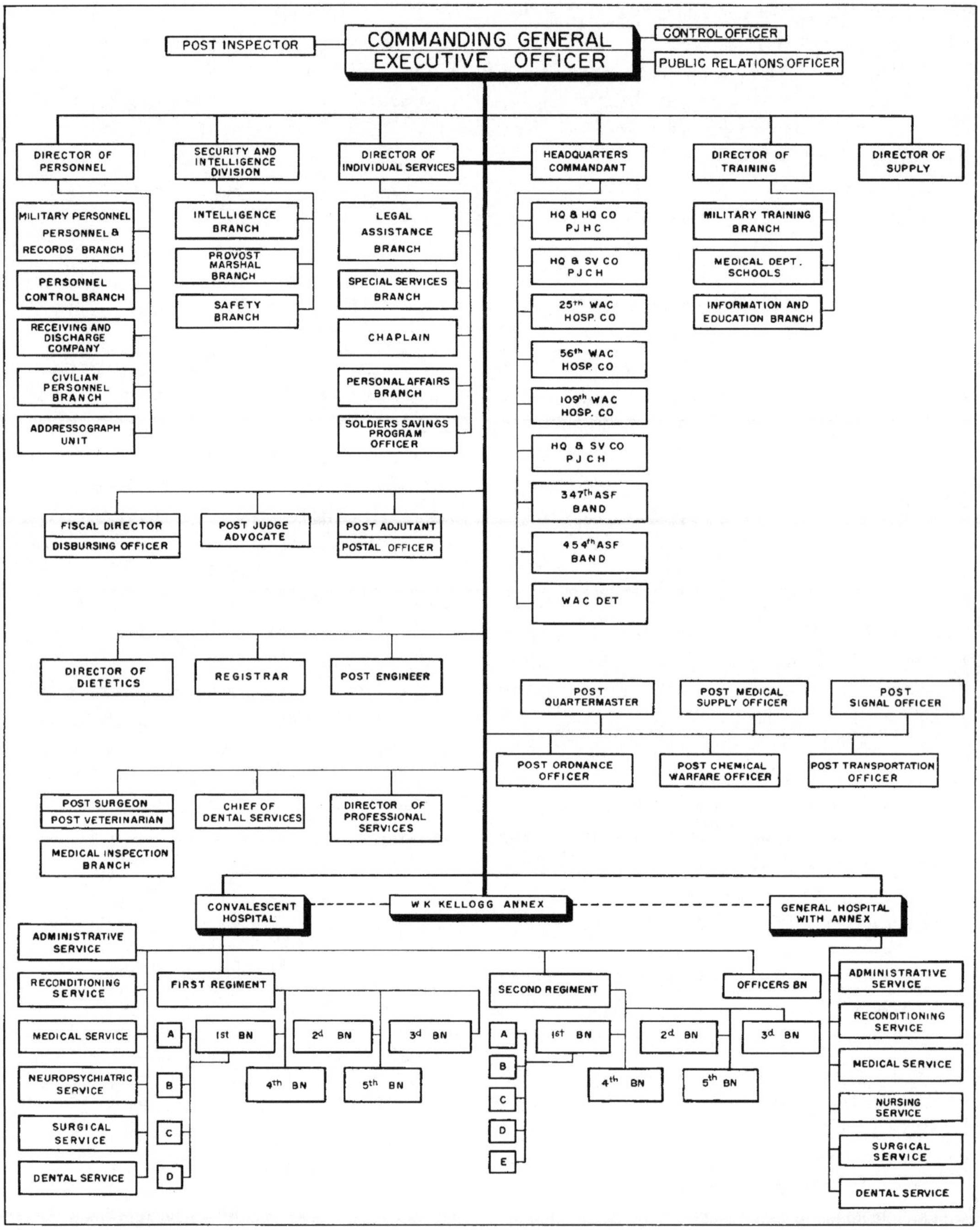

CHART 16—STANDARD PLAN FOR ORGANIZATION OF A HOSPITAL CENTER (ZI), 1945

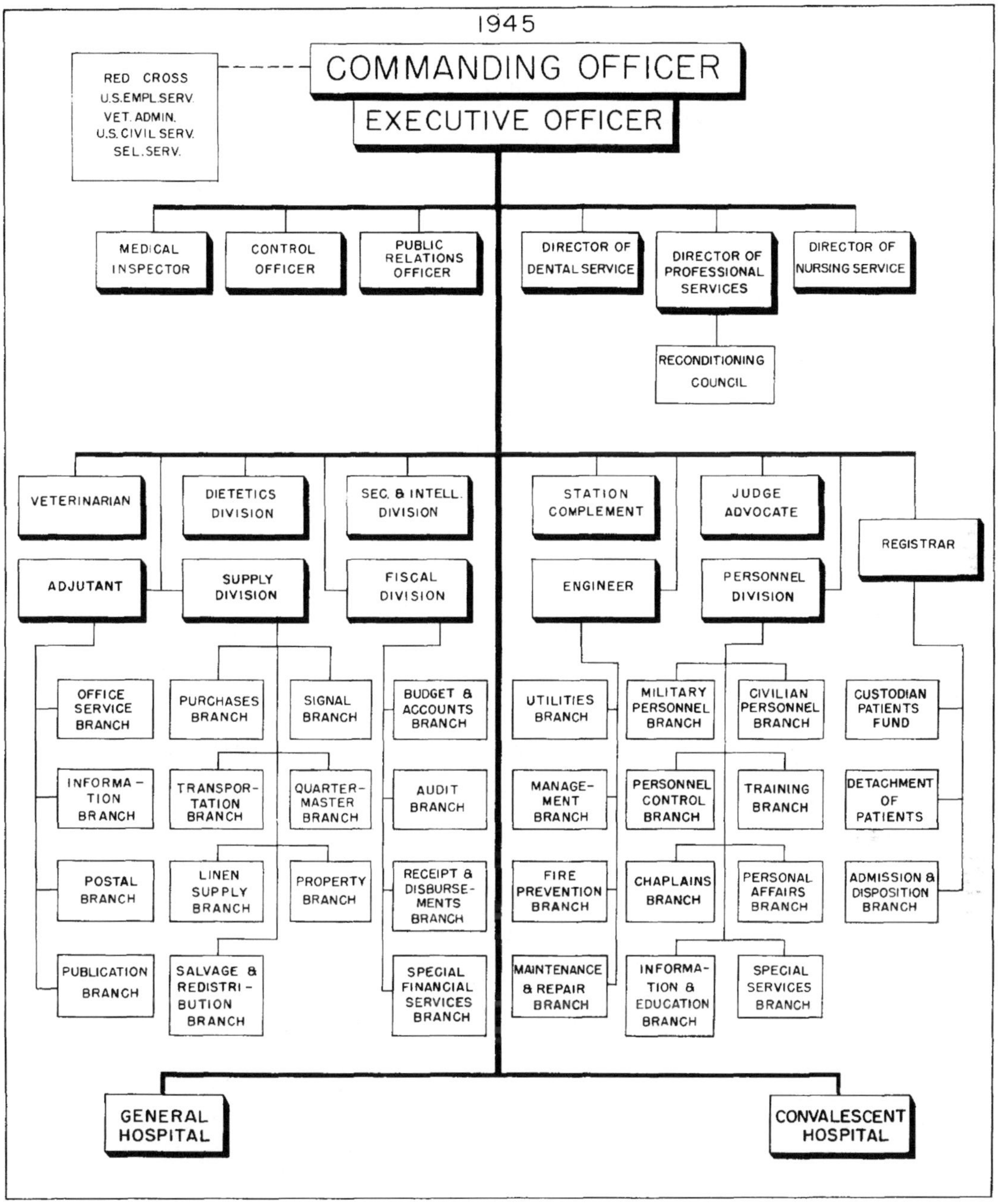

and service command surgeons.[61] Following receipt of their replies, that Office by the beginning of 1946 developed a standard plan for the organization of hospital centers. Although never published, it was significant because it represented The Surgeon General's idea of what the organization of a hospital center should be. Of prime importance was the fact that center headquarters was to be operational and was to perform for general and convalescent hospitals the administrative services that were common to both. Hence, the center commander's immediate staff and the administrative staff divisions of hospital centers were to be essentially the same as those found in both general and convalescent hospital organization charts. To assist a center commander in supervising and co-ordinating the professional activities of hospitals under his control, his immediate staff was to contain a director of dental services, a director of professional services, and a director of nursing services. General and convalescent hospitals, minus the staff and administrative divisions of center headquarters, were to be under separate commanders, each of whom reported directly to the center commander and had an administrative assistant to provide the few administrative activities that could not be concentrated under center headquarters.[62] *(See Charts 15, 16.)*

A significant feature of the hospital organization plans just discussed was their attempted conformity with the standard plan for the organization of ASF posts. While there were perhaps enough similarities between the functions of posts and those of hospitals to warrant such conformity, one may question whether it was altogether desirable or would have been required if standard plans emphasizing the peculiar functions of medical installations had been issued earlier. Certainly the Medical Department would have benefited from having such plans available when the hospital expansion program first began. Moreover, they would have made easier the task of simplifying and standardizing hospital administrative procedures. While accomplishments in this field were substantial, it was unfortunate that they came so late in the war. Offsetting this delay, perhaps, was the fact that management control became an established function in all large Army hospitals by the end of the war.

[61] For example, see: Ltr, SG to CG 9th SvC attn SvC Surg, 9 Jul 45, sub: Standard Orgn Charts for Hosps. SG: 323.3 (9th SvC)AA. Similar letters were sent to other service commands.

[62] Morgan and Wagner, *op. cit.*, pp, 156–64.

CHAPTER XVI

Changes in the Organization and Equipment of Hospital Units Prepared for Overseas Service

Since hospitals operating in overseas theaters were less subject to The Surgeon General's authority than those in the zone of interior, they were largely unaffected by the movement, discussed in the foregoing chapter, to standardize organization and simplify administrative procedures. Nevertheless, certain changes in their organization and equipment were made before they left the United States. Changes in organization were primarily of two types: the creation of units that would supply larger numbers of beds without corresponding increases in personnel and the reduction of personnel authorized for hospitals of different types.

Trend Toward Use of Larger Units

One method of supplying greater numbers of beds to theaters without proportionately increasing the number of personnel was to emphasize the use of larger hospital units.[1] Tables of organization for various sizes of station hospitals, ranging in capacity to 900 beds, had been developed during the early war years; but until the middle of 1944 a general hospital of only one size (1,000-bed capacity) was authorized. During the winter of 1943–44 the Technical Division of the Surgeon General's Office developed tables of organization, published in July 1944, for 1,500- and 2,000-bed general hospitals.[2] Another method of supplying more beds with limited amounts of personnel—the use of convalescent facilities to receive the convalescent patients of general hospitals—was employed successfully in the United States and needed to be extended, in the opinion of the Surgeon General's Office, to theaters of operations. Tables of organization for 1,000-bed convalescent camps and 3,000-bed convalescent centers were developed, but the General Staff would not include such units in the troop basis without requests from theaters. The latter were reluctant to requisition them because their capacities counted against fixed-bed quotas while their staffs were meager as compared to those of general

[1] See above, pp. 218–19.

[2] (1) T/O&E 8–550, Gen Hosp, 3 Jul 44. (2) An Rpt, Tec Div Oprs Serv SGO, FY 1945. HD.

hospitals with equal numbers of beds.[3] As a result, such units were not used widely, only four of each being activated in theaters and none in the United States. Instead, theaters requisitioned station and general hospital units to meet authorized quotas of beds and established convalescent facilities with personnel available from other sources.[4]

Cuts in Personnel of Hospital Units

As in zone of interior hospitals, reductions were made in the staffs of numbered hospitals. In compliance with a G–1 directive, the Surgeon General's Office in March 1944 reduced the ratio of nurses in station and general hospital units from 1 for every 9 or 10 beds to 1 for every 12. Thus the number authorized for a 1,000-bed general hospital was lowered from 105 to 83 and for a 750-bed station hospital from 75 to 63.[5] Also in March, in consonance with the general policy of replacing physicians with administrative officers wherever possible, a War Department circular directed that both the executive officers and registrars of station and general hospitals should be Medical Administrative Corps officers. The Surgeon General protested that executive officers, who served as commanding officers in the absence of their superiors, needed professional training in medicine, and subsequently the General Staff amended the announced policy to permit Medical Corps officers to continue serving as executive officers of general hospitals.[6] Meanwhile, the Surgeon General's Office was revising the tables of organization of both station and general hospitals, in order to reduce the number of Medical Corps officers and to increase the number of Medical Administrative Corps officers authorized for such units.[7] In July 1944 the number of physicians in a 1,000-bed general hospital was reduced from 37 to 32. Three months later the number of Medical Corps officers in station hospitals was also reduced, that for a 250-bed station hospital, for example, dropping from 13 to 10 and for a 750-bed station hospital from 23 to 20. At the same time, the number of Medical Administrative Corps officers assigned to these units was increased, the number in a 1,000-bed general hospital rising from 7 to 10 and in a 750-bed station hospital from 10 to 12.[8] No significant

---

[3] (1) Memo, SG for Dir Mil Pers Div ASF, 4 Aug 43, sub: Conv Cps. SG: 322.15–1. (2) T/O&E 8–595, Conv Cps (1,000-bed), 12 Jun 44. (3) T/O&E 8–591T, Conv Ctr (3,000-bed), 12 Jun 44. (4) Interv MD Historian with Col Arthur B. Welsh, 27 Dec 50. HD: 000.71. (5) Telewriter conv between Surg ETO and SG, 22 Oct 43. SG: 337.–1.

[4] An Rpt, MOOD SGO, FY 1945. HD.

[5] (1) DF WDGAP 320.21, ACofS G–1 WDGS to MPD ASF and SG, 8 Jan 44, sub: Nurse Pers Reqmts. HD: 211 (Nurse Reqmts). (2) T/O 8–550, Gen Hosp, C 3, 4 Mar 44. (3) T/O 8–560, Sta Hosp, C 3, 4 Mar 44.

[6] (1) WD Cirs 99, 9 Mar; 122, 28 Mar; and 152, 17 Apr 44. (2) Memo WDGCT 320.3 (11 Mar 44), ACofS G–3 WDGS for CG ASF, 25 Mar 44, sub: T/O&E 8–500 and T/O&E 8–550, with 4 inds. SG: 320.3–1.

[7] Ltr, SG to CG ASF, 17 Mar 44, sub: Revision of T/O&E 8–560, Sta Hosp, and Revision of T/O&E 8–550, Gen Hosp. SG: 320.3–1.

[8] (1) T/O 8–550, Gen Hosp, 1 Apr 42; C–2, 5 Oct 42; and T/O&E 8–550, Gen Hosp, 3 Jul 44. (2) T/O 8–560, Sta Hosp, 22 Jul 42, and T/O&E 8–560, Sta Hosp, 28 Oct 44. In 1948 the wartime chief of the Surgeon General's Mobilization and Overseas Operations Division stated that these cuts of Medical Corps officers had been too great. (Ltr, Col Arthur B. Welsh, MC, USA, 19 Apr 48, quoted in Rpt, Subcmtee on Employment of Med Resources, "Use of Med Resources," Cmtee on Med and Hosp Serv of Armed Forces, Off SecDef, 25 May 48. HD.) Several years later the number of Medical Corps officers in a 1,000-bed general hospital unit was further reduced to 28. (T/O&E 8–551, Gen Hosp, 3 Jul 50.) This final cut in physicians in general hospital units after the war represented a reduction of over 50 percent in the number of doctors authorized for a 1,000-bed general hospital in 1940.

reductions were made in the latter half of the war in the number of Medical Corps officers or nurses authorized for evacuation hospitals.[9]

In the spring of 1944 the General Staff directed reductions in the number of enlisted men in hospital units, as well as in those of units of other technical services.[10] The Technical Division of the Surgeon General's Office complied with this directive by reducing in the table of organization of general hospitals the number of men who performed housekeeping functions. It overcompensated for that reduction by providing for the attachment to hospitals of personnel from other technical services.[11] This meant that the number of enlisted men authorized for assignment to a 1,000-bed general hospital was reduced from 500 to 450, but that additional men could be supplied by attaching teams from nonmedical services, such as a Signal Corps team to operate communications systems and a Military Police team to supply interior and exterior guards.[12] Subsequently, in the fall of 1944 cuts were made also in the number of enlisted men authorized for station hospital units but, as in the case of general hospitals, provision was made for the attachment of teams of men from other technical services.[13] While this change did not necessarily mean that the total number of men working in and around a hospital plant was always reduced, it actually had that effect in many instances because some theater commanders did not approve the use of the teams authorized by the War Department and desired by theater surgeons. As a result, the change was unpopular with many Medical Department officers, especially those in theaters who wished the personnel needed to perform station services for hospitals to be organic elements of hospital units and not dependent upon decisions and actions of theater staff officers. In this connection, it is significant that the chief complaint which theater Medical Department officers made about cuts in both enlisted and commissioned personnel in hospital units was not that they would endanger the care of patients but that they would reduce the ability of hospitals to expand beyond table-of-organization capacities.[14]

Another change designed to save personnel was made in the organization of the hospital-center unit. This unit, intended to operate a 1,000-bed convalescent camp and to perform certain administrative services common to all hospitals in a center, was authorized 29 officers, 4 warrant officers, 1 nurse, and 255 enlisted

[9] Compare T/O&E 8-581, Evac Hosp, Semimobile, dated 26 Jul 43 with that dated 25 Mar 44, and T/O 8-580, Evac Hosp, 23 Apr 43, with T/O&E 8-580, Evac Hosp, 31 Jan 45.

[10] Memo, Dir Tec Div SGO for Chief Oprs Serv SGO, 17 Apr 44, sub: T/O&E 8-550, Gen Hosp. SG: 320.3-1.

[11] Memo, Dir Tec Div SGO for SG thru Chief Oprs Serv, 20 Apr 44, with incl. SG: 320.3-1.

[12] (1) T/O 8-550, Gen Hosp, C 4, 16 May 44. (2) WD Cir 256, 16 Oct 43.

[13] Ltr, SG to CG ASF, 21 Jul 44, sub: Revision to T/O&E 8-550, Sta Hosp. SG: 320.3-1. Compare T/O&E 8-560, Sta Hosp, 28 Oct 44, with T/O 8-560, Sta Hosp, 22 Jul 42.

[14] (1) Memo, Off Chief Surg Hq ETO for SG, 14 Jul 44, sub: Difficulties Presently Being Encountered in the Med Serv, ETO. HD: MOOD "ETO." (2) Memo, Dep Chief Plans and Oprs SGO for Dir Tec Div SGO, 21 Sep 44, with routing slip. SG: 320.3-1. (3) Ltr AG 320.3(14 Aug 44) OP-I-WDGCT-M, TAG to COs and CGs in TofOpns, 28 Nov 44, sub: Revised T/O&E 8-560, Sta Hosp. SG: 320.3-1. (4) Memo, Plans and Oprs MTO for Maj Gen [Morrison C.] Stayer, 25 Dec 44, sub: Memo for Dir Hosp Div SGO, 31 Oct 44, with incl. SG: 320.3 "T/Os Apr-Jun 45." (5) Memo, Dep Dir MOOD SGO for Insp Br SGO, 14 Aug 45, sub: Comments on Rpt by Col [Floyd L.] Wergeland and Lt Col Moorhead ref their visit to SWPA and POA. HD: MOOD "Pacific." (6) Rpt, Gen Bd USFET, "Orgn and Equip of Med Units," Study No 89. HD: 334 (ETO).

men until the early part of 1944.[15] During that year the belief developed that no saving in personnel was gained by concentrating hospitals and then providing them with increased overhead personnel.[16] Furthermore, separate tables of organization had been developed for convalescent camps and convalescent centers. The old table of organization for hospital centers, in consequence, was superseded in April 1944 and a hospital center headquarters, consisting of 7 officers, 1 warrant officer, 1 nurse, and 23 enlisted men, was authorized.[17] This headquarters was not expected to operate a convalescent camp and it was to borrow any additional personnel it needed for the performance of its functions from general hospitals located in the center. Only two of the hospital centers activated under the old table of organization were sent overseas. The other eight were inactivated and their personnel used in units of other types.[18] Toward the end of the war, six hospital center headquarters were activated under the new table of organization in the Southwest Pacific and sixteen in the European theater.[19]

New Hospital Units

Although emphasis in the latter half of the war was less upon the development of new hospital units than upon the use—through improvisation, if necessary—of Medical Department units already available, two new hospital units were developed and a third was proposed. In response to a request from the chief surgeon of the European theater for a hospital that would specialize in the treatment of neuropsychiatric cases, the Surgeon General's Office developed a table of organization in the latter half of 1943 for a neuropsychiatric general hospital. It was published in October.[20] The second hospital developed was for use in forward areas. In the absence of small surgical hospitals that were highly mobile, the need to treat and hold near the front lines nontransportable casualties (those who could not be moved immediately without danger to their lives) was met throughout most of the war by improvisation. During 1945 the Ground Surgeon and surgeons of some forces in combat zones proposed publication of a table of organization for a unit to meet this need. The Surgeon General opposed this development, believing that the reinforcement of available units—such as platoons of field hospitals—with surgical teams met the need adequately and at the same time promoted flexibility in the use of scarce categories of officers. The former view finally prevailed and on 23 August 1945 a table of organization for a 60-bed mobile army surgical hospital was published.[21] The third hospital, proposed but not developed, was also intended for use

[15] T/O 8-540, Hosp Ctr, 1 Apr 42.

[16] Speech, Med Hosp, Evac, and Sanitation, by Maj John S. Poe, MC, SGO, 11 Feb 44. HD: 322 (Hosp).

[17] T/O&E 8-500, MD Serv Orgn, 23 Apr 44.

[18] The 12th and 15th Hospital Centers were shipped to the European theater; the 9th, 10th, 11th, 16th, 17th, 18th, 19th, and 24th were inactivated. An Rpts. HD.

[19] (1) Quarterly Rpts, 1945, 26th, 27th, 28th, 29th, 30th, and 31st Hosp Ctrs. HD. (2) An Rpts, 1945, 801st, 802d, 803d, 804th, 805th, 806th, 807th, 808th, 809th, 812th, 813th, 814th, 815th, 818th, 819th, and 820th Hosp Ctrs. HD.

[20] (1) Telewriter conv, Surg ETO and SGO, 9 Aug and 22 Oct 43. SG: 337.-1. (2) Memo, CG ASF for AG, 26 Oct 43, sub: T/O&E 8-550S, Gen Hosp (1,000-bed) NP, ComZ, with Memo for Record. AG: 320.2 (13 Jul 43)(4). (3) T/O&E 8-550S, Gen Hosp, NP, 26 Oct 43.

[21] (1) Memo, Lt Col C[lifton] F. Von Kann for ACofS G-4 WDGS, 11 Aug 45, sub: Conf Rpt, Proposed Mobile Army Surg Hosp, T/O&E 8-571. HRS: G-4 files, "Hosp, vol. IV." (2) T/O&E 8-571, Mobile Army Surg Hosp, 23 Aug 45. Additional documents on this subject are on file in SG: 320.3.

in forward areas. Both in theaters of operations and in the Surgeon General's Office there was a belief that a small hospital was needed near the front lines to treat neuropsychiatric casualties who could be salvaged for further duty. A table of organization for such a unit was never published and theaters met this need by improvisation.[22]

Changes in Supplies and Equipment

During the latter part of the war changes occurred in both the medical and nonmedical equipment of hospitals. As a result of changes and improvements in pharmaceuticals and biologicals and of the accumulation of experience in the operation of hospitals under various sets of conditions in different parts of the world, the Surgeon General's Office made three complete revisions and several partial revisions of Medical Department equipment lists between the middle of 1943 and the end of 1945. Revision of these lists involved the selection of types and amounts of pharmaceuticals and biologicals, of surgical instruments and other operating room equipment, of X-ray and laboratory equipment, of ward equipment, and of other Medical Department items needed by hospitals of different types for the performance of their missions. These revisions, made by the Surgeon General's Organization and Equipment Allowance Branch, were based on combat experience as revealed by reports of essential technical medical data (ETMD's), interviews with officers who served overseas, and inspections of theater medical services; on changes in the size and personnel of units; and on the advice and recommendations of the Professional and Preventive Medicine Services of the Surgeon General's Office, the Army Medical Center, and the National Research Council. A significant administrative feature of these revisions was the consolidation and publication during 1944 and 1945 of equipment lists as parts of the medical section of the ASF supply catalog and their distribution by the Adjutant General's Office. Until that time, such lists had been issued in mimeograph form by the Medical Department alone. Items added to them made available to hospitals the newer drugs and biologicals and improved items of equipment developed during the war.[23]

Changes in the nonmedical equipment of hospital units revolved around the problem of supplying items of equipment necessary for station services, or housekeeping functions. The chief question was whether such equipment would be included in tables of equipment of hospitals, and therefore supplied automatically, or whether it would not be included, and supplied only when and if theater commanders requested it. Types of nonmedical equipment which demanded the attention of the Surgeon General's Office were those needed for such station services as laundries, electric lighting systems, and telephone communications systems.

Inspections of theater medical services by Surgeon General Kirk and his chief of Professional Services in the middle of 1943 revealed what they considered to be inadequate laundry service for hospitals in both the North African and Southwest

[22] (1) Ltr, Surg Fifth Army to SG thru Surg MTOUSA, 22 Jun 45, sub: Mobile Med Hosp. SG: 320.3. (2) An Rpt, NP Consultants Div SGO, FY 1945. HD.

[23] (1) History of Organization and Equipment Allowance Branch [SGO], 1939–44. HD. (2) An Rpt, Sup Serv SGO, FY 1944. HD. (3) An Rpt, Orgn and Equip Allowance Br Oprs Serv SGO, FY 1944. (4) An Rpt, Tec Div Oprs Serv SGO, FY 1945. Copies of the Equip Lists are on file, HD.

Pacific theaters. In their opinion this resulted from lack of sufficient numbers of laundries and from the use of improper types of laundry equipment. On 5 June 1943 The Surgeon General informed ASF headquarters of the improvements he considered necessary.[24] As a result, the offices of The Quartermaster General and The Surgeon General collaborated in changing washing formulae and laundry equipment to improve the quality of service which laundries afforded hospitals.[25]

The provision of adequate amounts of laundry equipment and of sufficient numbers of laundry operators was more complicated. On 1 July 1943 The Quartermaster General informed ASF headquarters that there was sufficient laundry equipment in this country to meet the needs of theaters, provided the latter requested its shipment.[26] Theater opinions of what constituted an adequate laundry service differed from The Surgeon General's, for theaters accepted lower standards of service than he considered desirable.[27] He wished, therefore, to find some way to assure that sufficient laundry equipment and personnel would be shipped with each hospital unit. The director of the ASF Planning Division, on the other hand, felt that theater commanders, with the advice and help of their surgeons, should determine the laundry services needed and request the War Department to supply the necessary equipment and personnel.[28] The ASF view prevailed and in August 1943 theater commanders were reminded of the necessity of planning in advance for the laundry service of hospitals but were informed that the War Department would not supply them with laundry equipment and personnel unless such were requested.[29] During the following year, after the General Staff authorized the attachment of technical-service teams to units of other technical services, revised tables of organization and equipment of hospital units carried a statement that Quartermaster Corps laundry teams were authorized for attachment to hospitals when theater commanders requested them.[30] Although this served as a reminder to theater staffs that they had to make specific provisions for hospital laundry services, it left to theaters considerable discretion in the matter and the Surgeon General's Office continued its unsuccessful attempt to have laundry equipment and personnel made integral parts of numbered hospitals.[31]

---

[24] (1) Ltr, SG to CG ASF, 5 Jun 43, sub: Laundry Fac in TofOpns. SG: 486.3. (2) Memo, Col R[obert] B. Skinner for the Record, 8 Jul 43, sub: Gen [Charles C.] Hillman's Trip to SWPA. Ground Med files, Chronological file (Col Skinner). (3) Memo, SG for CG ASF, 10 Aug 43, sub: Interim Progress Rpt: Steps Taken During First Sixty Days Since Apmt as SG. SG: 024.-1.

[25] Ltr, SG to CG ASF, 5 Jun 43, sub: Laundry Fac in TofOpns, with 1st, 2d, and 4th inds. SG: 486.3.

[26] Memo SPAOG 331.5, Dir Oprs ASF for Dir Planning Div ASF, 23 Jun 43, sub: Laundries and Laundry Equip, with 1st ind. HD: Wilson files, "Day File, Jul 43."

[27] (1) Memo, Col Arthur B. Welsh, MC for Dep SG, 13 Aug 43, sub: Data for Gen Somervell. SG: 486.3. (2) Memo, Dep SG for CG ASF, 16 Aug 43, sub: Interim Progress Rpt. HRS: ASF Control Div, 319.1 "SGs Interim Rpt, G-56."

[28] (1) Memo, Col Arthur B. Welsh, MC for Dep SG, 1 Jul 43, sub: Laundry for Overseas Hosps. SG: 331.5. (2) Memo, Maj John S. Poe for Col [Howard T.] Wickert, 16 Jul 43. SG: 414.4-5. (3) Historical Record, Laundry Section, Hospital Division [SGO], 1 July 1944, p. 18. HD: 024.

[29] Memo SPOPP 008, CG ASF for TAG, 3 Aug 43, sub: Aux Fac for Fixed Hosps. SG: 632.-1.

[30] (1) T/O&E 8-581, Evac Hosp (400-bed), 25 Mar 44. (2) T/O&E 8-550, Gen Hosp, 3 Jul 44. (3) T/O&E 8-560, Sta Hosp, 28 Oct 44. (4) T/O&E 8-580, Evac Hosp (750-bed), 31 Jan 45.

[31] Ltr, SG to CG ASF attn Dir Mob Div, 10 May 45, sub: Tables of Orgn and Equip. SG: 320.3. Success came after the war. For example, see T/O&E 8-566, Sta Hosp, 500-bed, ComZ, and T/O&E 8-551, Gen Hosp, 1,000-bed, ComZ. Reviewing the experi-

A similar problem arose in connection with electric lighting equipment. The Surgeon General's Office recommended that such equipment, including electric generators, should be specifically listed in tables of equipment of hospital units to insure its being provided for each.[32] During 1944 and 1945 this action was taken for field and evacuation hospital units; but electric lighting equipment was not included during the war in tables of equipment for general and station hospitals, convalescent hospitals, and convalescent camps and centers. Instead, a War Department memorandum placed upon the Chief of Engineers responsibility for furnishing electric lighting equipment, including generators, to such units when they received orders to move to theaters.[33]

At the beginning of the war the table of basic allowances for the Medical Department authorized telephone and switchboard equipment for the 750-bed evacuation hospital only. During the early part of the war, the tables for general and convalescent hospitals were revised to include that equipment. Similar action was taken for station and 400-bed evacuation hospitals during the latter part of the war.[34]

Other significant changes in the equipment of hospital units were additions of tool chests of various sorts. Experience showed that hospital personnel in many instances had to perform much maintenance work and that the number of tool chests previously provided was insufficient. Consequently, in successive revisions of tables of equipment of hospital units there were added tool chests for carpenters, refrigeration mechanics, electricians, plumbers, automobile mechanics, and the like.[35]

ences of World War II several years after its end, the former chief of the Surgeon General's Mobilization and Overseas Operations Division pointed out the failure to solve this problem. (Extract from Ltr, Col Arthur B. Welsh, MC, 19 Apr 48, quoted in "Use of Med Resources," Rpt by Subcmtee on Employment of Mil Med Resources to Hawley Bd, 25 May 48, p. 348. HD: 334.)

[32] An Rpt, Tec Div Oprs Serv SGO, FY 1945. HD.

[33] (1) T/O&E 8-510, Fld Hosp, C 3, 24 Mar 44. (2) T/O&E 8-581, Evac Hosp (400-bed), 25 Mar 44. (3) T/O&E 8-580, Evac Hosp (750-bed), 31 Jan 45. (4) WD Memo W 100-44, 9 May 44. HD: 412.-1. (5) WD Memo 100-45, 31 Mar 45. AG: 412 (5 May 44)(1).

[34] (1) T/BA 8, MD, 1 Oct 41. (2) T/BA 8, MD, 15 Jul 42; C 1, 29 Aug 42. (3) T/O&E 8-560, Sta Hosp, 28 Oct 44. (4) An Rpt, Strategic and Logistic Planning Sec MOOD SGO, 5 Jun 45 (HD), stated that switchboards and communications equipment had been provided for 400-bed evacuation hospitals. However, a search of the T/O&E for this hospital does not disclose such authorization until publication of T/O&E 8-581 on 11 January 1949.

[35] For example, see (1) T/E 8-560, Sta Hosp, 28 Dec 43. (2) T/O&E 8-581, Evac Hosp (400-bed), 25 Mar 44. (3) T/O&E 8-510, Fld Hosp, 31 Mar 44. (4) T/O&E 8-550, Gen Hosp, 3 Jul 44. (5) T/O&E 8-560, Sta Hosp, 28 Oct 44. (6) T/O&E 8-580, Evac Hosp (750-bed), 31 Jan 45.

CHAPTER XVII

Hospital Construction and Maintenance

Emphasis in the Medical Department construction program in the United States in the latter part of the war was on expanding and improving existing hospital plants rather than on the construction or acquisition of new ones. It will be recalled that ASF headquarters considered the hospital construction program substantially complete by the middle of 1943. At that time forty general hospitals were in operation and eighteen others were under construction. Afterwards, only eight additional general hospitals were authorized, and they were located in buildings which the Army already had. Moreover, the closure of station hospitals as troops moved overseas made it unnecessary, except in a few instances, either to build or to acquire new station hospital plants.[1] Despite this apparent completion of the hospital building program, there was feverish construction activity at many Medical Department installations. Mounting bed requirements in the first half of 1945 made it necessary to provide housing in general and convalescent hospitals for additional beds equal in number to 80 percent of those accumulated in general hospitals during the previous four years. Changes in concepts of patient treatment, patient welfare, and hospital administration created needs for facilities not available in hospital plants already built. Finally, The Surgeon General took advantage of the passing of the initial phase of the Army's construction program and of the increasing availability of scarce materials to press for improvements and refinements in existing plants in order to bring them up to the standards of peacetime civilian hospitals.

In expanding and improving hospital plants, The Surgeon General continued to have only partial responsibility and authority. He was dependent upon ASF headquarters for approval of all major projects and upon the Engineers for all construction work. They, in turn, continued to be subject to decisions and policies made by the General Staff. The Surgeon General's Hospital Construction Branch developed general programs and standard criteria for hospital expansions and improvements, and insisted, as before, upon an opportunity to approve or disapprove construction which changed either the capacities of hospital plants or the primary professional functions of any of their buildings. In general, that Branch tended to rely more than before on service command surgeons and ASF hospital commanders

[1] (1) Memo, Chief Cons Br SGO for HD SGO, 1 Nov 46, sub: Record of Expansion and Contraction, Hosps, ZI, and Hosp Ships. HD: 632. (2) See Table 14.

for assistance in planning and initiating programs for expansions, additions, and improvements. There were several reasons for this development. The expansion of existing hospital plants required individual attention and planning in order to make maximum use of available housing and to fit additional facilities into plants already constructed. Furthermore, many hospital commanders showed that they could secure additional facilities as gifts from civilian groups without assistance from the War Department. Finally, under prevailing War Department construction policies, requests for all but major construction projects had to be initiated in the field and not in the offices of the chiefs of technical services in Washington.[2] Over Air Forces hospital construction the Surgeon General's Office exercised less supervision than it had during the early part of the war. Complying with a request of the Air Surgeon and reflecting perhaps the growing independence of the Air Forces, The Surgeon General on 22 January 1944 delegated to the Air Surgeon authority to act as his representative in that field.[3]

Providing Housing for Additional Beds in General and Convalescent Hospitals in the United States

The primary method of obtaining housing for additional beds was to use existing buildings, whether for newly established hospitals or the expansion of those already in operation. This method was adopted because of restrictions on new construction imposed by ASF headquarters under policies of the General Staff.[4] When ASF approved the establishment of convalescent annexes for general hospitals in June 1943, it announced that new construction, except for gymnasiums, was not authorized. Existing Army housing or leased civilian buildings were to be used instead.[5]

During 1943, 1944, and 1945, on The Surgeon General's recommendation the Service Forces acquired through lease or transfer eighteen pieces of real estate, including schools, hotels, and National Youth Administration buildings, with enough space to house beds for 9,322 convalescent patients at a number of general hospitals. Other general hospitals established annexes in vacant Army buildings located near by.[6] After approving the establishment of convalescent centers for 25,000 patients early in 1944, ASF headquarters turned over to the Medical Department vacant barracks on Army posts. Meanwhile, the Air Forces followed the same procedure in setting up convalescent hospitals.[7] In most instances existing buildings were used during 1944 without

[2] WD Cir 58, 19 Dec 43.

[3] (1) Memo, Dep Air Surg for Chief Hosp Admin Div SGO, 14 Oct 43, sub: Processing of Recomds for AAF Hosp Cons, Maintenance, and Repair. SG: 632.-1. (2) Ltr, CG AAF (Air Surg) to SG, 10 Jan 44, sub: Delegation of Auth to CG AAF, the Air Surg, for Operational Control at AAF Hosp, with 1st ind, SG to CG AAF thru CG ASF, 22 Jan 44. SG: 323.7-5.

[4] ASF Cirs 78, 18 Mar 44; 178, 13 Jun 44; and 168, 11 May 45.

[5] 1st ind SPRMC 322 (18 Jun 43), CG ASF to SG, 22 Jun 43, sub: Conv Ctrs, on unknown basic ltr. SG: 632.-1.

[6] (1) Ltr, SG to COs of Gen Hosps, 3 Aug 43, sub: Estab of Conv Retraining Unit. SG: 632.-1. (2) Memo, SG for Reqmts Div ASF, 3 Sep 43, sub: Conv Fac. Off file, Gen Bliss' Off SGO, "Med Clarification of Disposition Policy." (3) Diary, Hosp Cons Br SGO, 13 Mar, 4 Apr, and 18 Aug 44. HD: 024.7-3. (4) Memo, Chief Cons Br SGO for HD SGO, 1 Nov 46, sub: Record of Expansion and Contraction, Hosps, ZI, and Hosp Ships. HD: 632.

[7] (1) Memo SPMOC 532 (3 Jun 44), CG ASF for SG, 29 Jun 44, sub: Housing Fac for Convs. Off file, Gen Bliss' Off SGO, "Med Clarification of Disposition Policy." (2) AAF Memo 20-12, 18 Sep 43, sub: Orgn AAF Conv Ctrs. HD.

extensive alterations and with little additional construction.[8]

The major hospital expansion program of the later war years came during the first six months of 1945, after G–4 approved additional beds to meet the estimated peak load of patients. For this expansion the War Department followed the same method—the use of existing buildings—but permitted more improvements and alterations than before. Both general and convalescent hospitals were expanded. Medical detachment barracks at general hospitals, which The Surgeon General early in the war had successfully insisted should be parts of hospital plants and of the same types and quality of construction, were converted into wards. Some convalescent annexes were made into wards and some nonhospital barracks were converted into housing for ambulatory patients. Four station hospital plants supplemented by near-by barracks were converted into general hospitals. Several staging area hospitals were modified to serve as debarkation hospitals. And additional barracks on posts where convalescent hospitals were located were turned over to them. These changes involved chiefly improvements, already authorized late in 1944 for general and convalescent hospital plants, such as sealing inside walls, painting and reflooring, installing sprinkler systems and fire escapes in converted wards, and inclosing the covered walkways connecting those wards with the rest of the hospital plant. In general, the erection of new buildings was avoided but in some places no post housing was available for medical enlisted men and Wacs. In these instances theater-of-operations-type barracks, along with buildings for detachment and company administration, recreation, supply, and messing, were constructed to house the men displaced from hospital barracks and the Wacs sent to hospitals to help with increased patient loads.[9]

Initiation and completion of this program represented co-ordinated efforts of the Surgeon General's Hospital Construction Branch, the Chief of Engineers' Office, ASF headquarters, and their field officers. Even before G–4 authorized the additional beds, the Surgeon General's Construction Branch collaborated with service command surgeons in making preliminary plans for hospital expansions, determining the number of additional beds that could be provided, and establishing general criteria for conversion work.[10] Meanwhile, the Chief of Engineers' Office called upon division engineers, by telephone, for preliminary layout plans and cost estimates. As a result, within forty-eight hours after that Office received a directive to proceed with the program, it authorized division engineers to begin work.[11] To achieve speed in the expansion, ASF headquarters per-

[8] (1) Tynes, Construction Branch. (2) Interv, MD Historian with Col Achilles L. Tynes, formerly Chief Hosp Cons Br SGO, 24 Apr 50. HD: 000.71.

[9] (1) Ltr, SG to CofEngrs, 13 Jan 45, sub: Emergency Expansion of Gen Hosps. SG: 322 "Hosp." (2) Memo SPMOC 632, CG ASF for CofEngrs, 22 Jan 45, sub: Prov of Add Hosp Fac for Gen Hosp Syst. CE: 683 Pt I. (3) Ltr, CofEngrs to Div Engrs, 2 Feb 45, same sub. SG: 632. (4) Engr Cons Directives, of various dates. Same file. (5) An Rpts, 1945, Birmingham, Battey, and Cp Butner Gen Hosps, and Cp Carson Hosp Ctr. HD.

[10] (1) Memo, Dir Hosp Div for Chief Hosp Cons Br, 19 Dec 44. SG: 632. (2) Memo, same for same, 6 Jan 45, sub: Ests of Cons Needs. Same file. (3) Off Memo, by Chief Hosp Cons Br, 12 Jan 45, sub: 6th SvC. Same file. (4) Ltr, SG to CofEngrs, sub: Emergency Expansion of Gen Hosps. SG: 322 "Hosp."

[11] 1st ind CE SPEMT 683, CofEngrs to CG ASF thru SG, 22 Feb 45, on Memo SPMOC 600.1, CG ASF for CofEngrs and SG in turn, 7 Feb 45, sub: Conversion, New Cons, and Preferred Maintenance at Gen and Conv Hosps. CE: 683 Pt I.

mitted The Surgeon General and the Chief of Engineers to make minor changes in the approved program, particularly in the number of beds for which housing was to be provided at each hospital.[12] In turn, they delegated similar authority to local engineer and medical officers, and the Chief of Engineers directed division engineers to settle layout plans locally and to secure The Surgeon General's approval by telephone.[13] Finally, both the Chief of Engineers and ASF headquarters instructed representatives in the field to cooperate fully with each other in pushing the program to completion.[14]

None of these measures would have been sufficient to assure the expansion of hospital housing capacity in time for the peak load if a solid foundation for it had not already been established. The existence at hospital plants of barracks similar in type to ward buildings made their conversion to wards relatively simple. Furthermore, establishment of convalescent hospitals during 1944, without G-4 approval and in the face of attempts of the Staff to reduce the number of general and convalescent beds, meant that a considerable portion of the housing needed for the additional beds authorized in November 1944 and January 1945 had already been provided.[15]

Construction of Additional Facilities at Existing Hospital Plants

In the latter half of the war the Medical Department also had to request additional facilities that had not been planned when hospitals were built because the need for them had not been anticipated. The extension of specialization in general hospitals during 1944 and 1945 required additional clinical facilities. For example, vascular centers needed constant-temperature rooms; orthopedic centers needed brace shops, plaster and dressing rooms, and extra X-ray facilities; and centers for the deaf, acoustic clinics.[16] Since the construction of such buildings could not normally be classified as "major" projects, local hospital commanders had to submit formal requests for each. As a rule, the professional consultants of the Surgeon General's Office worked closely with the Hospital Construction Branch and with hospital commanders, informing both of what was needed. For example, an orthopedic consultant recommended the construction of an orthopedic clinic at Fort George G. Meade (Maryland) Regional Hospital in June 1944, and a few months later an ophthalmology consultant recommended an acrylic eye laboratory and an eye clinic for Dibble General Hospital.[17] Generally, the Medical Department encountered little if any opposition in securing the approval of the Engineers and ASF headquarters for the construction of special clinical buildings. Perhaps this circumstance was due to the fact that their

[12] Memo SPMOC 632, CG ASF for CofEngrs, 22 Jan 45, sub: Prov of Add Hosp Fac for the Gen Hosp Syst. CE: 683 Pt I.

[13] Ltr, CofEngrs to Div Engrs, 2 Feb 45, sub: Prov of Add Hosp Fac for Gen Hosp Syst. SG: 632.

[14] (1) Ltr cited above. (2) Ltr SPMOC 632, CG ASF to CGs SvCs, 3 Feb 45, sub: Prov of Add Hosp Fac for Gen Hosp Syst. AG: 323.3 (4 Sep 44)(1).

[15] (1) See above, p. 202. (2) An Rpt, FY 1945, Hosp Cons Br SGO. HD.

[16] (1) Memo, Capt A. W. Clark for Col A[lbert] H. Schwichtenberg, 1 Feb 45, sub: Constant-Temperature Rooms. SG: 632. (2) Memo, Col Leonard T. Peterson, Chief Orthopedic Br SGO for Dir Hosp Div SGO, 26 Mar 45, sub: Orthopedic Clinic. Same file. (3) Diary, Hosp Cons Br SGO, 29 Feb and 6 Mar 44. HD: 024.7-3.

[17] (1) Ltr, Col Leonard T. Peterson to SG, 24 Jun 44, sub: Rpt of Visit to Ft George G. Meade Regional Hosp. HD: 333.-3. (2) Memo, Maj Middleton E. Randolph for SG, 27 Nov 44, sub: Rpt of Trip to Dibble Gen Hosp. HD: 333.-2.

use was so obviously a part of the professional care of patients. In the case of other special buildings less evidently needed for professional care but appropriate to almost all general hospitals, the Surgeon General's Office had to request ASF headquarters to establish a general policy permitting their construction. This occurred in the case of occupational therapy clinics, which were needed after The Surgeon General began to emphasize occupational therapy in all general hospitals, and in the case of neuropsychiatric social therapy clinics, which were needed after neuropsychiatric centers were established in many general hospitals. In October 1943 ASF headquarters approved the construction of occupational therapy clinics; about a year later, of neuropsychiatric social therapy clinics.[18] The provision of special clinical facilities continued even after the Medical Department began to contract the general-convalescent hospital system. As late as September 1945, for example, when specialized centers were being relocated because some hospitals were being closed, the Surgeon General's Office requested the construction of special buildings for centers for rheumatic fever, deaf, paraplegic, neuropsychiatric, and plastic surgery patients in hospitals that were expected to remain open for long periods of time.[19]

Development of the convalescent reconditioning program called for additions to hospital plants which were generally authorized less readily than special clinical buildings. Among them were recreational facilities, such as theaters, gymnasiums, swimming pools, ball fields, and bowling alleys; instructional facilities, such as classrooms and prevocational training shops; and others that could be used for both recreational and educational purposes, such as libraries and radio systems.

In the second half of 1943, with the inauguration of the reconditioning program and the growing belief that patients recuperated more rapidly if kept occupied physically and mentally to the maximum extent consistent with their degree of recovery, hospital commanders began to request appropriate facilities.[20] At that time The Surgeon General was reluctant to support requests for "elaborate and costly" additions, such as swimming pools; but he urged the construction at general hospitals of buildings normally erected on Army posts, such as gymnasiums, libraries, and theaters.[21] ASF headquarters approved the construction of gymnasiums and theaters in June and December 1943, respectively.[22]

As materials became more plentiful and the prospective load of battle casual-

[18] (1) Ltr, SG to CG ASF, 22 Oct 43, sub: Occupational Therapy Instls, with 1st ind SPRMC 632 (22 Oct 43), CG ASF to CofEngrs thru SG, 26 Oct 43. SG: 632.1 (2) Memo, Dir Hosp Div SGO for Chief Hosp Cons Br SGO, 28 Nov 44, sub: Rooms for Visiting with Relatives at NP Ctrs, with 1st ind, Chief Hosp Cons Br SGO to Dir Hosp Div SGO, 30 Nov 44. SG: 632. (3) Ltr. SG to CofEngrs, 13 Dec 44, sub: NP Social and Occupational Therapy Bldg, with 4 inds. Same file.

[19] Memo, Dep SG for CofEngrs, 11 Sep 45, sub: Engr Serv, Army—Project No 200 (Cons) Revised Estimates, FY 1946. SG: 632.

[20] For example: (1) Diary, Hosp Cons Br SGO, 17 Feb and 28 Mar 44. HD: 024.7-3. (2) An Rpts, 1943, Baxter, Billings, Bushnell, Hoff, and Kennedy Gen Hosps. HD. (3) Memo, Chief Hosp Cons Br SGO for Chief Prof Serv SGO, 21 Apr 44. SG: 631.

[21] (1) Memo, Brig Gen C[harles] C. Hillman, Chief Prof Serv SGO for Chief Hosp Admin Div SGO, 16 Dec 43, sub: Cons of Hosp Fac. SG: 631. (2) Memo, SG for Reqmts Div ASF, 5 May 43, sub: Recreational Fac in Army Hosps. Same file.

[22] (1) 1st ind SPRMC 322 (18 Jun 43), CG ASF to SG, 22 Jun 43, sub: Conv Ctrs, on unknown basic ltr. SG: 632.-1. (2) 1st ind, CG ASF to SG, 8 Dec 43, on Memo, SG for CG ASF, 22 Nov 43, sub: Theaters for Gen Hosps. SG: 631.

ties more imminent during 1944, The Surgeon General broadened his program.[23] In that year the construction at general hospitals of libraries, swimming pools, and athletic fields was approved by ASF headquarters.[24] Early in 1945, after the Reconditioning Consultant's Division published an elaborate convalescent-reconditioning program and the President gave it his blessing, The Surgeon General pressed for buildings and equipment of all types for use in that program. In February 1945 ASF headquarters approved the installation of four-channel, program-distribution (or radio) systems in general hospitals.[25] Two months later the General Staff approved a construction program for convalescent hospitals which included shops for machine work, welding, automobile repairs, woodwork, photography, electrical work, and the like; classrooms for general academic courses, business administration, and music appreciation; athletic facilities such as bowling alleys, stables, tennis courts, baseball and softball diamonds, archery ranges, golf courses, skeet ranges, and football fields; and theaters, libraries, clubhouses, and other recreational buildings.[26]

In securing eventual approval for such facilities, The Surgeon General encountered difficulties and delays. ASF headquarters would authorize only those which appeared necessary for the treatment and recovery of patients, and The Surgeon General therefore had to justify each request by explaining the therapeutic benefits additional facilities would afford.[27] Furthermore, ASF tended to limit programs which it approved to general hospitals that were expected to remain in operation during the postwar years.[28] The Surgeon General agreed that extra facilities should be provided first for general hospitals in which overseas patients were treated; but he wanted them later for regional and station hospitals also. He resisted attempts to limit reconditioning facilities to hospitals that would be used for the postwar period, arguing that they were needed for all patients of World War II, whether in hospitals that would be closed or in others that would be kept open after the war.[29] ASF headquarters sometimes encountered difficulties in getting money appropriated for the extra construction which The Surgeon General wanted. For example, the opposition of the Bureau of the Budget to the appro-

[23] For example, see: (1) Ltr, SG to CG ASF, 8 May 44, sub: Cons of Swimming Pools. SG: 631. (2) Memo, SPMC 631.-1, SG for Dir Spec Serv Div ASF, 10 May 44, sub: Bowling Alleys. Same file. (3) Diary, Hosp Cons Br SGO, 26 Feb 44. HD: 024.7-3. (4) Memo, SG for CofEngrs, 16 Mar 44, sub: Budget Def for Nurses Call Systs and Libraries for Army Hosps. SG: 632.-1.

[24] (1) 1st ind SPMOC 632 (9 Sep 44), CG ASF to CofEngrs, 23 Sep 44, on DF G-4 2623, ACofS G-4 WDGS to CG ASF, 8 Sep 44, sub: Libraries for Army Gen Hosps. (2) 1st ind SPRMC 631 (8 May 44), CG ASF to SG, 16 May 44, on Ltr SPMCH, SG to CG ASF, 8 May 44, sub: Cons of Swimming Pools. (3) Memo, SPMOC 600.1 (21 Sep 44), CG ASF for CofEngrs, n d, sub: Outdoor Recreational Fac for Conv Soldiers at Gen and Conv Hosps. All in SG: 631.

[25] 3d ind SPRLR 413.45 (3 Feb 45), CG ASF to Chief Sig Off, 16 Feb 45, on Ltr, Dep SG to CG ASF, 3 Feb 45, sub: Funds for Instl of PA Systs in Gen Hosps. SG: 413.47.

[26] Memo SPMOC 632 (29 Apr 45), CG ASF for CofEngrs, sub: Conv Hosps, with incl, Criteria for Providing and Maintaining Fac at AAF and ASF Conv Hosps. SG: 322 (Conv Hosp).

[27] (1) Diary, Hosp Cons Br SGO, 8 Mar, 22 Apr, and 4 Sep 44. HD: 024.7-3. (2) Ltr, SG to CG ASF, 8 May 44, sub: Cons of Swimming Pools. SG: 631. (3) Memo SPMCH 632, SG for CG ASF, 8 Dec 44. Same file.

[28] For example, see: 4th ind, CG ASF to SG, n d, on Ltr, SG to CG ASF, 8 May 44, sub: Cons of Swimming Pools. SG: 631.

[29] Memo, SG for CG ASF, 18 Oct 44, sub: Cons of Swimming Pools at Gen Hosps, with 2d ind, Dep SG to CG ASF, 9 Nov 44. SG: 631.

priation of money for the building of libraries delayed that program for several months during 1944.[30] In instances where lack of appropriated funds prevented ASF headquarters from approving additional construction or where those funds were sufficient to provide facilities for only a limited number of hospitals, ASF headquarters and the Surgeon General's Office approved, as a rule, the use of nonappropriated funds to construct them.[31] As a result of that policy and of generous gifts by civilians, some hospitals got such additions as swimming pools, bowling alleys, and radio systems before the use of War Department funds for such purposes was approved.[32] Others were not so fortunate. Furthermore, because of delays in getting ASF and G-4 approval, some hospitals never got to use the extra facilities authorized, for the war ended and their construction had to be canceled.[33]

Concurrently with the addition to hospitals of clinical and reconditioning facilities, the increase in administrative activities and the development of new operational procedures created needs for additional or enlarged administrative buildings. During the early war years several hospitals had begun to operate central service systems similar to those found in large civilian hospitals.[34] Such systems permitted the centralized maintenance, storage, preparation (including sterilization), and issuance of supplies and equipment which were used for certain diagnostic and therapeutic procedures in all wards but which were not needed in wards at all times. Among such items were those used for transfusion and intravenous medication, wound dressing, spinal puncture, thoracentesis, catheterization, gastric lavage and gastroduodenal suction, and oxygen administration.[35] In the last half of 1943 the Surgeon General's Office developed standard operating procedures for central service systems and prepared typical layouts for buildings to house them.[36] By January 1944 it decided that all hospitals with capacities of 750 or more beds should have such systems.[37] Their use would save both personnel and equipment, would achieve uniformity in sterilization techniques, and would insure the ready availability of all items needed

[30] (1) Memo, WD Budget Off for ACofS G-4 WDGS, 18 Jul 44, sub: Libraries for Army Gen Hosps. SG: 631. (2) 1st ind SPMOC 632 (9 Sep 44), CG ASF to CofEngrs, 23 Sep 44, on DF G-4 2623, ACofS G-4 WDGS to CG ASF, 8 Sep 44, same sub. Same file.

[31] For example, see: (1) Diary, Hosp Cons Br SGO, 16 and 19 Aug 44, 25 Nov 44, and 27 Jul 45. HD: 024.7-3. (2) 1st ind, CofEngrs to CG ASF, 21 Jun 44, on Memo SPRMC 631 (13 Jan 44), CG ASF for CofEngrs, 13 Jun 44, sub: Libraries at Gen Hosps. SG: 631.

[32] (1) Memo, SG for CG ASF, 18 Oct 44, sub: Cons of Swimming Pools at Gen Hosps. SG: 631. (2) Comments by Col A. L. Tynes, Chief Hosp Cons Br SGO at Conf of SvC Surgs, 12 Dec 44. SG: 632. (3) Diary, Hosp Cons Br SGO, 29 Mar 45. SG: 024.7-3. (4) Ltr, Dep SG to CG ASF, 3 Feb 45, sub: Funds for Instl of PA Systs in Gen Hosps. SG: 413.47.

[33] (1) Memo, Chief Hosp Cons Br SGO for Chief Oprs Serv SGO, 22 Aug 45, sub: Reduction of Cons Reqmts and Concurrent Changes in Budget. SG: 632. (2) Ltr SPMCH 632, SG to CG ASF, 17 Sep 45, sub: Cancellation and Reinstatement of Comd Cons Projects, ZI Gen Hosps. CE: 632 (Hosp). (3) Memo, CofEngrs for CG ASF, 9 Oct 45. Same file.

[34] An Rpt, 1941, Sta Hosp, Ft Bragg; and An Rpts, 1942, Percy Jones Gen Hosp and Sta Hosp Cp Butner. HD.

[35] WD Memo W 40-44, 12 Apr 44, sub: Central Serv Syst in Army Hosps. SG: 300.6.

[36] (1) Memo, Maj Michael E. DeBakey for Brig Gen C. C. Hillman, 20 Jul 43, sub: Central Serv. SG: 632.-1. (2) Memo, Chief Hosp Cons Br SGO for Dir Surg Div SGO, 21 Oct 43, sub: Central Serv Fac. Same file.

[37] Memo, Maj Edwin M. Loye for Lt Col A. L. Tynes, 20 Jan 44, sub: Discussion of Central Serv . . . in Gen Hillman's Off. . . . SG: 632.-1.

by doctors in wards.[38] ASF headquarters therefore authorized the Engineers to provide buildings for such services, either by new construction or by the alteration of existing buildings, wherever they were requested and justified by hospital commanders.[39] Thereafter, during 1944 and 1945 central service buildings were provided for all general and regional hospitals.[40]

In getting other administrative buildings, the Surgeon General's Office was less successful. One fault with hospital plants already constructed was that they lacked rooms for clinical conferences.[41] Moreover, the addition to general hospitals of functions and activities not common in peacetime increased the need for more administrative space. Special services officers, reconditioning officers, personal affairs officers, Veterans Administration representatives, and United States Employment Service representatives often had to set up offices in wards, barracks, and storerooms. Consequently, on 28 July 1944 The Surgeon General requested the enlargement of hospital administrative buildings. Before granting approval, ASF headquarters required him to collaborate with the Chief of Engineers in a detailed study of office-space requirements.[42] By the time it was completed in February 1945 the general-convalescent hospital expansion program had increased even more the need for administrative space.[43] On 3 April 1945 The Surgeon General again urged that it be authorized, and finally, on 25 April 1945, ASF headquarters instructed the Engineers and The Surgeon General to collaborate in planning whatever construction was needed to bring existing hospital plants up to the standards set by their joint study.[44] Surveys by service command surgeons of existing administrative space and of the additional amount required delayed the beginning of work on this program until hospitals began to close. It was then largely abandoned.[45]

Improvements in Existing Hospital Plants

At the same time hospital plants were being expanded and improved to meet needs that had developed during the war, the Surgeon General's Office was attempting to correct constructional defects and to bring the Army's hurriedly erected hospital buildings up to the standards of finish, appearance, and equipment of civilian institutions. During 1944 the reflooring program was continued,[46] and defects in hospital construction revealed by inspections made by the War Projects

[38] Ltr, SG to CofEngrs, 21 Jan 44, sub: Central Serv Bldg at Cushing Gen Hosp. SG: 632 (Cushing GH)K.

[39] Memo, CofEngrs for SG, 2 Feb 44, sub: Central Serv Bldgs at Gen Hosps. SG: 632.-1.

[40] (1) An Rpt, FY 1944 and 1945, Hosp Cons Br SGO. HD. (2) Memo, SG for CofEngrs, 10 Mar 45. SG: 632.

[41] 1st ind, SG to CofEngrs, 7 Mar 44, on Ltr, CO McGuire Gen Hosp to SG, 10 Feb 44, sub: Cons of Add Clinic-Type Bldg. SG: 632.-1 (McGuire GH)K.

[42] 1st ind SPMOC 632 (31 Jul 44), CG ASF to CofEngrs, 3 Aug 44, and 2d ind, CofEngrs to SG, 7 Aug 44, on Ltr SPMCH 632, Dep SG to CG ASF, 28 Jul 44, sub: Admin Space in Gen Hosps. CE: 683 Pt I.

[43] Ltr SPMCH 632, SG to CG ASF thru CofEngrs, 8 Jan 45, sub: Admin Space in Gen and Regional Hosps, with 1st ind, CofEngrs to CG ASF thru SG, 24 Feb 45. CE: 683 Pt I.

[44] 2d ind SPMCH 632, SG to CG ASF, 3 Apr 45, and 3d ind SPMOC 632 (3 Apr 45), CG ASF to CofEngrs thru SG, 25 Apr 45, on Ltr SPMCH 632, SG to CG ASF thru CofEngrs, 8 Jan 45, sub: Admin Space in Gen and Regional Hosps. CE: 683 Pt I.

[45] Diary, Hosp Cons Br SGO, 18 Sep 45. HD: 024.7-3.

[46] (1) See above, p. 96. (2) Diary, Hosp Cons Br SGO, 9 and 20 Jun 44. HD: 024.7-3.

Unit of the Bureau of the Budget were corrected by the Engineers.[47] In the opinion of the Surgeon General's Hospital Construction Branch a broader program of more general application was needed. Therefore, late in the summer of 1944, when ASF headquarters began to plan for the improvement of Army installations that would be selected for postwar use,[48] Surgeon General Kirk secured the personal backing of General Somervell for a relaxation of the War Department's policy of "Spartan simplicity" in order to permit higher maintenance standards for hospitals.[49] About the same time, Congressional criticism of Army hospital construction and maintenance apparently spurred ASF headquarters to more "aggressive action in increasing the maintenance program for hospitals."[50] At any rate, during September and October 1944 the ASF Command Installation Branch and offices of The Surgeon General and the Chief of Engineers agreed upon a program for improving ASF hospitals. It included covering floors in corridors and administrative buildings, as well as in wards and clinics, with linoleum over plywood; sealing exposed framing in corridors and nurses' quarters; inclosing all corridors used by patients; painting both exteriors and interiors to conform to peacetime standards, including the use of pastel colors for interiors; replacement of "victory-grade" with standard hardware and fittings; and the planting and proper maintenance of lawns and grounds.[51] In approving this program G–4 stipulated that it should be carried out only partially in hospitals that the Army would not retain after the war.[52] ASF headquarters decided therefore to limit the program to general and convalescent hospitals that would be retained in the postwar period and to delay its extension to regional and station hospitals until a later time.[53] The Surgeon General repeatedly protested against both the G–4 and ASF limitations, but was unsuccessful in getting them removed during the war.[54]

---

[47] For example, see: (1) Ltr SPMCH 632, SG to CofEngrs, 19 Aug 44, sub: Transmittal of Comments on Sta Hosp Cons Rptd to SG by War Projects Unit, Bu of Budget. CE: 632 (Hosp)No. 1. (2) Memo, CofEngrs for SG, 12 Oct 44, sub: Comments on Gen Hosp Cons. Same file. (3) Ltr SPMCH 632, SG to CofEngrs, 25 Nov 44, sub: Transmittal of Comments on Army Hosp Cons Rptd to SG by War Projects Unit, Bu of Budget. Same file. (4) Ltr SPEMY 632, CofEngrs to SG, 18 Apr 45, sub: Comments on Army Hosp Cons. SG: 632.

[48] 1st ind SPMOC 600.1 (18 Aug 44), CG ASF to CofEngrs, 25 Aug 44, on unknown basic ltr. CE: 632.

[49] Comments by Col A. L. Tynes, Chief Hosp Cons Br SGO at Conf of SvC Surgs, 12 Dec 44. SG: 632.

[50] (1) Memo, Dir Plans and Oprs ASF for Dir Mob Div ASF, 17 Sep 44. HRS: Maj Gen LeRoy Lutes' files, "Hosp and Evac, Jun 43–Dec 46." (2) Memo, Chief Hosp Cons Br SGO for Dep SG, 2 Sep 44, sub: Comments Relative to Rptd Defects in Hosp Cons. SG: 632. (3) *Investigations of the National War Effort, Report, Committee on Military Affairs, House of Representatives, 78th Cong, 2d sess, pursuant to* H. Res. 30 (Washington, 1944).

[51] (1) Memo, SG for CG ASF, 6 Sep 44, sub: Suggested Remedial Measures, Hosp Cons, ZI, in Tynes, Construction Branch. (2) Memo, CofEngrs for CG ASF, 18 Sep 44, sub: Preferred Maintenance for Post War Use Instls. CE: 632 (Hosp). (3) Memo, CofEngrs for CG ASF, 30 Sep 44, sub: Suggested Remedial Measures, Hosp Cons in ZI. CE: 600.18. (4) Memo, CofEngrs for CG ASF, 14 Oct 44, sub: Preferred Maintenance for Gen Hosps. Same file. (5) Diary, Hosp Cons Br SGO, 3 Oct 44. HD: 024.7–3.

[52] DF WDGDS 4031, ACofS G–4 WDGS to CG ASF, 27 Oct 44, sub: Increased Maintenance at Gen and Conv Hosps. HRS: G–4 file, 600.3 (I).

[53] Memo SPMOC 632, CG ASF for CofEngrs, 31 Oct 44, sub: Increased Maintenance at Gen and Conv Hosps, in Tynes, Construction Branch.

[54] (1) Memo, Dep SG for CG ASF, 10 Nov 44, sub: Increased Maintenance at Gen and Conv Hosps, with 1st ind SPMOC 632 (10 Nov 44), CG ASF to SG, 16 Nov 44, in Tynes, Construction Branch. (2) Memo, SG for CofEngrs, 11 Jul 45, sub: Increased Standards of Maintenance at Regional Hosps, with 3d ind SPMOC 423.3 (1 Aug 45), CG ASF to CofEngrs, 10 Aug 45. SG: 323.3 (Hosp).

Finally, in June 1946, the General Staff sanctioned the program, within the limits of funds available, for regional and station hospitals to be kept for the postwar Army.[55] Meanwhile, in March 1945, after representatives of G–4 suggested that the staging area hospitals being converted into debarkation hospitals should be "dressed-up" for the reception of returning war casualties, ASF headquarters authorized the application of the higher standards of maintenance to those hospitals.[56]

Although improvement of general and ASF convalescent hospitals was authorized in October 1944, it did not get started until early in 1945. Causes for delay during that period and later were numerous: the controversy over whether to limit the program to postwar hospitals; the tardiness of service commands, which under existing procedures had to initiate the requests for improvements; the time spent by the offices of The Surgeon General and the Chief of Engineers in deciding on colors of interior paint; the confusion in the field that arose from carrying on two projects at once—the improvements program and the hospital expansion program; the extension of the project to cover barracks and other buildings newly converted to hospital use; the effort to interfere as little as possible with the normal operation of the hospitals; and the hindrance of winter weather to the planting of lawns and the painting of exteriors. In view of such factors the Engineers estimated in February 1945 that the maintenance program would not be entirely completed until the end of 1945, but that the greater portion of it would be finished by the end of July.[57]

Another aspect of the general movement to raise the standards of Army hospital plants was extension of the program of installing air-conditioning or ventilating equipment and inauguration of a program of installing nurses' call systems. The Surgeon General's Office wanted the existing air-cooling program expanded. During the last six months of 1943 and the early part of 1944 the Hospital Construction Branch sought approval for the installation of air-conditioning equipment in the operating rooms of all general hospitals, whether they were located in areas with July temperatures above 75 degrees Fahrenheit or not, and in dental clinics in certain areas that had hot summers. It also requested that either mechanical-ventilating or evaporative-cooling equipment be permitted in some storerooms and in patients' recreation buildings.[58] A revision of policy by ASF headquarters in April 1944 permitted the installation of air-conditioning equipment in dental clinics in the South and of either mechanical-ventilating or evaporative-cooling

[55] Ltr SPMCH 600.3, SG to CG ASF thru CofEngrs, 4 Jun 46, sub: Increased Maintenance at Regional and Sta Hosps, with 1st ind, CofEngrs to Dir SS&P WDGS, 19 Jun 46, and 2d ind, Dir SS&P WDGS to SG thru CofEngrs, 26 Jun 46. SG: 600.3.

[56] (1) Memo SPMOC 632 (9 Mar 45), CG ASF for CofEngrs, 9 Mar 45, sub: Improvement of Debarkation Hosps. SG: 632. (2) Memo, Col L[loyd] E. Fellenz, GSC, G–4 Div for ACofS G–4 WDGS, 14 Mar 45, sub: Improvements at Debarkation Hosps. HRS: G–4 file, "Hosp and Evac Policy."

[57] Memo SPMOC 600.1, CG ASF for CofEngrs and SG in turn, 7 Feb 45, sub: Conversion, New Cons, and Preferred Maintenance at Gen and Conv Hosps, with 1st ind, CofEngrs to CG ASF thru SG, 22 Feb 45. CE: 683 Pt. I.

[58] (1) Memo, SG to CG ASF, 28 Jul 43, sub: Ventilative Treatment for Hosp Storehouses. (2) Memo, SG for CG ASF, 28 Aug 43, sub: Air Conditioning, Surgeries. (3) Memo, SG for CG ASF, 12 Oct 43, sub: Proposed Changes in WD Policy Governing Air Conditioning, Ventilation, and Cooling in ZI Hosps. (4) Memo, SG for CG ASF, 12 Feb 44, sub: Air Conditioning for Dental Clinics. All in SG: 673.–4.

equipment in patients' recreation buildings, but not in storehouses, in areas where the July temperatures exceeded 75 degrees Fahrenheit.[59] Soon afterward, as the closure of station hospitals began to make equipment in those plants available for other uses, The Surgeon General again requested an extension of the program, and on 13 July 1944 ASF headquarters approved the installation of air-conditioning equipment in operating rooms and of either air-conditioning or ventilating equipment in X-ray clinics and recovery wards of general and regional hospitals anywhere in the United States, regardless of average July temperatures. The installation of such equipment in station hospitals was still limited to those located in southern areas of the country.[60]

As in the case earlier of air-cooling equipment, a shortage of critical materials delayed initiation of a nurses' call-system program. During the winter of 1943–44 some hospitals nevertheless succeeded in procuring equipment and in having such systems installed with nonappropriated funds.[61] When equipment became more plentiful in the spring of 1944, ASF headquarters authorized the use of appropriated funds to install nurses' call-systems in all general hospitals and to some extent in others.[62] Because the amount of money set aside for this purpose was limited, The Surgeon General decided that, in general, only wards used for nonambulatory patients would get the equipment and general hospitals would get it before regional hospitals.[63] By March 1945 all general hospitals and all but thirty-one regional hospitals had had nurses' call systems installed. At that time ASF headquarters approved the Engineers' request for sufficient additional funds to complete the installation of such systems in all regional hospitals.[64]

Housing for Hospitals in Theaters of Operations

In the middle of 1943 Surgeon General Kirk and his chief of Professional Services had the problem of housing for hospitals in theaters called forcibly to their attention during visits to North Africa and the Southwest Pacific. According to plans at the beginning of the war, hospitals in theaters of operations were to be housed in tents, in existing buildings wherever they were available, or in buildings erected by the Engineers with either native or imported building materials according to standard plans for theater-of-operations-type construction. None of these means of housing had proved universally satisfactory. In some areas, such as North Africa, tentage was too hot. In others, such as the Pacific, it not only was too hot but it mildewed, rotted, and disintegrated within

[59] (1) Memo, CG ASF for SG, 14 Mar 44, sub: Proposed Revision of WD Memo W 100–4–43, with incl, draft of memo. SG: 300.6. (2) WD Cir 148, 14 Apr 44.

[60] (1) Ltr, SG to CG ASF, 19 Jun 44, sub: Air Conditioning in Gen and Regional Hosps, with 2d ind, CG ASF to CofEngrs, 13 Jul 44. (2) OCE Cir Ltr 3457 (Repairs and Utilities No 10), 19 Dec 44, sub: Refrigeration and Ventilation—Revision of Policy for Air-conditioning in Gen, Regional and Sta Hosps. Both in CE: 673.

[61] Ltr, SG to CofEngrs, 16 Mar 44, sub: MD Cons Reqmts for FY 1945. SG: 632.-1.

[62] Memo, CG ASF for SG, 1 Apr 44, referred to in 1st ind SPMCH 676, SG to CofEngrs, 26 Aug 44, on Memo, CofEngrs for SG, 23 Aug 44, sub: Nurses' Signaling Fac. SG: 413.45.

[63] 1st ind SPMCH 676, SG to CofEngrs, 26 Aug 44, on Memo, CofEngrs for SG, 23 Aug 44, sub: Nurses' Signaling Fac. SG: 413.45.

[64] Memo, CofEngrs for CG ASF, 25 Mar 45, sub: Nurses' Call Systs, with 1st ind SPMOC 676.1 (25 Mar 45), CG ASF to CofEngrs, 2 Apr 45. SG: 413.45.

about six months. In addition, the use of tentage made more difficult the control of mosquitoes in malarious areas. In some of the places where tentage was unsuitable for housing hospitals, there were no available existing buildings. Moreover, the Medical Department often encountered difficulties in getting theater-of-operations-type housing constructed because of shortages of lumber in theaters and of competition for Engineer services with such high-priority projects as the construction of harbors, docks, piers, airstrips, and essential roads. Beginning in the latter half of 1943 the Surgeon General's Office turned its attention to these problems.[65]

The problem of modifying tentage so that interior temperatures were lowered was relatively simple to solve. Late in July 1943 representatives of The Surgeon General and The Quartermaster General found that the British used a fly with their tents.[66] Suspended on poles above a tent, it provided shade for the tent roof and also retained an insulating layer of air, thereby reducing the temperature inside by about 20 degrees in the summer sun. After suitable tests, the Quartermaster Technical Committee in the summer of 1943 approved the use of flies with hospital tents. Plans were then made to procure 30,000, and subsequently tent flies were included in revised tables of equipment for hospital units. Thus a large existing stock of hospital ward tentage was adapted to use in tropical climates of low humidity.[67]

Meanwhile the Quartermaster Corps had begun a more extensive project—the development of a new type of hospital tent. Called a sectional hospital tent, it had two distinguishing characteristics. A white liner made of cotton sheeting covered the entire inside of the tent, lowering temperatures and promoting cleanliness. This tent was so constructed that a complete end section could be detached from the main body and additional center sections added to extend its length as desired. It was standardized in July 1944 and, as tables of organization and equipment of hospital units were subsequently revised, was included as a replacement for ward tents with flies. Some were issued for overseas use before the end of the war.[68]

The problem of providing housing in hot humid areas that had little lumber and no buildings was more difficult. During the early part of the war the Southwest

[65] (1) Memo, SG for CG ASF, 10 Aug 43, sub: Interim Progress Rpt. SG: 024.-1. (2) An Rpt, Chief Surg SWPA, 1942. HD. (3) Ltr, Hq USASOS SWPA to CG ASF thru CG SWPA, 16 Sep 44, sub: Rpt of Trip to SWPA. . . . SG: 333.1-1 (Aust)F. (4) Ltr, SG to CG ASF, 28 Nov 44, Hosp Fac in TofOpns. HD: 632.-1 (Hosp Fac in POA). (5) Memo SPMCP 632 (Aust)F, SG for CG ASF, 29 Dec 44, sub: Hosp Cons, SWPA. HRS: ASF Hq Somervell files, "SG, 1944."

[66] The United States Army used flies with small tents but had made no provision for their use with the much larger hospital ward tents. Information supplied by Dr. Irving G. Cheslaw, Historian, OQMG.

[67] (1) Memo SPOPI 424.1, Col Robert C. McDonald, MC, Chief Hosp and Evac Sec Planning Div Oprs ASF for Gen Lutes, 21 Jul 43, sub: Improvement in Tentage and Laundries for the MD. HD: Wilson files, "Day File, Jul 43." (2) Inf note, W. D. Styer to Col Smith, ca. 17 Aug 43. HRS: ASF Control Div, 319.1 "SGs Interim Rpt, G-56." (3) Memo, Col [Robert C.] McDonald for Col F. M. Smith, 17 Aug 43, sub: Shelter for Overseas Hosps. Same file. (4) Memo, Dep Dir Oprs ASF for CofS ASF, 31 Aug 43, sub: SGs Interim Progress Rpt, with 6 incls. Same file. (5) T/O&E 8-550, Gen Hosp, C 2, 16 May 44. (6) T/O&E 8-581, Evac Hosp SM (400-bed), 25 Mar 44.

[68] (1) Erna Risch, *The Quartermaster Corps: Organization, Supply, and Services* (Washington, 1953), p. 171, in UNITED STATES ARMY IN WORLD WAR II. (2) T/O&E 8-560, Sta Hosp, 28 Oct 44. (3) T/O&E 8-580, Evac Hosp, 31 Jan 45. (4) Information supplied informally by Dr. Risch on 30 November 1953.

Pacific theater had developed plans for partially prefabricated buildings and had arranged with the Australians for their manufacture. Constructed of corrugated sheets of iron, floored with wood or concrete, screened, and provided with wide overhanging eaves for protection against tropical rains, buildings of this type—called "Australian cowsheds"—had been satisfactory. By the middle of 1943, the demand for them threatened to exceed the Australian supply and the theater called upon the zone of interior to furnish prefabricated buildings to house 22,000 beds in 44 hospitals.[69] As a result, the offices of The Surgeon General and the Chief of Engineers worked on improvements in plans for overseas hospitals and on the provision of prefabricated buildings.[70] The term "prefabricated" was used loosely by both offices and apparently meant different things to different people, for in September 1943 the Surgeon General's Construction Division was surprised when it discovered that the Engineers were planning precut but not prefabricated buildings.[71] The Surgeon General protested against the adoption of precut construction, but because of the urgent need for hospital buildings in the Pacific, ASF headquarters, the Engineers reported, directed them to fill the theater's requisition.[72] In conferences with representatives of the Surgeon General, the Chief of Engineers agreed that truly prefabricated steel buildings would be preferable to those of precut wood, but pointed to restrictions upon the use of steel as the major reason for not planning its use in hospital buildings. The Surgeon General's Office then prepared an urgent request to ASF headquarters for steel, and the ASF Matériel and Production Division decided that, as a result of the cancellation of drum plate commitments, it could be supplied for buildings for twenty of the forty-four hospitals requested by the Pacific.[73] Subsequently, the Surgeon General's Office and the Engineers engaged in a revision of plans for the types, sizes, and internal arrangements of hospital buildings, to correct defects that had been revealed by experience in using theater-of-operations-type construction in the Desert Training Center in the United States.[74]

The plans for precut hospital buildings developed by the Office of the Chief of Engineers failed to meet the approval of theater headquarters. In the first place, the Southwest Pacific theater believed that they would not solve the engineering problem, for to erect them would require more construction personnel than would

[69] Office of the Chief Engineer, General Headquarters Army Forces, Pacific, *Engineers in Theater Operations,* in ENGINEERS OF THE SOUTHWEST PACIFIC 1941–45, vol. I (1947), pp. 127–28. Reference to a requisition dated 19 July 1943, which had not been located, is made in Ltr, CG USASOS SWPA to CG ASF thru CG USAFFE, 28 Apr 44, sub: Prefabricated Hosps. CE: 632 "Vol. 4."

[70] Memo, CofEngrs for SG, 19 Aug 43, sub: Proposed Plans for . . . Tropical Hosps . . . Prefabricated All Wood Bldgs, with 3 inds. SG: 632.–1 (Gen).

[71] Memo, CofEngrs for SG, 23 Sep 43, sub: Prefabricated Tropical Hosps, with 1 ind and 3 incls. CE: 632 "Vol. 4."

[72] (1) Memo, CofEngrs for SG, 13 Oct 43, sub: Structures for Tropical Hosps. SG: 632.–1 (Gen). (2) Memo, Maj Edwin M. Loye, SGO for Lt Col A. L. Tynes, SGO, 15 Oct 43, sub: Mtg . . . Regarding Prefabricated Steel and Stock Precut Wood Hosp Bldgs. Same file.

[73] (1) Ltr, Act SG to Mat Div SOS, 18 Oct 43, sub: Steel Hosp Bldgs. SG: 632.–1. (2) 1st ind, CG ASF to CofEngrs, 23 Oct 43, sub: Steel Hosp Bldgs, on unlocated basic Ltr. SG: MOOD "Pacific."

[74] (1) Memo, Chief Hosp Cons Br SGO for SG, 21 Feb 44, sub: Insp of TofOpns Type Hosp Facs in the C–AMA. SG: 632.–1. (2) Ltr, SG to CofEngrs, 24 Apr 44, sub: Modifications of TofOpns Specifications for Hosp Cons. Same file. (3) Rpt of Conf, CofEngrs to SG, 19 May 44. HD: 632.–1.

be available. In the second place, hospitals planned for precut construction were more elaborate than the theater thought necessary. For example, floor space per bed in wards was greater than in Australian prefabricated buildings, services and utilities were considered excessive, and certain buildings such as fire stations, guardhouses, and quarters for officers and enlisted men were considered unnecessary. War experience in the Pacific had dictated austerity in hospital housing which the Surgeon General's Office was unwilling to approve. The Southwest Pacific agreed to accept the hospital buildings being prepared for shipment from the United States "on the score of expediency," but requested that they be held until called for.[75] Meanwhile, the Southwest Pacific continued to use "Australian cowsheds" and the Central Pacific to use Quonset huts supplied by the Navy.[76] When precut hospital buildings did arrive in the Pacific, theater headquarters found them, for the reasons expected, unsatisfactory.[77] During the rest of 1944 and the early part of 1945 the Offices of The Surgeon General and the Chief of Engineers continued attempts to provide prefabricated hospitals that would meet the needs of the Pacific, but the war ended before they could achieve success.

---

[75] (1) Ltr, CG USASOS (SWPA) to CG ASF thru CG USAFFE, 28 Apr 44, sub: Prefabricated Hosps, with 7 inds. CE: 632 "Vol. 4." (2) Ltr, SG to CofEngrs, 29 May 44, sub: Prefabricated Hosps. SG: 632.-1. (3) Memo, Chief Theater Br SGO for Col Welsh, 29 Sep 44, sub: Housing for Hosps. SG: MOOD "Pacific."

[76] (1) Memo, Chief Theater Br SGO for Col [Arthur B.] Welsh SGO, 13 Sep 44, sub: Housing for Hosps in SWPA. SG: MOOD "Pacific." (2) Rad CM-IN-10289, CG USAFPOA to CG PE, Ft Mason, Calif, 8 Dec 44. SG: 632 "Hosp Misc 1944."

[77] (1) Memo, Chief Hosp Cons Br SGO for Dir Hosp Div SGO, 2 Sep 44. (2) Memo, Lt Col [Douglas B.] Kendrick, [Jr.] MC for SG, 2 Sep 44, sub: Rpt of Trip to SPA, SWPA, and CPA, 6 Jun-8 Aug 44. (3) Tel conv, Lt Col R. A. Lewis, OCE and Col Tynes, MC, SGO, 2 Sep 44, sub: Prefabricated Hosp Bldgs for Pacific Theater. All in SG: MOOD "Pacific." (4) Ltr, CG Hq Island Comd Saipan to CG POA, 17 Jan 45, sub: Deficiencies of Bks—Precut Ptbl Wood, for Hosp Usage, with 2 inds. CE: 632 (USAFPOA).

CHAPTER XVIII

Return to a Peacetime Basis

With the war's end, first in Europe and then in the Pacific, pressure to return to a peacetime basis was so great that hospital resources built up over a period of more than five years were liquidated in little over a year. This process was first completed in overseas theaters.

Redeployment and Demobilization of Numbered Hospital Units

The peak of hospital beds in overseas theaters was reached in May 1945, when there were in all theaters 343,975 fixed hospital beds and 85,975 mobile hospital beds. Of these, the greatest number were in the European theater, which at that time had 200,350 fixed beds and 58,200 mobile beds.[1] With the approach of V-E Day, the War Department placed emphasis upon evacuating as many patients as possible from both the European and Mediterranean theaters, in order to make full use of shipping space that would later be diverted to the Pacific and to free as many hospital units as possible for redeployment after the defeat of Germany.[2] In April 1945 the 60-day evacuation policy which Europe had been following on a *de facto* basis for several months was made official for both the European and Mediterranean theaters.[3] After V-E Day, as both troops and patients were moved out of these theaters, plans were made to ship some of their hospital units direct to the Pacific, some to the United States for later shipment to the Pacific, and some to the United States for inactivation.[4] As a result, by August 1945 the number of fixed beds in the European theater decreased to 141,850 and of mobile beds to 50,775.[5] In that month it was possible to place both the European and Mediterranean theaters on an inactive basis—that is, to reduce their establishments to the requirements of occupation forces. Their evacuation policies were therefore set at 120 days and their fixed-bed ratios at 4 percent.[6]

---

[1] Statistics Branch, Control Division, Hq. ASF, *Statistical Review, World War II: A Summary of ASF Activities* (n d), App R, p. 243 (cited hereafter as *Statistical Review, World War II*).

[2] (1) Ltr WDGDS 10303, Dep ACofS G-4 WDGS to CofSA, 17 Mar 45, sub: Evac of Pnts from ETO, with 3 incls. HRS: G-4 files, "Hosp, vol. III." (2) Cablegram CM-OUT-65962, WD to Hq ComZ ETO, 10 Apr 45. Same file. (3) Memo, SG for ACofS G-4 WDGS, 11 Apr 45, sub: Evac Policy with Spec Ref to ETO. SG: 705.

[3] S/S WDGDS 11921, ACofS OPD WDGS to CofSA, 18 Apr 45, sub: Proposed Change in Evac Policy for ETO and MTO. HRS: G-4 files, "Hosp, vol. III."

[4] (1) ASF Monthly Progress Rpt, Sec 7. *Health*, 30 Jun 45, p. 34. (2) ASF Monthly Progress Rpt, Sec 7, *Health*, 31 Jul 45, p. 29.

[5] *Statistical Review, World War II*, App R, p. 243.

[6] (1) Rad CM-IN-19035 (19 Jul 45), TERMINAL to WD, 19 Jul 45. SG: 705. (2) Memo, Lt Col E[dward] C. Spaulding, GSC for ACofS G-4 WDGS, 27 Jul 45, sub: Reduction of Fixed Hosp Bed Basis in ETO. HRS: G-4 files, "Hosp, vol. IV." (3) Memo, SG for ACofS G-4 WDGS, 10 Sep 45, sub: Recommended Reduction in Fixed Beds in ETO and MTO to 4 percent. SG: 632.2. (4) Rad CM-OUT-63182, WAR to CG ETO and MTO, 12 Sep 45. HRS: G-4 files, "Hosp, vol. IV." (5) Memo SPOPP 370.05, Act Dir Plans and Oprs ASF for SG and CofT, 24 Jul 45, sub: Evac Policy ETO. SG: MOOD "ETO." (6) Rad CM-OUT-46451 (Aug 45), COMGENSERV to CG USAF MTO, 8 Aug 45. SG: 705.

With redeployment, the number of fixed and mobile beds in the Southwest Pacific increased from 67,250 in May 1945 to 82,700 in August 1945. Meanwhile, the number of beds in other areas of the Pacific declined from 37,600 to 32,700.[7] The surrender of Japan in August heralded a cancellation of the shipment of further hospital units to the Pacific[8] and a repetition of the process that had been followed in Europe of clearing hospitals of patients by evacuating them to the United States. Early in August, the War Department directed the Pacific—which in April had been placed under a single command—to use all evacuation facilities available, reducing the evacuation policy to 60 days if necessary.[9] The next month it was possible to plan to place that area on an inactive basis. The War Department therefore directed it to return to a 120-day policy effective 1 December 1945 and to comment on a proposed reduction of its bed ratios to 4.8 percent.[10] Before this reduction was actually made, the Surgeon General's Office and the General Staff turned to re-examining the needs of all theaters.

By the end of October 1945 the number of beds in fixed hospitals in theaters of operations had been reduced, through the inactivation of some units in theaters and the return of others to the United States, from a peak of 343,975 in May 1945 to 236,050.[11] This reduction was not great enough to return physicians, dentists, and nurses to civilian life as rapidly as the public and the Congress desired, and in November 1945 both the Secretary of War and the Chief of Staff of the Army took personal interest in speeding that process. Consequently, G–1 called a conference of representatives of other General Staff divisions, of AAF, AGF, and ASF headquarters, and of the Surgeon General's Office. At this conference it was agreed that the Surgeon General's Office would make studies of the requirements of various theaters for beds during demobilization and would submit recommendations for changes in authorized ratios.[12] During November and December 1945 such studies were completed and the General Staff requested theaters to comment on the proposals of The Surgeon General. Aside from a recommendation that the authorized bed ratio of each theater be reduced, his most important proposal was the application of that ratio to beds not only in fixed hospitals but also in mobile hospital units that retained professional staffs of physicians, dentists, and nurses. The reason that The Surgeon General now proposed what he had protested against in August 1943—that is, the use of a single ratio for authorizing beds in both fixed and mobile hospitals—was that the need for mobile hospitals to support troops in combat had vanished with the cessation of hostilities. The only possible excuse for a theater's keeping professional staffs in the mobile units left there was to use these units as fixed hospitals. The Surgeon General's proposals were approved and as a result of studies by his Office and

[7] *Statistical Review, World War II,* App R, p. 243.

[8] ASF Monthly Progress Rpt, Sec 7, *Health,* 31 Aug 45, p. 13. HD.

[9] Memo, C. M. Ankcorn for ACofS G–4 WDGS, 10 Aug 45, sub: Evac from Pacific Theater. HRS: G–4 files, "Hosp, vol. IV."

[10] (1) Memo, Dir MOOD SGO for Record, 24 Sep 45. SG: MOOD "Pacific." (2) Rad CM–OUT–70899 (Sep 45), WARGFOUR to CINCAFPAC, 27 Sep 45. SG: 705. (3) Rad CM–IN–2145, CINCAFPAC to WD, 4 Oct 45. HRS: G–4 files, "Hosp, vol. IV."

[11] Statistical Health Rpts. Off file, Health Rpts Br Med Statistics Div, SGO.

[12] Memo, Lt Col Johnnie R. Dyer, GSC for ACofS G–4 WDGS, 26 Nov 45, sub: Delays in Discharge of Doctors and Dentists. HRS: G–4 files, "Hosp, vol. IV."

of comments by theaters, the General Staff in December 1945 authorized a bed ratio of 4 percent for all theaters except the American, which was to continue on a 3 percent basis.[13] In consequence, the number of beds in fixed hospitals and professionally staffed mobile hospitals decreased rapidly until by the end of May 1946 there were only 42,100 such beds in all theaters.[14]

Contraction of the Zone of Interior Hospital System

Soon after V-E Day G–4 began to put considerable pressure upon ASF, and that headquarters in turn upon the Surgeon General's Office, to estimate general and convalescent hospital requirements in the United States through the first quarter of 1946 and to make plans to reduce the number of beds accordingly.[15] Emphasis was placed upon planning for the contraction of the general-convalescent hospital system because the reduction and closure of station and regional hospitals, dependent primarily upon the reduction and closure of posts where they were located, had already begun and would continue under established procedures. After V-E Day, G–4 called for revised estimates of requirements and The Surgeon General projected forward to the end of 1946 his plans for shrinking the general-convalescent hospital system.[16]

In estimating bed requirements at this time, there still were uncertainties to contend with. Before V-J Day the number of battle casualties that would occur and the number of patients to be evacuated monthly from the Pacific were of course unknown. In addition, there was uncertainty about the amount and rate of redeployment of troops to the Pacific through the United States and the speed with which German prisoners of war would be repatriated.[17] After V-J Day some of these difficulties vanished but additional factors appeared. Among them were the rate at which the Army would be demobilized; the time required to treat patients for secondary diagnoses; the number of soldiers that would be found at separation centers to need hospitalization, especially for tuberculosis and deafness, before their discharge from the Army; and delays that the shortage of specialists might occasion in the disposition of patients already under treatment, particularly plastic surgery and amputation cases.[18]

In view of these uncertainties and difficulties, the Resources Analysis Division of the Surgeon General's Office presented to G–4 "conservative" estimates of the number of beds that could be eliminated each quarter, in order to protect the Medical Department against the possibility of having too few beds for any reason. For example, the number of patients who would

[13] ASF Monthly Progress Rpt, Sec 7, *Health*, 31 Dec 45, p. 17, HD. The studies made by the Surgeon General's Office, the comments of theaters, and the documents in which the Staff authorized new bed ratios are filed in HRS: G–4 files, "Hosp, vol. V."

[14] ASF Monthly Progress Rpt, Sec 7, *Health*, 31 May 46, p. 22. HD.

[15] (1) Diary, Resources Anal Div SGO, 16 Jun 45. HD: 024.7–3. (2) DF WDGDS 15204, ACofS G–4 WDGS to CG ASF, 23 Jun 45, sub: ZI Hosps. HRS: Hq ASF Planning Div file, 700 "ZI Hosp." (3) T/S SPOPP 702 (25 Jun 45), CG ASF to SG, 27 Jun 45, sub: ZI Hosps. Same file.

[16] (1) DF WDGDS 2399, ACofS G–4 WDGS to CG ASF attn SG, 18 Aug 45, sub: ZI Hosps. SG: 322 "Hosp." (2) Memo, SG for ACofS G–4 WDGS thru CG ASF, 14 Sep 45, sub: Cut-back in Gen and Conv Hosp Fac. Same file.

[17] Memo, SG for ACofS G–4 WDGS, 8 Jun 45, sub: Hosp Fac. SG: 322 "Hosp."

[18] 1st ind, SG to CG ASF, 28 Nov 45, on Memo SPOPP 705, CG ASF for SG, 9 Nov 45, sub: Cut-back in Gen and Conv Hosp Fac, ZI. SG: 323.3 (Gen Hosp).

need beds in November was used as the number who would need them in December, and to this number were added additional beds that would be vacant either because of dispersion or because some patients were absent from hospitals on leave and furlough.[19] On 14 September 1945 The Surgeon General informed G–4 that the capacities of general hospitals could be reduced by 40,000, 38,000, and 39,000 beds and of convalescent hospitals by 21,000, 14,000, and 8,000 beds during the last quarter of 1945 and the first two quarters of 1946, and that 16,000 additional general hospital beds could be eliminated during the last half of 1946. In December this program was revised, chiefly to speed the liquidation of the convalescent hospital system.[20]

Soon after V-E Day the Resources Analysis Division had established a procedure for reducing the number of beds in general and convalescent hospitals. It involved closing entire hospitals rather than parts of all of them, in order to free more physicians for return to civilian life—a matter that was to assume increasing importance as the press, the public, and the Congress continued to clamor for their release. For example, a reduction of the capacities of five 2,500-bed hospitals by 500 beds each would release only 25 physicians while the closure of one 2,500-bed hospital would release 60.[21] This decision having been made, the Division established certain broad principles to govern the selection of particular hospitals for closure during successive quarters. They were as follows: leased buildings should be returned to their owners, and hospitals needed by other government agencies, such as the Veterans Administration, should be transferred to these agencies as soon as possible; hospitals in heavily populated areas should be retained to permit the hospitalization of patients near their homes; hospitals that were less desirable because of climate and construction should be closed before others; hospitals needed for the postwar Army and for station hospital purposes should be retained; and hospitals designated as specialized centers for long-term cases, such as amputation and neurosurgery cases, should be retained as long as possible in order to keep to a minimum the transfer of those patients to other hospitals.

In some instances, these principles conflicted with one another. For example, Halloran and Mason General Hospitals were located in leased buildings and McGuire and Vaughan were desired by the Veterans Administration, but they were also situated in areas of dense population where many beds were needed. Lovell and Tilton General Hospitals were of poor construction, being among the first of the cantonment-type general hospitals constructed during World War II, but were located on Army posts and might be needed for station hospital use. These con-

[19] (1) Statement by Eli Ginzberg, Dir Resources Anal Div SGO, in Notes on Morning Sess of SvC Surgs Conf, 27 Sep 45. HD: Resources Anal Div files, "Hosp." (2) Memo, Dir Resources Anal Div SGO for Chief Oprs Serv SGO, 7 Jun 45, sub: Criteria for Reduction in Hosp Fac. SG: 323.3 (Hosp).

[20] (1) Memo, SG for ACofS G-4 WDGS thru CG ASF, 14 Sep 45, sub: Cut-back in Gen and Conv Hosp Fac. SG: 322 "Hosp." (2) Memo, SG for ACofS G-4 WDGS thru CG ASF, 21 Dec 45, same sub. SG: 323.3 (Hosp).

[21] (1) Memo, Dir Resources Anal Div SGO for Chief Oprs Serv SGO, 7 Jun 45, sub: Criteria for Reduction in Hosp Fac. SG: 323.3 (Hosp). (2) Statement by Eli Ginzberg, Dir Resources Anal Div SGO, in Notes on Morning Sess of SvC Surgs Conf, 27 Sep 45. HD: Resources Anal Div file, "Hosp." (3) Ltr, SG to CGs SvCs attn Surg, 20 Dec 45, sub: Comparative Studies of Gen-Conv and Sta-Regional Hosp Systs. SG: 323.3 (Hosp).

TABLE 15—U. S. ARMY GENERAL HOSPITALS IN THE UNITED STATES DURING WORLD WAR II

Name of hospital	War Department directive naming or designating hospital	Person for whom named	Location	Population of town or city according to 1940 census	Type of construction	Date ready for or received first patient	Authorized bed capacity as of April 1945	Specialties as of April 1945	Date of disposition of last general hospital patient up to 31 Dec. 1946	Disposition as listed by Army 31 July 1951
Army and Navy	WDGO 36 4 Jun 86	....	Hot Springs, Ark.	21, 370	Multi-story permanent (brick)	17 Jan. 1887	1, 220	General medicine; arthritis; deep x-ray therapy; radium therapy	....	Active 1951; retained for Regular Army
Ashburn	WDGO 68 16 Dec 42	Percy Moreau Ashburn (1872–1940), Col., MC, USA	McKinney, Tex.	8, 555	Special type resembling type A (tile)	15 Jun. 1943	1, 592	General medicine; arthritis	18 Dec. 1945	Transferred to Vet. Admin.
Ashford	WDGO 64 24 Nov 42	Bailey Kelley Ashford (1873–1934), Col., MC, USA	White Sulphur Springs, W. Va.	2, 093	Multi-story permanent (brick) (converted hotel)	14 Nov. 1942	2, 025	General medicine; neurology; neurosurgery; vascular surgery	15 Jun. 1946	Transferred to town of White Sulphur Springs, W. Va.
Barnes	Ltr AG 322.3 Gen Hosp (1–9–41)M (Ret) M–C, 11 Feb 41	Joseph K. Barnes (1817–83), Surgeon General, USA, 1864–82	Vancouver, Wash.	18, 788	Cantonment (wood)	16 Apr. 1941	1, 547	General and orthopedic surgery	14 Dec. 1945	Transferred to Vet. Admin.
Battey	WDGO 23 15 May 43	Robert Battey (1828–95), Surgeon, Confederate Army	Rome, Ga.	26, 282	Type A (brick)	7 Nov. 1943	1, 826	General medicine; general and orthopedic surgery; psychiatry	15 Dec. 1945	Transferred to State of Georgia
Baxter	WDGO 64 24 Nov 42	Jedediah Hyde Baxter (1837–90), Surgeon General, USA, 16 Aug. to 4 Dec. 1890	Spokane, Wash.	122, 001	Cantonment (wood)	24 Jun. 1943	2, 001	General medicine; general and orthopedic surgery; thoracic surgery	8 Nov. 1945	Transferred to Vet. Admin. and Navy Dept.
Billings	Ltr AG 322.3 Gen Hosp (1–9–41)M (Ret) M–C, 11 Feb 41	John Shaw Billings (1838–1913), Lt. Col., MC, USA	Fort Benjamin Harrison (Indianapolis, Ind.)	386, 972	Cantonment (wood)	15 Jul. 1941	1, 510	General and orthopedic surgery	15 Mar. 1946	Transferred to Vet. Admin.

Birmingham	WDGO 48 24 Aug 43	Henry Patrick Birmingham (1854–1932), Brig. Gen., MC, USA	Van Nuys, Calif. (Los Angeles)	1, 504, 277	Type A (stucco)	25 Feb. 1944	1, 777	General medicine; CNS syphilis; rheumatic fever; psychiatry	31 Mar. 1946	Transferred to Vet. Admin.
Borden	WDGO 64 24 Nov 42	William Cline Borden (1858–1934), Lt. Col, MC, USA	Chickasha, Okla.	14, 111	Cantonment (wood)	12 Mar. 1943	1, 400	General and orthopedic surgery; deaf	20 Sep. 1946	Assumed by War Assets Admin.
Brooke	WDGO 58 29 Oct 42	Roger Brooke (1878–1940), Brig. Gen., MC, USA	Fort Sam Houston (San Antonio, Tex.)	253, 854	Multi-story permanent (brick and tile)	4 Sep. 1942	3, 071	General medicine; trench foot; thoracic surgery; psychiatry	....	Active 1951; retained for Regular Army
Bruns	WDGO 67 14 Dec. 42	Earl Harvey Bruns (1879–1933), Col., MC, USA	Santa Fe, N. Mex.	20, 325	Cantonment (wood and asbestos shingle)	19 Apr. 1943	1, 575	General medicine; tuberculosis	14 Dec. 1946	Transferred to Atomic Energy Commission and Christian Brothers College
Bushnell	WDGO 64 24 Nov 42	George Ensign Bushnell (1853–1924), Col., MC, USA	Brigham City, Utah	5, 641	Two-story semipermanent (brick)	10 Oct. 1942	3, 377	Neurology; amputations; neurosurgery; deep x-ray therapy; psychiatry	28 Jun. 1946	Assumed by War Assets Admin.
Crile	WDGO 48 24 Aug 43	George Washington Crile (1864–1943), Brig. Gen., MC, Res., USA	Cleveland, Ohio	878, 336	Type A (brick)	8 Apr. 1944	1, 867	General and orthopedic surgery; plastic surgery; ophthalmologic surgery; psychiatry	25 May 1946	Transferred to Vet. Admin.
Cushing	WDGO 48 24 Aug 43	Harvey Cushing (1869–1939), Col., MC, Res., USA	Framingham, Mass.	23, 214	Type A (brick)	27 Feb. 1944	1, 800	Neurology; plastic surgery; ophthalmologic surgery; neurosurgery; psychiatry	30 Sep. 1946	Transferred to Vet. Admin.
Darnall	WDGO 15 29 Dec 41	Carl Rogers Darnall (1867–1941), Brig. Gen., MC, USA	Danville, Ky.	6, 734	Multi-story permanent (brick) (converted civilian hospital)	24 Mar. 1942	921	Psychiatry	15 Dec. 1945	Returned to State of Kentucky

TABLE 15—U. S. ARMY GENERAL HOSPITALS IN THE UNITED STATES DURING WORLD WAR II—Continued

Name of hospital	War Department directive naming or designating hospital	Person for whom named	Location	Population of town or city according to 1940 census	Type of construction	Date ready for or received first patient	Authorized bed capacity as of April 1945	Specialties as of April 1945	Date of disposition of last general hospital patient up to 31 Dec. 1946	Disposition as listed by Army 31 July 1951
Deshon	WDGO 64 24 Nov 42	George Durfee Deshon (1865–1917), Lt. Col., MC, USA	Butler, Pa.	24, 477	Multi-story permanent (brick) (converted civilian sanitorium)	1 Dec. 1942	1, 774	General and orthopedic surgery; deaf	29 Apr. 1946	Transferred to Vet. Admin.
DeWitt	WDGO 48 24 Aug 43	Calvin DeWitt (1840–1908), Brig. Gen., MC, USA	Auburn, Calif.	4, 013	Type A (tile)	27 Feb. 1944	1, 852	General medicine; neurology; neurosurgery; vascular surgery; psychiatry	30 Dec. 1945	Transferred to State of California
Dibble	WDGO 48 24 Aug 43	John Dibble (1890–1943), Col., MC, USA	Menlo Park, Calif.	3, 258	Type A (stucco)	22 Feb. 1944	1, 868	Plastic surgery; ophthalmologic surgery; blind; psychiatry	15 Jun. 1946	Transferred to Federal Public Housing Authority
England (Thomas M. England after 14 Nov. 1944)	WDGO 57 21 Sep 43	Thomas Marcus England (1876–1943), Lt. Col., MAC, USA	Atlantic City, N. J.	64, 094	Multi-story permanent (brick) (converted hotels)	15 Aug. 1943	3, 650	Neurology; amputations; neurosurgery	7 Jun. 1946	Leases canceled; returned to owners.
Finney	WDGO 67 14 Dec 42	John Miller Turpin Finney (1863–1942), Brig. Gen., MC, Res., USA	Thomasville, Ga.	12, 683	Cantonment (tile and gypsum board)	5 Jun. 1943	1, 994	General medicine; CNS syphilis; general and orthopedic surgery; psychiatry	15 Dec. 1945	Transferred to Vet. Admin.
Fitzsimons	WDGO 40 26 Jun 20	William Thomas Fitzsimons (1889–1917), 1st Lt., MC, Res., USA	Denver, Colo.	322, 412	Multi-story permanent (brick)	13 Oct. 1918	3, 417	General medicine; tuberculosis; general and orthopedic surgery; thoracic surgery; deep x-ray therapy; psychiatry	....	Active 1951; retained for Regular Army

Fletcher	WDGO 67 14 Dec 42	John Pierpont Fletcher (1884–1941), Col., MC, USA	Cambridge, Ohio	15,044	Cantonment (brick)	26 Jun. 1943	1,670	General medicine; general and orthopedic surgery	29 Mar. 1946	Transferred to State of Ohio, Department of Public Welfare
Foster	WDGO 67 14 Dec 42	Charles Lovelace Foster (1871–1941), Col., MC, USA	Jackson, Miss.	62,107	Special type resembling type A (tile and brick)	11 Sep. 1943	1,905	General medicine; rheumatic fever; general and orthopedic surgery	15 Dec. 1945	Transferred to Vet. Admin.
Gardiner	WDGO 63 1 Oct 43	Ruth Mabel Gardiner (1914–43), 2d Lt., ANC, USA	Chicago, Ill.	3,396,808	Multi-story permanent (brick) (converted hotel)	1 Oct. 1943	1,061	General and orthopedic surgery	21 Jun. 1946	Transferred to Fifth Army headquarters
Glennan	WDGO 23 15 May 43	James Denner Glennan (1862–1927), Brig. Gen., MC, USA	Okmulgee, Okla.	16,051	Type A (brick)	17 Dec. 1943	1,690	Prisoners of war	2 Dec. 1945	Transferred to Oklahoma A. and M. College
Halloran	WDGO 53 14 Oct 42	Paul Stacy Halloran (1874–1931), Col., MC, USA	Willowbrook, Staten Island (Richmond), N. Y.	174,441	Multi-story permanent (brick) (converted civilian buildings)	5 Nov. 1942	5,350	Neurology; general and orthopedic surgery; neurosurgery	31 Dec. 1946	Leases canceled; returned to owners
Hammond	WDGO 64 24 Nov 42	William Alexander Hammond (1828–1900), Surgeon General, USA, 1862–63	Modesto, Calif.	16,379	Cantonment (wood)	24 Oct. 1942	2,540	Neurology; general and orthopedic surgery; neurosurgery; psychiatry	20 Dec. 1945	Transferred to State of California
Harmon	WDGO 64 24 Nov 42	Daniel Warwick Harmon (1880–1940), Col., MC, USA	Longview, Tex.	13,758	Cantonment (wood)	9 Dec. 1942	2,218	General medicine; CNS syphilis; tropical disease; general and orthopedic surgery; psychiatry	6 Dec. 1945	Transferred to Le Tourneau Foundation
Hoff	Ltr AG 322.3 Gen Hosp (1–9–41) M (Ret) M–C, 11 Feb 41	John Van Rensselaer Hoff (1848–1920), Col., MC, USA	Santa Barbara, Calif.	35,958	Cantonment (wood)	12 Jun. 1941	1,141	General and orthopedic surgery; deaf	10 Nov. 1945	Assumed by Federal Public Housing Authority

TABLE 15—U. S. ARMY GENERAL HOSPITALS IN THE UNITED STATES DURING WORLD WAR II—Continued

Name of hospital	War Department directive naming or designating hospital	Person for whom named	Location	Population of town or city according to 1940 census	Type of construction	Date ready for or received first patient	Authorized bed capacity as of April 1945	Specialties as of April 1945	Date of disposition of last general hospital patient up to 31 Dec. 1946	Disposition as listed by Army 31 July 1951
Kennedy	WDGO 64 24 Nov 42	James Madison Kennedy (1865–1930), Brig. Gen., MC, USA	Memphis, Tenn.	292,942	Two-story semipermanent (brick)	1 Jan. 1943	4,387	Neurology; general and orthopedic surgery; thoracic surgery; neurosurgery psychiatry	23 Jun. 1946	Transferred to Vet. Admin.
LaGarde	Ltr AG 322.3 Gen Hosp (1–9–41) M (Ret) M–C, 11 Feb 41	Lewis Anatole LaGarde (1849–1920), Col., MC, USA	New Orleans, La.	494,537	Cantonment (wood)	14 Jun. 1941	1,176	General and orthopedic surgery; psychiatry	7 Dec. 1945	Transferred to Vet. Admin.
Lawson	Ltr AG 322.3 Gen Hosp (1–9–41) M (Ret) M–C, 11 Feb 41	Thomas Edwin Lawson (1793–1861), Surgeon General, USA, 1836–61	Atlanta, Ga.	302,288	Cantonment (wood)	22 Jul. 1941	2,514	Neurology; amputations; neurosurgery; deep X-ray therapy	25 Jun. 1946	Transferred to Vet. Admin. and Federal Public Housing Authority
Letterman	WDGO 152 23 Nov 11	Jonathan Letterman (1824–72), Surgeon Major, USA	San Francisco, Calif.	634,536	Multi-story permanent (concrete, brick and tile, with stucco finish)	27 Jul. 1899 (Called U. S. Army General Hospital, Presidio of San Francisco, until 1911)	3,500	Deep X-ray therapy; radium therapy	....	Active 1951; retained for Regular Army
Lovell	Ltr AG 322.3 Gen Hosp (1–9–41) M (Ret) M–C, 11 Feb 41	Joseph Lovell (1788–1836), Surgeon General, USA, 1818–36	Ayers, Mass.	3,572	Cantonment (wood)	20 Jun. 1941	4,000	General medicine; CNS syphilis; general and orthopedic surgery	24 Jun. 1946	Redesignated as Station Hospital, Fort Devens, Mass.
Madigan	WDGO 76 22 Sep 44	Patrick Sarsfield Madigan (1887–1944), Col., MC, USA	Tacoma, Wash.	109,408	Type A (brick)	22 Aug. 1944 (Formerly an ASF station hospital)	4,300	General medicine; general and orthopedic surgery	....	Active 1951; retained for Regular Army

Mason	WDGO 48 24 Aug 43	Charles Field Mason (1864–1922), Col., MC, USA	Brentwood, L. I., N. Y.	568	Multi-story permanent (brick) (converted civilian hospital).	5 Jul. 1943	3,032	Psychiatry	20 Dec. 1946	Leases canceled; returned to owners
Mayo	WDGO 48 24 Aug 43	William James Mayo (1861–1936), Brig. Gen., MC, Res., USA and Charles Horace Mayo (1865–1939), Brig. Gen., MC, Res., USA	Galesburg, Ill.	28,876	Type A (brick)	1 Feb. 1944	1,855	General medicine; neurology; neurosurgery; vascular surgery	15 Sep. 1946	Transferred to State of Illinois
McCaw	WDGO 64 24 Nov 42	Walter Drew McCaw (1863–1939), Brig. Gen., MC, USA	Walla Walla, Wash.	18,109	Cantonment (wood)	5 Mar. 1943	1,502	Neurology; general and orthopedic surgery; neurosurgery; psychiatry	25 Nov. 1945	Transferred to Vet. Admin.
McCloskey	WDGO 64 24 Nov 42	James Augustus McCloskey (1909–41), Maj., MC, USA	Temple, Tex.	15,344	Two-story semipermanent (brick)	20 Oct. 1942	3,454	Neurology; amputations; neurosurgery; psychiatry	31 Mar. 1946	Transferred to Vet. Admin.
McGuire	WDGO 48 24 Nov 43	Hunter Holmes McGuire (1835–1900), Medical Director, Second Army Corps, Army of Northern Virginia, Confederate Army	Richmond, Va.	193,042	Type A with VA-type buildings (brick)	29 Jul. 1944	1,765	Neurology; amputations; neurosurgery	31 Mar. 1946	Transferred to Vet. Admin.
Moore	WDGO 64 24 Nov 42	Samuel Preston Moore (1813–89), Surgeon General, Confederate Army	Swannanoa, N. C. (Asheville).	51,310	Cantonment (wood)	2 Dec. 1942	2,605	General medicine; tropical disease; general and orthopedic surgery; psychiatry	15 Nov. 1946	Transferred to Vet. Admin.
Newton D. Baker	WDGO 15 23 Mar 43	Newton Diehl Baker (1871–1937), Secretary of War, World War I	Martinsburg. W. Va.	15,063	Type A (brick)	28 Jan. 1944	1,806	Neurology; plastic surgery; ophthalmologic surgery; neurosurgery; psychiatry	20 Jun. 1946	Transferred to Vet. Admin.

TABLE 15—U. S. ARMY GENERAL HOSPITALS IN THE UNITED STATES DURING WORLD WAR II—Continued

Name of hospital	War Department directive naming or designating hospital	Person for whom named	Location	Population of town or city according to 1940 census	Type of construction	Date ready for or received first patient	Authorized bed capacity as of April 1945	Specialties as of April 1945	Date of disposition of last general hospital patient up to 31 Dec. 1946	Disposition as listed by Army 31 July 1951
Nichols..........	WDGO 64 24 Nov 42	Henry James Nichols (1877–1927), Lt. Col., MC, USA	Louisville, Ky.	319,077	Cantonment (wood)	11 Dec. 1942	1,717	Neurology; general and orthopedic surgery; neurosurgery	29 Mar. 1946	Transferred to Vet. Admin.
Northington......	WDGO 23 15 May 43	Eugene Garland Northington (1880–1933), Lt. Col., MC, USA	Tuscaloosa, Ala.	27,493	Type A (tile and brick)	5 Sep. 1943	2,131	Neurology; plastic surgery; ophthalmologic surgery; neurosurgery; psychiatry	5 Apr. 1946	Transferred to city of Tuscaloosa, Ala.
Oliver..........	WDGO 64 24 Nov 44	Robert T. Oliver (1868–1937), Col., DC, USA	Augusta, Ga.	65,919	Multi-story permanent (brick) (converted hotel)	28 Jan. 1943	2,240	General medicine; general and orthopedic surgery	....	Inactive under 3d Army except for 500 beds transferred to VA.
O'Reilly..........	Ltr AG 322.3 Gen Hosp (1–9–41) M (Ret) M–C, 11 Feb 41	Robert Maitland O'Reilly (1845–1912), Surgeon General, USA, 1902–09	Springfield, Mo.	61,238	Cantonment (wood)	7 Nov. 1941	3,232	Neurology; plastic surgery; ophthalmologic surgery; neurosurgery	23 Sep. 1946	Transferred to Vet. Admin.
Percy Jones.......	WDGO 64 24 Nov 42	Percy Lancelot Jones (1875–1941), Col., MC, USA	Battle Creek, Mich.	43,453	Multi-story permanent (brick) (converted civilian sanitarium)	15 Jan. 1943	3,414	Neurology; amputations; neurosurgery; deep x-ray therapy	....	Active 1951; retained for Regular Army
Prisoner of War, No. 2.	WDGO 88 23 Nov 44	....	Camp Forrest (Tullahoma, Tenn.)	4,549	Cantonment (wood)	21 Oct. 1944 (Formerly an ASF station hospital).	2,500	Prisoners of war	15 Dec. 1945	Reverted to Station Hospital, Camp Forrest, Tenn. Later assumed by War Assets Admin.

Ream	WDGO 63 1 Oct 43	William Roy Ream (1877–1918), Maj., MC, USA	Palm Beach, Fla.	3,747	Multi-story permanent (brick) (converted hotel)	10 Sep. 1943 (Formerly an AAF station hospital)	...	...	21 Jul. 1944	Leases canceled; returned to owners
Rhoads	WDGO 67 14 Dec 42	Thomas Leidy Rhoads (1870–1940), Col., MC, USA	Utica, N. Y.	100,518	Cantonment (wood)	25 Aug. 1943	2,000	General medicine; general and orthopedic surgery	30 Jun. 1946	Transferred to State of New York
Schick	WDGO 64 24 Nov 42	William Rhinehart Schick (1910–41), 1st Lt., MC, Res., USA	Clinton, Iowa	26,270	Two-story semipermanent (brick)	12 Feb. 1943	2,014	General medicine; CNS syphilis; general and orthopedic surgery; psychiatry.	25 Feb. 1946	Transferred to Vet. Admin.
Stark	Ltr AG 322.3 Gen Hosp (1–9–41) M (Ret) M–C, 11 Feb 41	Alexander Newton Stark (1869–1926), Col., MC, USA	Charleston, S. C.	71,275	Cantonment (wood)	18 May 1941	2,400	General and orthopedic surgery.	23 Oct. 1945	Transferred to Charleston (S. C.), County Board of Control
Thayer	WDGO 23 15 May 43	William Sydney Thayer (1864–1932), Brig. Gen., MC, Res., USA	Nashville, Tenn.	167,402	Cantonment (cinder block)	4 Oct. 1943	1,867	General medicine; CNS syphilis; general and orthopedic surgery.	18 Dec. 1945	Transferred to Vet. Admin.
Tilton	Ltr AG 322.3 Gen Hosp (1–9–41) M (Ret) M–C, 11 Feb 41 and WDGO 64 24 Nov 42	James Tilton (1745–1822), Surgeon General, USA, 1813–15	Fort Dix (Wrightstown, N. J.).	241	Cantonment (wood)	14 Jul. 1941	3,700	General medicine; general and orthopedic surgery; psychiatry.	...	Redesignated station hospital 30 June 1949.
Torney	WDGO 64 24 Nov 42	George Henry Torney (1850–1913), Surgeon General, USA, 1909–13	Palm Springs, Calif.	3,434	Permanent (stucco) (converted hotel)	5 Aug. 1942	1,600	General medicine; rheumatic fever; general and orthopedic surgery.	22 Nov. 1945	Assumed by Federal Works Admin.
United States Army General Hospital, Camp Butner, N. C.	WD Cir 36 30 Jan 45	...	Wilkins, N. C. (Durham)	60,195	Two-story semipermanent (brick)	30 Jan. 1945 (Formerly an ASF station hospital)	2,900	General medicine; trench foot; psychiatry	29 Mar. 1946	Reverted to Camp Butner. Later transferred to State of N. C.

TABLE 15—U. S. ARMY GENERAL HOSPITALS IN THE UNITED STATES DURING WORLD WAR II—Continued

Name of hospital	War Department directive naming or designating hospital	Person for whom named	Location	Population of town or city according to 1940 census	Type of construction	Date ready for or received first patient	Authorized bed capacity as of April 1945	Specialties as of April 1945	Date of disposition of last general hospital patient up to 31 Dec. 1946	Disposition as listed by Army 31 July 1951
United States Army General Hospital, Camp Carson, Colo.	WD Cir 36 30 Jan 45	....	Colorado Springs, Colo.	36,789	Two-story semipermanent (cinder block)	30 Jan. 1945 (Formerly an ASF station hospital)	3,000	General medicine; trench foot; psychiatry	5 to 12 Apr. 1946	Reverted to Camp Carson, Colo.
United States Army General Hospital, Camp Edwards, Mass.	WD Cir 36 30 Jan 45	....	Falmouth, Mass.	6,878	Cantonment (wood)	30 Jan. 1945 (Formerly an ASF station hospital)	3,200	General and orthopedic surgery; psychiatry	15 Mar. 1946	Reverted to Camp Edwards, Mass.
United States Army General Hospital, Camp Pickett, Va.	WD Cir 36 30 Jan 45	....	Blackstone, Va.	2,699	Cantonment (wood)	30 Jan. 1945 (Formerly an ASF station hospital)	2,700	General medicine; general and orthopedic surgery; psychiatry	15 Dec. 1945	Reverted to Camp Pickett, Va.
Valley Forge......	WDGO 64 24 Nov 42	....	Phoenixville, Pa.	12,282	Two-story semipermanent (brick)	12 Mar. 1943	2,509	Plastic surgery; ophthalmologic surgery; blind; psychiatry	....	Active 1951; retained for Regular Army.
Vaughan..........	WDGO 48 24 Aug 43	Victor Clarence Vaughan (1851–1929), Col., MC, Res., USA	Hines, Ill. (Chicago)	3,396,808	Type A with VA-type buildings (brick)	1 Aug. 1944	1,900	General medicine; general and orthopedic surgery; psychiatry	1 Apr. 1946	Transferred to Vet. Admin.
Wakeman.........	WDGO 34 25 Apr 44	Frank Bolles Wakeman (1896–1944), Col., MC, USA	Camp Atterbury (Columbus, Ind.)	11,738	Two-story semipermanent (cinder block)	5 Apr. 1944 (Formerly an ASF station hospital)	2,700	Neurology; plastic surgery; ophthalmologic surgery; neurosurgery	31 Dec. 1946	Redesignated as Station Hospital, Camp Atterbury
Walter Reed......	WDGO 83 2 May 06	Walter Reed (1851–1902), Maj., MC, USA	Washington, D. C.	663,091	Multi-story permanent (brick)	May 1909	3,000	General medicine; thoracic surgery; amputations; deep x-ray therapy; radium therapy; psychiatry	....	Active 1951; retained for Regular Army.

William Beaumont.	WDGO 40 26 Jan 20	William Beaumont (1785–1853), Surgeon Major, USA	El Paso, Tex.	96,810	Two-story permanent (tile with stucco finish)	1 Jul. 1921	4,000	General medicine; general and orthopedic surgery; plastic surgery; ophthalmologic surgery; deep x-ray therapy; psychiatry	....	Active 1951; retained for Regular Army
Winter..........	WDGO 67 14 Dec 42	Francis Anderson Winter (1867–1931), Brig. Gen., MC, USA	Topeka, Kans.	67,833	Cantonment (brick)	5 Jul. 1943	1,771	General medicine; general and orthopedic surgery; psychiatry	25 to 30 Nov. 1945	Transferred to Vet. Admin.
Woodrow Wilson..	WDGO 64 24 Nov 42	Thomas Woodrow Wilson (1856–1924), President of US, World War I	Staunton, Va.	13,337	Cantonment (brick)	6 Jun. 1943	1,565	General medicine; CNS syphilis; general and orthopedic surgery	31 Mar. 1946	Transferred to Augusta County, Commonwealth of Virginia

Sources: (1) An Rpts, Hosps listed. HD. (2) Weekly Health Rpts, 1943–44. AML. (3) Weekly Hosp Rpts, 1945–46. HD. (4) Chart, Occupancy and Operating Pers Data for the General-Convalescent Hosp Syst, by SvC and Hosp, end of Apr 45. HD:322. (5) Program of Instls, vol. I, 31 Jul 51, Dept of Army. SG: 319.26. (6) *Hammond's Library Atlas of the World* (New York, 1943). (7) Interv, MD Historian with Harvey J. Hall, Med Fac Planning Br, Med Plans and Oprs Div, SGO, 11 Mar 52. HD: 000.71. (8) AG files: 322.3, 323.3, 600.05, and 680.9. (9) SG files: 323.3, 705, and 633–99.

flicts complicated the selection of hospitals to be closed.[22]

In addition, the needs of both the Veterans Administration and the postwar Army had not been fully determined.[23] Finally, local citizens sometimes protested the closure of hospitals, and service command surgeons, because of local conditions, disagreed with some of the decisions made in the Surgeon General's Office.[24] Despite these difficulties, the program for closures drawn up in the fall of 1945 was followed with comparatively few changes.

The actual process of closing hospitals was a responsibility of service command officials until April 1946, when general hospitals were placed again, as they had been before the war, under the direct command of The Surgeon General. ASF headquarters informed service commanders of the hospitals that would be closed each quarter; the Surgeon General's Office decided the particular dates on which they would be closed; and several months prior to those dates the Medical Regulating Officer "blocked" those hospitals—that is, permitted no more patients to be sent to them. After hospitals were blocked, service commanders were required to revise authorized bed capacities twice monthly and to reduce personnel in accordance with these revisions. Hospital commanders submitted information which higher authorities needed in order to declare as surplus the property no longer required by the Army. They also disposed of hospital personnel, supplies, and equipment under procedures established by ASF headquarters. After hospital buildings were declared surplus, the Medical Department lost all control over them and they were disposed of by other government agencies.[25] In order to assure the reduction and closure of hospitals according to schedule, the Surgeon General's Resources Analysis Division each month analyzed hospitalization reports from service commands and called the attention of local Army authorities to any failures in making reductions.[26] Beginning in July 1945, in compliance with instructions from G–4, The Surgeon General reported monthly to that Division the progress made in contracting the hospital system.[27]

Under these procedures the Medical Department moved from a wartime to a peacetime basis for hospitalization in the United States in approximately a year's time. By July 1946 all of the convalescent hospitals but one, the Old Farms Convalescent Hospital for the blind, had been closed.[28] By December of that year all regional hospitals either had been closed or

[22] Memo, Dir Resources Anal Div SGO for Chief Oprs Serv SGO, 4 Sep 45, sub: Plan for Post V-J Day Reduction in Gen Hosp Fac. SG: 323.3 (Gen Hosp).

[23] (1) Ltr, Dep SG to VA, 29 Dec 45. SG: 323.3 (Gen Hosp). (2) Memo, SG for ACofS G–4 WDGS thru CG ASF, 5 Sep 45, sub: Comd Instls for Retention in Post-War Mil Estabs. SG: 370.01.

[24] (1) Ltr, SG to Hon Francis J. Meyers, 28 Jan 46. SG: 323.3 (Hosp). (2) Ltr, SG to Mrs Dorothy Finn, Stockton, Calif, 15 Jan 46. Same file. (3) Statements by SvC Surgs in Notes on Morning Sess of SvC Surgs Conf, 27 Sep 45. HD: Resources Anal Div file, "Hosp."

[25] (1) Memo, SG for Dir Mob Div ASF, 24 Sep 45, sub: Closure of ZI Gen Hosps. SG: 322 "Hosp." (2) Ltr SPMOC 632, CG ASF to Serv Comdrs, 2 Oct 45, sub: Closure of Gen Hosps. Same file. (3) Diary, Resources Anal Div SGO, 13 Dec 45. HD: 024.7–3. (4) Notes on Morning Sess of SvC Surgs Conf, 27 Sep 45. HD: Resources Anal Div file, "Hosp."

[26] Ltr, SG to CGs SvCs attn Surg, 7 Nov 45, sub: Comparative Studies of Gen-Conv and Sta-Regional Hosp Systs. SG: 323.3 (Hosp). Similar letters for other months are found in the same file.

[27] Memo, SG for ACofS G–4 WDGS, 15 Jul 45, sub: Hosp Fac. HRS: G–4 files, 334 vol. II. Similar letters for other months are found in this same file and in SG: 322 (Hosp).

[28] Weekly Hosp Rpt, vol. II, No 27, for week ending 5 Jul 46. Off file, Med Statistics Div SGO.

had reverted to station hospitals.[29] By the beginning of 1947 the Army (including the Air Forces) had only 54 station hospitals with 15,715 beds, only 14 general hospitals with 34,846 beds, and only 1 convalescent hospital (Old Farms) with 100 beds.[30] A comparison of bed authorizations for general and convalescent hospitals during successive quarters of 1945 and 1946 with the program for bed reductions prepared by the Surgeon General's Office in the fall of 1945 shows that the program was followed closely. The chief deviation occurred in a more rapid liquidation of convalescent hospitals than had been anticipated. A comparison of "patients remaining" in general and convalescent hospitals with authorized beds shows a close correlation between reductions in the patient-load and in hospital beds. As in earlier months, the number of beds occupied continued to be considerably smaller than either the number of beds authorized or the number of patients remaining.[31] *(See Table 15; also Chart 10.)*

[29] (1) Weekly Hosp Rpt, vol. III, No 49, for week ending 6 Dec 46. Off file, Med Statistics Div SGO. (2) WD GO 148, 11 Dec 46.

[30] Information furnished by Resources Analysis Division, SGO, 4 Dec 50. The fourteen general hospitals were Army and Navy, William Beaumont, Fitzsimons, Letterman, Walter Reed, Brooke, Madigan, Oliver, Percy Jones, Tilton, Valley Forge, McCornack, Murphy, and Pratt. The last three had been designated general hospitals in May 1946 by WD GO 45, 15 May 46.

[31] (1) Memo, SG for ACofS G-4 WDGS thru CG ASF, 14 Sep 45, sub: Cut-Back in Gen and Conv Hosp Fac. SG: 322 "Hosp." (2) Memo, SG for ACofS G-4 WDGS thru CG ASF, 21 Dec 45, same sub. SG: 323.3 "Hosp." (3) Weekly Hosp Rpts, vol. II, No 52, for week ending 28 Dec 45; vol. III, No. 13, for week ending 29 Mar 46; vol. III, No 26, for week ending 28 Jun 46; and vol. III, No 52, for week ending 27 Dec 46. Off file, Med Statistics Div SGO.

PART FOUR

EVACUATION TO AND IN THE ZONE OF INTERIOR

Introduction

The evacuation of patients from theaters of operations to the zone of interior and from one point to another in the United States was an intricate operation, involving not only the transportation but also the care en route of patients suffering from all kinds of diseases and injuries. It was complicated by many factors, among them the means employed. Various types of transportation facilities were used—motor vehicles, trains, ships, and airplanes. Each of these had subtypes. For example, both hospital and transport ships returned patients from theaters. Various kinds of personnel, civilian and military, were employed to operate transportation facilities and care for patients aboard them—doctors, nurses, technicians, pilots, and many others. Moreover, equipment and supplies needed to care for patients in transit were extensive and sundry, ranging from aspirins to operating tables. To some degree personnel and equipment required were governed by transportation facilities employed, because hospital ships, for instance, needed more elaborate equipment and larger staffs than did airplanes.

Evacuation was further complicated by its interrelationship with plans, policies, and procedures for hospitalization. For example, the division of general hospital beds between the theaters and the zone of interior was determined by—among other factors—the evacuation facilities expected to be available. On the other hand, the number of beds supplied to theaters influenced the number of patients to be transferred to the zone of interior, and hence the transportation facilities that would be required. Successful operation of the specialized hospital system in the United States and observance of a policy of hospitalizing patients as near their homes as possible depended upon the evacuation system.[1]

To co-ordinate evacuation with hospitalization and to use all available means—transportation facilities, personnel, and equipment—in such a way that large numbers of patients would be moved as safely and expeditiously as possible required a highly organized operational system. Its development and conduct were complicated not only by the divers means employed but also by the distances traversed and the agencies involved. Patients traveling by land, air, and sea from hospitals in theaters of operations to those in the zone of interior were the responsibility of successive military agencies. Among them were the bases and headquarters of theaters of operations; the Air Transport Command with its overseas wings; the Transportation Corps with its ports of embarkation and debarkation in the United States; the Offices of the Chief of Transportation, The Surgeon General, and the Air Surgeon; service and air commands in the United States; and the headquarters of both the Air and Service Forces.

Involvement of so many agencies made it important to define their respective areas of responsibility—particularly after

[1] Interrelationships between hospitalization and the policies and processes of evacuation have been discussed at various points in preceding chapters and will be referred to again from time to time.

the War Department reorganization in March 1942. On recommendation of SOS headquarters, this was done for major agencies the following June. The commanding general, Army Air Forces, was charged with development and operation of air evacuation. Commanders of theaters of operations and of major commands in the United States were declared responsible for the movement of patients within their own commands. The commanding general, Services of Supply, was charged with evacuating patients from all major commands—those overseas as well as in the United States—and of co-ordinating all plans of such commands for the evacuation of sick and wounded to be delivered to his control.[2] To assist him in this function, various responsibilities (which will be discussed later) were assigned to the Chief of Transportation, The Surgeon General, and port and corps area commanders. In the early part of the war their activities were closely supervised and coordinated by the SOS Hospitalization and Evacuation Branch.

Beginning in 1943 a series of events transferred that Branch's responsibility and authority for evacuation to The Surgeon General and the Chief of Transportation. Early that year, it will be recalled, ASF (formerly SOS) headquarters began to return to The Surgeon General some of the functions it had assumed earlier in hospitalization and evacuation operations. Some of the officers of its Hospitalization and Evacuation Branch were transferred to the Surgeon General's Office after the Branch was reduced in status to a section of another branch in ASF headquarters. One of them was Lt. Col. John C. Fitzpatrick, who had been active in sea evacuation operations while in ASF headquarters. Soon afterward, The Surgeon General and the Chief of Transportation decided that the latter would need constant technical advice from the Medical Department on matters of evacuation that concerned him and that the former would need a means of exercising technical supervision over evacuation operations. Accordingly The Surgeon General in June 1943 assigned Colonel Fitzpatrick as his liaison officer with the Chief of Transportation, who gave him office space for a Transportation Liaison Unit. In this capacity Colonel Fitzpatrick assisted the Chief of Transportation in estimating evacuation requirements and in planning and supervising the transportation of patients by water and rail.

In the spring of 1944, in anticipation of the patient load expected as a result of aggressive combat operations, the unit headed by Colonel Fitzpatrick was increased in size and given additional authority and responsibilities. In May, it will be recalled, The Surgeon General removed the Evacuation Branch from his Hospital Division and merged it with the Transportation Liaison Unit to form a Medical Regulating Unit. This step combined the function of regulating the flow of patients from ports to hospitals of definitive treatment with that of providing for their transportation. Thus one office, representing The Surgeon General and belonging to his Operations Service but located in and working as a part of the Movements Division of the Office of the Chief of Transportation, assumed responsibility in the latter half of the war for supervising all evacuation operations ex-

[2] (1) Ltr AG 704 (6-17-42) MB-D-TS-M, TAG to CGs AGF, AAF, SOS, *et al.*, 18 Jun 42, sub: WD Hosp and Evac Policy. (2) Ltr SPOPM 322.15, CG SOS to CGs and COs of CAs, PEs, Gen Hosps, and SG, 18 Jun 42, sub: Opr Plans for Mil Hosp and Evac. Both in AG: 704(6-17-42).

cept the movement of patients by air. The Air Forces Medical Regulating Service in the Air Surgeon's Office controlled the transfer of patients between AAF hospitals and supervised air evacuation operations. Collaborating closely with the ASF Medical Regulating Unit, the Air Regulating Office followed the pattern of the ASF office both in its development and in its procedures.[3]

In contrast with wartime operations, evacuation of patients from overseas areas and within the United States in peacetime had been a small-scale affair. The few troops who were in overseas areas were not engaged in combat activities; and therefore the number of patients who needed to be returned to the United States for hospital care was not large. General hospitals in this country were located in relation to troop density and served on a regional basis to treat complicated cases of all types rather than on a specialized basis to treat few types of cases from wide areas; and therefore the movement of patients from station to general hospitals was also a relatively simple procedure.

The primary means of transporting patients from overseas areas was by troop transports. No hospital ships were available, and the movement of patients by air was still in the experimental stage. Transports delivering troops and supplies at overseas ports took aboard patients for return trips and transport surgeons cared for them in ships' hospitals or in ships' quarters.[4] Before arrival in the United States, transport surgeons radioed to ports of debarkation lists of patients aboard, with their diagnoses and proposed dispositions. Ports receiving such information arranged with the corps area (later called service command) in which they were located for the transportation of patients being evacuated. Upon arrival of transports, port commanders issued orders transferring patients to general hospitals in which ports had bed credits and then informed The Surgeon General of the number received and of the hospitals to which they had been transferred. The New York Port, for example, had bed credits in both Tilton and Lovell General Hospitals and transferred patients within the limit of its allotments to these hospitals. Because the nearest meant an ambulance trip of more than two hours, the port occasionally kept in its station hospital for short periods of time patients who needed rest before further travel. Personnel both for transports and for the debarkation of patients was supplied by ports from their bulk personnel allotments or was borrowed from corps areas.[5]

Within the United States patients were moved from ports to hospitals, or from one hospital to another, by ambulance, by trains, and by airplanes. Ambulances available to all hospitals were used, as hospital commanders directed, for short trips. Accommodations for patients aboard regularly scheduled passenger trains were

[3] (1) Ltr, SG to CG ASF thru CofT, 17 Apr 43, sub: Coord Med Serv for PE, with 2 inds. HD: Wilson files, "Book IV, 16 Mar 43–17 Jun 43." (2) ASF Cir 147, 19 May 44. (3) WD Cir 140, 11 Apr 44. (4) AAF Reg 25–17, 7 Feb and 6 Jun 44. (5) An Rpt, FY 1944 and 45, Oprs Serv SGO. HD. (6) An Rpt, FY 1944, Oprs Div Off Air Surg. HD. (7) Ltr, Dr. Richard L. Meiling to Col Calvin H. Goddard, 30 Jun 52. HD: 314 (Correspondence on MS) XI.

[4] Reports of transport surgeons, required as a part of each voyage report by AR 30–1150, 19 September 1941, were submitted through port surgeons to Army Transport Service. For surgeon's reports see files SG: 721.5, QM or TC: 569.1 under name of Army transport.

[5] (1) AR 40–1025, 12 Oct 40. (2) WD Cir 120, 21 Jun 41. (3) An Rpt, NYPE, 1943, contains an account of activities before 1943. HD.

arranged by corps area officers with local agents of carriers involved. Normally, transfers were made without reference to such higher authority as the Surgeon General's Office, because station hospitals, corps area surgeons, and port commanders had general hospital beds set aside for their use by the bed-credit system.[6] Some airfields and air training centers converted airplanes available to them into airplane ambulances and used them to transfer patients from scenes of crashes to near-by hospitals or, in some instances, from one hospital to another. When airplane ambulances were not available, medical personnel on duty with the Air Corps made local and informal arrangements with Air Corps operations officers for the transportation of patients in operational planes.[7] Such an informal system worked well enough as long as the number of patients to be evacuated was small and the distances they were to be moved were short, but it was not easily adaptable to the movement of large numbers of patients over long distances. The way this system was transformed will be discussed later. It will be helpful, though, to consider first the magnitude of operations that made necessary such a transformation.

---

[6] An Rpts, Lovell and Tilton Gen Hosps, 1941. HD.

[7] (1) Ltr, Walter Reed Gen Hosp to SG, 11 Jan 41, sub: Airplane Trans of Pnts, with inds. SG: 580.-1 (Walter Reed GH)K. (2) Ltr, Hq West Coast ACTC to CofAC, 15 Aug 41, sub: Air Amb, with inds. AAF: 452.-1B (Amb Planes).

CHAPTER XIX

Estimated and Actual Requirements for Evacuation from Theaters of Operations

Estimating future evacuation requirements was primarily a matter of calculating the probable patient-load of theaters and of determining the part that would be transferred to the zone of interior under prevailing policies. Early in the war estimates of this kind were practically unnecessary because the number of patients to be evacuated was still comparatively small, combat operations were limited, and there was plenty of space for evacuees aboard returning transports. Meeting evacuation requirements amounted simply to insuring that transports had adequate hospital space, attendant personnel, and medical supplies, and that they were routed on return trips to places where patients had accumulated. In the latter half of the war this situation changed. The number of patients evacuated, which had been less than 1,000 a month before November 1942 and an average of about 3,300 from then until the middle of 1943, mounted steadily until it reached a peak of more than 57,000 in May 1945. *(Table 16)* Moreover, as the build-up of troops in theaters ceased, the number of returning transports declined. Under these circumstances estimates of the evacuation load had to be made so that enough transportation could be assembled to handle it; and estimates had to be made far enough in advance so that the use of transportation facilities—which came to include airplanes and hospital ships as well as troop transports—could be properly co-ordinated.

A study which the Surgeon General's Office made in the winter of 1943–44 of the patient load that would develop during 1944 evoked a critical appraisal early that year not only of plans for supplying the Army with hospitalization but also of plans for evacuating patients from theaters of operations.[1]

Whether plans for evacuation would be adequate depended upon the size of the evacuation load and upon the use to be made of transportation facilities. The Surgeon General's estimate of the potential load was questioned by ASF headquarters and the Chief of Transportation. Subsequently, as a result of additional information supplied by the European and Medi-

[1] See above, pp. 201–02. The following three paragraphs are based upon "Hospitalization and Evacuation: A Re-estimate of the Patient Load and Facilities," February 1944, and "Hospitalization and Evacuation, An Analysis," March 1944, together with memorandums and letters in ASF Planning Div Program Br files 370.05 and "Hosp and Evac, vol. 3."

TABLE 16—PATIENTS DEBARKED IN THE UNITED STATES, 1920–45

Date	Total Patients Debarked[a]	Returned by Water						Returned by air	
				Troop Transport		Hospital Ship			
		Number	Percentage of Total Patients Debarked	Number	Percentage of Total Patients Debarked	Number	Percentage of Total Patients Debarked	Number	Percentage of Total Patients Debarked
1920–40[b]	15, 846	....	....	....	....	....	....	....	....
1941[c]	2, 390	....	....	....	....	....	....	....	....
1942	9, 248	....	....	....	....	....	....	....	....
1943[d]									
January	2, 475	2, 442	98. 7	2, 442	98. 7	0	0	33	1. 3
February	2, 177	2, 136	98. 1	2, 136	98. 1	0	0	41	1. 9
March	2, 351	2, 300	97. 8	2, 300	97. 8	0	0	51	2. 2
April	4, 777	4, 712	98. 6	4, 712	98. 6	0	0	65	1. 4
May	5, 349	5, 242	98. 0	5, 242	98. 0	0	0	107	2. 0
June	6, 115	5, 971	97. 6	5, 222	85. 4	749	12. 2	144	2. 4
July	5, 735	5, 350	93. 3	5, 350	93. 3	0	0	385	6. 7
August	8, 183	7, 762	94. 9	7, 762	94. 9	0	0	421	5. 1
September	9, 425	9, 088	96. 4	9, 088	96. 4	0	0	337	3. 6
October	7, 469	6, 884	92. 2	6, 884	92. 2	0	0	585	7. 8
November	10, 604	10, 195	96. 1	8, 984	84. 7	1, 211	11. 4	409	3. 9
December	7, 163	6, 481	90. 0	6, 481	90. 0	0	0	682	10. 0
Total	71, 823	68, 563	95. 5	66, 603	92. 8	1, 960	2. 7	3, 260	4. 5
1944									
January	7, 724	7, 179	92. 9	6, 018	77. 9	1, 161	15. 0	545	7. 1
February	9, 763	9, 220	94. 4	9, 220	94. 4	0	0	543	5. 6
March	8, 894	8, 172	91. 9	6, 458	72. 6	1, 714	19. 3	722	8. 1
April	7, 082	6, 249	88. 2	4, 994	70. 5	1, 255	17. 7	833	11. 8
May	9, 652	7, 965	82. 5	4, 462	46. 2	3, 503	36. 3	1, 687	17. 5
June	9, 712	7, 532	77. 6	6, 125	63. 1	1, 407	14. 5	2, 180	22. 4
July	11, 593	7, 547	65. 1	4, 841	41. 8	2, 706	23. 3	4, 046	34. 9
August	14, 060	9, 708	69. 0	8, 044	57. 2	1, 664	11. 8	4, 352	31. 0
September	21, 383	15, 860	74. 2	11, 515	53. 9	4, 345	20. 3	5, 523	25. 8
October	20, 894	17, 085	81. 8	11, 530	55. 2	5, 555	26. 6	3, 809	18. 2
November	19, 700	16, 846	85. 5	11, 665	59. 2	5, 181	26. 3	2, 854	14. 5
December	32, 511	28, 115	86. 5	21, 393	65. 8	6, 722	20. 7	4, 396	13. 5
Total	172, 968	141, 478	81. 8	106, 265	61. 4	35, 213	20. 4	31, 490	18. 2
1945									
January	33, 382	29, 329	87. 9	26, 191	78. 5	3, 138	9. 4	4, 053	12. 1
February	38, 251	31, 989	83. 6	26, 814	70. 1	5, 175	13. 5	6, 262	16. 4
March	44, 854	36, 387	81. 1	31, 210	69. 6	5, 177	11. 5	8, 467	18. 9
April	43, 839	34, 650	79. 0	26, 982	61. 5	7, 668	17. 5	9, 189	21. 0
May	57, 030	46, 099	80. 8	36, 545	64. 0	9, 554	16. 8	10, 931	19. 2
June	45, 168	34, 228	75. 8	26, 778	59. 3	7, 450	16. 5	10, 940	24. 2
July	36, 873	24, 547	66. 6	15, 379	41. 7	9, 168	24. 9	12, 326	33. 4
August	26, 258	17, 469	66. 5	9, 575	36. 5	7, 894	30. 0	8, 789	33. 5
September	19, 780	12, 393	62. 7	8, 007	40. 5	4, 386	22. 2	7, 387	37. 3
October	19, 618	14, 944	76. 2	10, 081	51. 4	4, 863	24. 8	4, 674	23. 8
November	13, 138	11, 061	84. 2	3, 489	26. 6	7, 572	57. 6	2, 077	15. 8
December	7, 781	6, 121	78. 7	572	7. 4	5, 549	71. 3	1, 660	21. 3
Total	385, 972	299, 217	77. 5	221, 623	57. 4	77, 594	20. 1	86, 755	22. 5

[a] Figures through April 1943 include Army patients only; the remainder include in addition prisoner-of-war patients, some patients of Allied nations, and a few American Red Cross patients.

[b] Figures from *Annual Report . . . Surgeon General, 1920–41* (1920–41).

[c] Figures for 1941 and 1942 supplied by Medical Statistics Division, SGO.

[d] Figures for 1943–45 from History . . . Medical Regulating Service . . . They were compiled originally from monthly reports of patients debarked, now located in SG: 705 "Evac Reqmts, Books I and II."

terranean theaters, the Chief of Transportation decided to use lower figures. For example, The Surgeon General first estimated that 44,300 patients would be evacuated to the United States during September 1944, but the Chief of Transportation in March 1944 believed that the figure would be nearer 27,000. Neither considered that airplanes would supply any significant capacity for evacuation. Past performance indicated that few patients would be transported from theaters by air, and air travel—being subject to weather conditions—was considered uncertain at best. Both officers concentrated their attention, therefore, on surface vessels.

In determining patient capacities of transports and hospital ships expected to be available, two factors had to be considered. The use of hospital ships for intratheater evacuation, a matter which had not entered into considerations leading to their authorization, would reduce the number and therefore the total capacity of hospital ships for transporting patients from theaters to the United States. Also, capacities of transports would vary according to the standards set for lifeboats and other lifesaving equipment for patients. Under "desirable" standards, which were the highest in terms of lifesaving equipment, capacities would be least. If standards were lowered, capacities would be increased. Under "adequate" standards a transport was permitted to load more patients than it had spaces for in lifeboats, provided the latter could accommodate all litter and hospital ambulant patients. For others—mental and troop class patients—only flotation equipment was necessary. Under "acceptable" standards even litter and hospital ambulant patients could exceed accommodations for patients in lifeboats, though flotation equipment had to be provided for the excess in these categories as well as for all other patients aboard. Hence, greatest capacities could be achieved by evacuating patients under "acceptable" conditions.

Because of variations in standards of lifesaving equipment and in estimates of the evacuee load, opinions about the adequacy of planned shipping facilities differed. Both the Chief of Transportation and The Surgeon General agreed that hospital ships already authorized would be sufficient to evacuate to the United States only a portion of the "helpless fraction" (estimated to be about 60 percent of the total number) of patients. They disagreed about the adequacy of transports for the remainder of the load, including helpless patients who could not be accommodated aboard hospital ships. On the basis of his estimate The Surgeon General concluded that sufficient shipping would be available for evacuation from the Pacific but that, even under "acceptable" conditions, there would be barely enough space for patients from the European theater in hospital ships already authorized and in transports expected to be available. Nor would there be enough for patients from the Mediterranean. Using a lower estimate the Chief of Transportation decided that the space available under "acceptable" standards would be sufficient for the patients from all theaters. In view of this decision and the constant need for more troop ships, he advised against the procurement of additional hospital ships. By the end of March ASF headquarters adopted a middle-of-the-road course, accepting recommendations of the Transportation Corps but directing that plans for seven additional hospital ships be drawn to be used if needed, that provision be made for additional medical personnel for sea evacuation, and that more extensive use of air evacuation be arranged in order to reduce the number of patients carried by water and thus enable higher standards to be observed on ships.[2]

Events in 1944 justified the course adopted by ASF headquarters. As a result of co-operative efforts of the Army Service Forces, the Army Air Forces, the War Department General Staff, and overseas wings of the Air Transport Command, air evacuation increased. In the spring of 1944 the Air Forces estimated that 800 to 1,910 patients from the European theater and 300 to 1,350 from the Mediterranean could be evacuated monthly in transport planes without altering their accommodations and without interfering with normal high priority traffic. The installation of special equipment to support tiers of litters in aircraft cabins, it was anticipated, would raise these figures 50 percent. In May 1944 the Air Forces made plans for placing webbing-strap litter supports in sixty-five of the C-54A planes already in use and in all transport planes to be built subsequently, and the Air Transport Command directed its overseas wings to prepare for the evacuation of the number of patients planned.[3] In consequence, the proportion of the total monthly patient load evacuated by air increased from 11.8 percent in April to a peak of 34.9 percent in July 1944, and of the total annual load from 4.5 percent in 1943 to 18.2 percent in 1944. *(See Table 16.)*

Additional hospital ships became available during 1944—a cumulative total of 9 by the end of June, 16 by the end of July, and 22 by the end of September.[4] This number was insufficient to meet the demands of all theaters, because the ships had to be deployed in terms of world-wide shipping needs rather than according to the desires of theaters for accommodations for patients. Some were required for intra-theater evacuation; others for the transportation of patients to the United States.[5] As troop shipping to the Mediterranean declined during 1944, space for patients aboard transports returning to the United States became insufficient for the evacuee load and hospital ships had to be used to a greater extent for that theater than for others. Consequently, between March and December 1944 more patients were returned from the Mediterranean by hospital ship than by transport. The European theater, generously supplied with troop shipping because of its combat operations, received fewer hospital ships proportionately than did the Mediterranean and hence had enough for only a third of the patients evacuated by water from that theater between April and December 1944. Because of the need for hospital ships in the Atlantic and Mediterranean, only one of those built by the Army was sent to the Pacific before 1945, and not until the latter half of 1944 did the three ships built and operated by the Navy for the Army—the *Hope, Comfort,* and *Mercy*—go into service there. Evacuation by hospital ship from the Pacific during 1943 and

[2] See last note above.

[3] (1) Memo, SG for CG ASF (Plans and Oprs), 27 Feb 44, sub: Potentialities of Air Evac of Pnts for Overseas to US. SG: 580. (2) Rpt of Conf on Air Evac, 13 Apr 44. SG: 337.1. (3) Memo, CG ASF for ACofS OPD WDGS, 26 Apr 44, sub: Air Evac from Eur and NATO, with inds. OPD: 580.81. (4) Ltr, ATC to Eur Wing, NA Wing, Carib Wing, ATC, 11 May 44, sub: Air Evac from Eur and NATO. SG: 580. (5) Memo, CG ASF for CG AAF, 20 Jun 44, sub: Air Evac for CBI and Pac Areas. HRS: ASF Planning Div Program Br file, "Hosp and Evac."

[4] See pp. 405-10, and *Table 18*.

[5] (1) Rads, WD (init by Mvmt Div OCT) to CG NATO, 6 Oct 43, 12 Mar 44; NATO to AGWAR, 8 and 12 Oct, 18 Dec 43; Pacific to AGWAR, 28 Jan 44; ETO to AGWAR, 5 Feb 44; WD (init by Mvmt Div OCT) to CG SOS London, 11 Feb 44. SG: 560.1; 705.1 (N Africa), (Gr Brit), (Pac). (2) Ltr, CofT to CinC SWPA, 29 Jan 44, sub: Hosp Ships, with inds. SG: 560.2.

1944 was limited therefore to the return of three shiploads of patients—one by a Navy ship from the Central Pacific in November 1943, another by a Navy ship from the South Pacific in October 1944, and the third by the *Comfort* from the Southwest Pacific in December 1944. Despite the lack of enough hospital ships to meet the desires of all theaters, the proportion of patients evacuated from theaters to the United States aboard hospital ships increased, as those authorized became available, from 2.7 percent of the total in 1943 to 20.4 percent in 1944.[6] *(See Table 16.)*

Increased transportation of patients by airplane and hospital ship reduced the proportion of the total patient load evacuated by transports from 92.8 percent in 1943 to 61.4 percent in 1944. This reduction might have been smaller if theaters had evacuated as many patients by transport as zone of interior authorities considered proper. Failure to do so resulted in part from the lower estimates of capacity that theater officials used in figuring accommodations for patients aboard transports. To raise these estimates the Chief of Transportation in January 1944 began a survey of all transports to establish their official capacities under "adequate" standards.[7] Even after these capacities were set not all theaters used transports to the extent prescribed. Thus the European theater until the end of 1944 adhered rather closely to the recommendation of its chief surgeon, Maj. Gen. Paul R. Hawley, that helpless patients should be evacuated only by hospital ships, even though the War Department had stated early that year that helpless patients would have to be evacuated by transports as well. Although forced by circumstances—increases in the patient load resulting from the invasion of the continent, the need to vacate some of the beds in hospitals in the theater, and the lack of sufficient numbers of hospital ships—to return some helpless patients to the United States in transports during 1944, the European theater steadfastly refused to make full use of officially announced capacities.[8] As a result, patients accumulated in its hospitals while beds in general hospitals in the United States remained empty. Theaters in the Pacific complied more readily with War Department policy on the use of transports and therefore did not develop similar backlogs, but in the fall of 1944 a problem developed in the Southwest Pacific when the number of mental patients to be evacuated exceeded the capacities of returning transports for patients of that type. It was solved by evacuating mental patients by air (a practice formerly considered undesirable) and by increasing and improving accommodations aboard transports for mental patients.[9]

Toward the end of 1944 attention was focused upon estimates of the evacuation load for 1945 and upon an evaluation of

[6] (1) Study of Pnt Evac. HD: 705 (Evac). This study consists of work sheets on which the ASF Medical Regulating Unit listed monthly, by theater of operations, the transports and hospital ships evacuating patients and the number of patients, by transportation classification, on each. (2) Roland W. Charles, *Troopships of World War II* (Washington, 1947), pp. 327–51.

[7] (1) TC Cir 80–12, 22 Jan 44 and Misc Ltr 28, 14 Jul 44, sub: Capacity of Pers Trans. TC: 569.6. (2) Ltr, SG to South Pacific Base Comd attn Chief Surg, 25 Sep 44, sub: Pers Capacity of Trans. SG: 560. Similar letters were sent to the other theater commands.

[8] (1) Memo for Record, on draft Rad, WD to Hq ComZ ETO, 19 Sep 44. HD: 705 (MRO, Fitzpatrick Stayback, 1484). (2) Intcrv, MD Historian with Gen Hawley, 18 Apr 50. HD: 000.71.

[9] (1) Memo for Record, on draft Rad, WD (prepared by Mvmt Div OCT) for CinC SWPA, 9 Oct 44. HD: 705 (MRO, Fitzpatrick Stayback, 1496). (2) Memo for Record by Lt Col Lamar C. Bevil, MC (SGO), 1 Nov 44, sub: Conf Ref Evac of Disturbed Mental Pnts from SWPA. HD: MOOD "Pacific."

the means available or required to handle it. There were several reasons for the inquiry: first, the war was lasting longer than had been anticipated; second, the patient load in the European theater was becoming heavy because of a high incidence of trench foot, a larger number of casualties resulting from intensified combat activity, and failure to use fully the evacuation space available aboard transports; and third, the possibility of victory in Europe during 1945 made it necessary to plan for evacuation in terms of the redeployment of ships to the Pacific.

In a study prepared by the ASF Medical Regulating Unit, adopted by the Joint Logistics and Joint Military Transportation Committees, and submitted on 16 December 1944 to the Joint Chiefs of Staff, the number of patients who would need evacuation was estimated by class, by month, and by theater, for the period from December 1944 through December 1945. From these estimates were subtracted the numbers of patients of all classes who could be evacuated each month, from each theater, by troop transports and by airplanes. The remainder represented the number of patients who would have to be evacuated by hospital ships. Conclusions drawn from these calculations were that a peak load of more than 54,000 patients would require evacuation in August 1945, that hospital ships already authorized would not be able to transport all who could not be accommodated in transports and airplanes, and that an additional number of hospital ships ranging from two in January 1945 to twenty-eight in April would therefore be needed.[10]

This study led the Joint Chiefs of Staff on 21 December 1944 to approve the conversion of troop transports to ambulance-type hospital ships in sufficient numbers (later determined by the Joint Military Transportation Committee to be six) to provide additional carrying capacity for 5,500 patients.[11] While neither the Joint Committee nor the Joint Chiefs expected this action to eliminate entirely the shortage of space for evacuation, they anticipated that it would reduce the shortage to manageable proportions.

Steps taken to "manage" the shortage applied primarily, though not altogether, to the European theater, which was expected to have almost as many patients to evacuate early in 1945 as the Pacific and Mediterranean theaters combined. It already had a backlog of patients awaiting evacuation and therefore a shortage of hospital beds. Furthermore, the patients who had accumulated would need to be evacuated from Europe early in 1945 because redeployment of transports from Europe to the Pacific would reduce capacities for evacuation from the European theater later in the year.[12] Therefore, on 3 December 1944 the Chief of Staff, on the recommendation of the Medical Regulating Officer and the Office of the Chief of Transportation, overruled General Hawley's objections and ordered the European theater to exploit fully the normal patient capacity of transports, even though it

[10] (1) Memo, Joint Logistics Plans Cmtee for Lt Col J[ohn] C. Fitzpatrick, 15 Nov 44, sub: Hosp Ship Program. (2) Joint Logistics Cmtee (JLC 221/1), 7 Dec 44, Hosp Ship Program. (3) JCS/1199, 16 Dec 44, Hosp Ship Program, Rpt with Apps "A" to "N", 64 pp. All in SG: 560.2.

[11] Joint Mil Trans Cmtee, JMTC 89/1, 26 Dec 44, Hosp Ship Program. SG: 560.2 JMTC selected the *Saturnia*, *Republic*, *President Tyler*, *Athos II*, *Columbie*, and the USS *Antaeus* (ex *St. John*) for conversion. All but the last were to be converted, manned, and operated by the Army.

[12] Following series of files (1945) deal with evacuation requirements, adequacy of hospitalization both in theaters and zone of interior, and use of evacuation facilities: HRS: G-4 file, "Hosp, vol. II"; HRS: ASF Planning Div Program Br files, "Hosp and Evac"; and SG: 705.

might have to reduce its evacuation policy to 90 days to supply enough patients for this purpose.[13] Meanwhile, American and British officers, both in the zone of interior and in the theater of operations, were discussing more extensive use of some of the larger and faster British vessels for evacuation. Subsequently they agreed to arrangements for enlarging the capacities of the *Queen Mary* and *Queen Elizabeth* for litter and hospital ambulatory patients to 2,000 and 2,500 respectively and for troop class patients to 1,000 each. This agreement was approved by the Combined Military Transportation Committee on 16 January 1945.[14] A third step was to increase the evacuation of patients by air, for it had fallen from a peak of 2,846 patients returned from Europe in July 1944 to 987 in November. Again on the recommendation of the ASF Medical Regulation Officer, the Chief of Staff directed the European theater on 25 December 1944 to arrange to use air evacuation to "the fullest practical extent". Soon afterward, the theater Air Priorities Board agreed to allocate spaces on planes for the evacuation of 3,000 patients per month.[15] A fourth step was taken in March 1945 after a re-evaluation of the evacuation load indicated that estimates made in December for the Southwest Pacific and European theaters were perhaps too low. With the concurrence of The Surgeon General, the Chief of Transportation directed that restrictions imposed by lifeboat standards upon patient capacities should be waived, as they had been for the *Queens,* for seventeen Army transports and three Navy transports, and that those vessels should be prepared to carry "maximum" loads of patients.[16]

By these measures sufficient facilities were provided to meet evacuation requirements during the first half of 1945 and to carry a peak load of 57,030 patients in May, just after V–E Day. During this period the major portion of patients came from the European theater, which was most affected by the measures adopted. In compliance with the Chief of Staff's order of 3 December 1944, it began to use space aboard transports more fully, sending to the United States in transports during that month 15,682 patients as compared with 4,665 in November, and increasing the number steadily during the early part of 1945. The number of patients evacuated by air from the European theater also grew, rising from 987 in November 1944 to more than 2,500 in February 1945. By March, arrangements for enlarging the capacities of the *Queens* had been completed and each of those vessels returned as many as 2,000 to 3,000 patients per trip. Gradually, also, greater numbers of patients were evacuated aboard transports for which maximum loading was author-

[13] (1) Diary, ASF Planning Div, 2 Dec 44. HD: 705 (MRO, Fitzpatrick Stayback, 1584). (2) Interv, MD Historian with Col Fitzpatrick, 18 Apr 50. HD: 000.71. (3) Rad CM–OUT–72113 (3 Dec 44), WD (init by Mvmt Div OCT) to ComZ ETO. HRS: G–4 file, "Hosp, vol. III."

[14] (1) Tel Conv WD–TC–1367, Washington and London (OCT officials), 27 Nov 44. SG: 337. (2) Rad CM–OUT–76241 (12 Dec 44), WD (init by Mvmt Div OCT) to ETO ComZ. SG: 560.2. (3) Rad CM–IN–16292 (17 Dec 44), UK Base Sec to WD. SG: 705. (4) Memo CMT 67, 16 Jan 45, sub: Combined Mil Trans Cmtee, Return of Pnts and other Pers Westbound on the *Queen Elizabeth* and *Queen Mary*. Same file.

[15] (1) Ltr, CG AAF to CG ASF (SG), 4 Oct 44, sub: Air Evac, ETO. SG: 580 (Gr Brit). (2) Memo, SG for CG ASF, 23 Dec 44, sub: Evac of Pnts, ETO. Same file. (3) Memo, ASF Planning Div for ASF Plans and Oprs, 6 Feb 45, sub: Air Evac to ZI. SG: 580. (4) Rad CM–OUT–82083 (25 Dec 44), WD to Hq ComZ ETO. OPD: In and Out Messages.

[16] (1) Ltr, CofT for CGs BPE, NYPE, and HRPE, 5 Feb 45, sub: Pnt Capacities, Amer Trp Trans. SG: 705. (2) Memo, CofT for Naval Trans Serv, 22 Feb 45, sub: Pnt Capacity, *Mount Vernon, Wakefield,* and *West Point.* TC: 569.5. (3) Rads, CofT to PEs and ETO, 16 and 22 Mar 45. Same file.

ized, some carrying 2,000 or more patients per trip in May. In addition, some of the hospital ships which had been used in the Mediterranean were sent to the European theater, as were the last two of the twenty-four authorized in July 1943 and the first of the five authorized in December 1944. All of these were in service by April 1945. As a result, during the first half of 1945, seventeen hospital ships made from one to four trips each from Europe to the United States. The patient load from the Mediterranean theater, which was considerably smaller by the early part of 1945 than before, was carried in the hospital ships still assigned to that theater, and in transports and airplanes.[17] By April 1945, enough evacuation facilities were available for the War Department to decide, with the approach of V–E Day, to speed the flow of patients from both the European and Mediterranean theaters. Accordingly, in May it placed these theaters on 60-day evacuation policies.[18]

Evacuation from the Pacific continued to be primarily by transport. Although plans were made as early as April 1945 to transfer hospital ships from the Atlantic to the Pacific, only one Army hospital ship—sent to the Pacific in the latter half of 1944—made a trip carrying patients from that area to the United States in the first half of 1945. The number of patients evacuated by air from the Pacific rose from 2,763 in April 1945 to 4,665 the following June. From all theaters, 262,524 patients were evacuated to the United States during the first half of 1945. Of these, 19 percent were returned by air, 14.5 percent by hospital ship, and 66.5 percent by troop transport. *(See Table 16.)*

Evacuation requirements fell off during the last half of 1945 with the cessation of hostilities. By September the patient load of the European and Mediterranean theaters had been so reduced that it was possible for them to return to a normal 120-day evacuation policy and to send patients to the United States thereafter almost exclusively by either hospital ship or airplane. Since the Pacific had no great backlog of patients, evacuation from that area in 1945 caused no problem. In the latter half of 1945, Navy hospital ships, Army and Navy transports, airplanes, and the three hospital ships operated by the Navy for the Army evacuated large numbers of patients to the United States. To these were added ten Army hospital ships transferred from the Atlantic. Just before V–J Day space for evacuation from the Pacific was so ample that the War Department ordered a reduction in its evacuation policy to 60 days to provide enough patients to make full use of available transportation. After V–J Day the Pacific was ordered to return all of its patients as quickly as possible. The patient load was in consequence reduced by October to a point that it was possible for the theater to lower its ratio of beds to troop strength and to return to a 120-day evacuation policy.[19] *(See Table 14.)* During the latter half of 1945, of the 123,448 patients evacuated from all theaters, 29.9 percent returned to the United States by air, 31.9 percent by hospital ship, and 38.2 percent by transport. This represented a reversal of the situation during the first half of the year, when approximately two thirds of all patients were evacuated by transport. During the entire year, 385,792 patients were evacuated from all theaters: 22.5 percent by air, 20.1 percent by hospital ship, and 57.4 percent by transport. *(See Table 16.)*

[17] Study of Pnt Evac. HD: 705 (Evac).
[18] See p. 300.
[19] Study of Pnt Evac. HD: 705 (Evac). Also see p. 301.

CHAPTER XX

Development of Procedures for Evacuation from Theaters to the Zone of Interior

Before the patient load (described in the last chapter) could be transferred from theaters to general hospitals in the United States, policies and procedures to govern the entire operation had to be developed. Those established early in the war remained effective with minor modifications to its end.

Procedures for Sea Evacuation

SOS directives charged ports of embarkation, operating directly under the Chief of Transportation, with responsibility for the evacuation of patients from overseas areas to which they supplied war materiel. A basic prerequisite to the discharge of this responsibility was information about the kind and number of patients to be evacuated. Accordingly, in August 1942 SOS headquarters announced that patients would be classified for transportation purposes as mental, hospital, or troop class.[1] The next month these classes were increased to four by splitting the hospital class in two: hospital litter and hospital ambulant. Mental, or Class I, patients were those who required security accommodations aboard ships or trains to prevent them from injuring or destroying themselves. Hospital litter, or Class II, patients were those whose physical condition required them to remain in bed and be cared for entirely by others. Hospital ambulant, or Class III, patients were those who required medical care and service, even though they did not have to remain in bed at all times. Troop class, or Class IV, patients were those who needed little medical care en route and were able to care for themselves even in emergencies.[2]

In 1944 subdivisions were established for Class I, or mental patients. They were actually of three groups: those who were seriously disturbed and needed locked-ward accommodations in hospitals as well as on ships; those who were borderline cases and might or might not require locked-ward care on land but did require it aboard ships; and those who were only mildly disturbed and did not need to be

[1] Memo, CG SOS (init by Lt Col J[ohn] C. Fitzpatrick) for SG, 21 Aug 42, sub: Est of Reqmt for Sea Evac. SG: 560.-2.

[2] Ltr SPOPH 322.15, CG SOS to CGs and COs of SvCs and PEs and to SG, 15 Sep 42, sub: Mil Hosp and Evac Oprs. AG: 370.05.

placed under restraint in any event. Patients of the last type suffered from being quartered with the more serious mental cases and, if placed in locked wards, took up space needed for the latter. Yet, under existing regulations and classifications, transport surgeons and medical officers in charge of patients on hospital ships often treated all mental patients alike, regardless of the degree of their disability. To remedy this situation the War Department in June 1944 broke the classification for mental patients (Class I) into three parts—Class I A, Class I B, and Class I C—to conform with the three groupings just stated.[3] The Chief of Transportation then ordered hospital ship commanders and transport surgeons not to place Class I C patients in restrictive quarters but to evacuate them instead in accommodations used for troop class (Class IV) patients.[4]

To furnish ports in the United States with information about the number of patients of each type to be returned to the zone of interior, SOS headquarters in September 1942 devised a system of reports of "essential information concerning evacuation of sick and wounded from overseas." Offices of both The Surgeon General and the Chief of Transportation concurred in its establishment. Each overseas commander was required to report monthly to the port commander serving his area the following information: (1) the total number of patients awaiting evacuation, (2) the number in each of the four classes listed above who were awaiting evacuation at each port within the theater, and (3) the number in each class who were expected to require evacuation at the beginning of the following month. Upon embarkation of patients for the United States, each theater commander was required to report by air mail to port commanders in the United States the name of the ship upon which patients embarked, the number of patients of each class aboard the ship, and the expected date and port of arrival in the United States. Receipt of such information would supply a basis for the Transportation Corps to use in providing transportation and for the Medical Department to use in assuring the availability of sufficient numbers of vacant beds for patients being evacuated.[5]

Early in 1943 this system was slightly modified. In some instances embarkation reports failed to reach ports in the United States before the arrival of ships carrying patients. In others, theaters failed to submit such reports. In still others, they submitted incorrect reports. For example, on 9 December 1942, 788 patients arrived from the European theater at the port of Halifax in Canada. Although the theater had reported them all as ambulatory, it was discovered upon arrival that seven were litter and 104 mental patients who required attendants. Because of the erroneous report, insufficient medical personnel had been sent to Halifax to care for the patients received and their debarka-

[3] Ltr AG 704.11 (3 Jun 44) OB-S-E-SPMOT-M, TAG to CGs AAF, AGF, ASF, Base Comds, and TofOpns, 8 Jun 44, sub: Procedure for Evac of Pnts by Water or Air from Overseas Comds. SG: 705.-1.

[4] (1) Ltr, Hq ComZ ETO to CofT, 10 Jul 44, sub: Accommodations for Class I A Pnts on Trp Trans. TC: 569.6. (2) Telg, CofT (Mvmt Div) to CPE, 28 Jul 44. SG: 560.2. (3) Telg, CofT (Mvmt Div) to CGs PEs, 2 Sep 44. SG: 705. (4) Ltr, CofT (Mvmt Div) to PEs, 21 Sep 44, sub: Sea Evac of Mental Pnts. SG: 560.2.

[5] (1) Memo, CG SOS for ACofS OPD WDGS, 3 Sep 42, sub: Essential Inf Conc Evac of Sick and Wounded from Overseas. OPD: 370.05. (2) Ltr AG 370.05 (9-15-42) MS-SPOPH-M, TAG to CGs Def Comds, TofOpns, and Base Comds, 16 Sep 42, same sub. SG: 705.-1.

tion was delayed.[6] To prevent similar occurrences, as well as the arrival of patients without prior arrangements for their reception, theaters were directed in January 1943 to exercise more care in making reports of embarkation and to transmit them by radio rather than by air mail.[7]

Another modification in the reporting system occurred as a result of increasing participation during 1942 of agencies other than the Army Transportation Corps in the evacuation of patients. Some were returned on British ships; others, by the Air Transport Command and the U. S. Navy. For example, by the end of 1942 most patients evacuated from the South Pacific area were returned by the Navy; and from Central Africa, by the Air Transport Command. Commanders of those areas considered it unnecessary to submit reports of patients awaiting evacuation, since they did not normally use Army ships. While failure to receive such reports did not interfere with the Chief of Transportation's efforts to supply sufficient transport lift for patients awaiting evacuation by sea, it did hamper planning for the reception of patients in the United States and for their further transportation, usually by rail, to hospitals of definitive treatment. Therefore, on 13 January 1943 the War Department directed theater commanders to report monthly, in addition to information already required, the number of patients awaiting evacuation by air, by Navy ships, and by any other means, as well as the number in each category who were expected to need evacuation at the end of the following 30 days.[8]

Further changes were made later in the war. Toward the end of 1944 the return of able-bodied men and officers on "rotation" complicated the problem of evaluating the adequacy of patient lift because such persons sometimes took up space on transports which the Medical Regulating Unit had considered available for patients. In August 1944, therefore, the War Department directed theater commanders to add to reports of patients all other military personnel awaiting transportation to the zone of interior.[9] Early in 1945, as the patient load mounted toward its peak, the Surgeon General's Resources Analysis Division requested additional information for planning purposes. As a result, the War Department directed theaters in March 1945 to report not only the patients awaiting evacuation and those expected to need evacuation at the end of the following month but also those that were expected to need evacuation at the end of the second and third months after the date of the report.[10]

To assure proper use of the information submitted by theaters, the SOS Hospitalization and Evacuation Branch prepared a directive in October 1942 for the Chief

[6] (1) Memo, Lt Col J. C. Fitzpatrick for Chief Hosp and Evac Br Plans Div Oprs SOS, 21 Dec 42, sub: Rpt on Temp Duty, Hq 2d SvC and Hq NYPE. HD: 705 (MRO, Fitzpatrick Daybook, Aug 42–Jun 43). (2) Memo, CG SOS for CofT, 3 Jan 43, sub: Reception of Pnts Evac by Sea from Overseas Comds. Same file.

[7] (1) Memo, CG SOS for TAG, 2 Jan 43, sub: Compliance with Directive. AG: 704 (1-2-43). (2) Rad CM-OUT-1128, AGWAR to ETOUSA, 3 Jan 43, HD: Wilson files, "Book III, 1 Jan 43–15 Mar 43."

[8] Ltr, TAG to CGs Def Comds, Depts, and Base Comds, 13 Jan 43, sub: Essential Info Conc Evac of Sick and Wounded from Overseas. AG: 370.05.

[9] OCM form, with message prepared by OCT for dispatch to CGs Def Comds, TofOpns, and PEs, 30 Aug 44, and with Memo for Record. TC: 370.05.

[10] (1) Memos, SG (Resources Anal Div) for ASF (Plans and Oprs), 21 and 27 Feb 45, sub: Rpt for Overseas Theaters. SG: 705. (2) Rad CM-OUT-55158, WD to all Overseas Comds, 17 Mar 45. TC: 370.05 (Monthly Rpt of Reqmts).

of Transportation to issue to port commanders.[11] It required them to transmit information received from theaters to the Office of the Chief of Transportation, to other interested port commanders, and to the commanding generals of service commands in which ports were located. Also, port commanders were to compare the number and types of patients to be evacuated during the following month with accommodations aboard transports scheduled to call at theater ports. If it appeared that there would be insufficient "lift"—that is, too few ships returning from theaters or unsuitable accommodations on available ships for different classes of patients—port commanders were to report this fact to the Chief of Transportation in order that additional lift might be provided. Finally, port commanders were to use information received in embarkation reports to plan transportation from ports in the United States to hospitals of definitive treatment.[12]

In the final months of 1942 transports arriving at overseas ports sometimes found more patients ready for evacuation than theaters had reported and hence had insufficient accommodations for all of them. This situation resulted from the temporary and sudden accumulation of patients, particularly of Class I (mental), after reports had been sent in, and from the preemption of all space on a transport by its first port of call to the detriment of ports of later call. Measures were taken to avoid such occurrences. Port commanders were required to submit their comparisons of evacuation requirements with scheduled sailings of transports to the Office of the Chief of Transportation for review. When that Office found that accommodations on transports scheduled for return trips from theaters were insufficient for patients needing to be evacuated, it directed port commanders to determine through direct communication with theater commanders what additional evacuation space was really necessary. The Chief of Transportation was then responsible for complying insofar as possible with desires of the theater commander. In addition, when transports sailed for a theater with several ports of call, port commanders in the United States were required to inform theater commanders of their capacities and theater commanders in turn were required to suballocate reported space among the several ports under their jurisdiction.[13]

Later in the war, the Medical Regulating Unit used information submitted in reports of patients being embarked and awaiting evacuation to plan the most effective use of all available evacuation facilities. Its Water Evacuation Section maintained at all times current records of patients needing transportation from different ports in the several theaters. Comparisons of such records with space for patients aboard scheduled transports revealed whether or not anticipated lift for a particular port or theater would be adequate. If not, the Medical Regulating Officer recommended steps to supply the required lift such as changes in the schedules of transports, increases in the number

[11] Memo, CG SOS (Hosp and Evac Br) for CofT, 10 Oct 42, sub: Sea and Port Evac Oprs. SG: 705.-1.

[12] Ltr SPTSM 370.05, CofT (Mvt Div) to CGs PEs, 23 Oct 42, sub: Sea and Port Evac Oprs, with incl. SG: 704.-1.

[13] (1) Ltr, Surg NOPE to CG SOS (Plans Div), 10 Feb 43, sub: Overseas Evac Plan Ships' Hosp Space Almt, with 5 inds. HD: 705 (MRO, Fitzpatrick Daybook, Aug 42–Jun 43). (2) Memo, Chief Hosp and Evac Sec Plans Div ASF for Col [Frank A.] Heileman, 22 Apr 43, sub: Sea Evac Oprs. HD: Wilson files, "Day File." (3) Memos, ACofS for Oprs ASF for SG and CofT, 9 May 43, sub: Hosp and Evac Oprs. Same file.

of patients to be evacuated by air, or the redeployment of hospital ships.[14]

While directives issued during 1942 charged the Chief of Transportation and port commanders under his control with evacuation from theaters of operations, they contained no demarcation of areas of responsibility of overseas commanders and the Chief of Transportation for transfer of patients from control of the former to the latter. To insure co-ordination between a theater and the zone of interior, such demarcation was necessary. Hence, early in 1943 the SOS Hospitalization and Evacuation Branch prepared a directive on "sea evacuation operations" which the War Department issued on 25 January 1943.[15] This directive detailed specifically for the first time the respective responsibilities of the Chief of Transportation, port commanders, and theater commanders.

The Chief of Transportation was charged with the care, treatment, and safety of patients after their ships had left overseas ports. Up to that point theater commanders were responsible. These commanders were charged with selecting patients to be evacuated, with concentrating them at or near ports of embarkation, and, in co-ordination with overseas port officials, with placing them on ships bound for the United States. They were responsible for insuring that patients were not placed on ships lacking suitable accommodations. For example, a theater commander was not to permit mental (Class I) patients to be embarked in excess of a ship's capacity for patients of that type. Furthermore, he was to prevent the loading of ships with more patients than could be "reasonably expected to be evacuated to lifeboats should it become necessary to abandon ship." This left the decision as to suitability of accommodations up to theaters. Eventually, though, they were forced to substitute the War Department's opinion of suitable accommodations for their own. As transportation and medical officials of ports in the zone of interior completed surveys of transports during 1944, theaters were expected to use officially announced capacities for patients of all classes.[16]

Theater commanders were also responsible for providing adequate medical personnel for patients embarked and for furnishing any additional medical supplies requested by transport surgeons. Personnel whom they placed on ships normally belonged to the Chief of Transportation and were supplied to theaters on an "attached" basis. Medical hospital ship platoons of various sizes were attached to United States ports by the Chief of Transportation. Port commanders then ordered them to temporary duty in theaters of operations. Only when such platoons were not available were theater commanders required to supply medical troops of their own. As with personnel, theater commanders were expected to furnish additional medical supplies to transports only in unusual or emergency circumstances. Normally port commanders in the United States placed aboard each transport enough medical supplies to care for all troops on its outbound voyage and for patients, on the inbound voyage,

[14] Examples of the records kept may be found in "Estimate of Evac Reqmts [Weekly]," Books 1 thru 8, 31 Jan 44–27 May 46, and "Evac Reqmts—Monthly Rpt," Books 1 and 2, Nov 43–May 46. SG: 705. Also see Study of Pnts Evac. HD: 705 (Evac).

[15] Ltr AG 370.05 (1–19–43) OB-S-SPOPH-M, TAG to CGs Theaters, Depts, Base Comds and Task Forces, and COs Base Comds and Task Forces, 25 Jan 43, sub: Sea Evac Oprs. AG: 704 (1–19–43).

[16] See above, p. 327.

equal in number to one fourth of the transport's troop capacity.

Theater commanders were given additional responsibilities in connection with sea evacuation operations in the latter part of the war. To reduce the medical personnel who would be needed for assignment to regularly organized medical hospital ship platoons, they were required after 8 June 1944 to form Medical Department officers, nurses, and enlisted men being returned to the United States on "rotation," into provisional medical hospital ship platoons. Regularly organized platoons were saved for use only when provisional platoons could not be formed. In the same month, theater commanders were directed to furnish transport surgeons and hospital ship commanders not only with evacuation orders but also with lists of patients showing diagnosis, transportation classification, and type of accommodation needed for each. Similar lists had formerly been prepared by transport surgeons and hospital ship commanders for submission to zone of interior port officials for use in debarkation activities. Now, their preparation by theaters saved time for medical officers aboard ships and assisted them in placing patients in suitable accommodations. Theater officials were expected, in addition, to assemble complete sets of records for each patient and to deliver them, along with patients' baggage and valuables, to ships upon which patients were embarked. When records were missing, theater commanders either had new ones prepared or submitted to ships' officers certified statements of those missing and of the reasons for their absence.[17] Near the end of the war an additional duty was placed on theater personnel. Up to that time debarkation tags containing information similar to that found on embarkation lists were prepared and attached to patients aboard ship.[18] In July 1945 a War Department circular required theater hospitals to prepare and attach identification tags to each patient before his embarkation. These tags were made of four perforated sections. The first three could be detached to serve theater ports, ships, and United States ports as records of patients handled. The last section, containing information about a patient's diagnosis, could be used by debarkation hospitals in assigning patients to wards.[19]

The directives just discussed served as a basis for co-ordination of activities of theaters and the zone of interior in the evacuation of patients by sea. A further step—the co-ordination of activities of transport surgeons with those of the ports of debarkation in the United States—was taken in 1943. In the spring the New York Port issued instructions for transport surgeons. In addition to describing the manifold duties and responsibilities of transport surgeons for sanitation aboard transports, for the care of outbound troops, and for the care and treatment of inbound patients, these instructions covered the duties of transport surgeons in the transfer of patients from ships to ports. Upon arrival at a zone of interior port, each transport surgeon was required to submit to a port surgeon's representative a list of all Army patients, showing for each a

[17] (1) Ltr AG 704.11 (3 Jun 44) OB-S-E-SPMOT-M, TAG to CGs AAF, AGF, ASF, Base Comds, and TofOpns, 8 Jun 44, sub: Procedure for Evac of Pnts by Water or Air from Overseas Comds. SG: 705.-1. (2) Ltr, CofT to CG NATOUSA, 13 Nov 43, sub: Embarkation of pnts. HD: 705 (MRO, Fitzpatrick Stayback, 493). (3) Ltr, Stark Gen Hosp to CG CPE, 10 Jan 44, sub: Pnt Lists for Hosp Ships, with 4 inds. SG: 705.-1. (BB).

[18] TC Cir 50-31, 30 May 44, sub: Use of Debarkation Tag (Manual for Trans Surg); (Revised 17 Jul 44). TC: 710.

[19] WD Cir 218, 20 Jul 45.

brief diagnosis, a classification (neuropsychiatric, medical, or surgical), and whether litter or ambulatory, along with records accompanying each patient. Each transport surgeon was required to submit a list of the baggage of patients and a list of patients' money and valuables in the surgeon's possession. Finally, he was to complete all entries on a debarkation tag for each patient and was to insure the attachment of such tags to the clothing of all except those who were neuropsychiatric. Tags for the latter were to be delivered to debarkation officers. These actions were designed to assist ports in planning the transfer of patients to general hospitals and to assist these hospitals in assigning them to proper wards.[20]

As experience accumulated and the evacuation load grew heavier, the Transportation Corps, assisted by the Medical Regulating Officer, supplied transport surgeons and hospital ship commanders with more specific instructions than formerly. Toward the end of 1943 the guide for transport surgeons which the New York Port had issued earlier was sent to other ports for transmission to the surgeons of transports which called at them.[21] About the same time, general regulations covering the sailing of hospital ships were published. Later, as the number of hospital ships in service increased, the Charleston Port, which had been designated as the home port for Army hospital ships serving the European and Mediterranean theaters, issued a sixty-one page manual of instructions for their commanders. It covered such subjects as reports and records, procedures in case of death, regulations for sanitation and hygiene, quarantine procedures, suggestions for the care of patients at sea, supplies and equipment, and the like.[22] Instructions issued to transport surgeons and hospital ship commanders also included procedures to be followed in preparing for debarkations at ports in the United States, but gradually many of their duties in this connection were transferred, as already described, to theater officials. As that happened medical officers on ships became responsible for checking for accuracy and completeness the embarkation lists and identification tags prepared in theaters.

Procedures for Air Evacuation

Though few patients were transported by air from theaters to the United States in the first year and a half of the war, such demands for air evacuation as were made resulted in the establishment during 1942 of a basic system of air evacuation.

Earliest requests for the evacuation of patients by air from outlying areas came particularly from the Alaska Defense Command. Before the war that Command had asked for airplane-ambulance service to the United States; in the first half of 1942 it renewed its requests, pointing out then and later that evacuation by sea was uncertain, delaying the movement of patients in some cases from two to four weeks and subject at all times to interruption by enemy activities.[23] To the demands of Alaska were added in July

[20] (1) Instructions for Transport Surgeons, Off Port Surg, NYPE, 26 May 43. HD: 560 (NYPE), (2) ARs 55-350, 14 Sep 42; 55-415, 11 Dec 42.

[21] Ltr, CofT (Mvmt Div) to CGs PEs, 9 Dec 43, sub: Guide for Trans Surgs. HD: 705 (MRO, Fitzpatrick Stayback, 583).

[22] (1) AR 55-530, 30 Dec 43. (2) CPE, Instructions (Med) to Hosp Ship Comdrs, 30 Aug 44. HD: 560 (CPE). (3) TCP 16, 4 Apr 45, US Army Hosp Ship Guide. HD: 560.

[23] (1) Gordon H. McNeil, History of the Medical Department in Alaska in World War II (1946), pp. 167-192. HD. (2) Ltrs, CG Alaska Def Comd to CG Western Def Comd and Fourth Army, 14 Jul and 6 Oct 42, sub: Aircraft Amb for Alaska. AG: 452. The 14 July 1942 letter cites earlier letters on the same subject dated 10 November 1941 and 6 April 1942.

1942 a request of the Newfoundland Base Command for air evacuation to New York. The Surgeon General's Office and SOS headquarters approved this request and passed it on to the Army Air Forces, which in June had been charged with responsibility for the development and operation of air evacuation.[24]

The Air Surgeon saw in these demands an opportunity to develop an air evacuation system,[25] but basic decisions had to be made first as to (1) who within the Army Air Forces would be responsible for planning and operating this system, (2) whether or not special airplane ambulances would be provided, and (3) the extent to which air evacuation would be encouraged or permitted. On 25 August 1942 the Air Surgeon foreshadowed the answer to the second question when he stated that "airplanes have not been produced in sufficient quantity to allot planes solely for ambulance use. . . ."[26] On the same day he recommended that the Air Transport Command be charged with planning, developing, and operating a system of air evacuation from outlying bases to the United States.[27]

Three days later the Air Staff announced its decisions. Special planes would not be provided for the evacuation of patients from overseas bases and theaters; but air evacuation would be carried out in connection with the routine operation of air transports. Since the Air Transport Command operated such transports, it would operate the air evacuation system. The Air Surgeon—not the Air Transport Command—would be responsible for planning and establishing policies for this system.[28] To discharge this responsibility, the Air Surgeon expanded his Office, assigning to it in September and October two officers—Maj. (later Col.) Richard L. Meiling and Col. Wood S. Woolford—who had already demonstrated an interest in air evacuation.[29]

Meanwhile the Air Surgeon had drafted a policy governing the extent of air evacuation. After approval by the Air and General Staffs it was announced to theaters by the Chief of Staff of the Army on 25 September 1942. Air evacuation would be accomplished "upon call" on the Air Transport Command, but such calls would be kept "to [a] minimum." Theater commanders would classify patients for air evacuation according to the following order of precedence: first, emergency cases for whom essential medical treatment was not available locally; second, cases for whom air evacuation was a "military necessity"; and third, cases—except psychotics—who required prolonged hospitalization and rehabilitation.[30]

[24] (1) Ltr, CG Eastern Def Comd and First Army to CG AAF, 31 Jul 42, sub: Air Amb Evac of Pnts from Newfoundland Base Comd, with 3 inds. SG: 705.-1 (Newfoundland)F.

[25] The chief of the SOS Hospitalization and Evacuation Branch gained this impression after conferring with representatives of the Air Surgeon. Diary, Hosp and Evac Br SOS, 12 Nov 42. HD: Wilson files, "Diary."

[26] 4th ind, CG AAF (Air Surg) to SG, 25 Aug 42, on Ltr, CG Eastern Def Comd and First Army to CG AAF, 31 Jul 42, sub: Air Amb Evac of Pnts from Newfoundland Base Comd. SG: 705.-1 (Newfoundland)F.

[27] Ltr, Air Surg to ACofAir Staff A-4, 25 Aug 42, sub: Evac of Casualties by Air. AAF: 370.05.

[28] (1) Memo, CG AAF (ACofAir Staff A-4) for CG ATC, 28 Aug 42, sub: Evac of Casualties by Air. (2) 1st ind, Same to Air Surg, 28 Aug 42, on Ltr Air Surg to ACofAir Staff A-4, 25 Aug 42, same sub. Both in AAF: 370.05.

[29] (1) An Rpt, FY 1943, Oprs Div ASO. USAF: SGO Hist Br. (2) Medical History, I Troop Carrier Command From 30 April 1942 to 31 December 1944, pp. 49-50. Same file. (3) Ltr, Dr. Richard L. Meiling to Col Calvin H. Goddard, 30 Jun 52. HD: 314 (Correspondence on MS) XI.

[30] (1) Rad CM-OUT-8628 thru 8637, Marshall to CGs Bases, Def Comds, and Theaters, 25 Sep 42. OPD: 704.1. These messages were all identical. (2) Memo, Lt Col Milton W. Arnold, AC, for Lt Col M. T. Stallter, 9 Sep 42, sub: Evac of Casualties by Air. AG: 580.-1.

After basic decisions were made about air evacuation from theaters, representatives of the Air Surgeon's Office, the SOS Hospitalization and Evacuation Branch, and the Air Transport Command collaborated in establishing operational procedures and delineating responsibilities of various participating commands. Whereas the Air Transport Command was responsible for equipment attached to planes, such as litter brackets, the Medical Department was to furnish all medical supplies and equipment used in the care of patients en route. Supplies such as litters and blankets were to be furnished by theaters, but were to be returned by the Services of Supply after patients arrived in the United States. Medical air evacuation transport squadrons, consisting of nurses and enlisted technicians, were to be assigned to the Air Transport Command to furnish attendants for patients aboard transport planes. Theater commanders were to transfer patients to points along regular ATC routes. They were also to co-ordinate plans for air evacuation to the United States with the commanders of ATC wings serving their respective areas, reporting to the latter daily the location and number of litter, hospital ambulant, and troop class patients who should be picked up. Flight surgeons alone would determine the suitability for flight of patients selected by theater commanders. Finally, the Air Transport Command would be responsible for the care and treatment of patients from the time it accepted them in theaters until it delivered them to SOS or AAF control in the United States.[31]

Although ATC medical officers alone could determine the final suitability of patients for flight, after the first half of 1944 theater medical authorities were responsible for establishing the general groups of patients to be transported by air. They agreed that litter patients should take precedence over the less serious cases. The chief surgeons of both the European and Mediterranean theaters considered patients requiring neurosurgery, maxillofacial surgery, and plastic surgery, as well as those who were blind, to be among those who should have priorities in air evacuation. Both believed that serious mental disturbances were a contraindication to transportation by air.[32] On the other hand, in the fall of 1944 the Southwest Pacific theater included mental patients among the groups to be evacuated by air as a regular procedure. Success in this practice resulted in the preparation in August 1945 of a standing operating procedure for the air evacuation of psychiatric patients.[33]

Early in 1943 the Air Priorities Division of the Air Transport Command determined the priority of patients designated for air transportation as against priorities already established for passengers and

[31] (1) Rpt, Mins of Mtg, ATC, 13 Oct 43, Air Evac of Wounded. AAF: 370.05. (2) Memo, CG SOS for CG AAF, 9 Nov 42, sub: Evac Oprs. AG: 704 (17 Jun 42)(1). (3) Memo, CG SOS for CG AAF, 12 Nov 42, sub: Status of Hosp Cons and Evac Fac for Alaska Sta. AG: 632. (4) 2d ind, CofSA to CG Alaska Def Comd, 21 Nov 42, on unknown basic Ltr. AG: 632. (5) Ltr, CG AAF to Surg 11th AF, 13 Dec 42, sub: Recommended Plan of Air Evac. AAF: 370.05. (6) Diary, SOS Hosp and Evac Br, 17 Dec 42. HD: Wilson files, "Diary."

[32] (1) *Logistical History of NATOUSA-MTOUSA, 30 November 1945* (Naples, Italy, 1945), pp. 328–29, HD: MTO, 314. (2) Off Chief Surg Hq ETO, Admin Memo 147, 2 Nov 44; Admin Memo 16, 23 Mar 45, and other correspondence dealing with selection of patients for air evacuation. HD: ETO, 370.05 (Evac Br Corresp 1944–45).

[33] History of the Medical Department, Air Transport Command, 1 January 1945–31 March 1946. HD: TAS. For a discussion of medical considerations involved in air evacuation, see Sidney Leibowitz, "Air Evacuation of Sick and Wounded," *The Military Surgeon*, vol. 99, No. 1 (July 1946), pp. 7–10.

cargo in general. Three degrees of precedence for the latter two were announced in January. Persons whose movement was required by an emergency so acute that any delay would seriously and directly impair the war effort were given a Class 1 priority. Passengers and cargo whose transportation by air was absolutely necessary for the accomplishment of a mission essential to the prosecution of the war were given a Class 2 priority. Class 3 priorities were given to passengers and cargo whose transportation by air was vital to the war effort but not of an extremely urgent nature.[34] In February 1943 ATC headquarters announced that patients would normally have Class 3 priorities but could not be displaced, or "bounced," once they were en route, except at the discretion of ATC flight surgeons at stopover points. In effect, this gave patients a Class 3 priority for loading but a Class 1 priority for the duration of flight. In emergencies, ATC announced, patients might be given initially the highest priority at a theater commander's disposal. Medical attendants were to travel under the same priorities as patients during flights to the United States; to insure their prompt return to theaters which supplied them, they were then to be given a Class 2 priority.[35]

An important change in the system of determining priorities was made in 1944. Beginning in April the Air Transport Command allocated transport space on a tonnage basis to each theater commander, and theater priorities boards then determined the amount of space that would be set aside for patients, for other personnel, and for cargo.[36] Among the obvious advantages of this system was the increased certainty with which both theater surgeons and Medical Regulating Officers in the United States could plan air evacuation.

The use of air evacuation necessitated a system by which airports in the United States and air bases along Air Transport Command routes could be informed of the arrival of patients by plane. In October 1943 the Air Transport Command issued a regulation making ATC officers responsible for the necessary reports. It required a base embarking patients for another to inform it by the fastest means of communication available. It also required the pilot of a plane carrying patients to report his cargo to the operations officer of the next stopping point thirty minutes before arrival. After planes landed in the United States, ports of aerial debarkation—using a code devised by the ASF Medical Regulating Unit—reported patients received to the Air Forces Regulating Officer.[37]

Procedures for Debarkation

Patients transported from theaters to the zone of interior by the Transportation Corps and the Air Transport Command had to be transferred soon after arrival to service commands for definitive treatment. It was necessary, therefore, to determine the point where responsibility for their transportation and care devolved upon service commands, and to establish procedures for their debarkation, their movement from ships and planes to near-by

[34] Air Priorities Div, ATC, Directive No 5, Priorities for Air Trans, 9 Jan 43. AAF: 580 "Air Trans."

[35] (1) Ltr AFATC 580.1, CG ATC to CGs Overseas Comds, Wing Comdrs, 26 Feb 43, sub: Air Priorities Instruction No 4. AAF: 370.05. (2) WD Memo 95-6-43, 26 Feb 43. AG: 580.81 (1-10-43).

[36] (1) WD Cir 130, 4 Apr 44. (2) AAF Reg 25-6, 29 Apr 44.

[37] (1) ATC Reg 25-6, 15 Oct 43. (2) AAF Ltr, 4 Oct 44, sub: Rpt of Pnts for Trf. (3) Comments by Brig Gen Richard L. Meiling USAF, 30 Jun 52. HD: 314 (Correspondence on MS) XI.

hospitals, and their reception and preparation for further transportation to hospitals of definitive treatment. Problems in this connection were not as great for air bases as for port commands because patients arrived by plane in smaller groups and fewer numbers than by ship.

In the early period of the war ports of embarkation were responsible for sending patients who arrived from theaters to general hospitals for further treatment.[38] This responsibility conflicted with a basic principle of Army evacuation, namely, that support was always from rear to front. According to it, responsibilities of ports for the movement of patients should have ended at their normal rear boundaries. Failure to observe this principle is perhaps accounted for by the lingering influence of peacetime practices. In peacetime the most common movement of patients in the United States was from station to general hospitals and in such instances station commanders were responsible for issuing orders and arranging transportation. So long as the number of evacuees arriving at ports was small, it was perhaps logical that port commanders should perform this service for them as well as for patients from port complements.

The practice of considering commanders of ports of embarkation responsible for transferring evacuees to general hospitals had to be partially modified after patients began to return to the United States by air. Under current regulations theater commanders issued orders directing them to report to commanders of seaports responsible for the supply and evacuation of respective theaters. As a result patients who traveled by air from the Caribbean, for example, landed in Florida with orders to report to the commander of the New Orleans Port of Embarkation. In such instances they had to be sent by rail from Miami to New Orleans for subsequent transfer to a general hospital, rather than directly to the general hospital which was nearest Miami (Lawson General Hospital, Atlanta, Ga.). This not only caused inconvenience to patients and delayed their treatment, but also added unnecessary burdens to transportation facilities that were already overtaxed. In February 1943 SOS Headquarters referred this problem to the Air Surgeon's Office. On the recommendation of the latter the War Department in May directed overseas commanders not to designate, in orders transferring patients to the United States, specific commanders to whom they were to report. At the same time air bases in the United States were granted authority to issue orders transferring patients to general hospitals for definitive treatment.[39]

Unlike port commanders, commanders of air bases serving as debarkation points operated debarkation hospitals or at least used station hospitals located on such bases for debarkation processing of patients. They were responsible for removing patients from airplanes and transporting them and their baggage to such hospitals. To discharge this responsibility they were required by ATC regulations to supply a team of at least one medical officer and four enlisted men to meet each plane bringing in patients. They did not assume the additional responsibility and authority of arranging for the transportation of patients from air debarkation hospitals to

[38] (1) AR 40–1025, 12 Oct 40; C 1, 21 Aug 42; C 4, 5 Jul 43. (2) WD Cir 64, 1 Jun 42. (3) WD Cir 316, 6 Dec 43.

[39] (1) Ltr, CG Trinidad Sector and Base Comd to CG NOPE, 27 Jan 43, sub: Designation of Specific Hosp in Evac Orders with 5 inds. AAF: 370.05 (Evac). (2) WD Cirs 119, 11 May 43, and 137, 16 Jun 43.

general hospitals. Instead they normally called upon service commands to perform this function, but in extreme emergencies might arrange locally, or apply to the Air Surgeon, for air transport.[40]

Early in the war commanders of ports of embarkation were responsible for removing patients from ships and also for transporting them to debarkation hospitals operated by service commands. By the middle of 1943 several developed "SOP" (Standing Operating Procedures) for this operation. The SOP for the New York Port, for example, explained procedures for the transfer of patients from transports to near-by hospitals. Upon arrival of a ship, a party from the port went aboard to verify the reported number and classification of patients and to receive from the transport surgeon his list of patients classified according to diagnosis (medical, surgical, or neuropsychiatric). This list was sent immediately to Halloran General Hospital, so that room in appropriate wards could be prepared. Ambulatory patients, the first to be debarked, were dispatched to Halloran in commercial buses in groups of ten, with two enlisted men as medical attendants for each group. Litter patients were placed in ambulances, each carrying four patients and one attendant. Finally, mental patients were consigned to ambulances, with necessary attendants. After patients were removed from a ship, their valuables were turned over to the boarding officer for transmission to the receiving hospital. Baggage of small groups was sent by the port direct to the hospital, while that of large groups was handled by the baggagemaster's section of the Army Transport Service or, later, the port's water division. Patients' records were put in proper order and transmitted to Halloran General Hospital. The port surgeon's office then sent reports of debarkation to the Chief of Transportation, The Surgeon General, the commander of the New York Port of Embarkation, and the surgeon of the Second Service Command.[41]

For debarking patients from ships and transporting them to general hospitals port commanders normally used personnel and vehicles belonging to installations under their control. For example, the Charleston Port trained as litter bearers enlisted men belonging to its own medical detachment and to port and service battalions in training or on duty in the area. It also used its own ambulances, trucks, and passenger cars to carry patients to Stark General Hospital, which was located near by.[42] This procedure sufficed when the number of patients received was small. When large-scale operations were expected, other arrangements had to be made. In the fall of 1942, for instance, to assist in the reception of casualties from the North African invasion the New York Port called upon the Second Service Command for both personnel and vehicles and used, in addition, an ambulance section of a Ground Forces medical regiment.[43] In

[40] (1) Memo, Air Surg for ACofAir Staff A-4, 24 Feb 43, sub: Air Evac Casualties, with draft of directive to all air commands in the United States. AAF: 370.05. (2) ATC Reg 25-6, 15 Oct 43 and 29 Apr 44; AAF Reg 25-17, 6 June 44; AAF Ltr 25-10, 11 Jul 44 and 9 Dec 44.

[41] Ltr, Surgs Br NYPE to Port Surg NYPE, 12 Jul 43, sub: SOP of Trans and Evac Off, with inds. HD: 370.05.

[42] (1) Ltr, Surg CPE to CofT, 19 Nov 42, sub: Overseas Evac Plans. SG: 705.-1. (2) An Rpt, 1943, Med Dept CPE. HD.

[43] (1) Mins. Conf on Evac of Mil Pers, 26 Oct 42. TC: 370.05. (2) Ltr, Surg NYPE to Col H. D. Offutt, SGO, 12 Nov 42, with incls. SG: 705 (NYPE). (3) Memo for Record, on 1st ind SPOPH 370.05 (11-24-42) Hosp and Evac Br SOS to CofT, 26 Nov 42, on unknown basic Ltr. HD: 705 (MRO, Fitzpatrick Daybook, Aug 42-Jun 43).

such instances ports actually controlled the movement to hospitals of only small numbers of patients, while they continued to be responsible for the larger groups moved in service command vehicles by service command personnel.

Early in 1944 this procedure was changed. To provide a clear-cut line of demarcation between responsibilities of ports and service commands and to simplify operations by having only one agency furnish vehicles and personnel for transportation from ports to hospitals, the Second Service Command proposed, and the commanding general of the Service Forces approved, a change in the transfer point.[44] After 11 April 1944 it was normally at shipside rather than in trains or hospitals.[45] In the case of New York this proved advantageous. The Second Service Command controlled a number of nearby medical installations upon which it could call for ambulances and personnel to move large shipments of patients to Halloran and Mason General Hospitals. In other instances this change introduced the very situation it was designed to correct. The Ninth Service Command, for example, had to call upon the San Francisco Port for twenty buses each capable of carrying thirty-seven ambulatory patients to assist in transporting patients from docks to the Letterman General Hospital. In any event the removal of patients from ships to debarkation hospitals required close co-operation between port and service command officials.[46]

For the transportation of patients from docks to hospitals, service commands used ambulances, buses, and trains, depending upon the physical condition of patients and the distances to be traveled. The Second Service Command, for example, transferred patients from piers located in Brooklyn, Staten Island, New Jersey, and the North River to service command debarkation hospitals by ambulance, government bus, commercial bus, and hospital train. During 1944 this Command called upon as many as twenty of its installations to supply vehicles and personnel for such movements. In a single day, it reported, more than 200 ambulances and 55 buses were used to move 3,000 patients received in one convoy. The First Service Command normally used trains to move patients from ships in the Boston harbor to Camp Edwards and Camp Myles Standish hospitals. The Fourth Service Command used motor vehicles almost exclusively to transport patients from the Charleston port to Stark General Hospital. In the Ninth Service Command patients were transported from the San Francisco port to Letterman General Hospital in buses and ambulances, but they were moved from the Seattle port to Madigan General Hospital in small groups by ambulance and in large groups by rail.[47]

Ports continued to be responsible for debarking patients from ships. Normally they used their own men, including specially trained port and sanitary companies, as litter bearers, but in some instances they

[44] (1) Rpt, Conf CGs of SvCs, Dallas, Tex, 17–19 Feb 44. HD: 337. (2) Memo, CG ASF (Control Div) for CofSA thru SG and CofT, 26 Feb 44, sub: Control of Med Serv at PE, with 3 inds. SG: 705. (3) Rpt, Conf to Discuss Proposed Changes in AR 170–10 and Cir 316, 6 Mar 44. SG: 337.-1. (4) Memo, Opns Div ASF for Planning Div ASF, 10 Mar 44, sub: Evac of Returning Casualties from Ports. TC: 370.05 (Evac of Pnts).

[45] ASF Cir 99, sec IV, pt 2, 11 Apr 44.

[46] An Rpts, 1944, Letterman Gen Hosp; NYPE; and 1st, 2d, 4th, and 9th SvCs. HD.

[47] An Rpts from SvCs, Ports, and Gen Hosp (Halloran, Hammond, LaGarde, Letterman, Lovell, Madigan, McGuire, Stark) and Sta Hosps (Cp Edwards, Cp Myles Standish) for 1944 and 1945 explain debarkation procedures and reception of patients by hospitals. HD.

still borrowed enlisted men from service command hospitals. To save personnel and speed operations the Boston Port used wheeled litters to move patients on its piers. Ports differed in the order in which they unloaded patients. Some unloaded mental patients first, and then ambulatory patients. Others reversed this order. Usually litter patients were debarked last because such preparations as transferring them to litters could be made while other patients were being debarked. As ports gained experience in operations and improved procedures, the time required to unload ships decreased. For example, the Charleston Port cut the time from five hours at the beginning of 1944 to two hours by the end of 1944 and then to one hour for a 600-patient hospital ship during 1945. The Boston Port reported that on one occasion in 1945 as many as 1,958 patients, among them 287 litter cases, were moved from a transport to near-by trains in two hours and twenty minutes.[48]

The manner in which general hospitals received evacuees differed from one to another. In May 1943 The Surgeon General directed hospitals receiving large numbers of patients from either ships or trains to admit them directly to wards, without "processing" them through hospital receiving offices. The reason was to avoid delays in giving patients needed food, rest, and treatment. Halloran General Hospital had developed a different system, and on request of the hospital and the Second Service Command, The Surgeon General approved its continued use. There, a receiving ward had been established to care for a large number of patients. It contained a mess hall for the prompt feeding of patients, space for the medical inspection of patients and for the care of those needing immediate medical treatment, bathing facilities, and a clothing room in which patients received fresh hospital clothes and stored their own clothing. There was also space for a battery of typists brought in to complete all of the paper work required for the admission of patients. The average length of time patients stayed in this building, before being admitted to wards, was reported to be 61 minutes.[49]

With the growth of the evacuee load in 1944 and 1945 debarkation hospitals had to transfer evacuees to other hospitals as rapidly as possible—normally within seventy-two hours—so as to keep enough beds vacant for large groups of new patients arriving in quick succession. With such a short period of time the medical and surgical care afforded evacuees had to be limited. They were given necessary medications and their dressings were changed, while a brief examination served to check the accuracy of the diagnosis carried in medical records and to determine their ability to undertake further travel. Primary emphasis was upon administrative matters. Records required for use in debarkation hospitals had to be prepared; reports of patients received had to be made to Washington; orders for their transfer to other hospitals had to be issued; patients had to be outfitted with complete

[48] (1) Files SG: 705 (ports or debarkation hospitals) contain correspondence dealing with debarkation difficulties and operational procedures; for example, Memo, CG 4th SvC for CG ASF, 13 Jun 44, sub: Evac of Overseas Casualties at Stark Gen Hosp. SG: 705 (Stark GH). (2) History of Stark General Hospital, Charleston, S. C., 1941–45. HD. (3) An Rpts, Boston, Charleston, Hampton Roads, New Orleans, New York, San Francisco, and Seattle PEs, 1944, 1945. HD.

[49] Ltr, Halloran Gen Hosp to SG, 19 May 43, sub: Admission of Pnts when Arriving in Convoy. SG: 705.1 (Halloran GH). (2) An Rpt, Halloran Gen Hosp, 1943. HD.

uniforms and given partial payments;[50] and arrangements had to be made for their transportation. The paper work thus required was voluminous. Beginning in the latter part of 1944 attempts were made to simplify it. Concurrently, it will be recalled, the Surgeon General's Office was engaged in a more general project to standardize and simplify administrative procedures in all hospitals. Changes that were made in debarkation procedures were of two types. In June 1944 the Control Divisions of Stark General Hospital and the Fourth Service Command proposed the elimination of records required for patients admitted to hospitals for definitive treatment but not needed for those in transit and the simplification of entries in other records. As a result, evacuees were not admitted to the registers of debarkation hospitals and their names were not entered on admission and disposition sheets. In addition, standard rubber stamp entries were authorized for use in patients' service and field medical records.[51] During the winter of 1944–45 another measure toward simplifying the work of debarkation hospitals was adopted: the installation of addressograph equipment. With this equipment hospitals prepared plates for use in making rosters and in issuing orders and thus eliminated the necessity of typing each separately.[52] Though seemingly small when considered individually, the significance of such measures can be judged more accurately if the total evacuation load of different hospitals is taken into account. Stark General Hospital, for example, admitted 44,003 patients in the nine-month period from 1 January 1945 to 30 September 1945, while Halloran admitted about 69,500 and Letterman about 73,000 during the entire year.[53]

[50] That is, partial payments of the pay and allowances due service men, made by the Army pending full settlement of their accounts.

[51] (1) Memo, CofT (Mvmt Div by Lt Col J. C. Fitzpatrick) for SG (Hosp Div), 23 May 44. TC: 370.05. (2) Memo, CG 4th SvC for CG ASF (Control Div), 13 Jun 44, sub: Evac of Overseas Casualties at Stark Gen Hosp, with inds. SG: 705 (Stark GH).

[52] (1) Memo, SG (Control Div) for QMG, 30 Aug 44, sub: Use of Addressograph and Embossing Equip in Debarkation Hosps. SG: 413.51. (2) Ltr, SG to CG 2d SvC, 20 Dec 44, sub: Admitting Off Procedure for Pnts Retd from Overseas. SG: 705 (2d SvC). (3) Memo, Hosp Div SGO for HD SGO, 18 Jun 45, sub: Add Mat for An Rpt for FY 1945. HD: 319.1-2. (4) Memo, NP Cons Div SGO for Hosp Div SGO, 14 May 45, sub: Procedure of Pnts Recd from Overseas thru Stark Gen Hosp. SG: 705 (Stark GH).

[53] An Rpts, Stark, Halloran, and Letterman Gen Hosps, 1945. HD.

CHAPTER XXI

Movement of Patients in the United States

The movement of patients in the United States, although fairly simple early in the war when it involved only the transfer of individuals or small groups from station to general hospitals, began to assume different characteristics about the middle of 1943. A steady increase in the number of evacuees received from theaters—from about 3,000 per month early in 1943 to a peak of more than 57,000 in May 1945—focused attention on the transportation of patients from debarkation to general hospitals. Meanwhile declining troop strength in the United States, along with establishment of regional hospitals to serve in lieu of general hospitals for patients from camps in surrounding areas, reduced to a trickle the transfer of zone of interior patients to general hospitals. Growth of the Army's fleet of hospital cars from 24 early in 1943 to 380 by the end of the war, along with a shortage of commercial sleepers and diners, meant that emphasis shifted from the transportation of patients on regular passenger trains to their movement on Army hospital trains. A change in Air Force policy in the spring of 1944, permitting certain planes to be assigned primarily to evacuation operations in the United States, resulted in a transition from sporadic to regular movement of patients by air. Finally, compliance with the policy established early in 1943 of transferring patients from debarkation hospitals to hospitals designated as specialized centers and located as near as possible to patients' homes complicated the problem of planning their transportation.

Regulating the Flow of Patients

Although The Surgeon General was designated by Army directives as the chief medical "regulator," in the early part of the war he exercised only a general influence over the distribution of patients among Army hospitals. His office granted ports unlimited bed credits in general hospitals located nearest them. Port commanders then transferred patients to such hospitals, reporting later to the Surgeon General's Office the number received from theaters, the date of their arrival, and the name of the hospital to which they had been transferred.[1] Station hospitals transferred patients to general hospitals in which they held bed credits. General hos-

[1] (1) WD Cir 120, 21 Jun 41. (2) An Rpt, 1943, NYPE, HD. (3) Ltr, SG to CG HRPE, 14 Aug 42, sub: Rpt of Pnts Arriving from Overseas. SG: 705.-1 (HRPE).

pitals normally did not hold bed credits in other general hospitals and hence had to request the Surgeon General's Office to authorize transfers and to designate receiving hospitals. In order to know which had vacant beds, The Surgeon General began in April 1943 to require all general hospitals to submit daily bed status reports to his Office.[2] When general hospitals requested the transfer of patients to other such hospitals in order to free beds for subsequent arrivals from near-by ports, his Office authorized the transfer of groups, sometimes as large as 250. Decisions as to particular patients to be transferred were left to hospital commanders. Normally, then, in the first part of the war the Surgeon General's Office authorized the transfer of patients in bulk and depended upon local commanders to request individual transfers to comply with the policy of hospitalizing patients near their homes and in specialized centers.[3]

Later in the war, as the movement of patients in the United States increased and grew more complex, a new procedure was developed to give the Surgeon General's Office greater control over the transfer of individual patients. It involved reports to the Medical Regulating Unit of patients received at debarkation hospitals and of vacant beds in general and convalescent hospitals. In May 1944 the Medical Regulating Officer established a system for debarkation hospitals to use in requesting the transfer of patients to other hospitals. Instead of asking for authority to transfer a certain number of patients without regard to disabilities or home locations, debarkation hospitals reported in coded teletype messages the geographical destination (home), diagnosis or special disability, sex and military status, and general physical condition (litter or ambulatory) of each patient received. For example, one male enlisted neurosurgical patient whose home was in Florida was reported as "6NCY"; ten such patients, as "6NCY10." In August 1944 this system was revised, and additional medical classifications or diagnoses were listed, along with more exact definitions of each. About the same time, the system of daily bed status reports was changed. In the fall of 1943 a code had been established for hospitals to use in reporting vacant beds. In August 1944 this code was modified so that hospitals reported vacant beds not in such general categories as medicine, surgery, and neuropsychiatry but in terms of the particular diseases or injuries for which they had been designated as specialized centers. For example, hospitals with vacant beds for male neurosurgical patients reported them under code "12TVKN." Early in 1945 both debarkation and bed status reports were further revised to reflect changes in specialty designations of hospitals and thereby to permit a greater degree of accuracy in sending patients to proper hospitals. Using both reports together, the Medical Regulating Unit was able to direct debarkation hospitals to transfer patients, in small groups or as individuals if necessary, to general hospitals that specialized in the diseases or injuries with which they suf-

[2] (1) AR 40-600, 6 Oct 42. (2) Ltr, SG to CO Billings Gen Hosp, 26 Apr 43, sub: Daily Bed Rpt. SG: 632.2 (Billings GH). By July 1943 the Hospitalization and Evacuation Division, SGO, was receiving daily reports from 28 hospitals, giving number of patients, number of medical, surgical, and neuropsychiatric beds, and number of patients transferred to and received from other general hospitals.

[3] Telegrams in which the Surgeon General's Office authorized the transfer of patients are filed in SG: 704.-1 and 705.-1. See also weekly diaries of the Hospital Administration Division. HD.

fered and that were located as near as practical to their home addresses.[4]

At first this system applied only to patients being transferred from debarkation hospitals to general hospitals of definitive treatment, but gradually it was extended to cover even the transfer of patients from station and regional hospitals to general hospitals. Because of crowded conditions of general hospitals in the populous northeastern part of the United States, in July 1944 The Surgeon General directed that no patients should be transferred to certain hospitals in that area without prior approval of the ASF Medical Regulating Officer. In effect, this directive canceled all bed credits which station or regional hospitals held in the hospitals listed. About two months later additional hospitals were placed in this category, raising the number thus restricted from thirteen to thirty-one. Ultimately, early in 1945 the system that originated as a means of authorizing the transfer of evacuees from debarkation to general and convalescent hospitals was formally extended to include all transfers to such hospitals.[5] The degree of control which the Medical Regulating Officer thus achieved over the use of beds in general and convalescent hospitals enabled him to authorize transfers of patients promptly and to use beds effectively when they were at a premium in the first half of 1945.

Centralized control over the transfer of patients to general and convalescent hospitals did not assure that policies on the hospitalization of patients near their homes and in specialized centers would be wholly complied with. Hospital beds in the United States were not distributed in proportion to density of population. Hence, early in 1945 when the patient load became great enough to fill general and convalescent hospitals, it was impossible for the Medical Regulating Officer to send all patients to hospitals located near their homes. Furthermore, the necessity of sending patients to specialized centers sometimes conflicted with and outweighed the desirability of sending them to hospitals near their homes. Finally, debarkation hospitals had time for little more than superficial examinations of patients before requesting their transfer to other hospitals. As a result, the medical classifications reported by debarkation hospitals were sometimes incorrect and patients were sent to general hospitals when they should have been sent to convalescent hospitals.[6]

Some idea of the complexity of the process of authorizing patient-transfers may be gained from the work load of the ASF Medical Regulating Unit. In the early part of 1945 it received bed status reports from 64 general, 12 convalescent, and 7 temporary debarkation hospitals. Information from these reports was posted daily to show at all times the ability of hospitals to accept patients. Each day the Unit received approximately 100 telegrams, 10 letters, and 25 telephone calls requesting the transfer of patients in small groups or as individuals. Every month it received in addition fifty to sixty coded

[4] (1) History . . . Medical Regulating Service. . . . (2) ASF Cirs 149, 20 May 44; 284, 30 Aug 44; 249, 4 Aug 44; and 89, 10 Mar 45. (3) Ltr, CG ASF (SG) to CO Billings Gen Hosp, 15 Oct 43, sub: Daily Bed Rpt. SG: 632.-2 (Billings GH)K. Identical letters were sent to other general hospitals. Telegrams and correspondence on bed capacities and patient transfers are filed in HD: 705 (MRO Staybacks), 705 (MRO Chart on Pnt Capacities in Hosps), and 705 (MRO Daily Diaries, Daily Bed Status).

[5] Telg SPMDD-DR, SG (MRO) to all SvCs, 3 Jul 44, 17 Sep 44, 21 May 45, 6 Sep 45. HD: 705 (Med Reg Unit book).

[6] See above, pp. 211-12, 240-41.

telegrams from debarkation hospitals requesting the transfer of patients to general hospitals; the typical request covered 500 patients who had to be transferred because of their diagnoses, home addresses, sex, and military status to an average of forty-five different hospitals.[7]

Procedures for Rail Evacuation

The principal method of moving patients in the United States—other than by ambulance—was by train—either regular passenger trains or hospital trains made up of Army hospital cars supplemented by commercial equipment. During most of 1942 patients were moved almost exclusively in Pullman cars of passenger trains, because the necessity of transporting large groups was practically nonexistent and the Army had only six hospital cars. For groups of patients and attendants numbering fewer than fifty, local transportation officers arranged with railroads for cars and routings. For larger groups, the Office of the Chief of Transportation made necessary arrangements, upon request of local transportation officers.[8]

Toward the end of the summer of 1942, SOS headquarters, the Chief of Transportation, and The Surgeon General began to plan for the operation of hospital trains. By that time the delivery of additional hospital cars—enough to serve as the nuclei of eight hospital trains—was expected, and an increase in the number of evacuees was impending. Since several agencies were involved, delineation of their responsibilities for the control and operation of hospital cars was complicated. Although hospital cars were procured by the Transportation Corps and used by the Medical Department, SOS headquarters decided with the approval of both The Surgeon General and the Chief of Transportation that they should be "attached" to (i.e., placed under the jurisdiction of) service commands. A service command hospital was being constructed near each port which lacked one, and it was anticipated that patients debarked at ports would be transported by motor vehicles to such hospitals and there turned over to service command control. Hence, ports would have no need for hospital cars. In addition, it was thought that service commands could furnish personnel and medical supplies for hospital trains more easily than could ports. Experience had already shown that service commands where ports were located would need hospital cars most, because general hospitals in such commands would receive large numbers of patients for transfer to hospitals further inland. Plans were therefore made to attach six hospital cars each to the Second, Fourth, and Ninth Service Commands, four to the Eighth, and two to the Sixth (for use in evacuating patients from areas in Canada), and service commands were directed to furnish supplies and medical attendants for hospital trains. Any of the hospital cars could be attached to or detached from service commands by the Chief of Transportation. Either one unit car and two ward cars, or one ward dressing car and two ward cars, were to form the nucleus of a hospital train. Supplemental Pullmans, diners, and other

[7] Memo, Dirs Hosp and Resources Anal Divs SGO for Dir HD SGO, 18 Jun 45, sub: Add Mat for An Rpt for FY 1945. HD: 319.1–2.

[8] (1) Memo, CofT for SG, 28 Mar 42, sub: Basic Plan for Evac of Sick and Wounded. HD: 705. (2) AR 30–925, C 2, 22 Aug 42. (3) WD Cir 192, 16 Jun 42. (4) Ltr SPOPH 322.15, CG SOS to CGs and COs of SvCs and PEs, and to SG, 15 Sep 42, sub: Mil Hosp and Evac Oprs, with incl. HD: 705.

rail equipment were to be used to complete it.[9]

After the decision to attach hospital cars to service commands was made, SOS headquarters issued directives establishing procedures for their use. The directives conflicted with one another and with Army regulations governing the transportation of personnel in general. As already noted, War Department regulations permitted local transportation officers to arrange with railroads for the transportation of groups of persons numbering less than fifty (after June 1943 less than forty), but provided that the Chief of Transportation would arrange for the transportation of all larger groups. This meant arranging with railroads for carrier-owned equipment and for routes and schedules.[10] On the other hand, SOS directives provided that local transportation officers could arrange for all routings of hospital cars within the boundaries of service commands to which they were attached. Another stated in contradiction that except in emergencies service commands would ask the Chief of Transportation for routing instructions to cover the movement of each hospital car. Two SOS directives stated that service command transportation officers would arrange with railroads for all supplemental rail equipment, while another limited them to arrangements for supplemental equipment needed when hospital cars were moved within service command boundaries. None of the SOS directives took account of Army regulations requiring the Chief of Transportation to arrange for equipment and routings for the movement of large groups.[11] Such conflicting instructions caused confusion about which both the Office of the Chief of Transportation and service commands complained.[12]

The feasibility of attaching cars to service commands and then attempting to divide authority for controlling their use was questioned in the winter of 1942 and again in the spring of 1943. The commanding general of the Eighth Service Command believed that hospital cars would be used most in the transportation of patients arriving from theaters of operations and proposed, therefore, that they should be controlled exclusively by the Transportation Corps and operated by ports.[13] The Chief of Transportation considered this possibility, but agreed with the SOS Hospitalization and Evacuation Branch to follow plans already made. Nevertheless, in preparation for the reception of casualties from the North African invasion, all hospital cars were temporarily transferred to the New York and Hampton Roads Ports and placed under their jurisdiction.[14] In December 1942 both the Chief of Transportation and the Hospitalization and Evacuation Branch agreed that they should be returned to

[9] (1) Memos, CG SOS for CGs 2d, 4th, 6th, 8th, and 9th SvCs, CofT, and SG, 18 and 26 Aug 42, sub: Location and Control of Hosp Tns. AG: 531.4. (2) Ltr, CofT to CGs PEs and SvCs, 9 Sep 42, sub: Control of Hosp Tns. TC: 531.4. For a discussion of different types of Army-owned hospital cars, see below, pp. 372–75, 381–83.

[10] (1) WD Cir 192, 16 Jun 42. (2) AR 55–130, 28 Dec 42, with C 2, 4 Jun 43.

[11] (1) Memos cited n. 9(1). (2) Ltr cited n. 8(4).

[12] (1) Ltr, CG Ft Sam Houston to CG NYPE, 27 Sep 42, sub: Control of Hosp Tns, with inds. HD: Wilson files, 531.4. (2) 3d ind, CG SOS to CG SFPE thru CG 9th SvC, 3 Nov 42, on telg (n d) from CG 9th SvC. AG: 322.38. (3) Memo, Tank Car Br OCT for Col William J. Williamson, OCT, 16 Nov 42, sub: Opr of Hosp Tn Cars. TC: 531.4.

[13] Rpt, Conf of CGs SvCs, New Orleans, La., 17 Dec 42. HD: 337.

[14] (1) Ltr, CG SOS to TAG, 31 Oct 42, sub: Hosp and Evac for Special Opr. TC: 531.4. (2) Memo, CG SOS for SG and CofT, 1 Nov 42, same sub. HRS: ASF Planning Div file, "Hosp and Evac No 15."

service commands.[15] In the spring of 1943, when plans were being made to receive ninety-six hospital cars ordered earlier, a representative of The Surgeon General suggested that it would be advantageous eventually, when large numbers of patients began to arrive from theaters of operations, to have service commands supply personnel for hospital trains but to place all hospital cars in pools under the exclusive control of the Chief of Transportation. Presumably such an arrangement would have promoted the more efficient use of cars, but the Transportation Corps preferred to continue the system of attaching cars to service commands in which ports were located, and The Surgeon General's representative concurred in plans for the allocations of 45 cars to the Second, 24 to the Third, and 27 to the Ninth Service Commands.[16]

Later in the war, when a shortage of carrier-owned equipment combined with a steadily increasing evacuation load to require the greatest possible use of Army hospital cars, centralized control was adopted, along with other measures, to achieve that goal. By the winter of 1943–44 it was widely recognized that maximum use was not being made of hospital cars. In many instances they returned empty to home stations after delivering patients to general hospitals. In others, service commands permitted hospital cars to stand idle while they arranged for carrier-owned equipment to transport patients. In February 1944 the Surgeon General's Office pointed to this situation and suggested again that better use could be achieved by centralizing control of hospital cars in the Office of the Chief of Transportation.[17]

Before this step was finally taken, a movement already begun to achieve closer co-operation between the Transportation Corps and the Medical Department had to be completed. Late in 1943 the Evacuation Branch of the Surgeon General's Office had agreed to supply the Office of the Chief of Transportation with copies of all messages authorizing general and debarkation hospitals to transfer patients to other hospitals, enabling the latter to anticipate requests from service commands for rail equipment. A short time later the Chief of Transportation established an evacuation unit in his Traffic Control Division. It collaborated with the Surgeon General's Office and service commands in planning rail movements, and for this purpose kept a current record of the location and use of each hospital car. In May 1944 the transfer (already mentioned) of the Surgeon General's Evacuation Branch to the Medical Regulating Unit, which was physically located in the Office of the Chief of Transportation, enabled medical officers who authorized the transfer of patients from debarkation to other hospitals to consult at all times with transportation officers as to the availability of Army hospital cars and carrier-owned equipment. Conversely, transportation officers had readily available information as to the lo-

[15] (1) Ltr, CofT to CGs NYPE and HRPE, 10 Dec 42, sub: Hosp Cars. TC: 531.4. (2) Diary, Hosp and Evac Br SOS, 22–23 Dec 42. HD: Wilson files, "Diary." (3) Memo, ACofT for CofT, 22 Dec 42, sub: Asgmt of Hosp Tn Cars. TC: 531.4.

[16] (1) Memos, Mtg, Off Chief Rail Div OCT, 22 Apr and 18 May 43. SG: 453.–1. (2) Ltr, CG ASF to CGs 2d, 3d, and 9th SvCs, 22 May 43, sub: Location of Add Hosp Cars. TC: 531.4. (3) Memo, Mvmt Div OCT for ACofT, 2 Jul 43, sub: Mtg of SvC Comdrs. Same file.

[17] (1) Memo for Record, on 3d ind, CG ASF to CofT, 10 Sep 43, on unknown basic ltr. HD: Wilson files, "Day File." (2) Ltr, Dir Hosp Admin Div SGO to Surg 9th SvC, 4 Dec 43. SG: 705.–1 (9th SvC)AA. (3) Hosp and Evac: Re-estimate of Pnt Load and Facs, pp. 25–26. HD: 705.–1. (4) Rpt, Conf CGs of SvCs, Dallas, Tex, 17–19 Feb 44. HD: 337.

cation, destination, number, and types of patients to be moved by rail.[18]

As the offices of The Surgeon General and the Chief of Transportation developed closer co-operation in planning the movement of patients by rail, measures were adopted to centralize the control of hospital cars. At the end of 1943, SOS directives that had caused confusion by attempting to divide responsibility for their use between service commands and the Office of the Chief of Transportation were superseded by a War Department circular which agreed in its provisions with general transportation regulations. The routing, including scheduling for train connections, of all hospital cars—whether empty or loaded and whether moving within or beyond service command boundaries—was centralized in the Office of the Chief of Transportation. Moreover, local transportation officers were specifically limited in the arrangements which they could make for supplemental rail equipment to instances when fewer than forty persons were to be carried on hospital trains. When larger groups were moved the Office of the Chief of Transportation alone could make all arrangements. For several months this Office was indulgent, accepting generally the recommendations of service commands as to dates of hospital train movements and the make-up (that is, the combination of Army-owned with carrier-owned cars) of hospital trains. Later, in the spring of 1944, it began to exercise its authority to arrange without consultation with service commands for the rail transportation of groups of patients numbering forty or more. Informed by the Medical Regulating Unit of the patients to be moved and of their destinations, the Traffic Control Division determined the make-up of hospital trains and set the dates of their departure. Upon the recommendation of the Medical Regulating Officer it diverted hospital cars to places where they were needed, informing service commands to which they were attached only if this action delayed their return to home stations for more than ten (later five) days. This meant, for example, that a car attached to the Second Service Command, carrying patients to a hospital in the Fifth Service Command, might be loaded with other patients at the latter place and diverted to a destination in the Fourth Service Command before being returned to its home station.[19]

Further centralization in rail evacuation operations and more extensive use of hospital cars was achieved during 1945 when the size of groups for which service commands might independently arrange commercial transportation was reduced from a maximum of thirty-nine to fourteen. As long as service commands could arrange for the movement of groups of patients that were large enough to warrant the addition of a special tourist or sleeping car to a regularly scheduled train (that is, any group of fifteen or more persons), it was possible for such a car to be procured to move patients along a route

[18] (1) Memo, CofT for SG, 23 Oct 43, sub: Opr of Hosp Tn Cars. SG: 453.-1. (2) Memo, Maj Samuel N. Farley, TC, for Lt Col I. Sewell Morris, TC, 27 Oct 43, sub: Conf in SGO re Better Util of Govt-Owned Hosp Cars. Off file, Hosp Evac Unit, OCT. (3) Memo, Same for Same, 17 Jan 44, sub: Functions of the Hosp Evac Unit. Same file.

[19] (1) Interv, MD Historian with Samuel N. Farley, 9 Oct 52. HD: 000.71. (2) WD Cir 316, 6 Dec 43. (3) ASF Cir 147, 19 May 44. (4) Memo, Lt Col John C. Fitzpatrick for Gen [Raymond W.] Bliss, 23 May 44, sub: Util of Hosp Tns. HD: 705 (MRO, Fitzpatrick Stayback, 1334). (5) Memo, SG for Fiscal Dir ASF, 26 Jul 44. SG: 322 (Hosp Tns). (6) ASF Cir 328, 30 Sep 44. (7) Transcript of Proceedings, Hosp Tn Conf, 15–16 Feb 45. HD: 531.4.

over which an Army hospital car—under orders of the Office of the Chief of Transportation—was traveling empty at approximately the same time. The Chief of Transportation therefore recommended in May 1945 that arrangements for the movement of all groups of patients and attendants numbering fifteen or more persons should be centralized in his Office. This recommendation was approved and in June 1945 local transportation officers were limited to making arrangements for the movement of individuals and of groups of patients and attendants numbering fourteen or less. Knowing the locations and routes of all Army hospital cars, the Chief of Transportation could then arrange to use them in moving some of the groups which service commands had formerly dispatched in extra sleeping and tourist cars of regularly scheduled passenger trains.[20]

Despite the fact that centralized control of hospital cars and hospital train movements was not wholly approved by service commands, the Surgeon General's Office considered such control essential. One service command surgeon felt that his lack of control over the personnel on hospital cars from other commands jeopardized the loading and care en route of patients whom he was transferring. A local transportation officer in another service command believed that he could expedite the movement of patients from the debarkation hospital which he served if he were permitted to arrange rail movements independently. Still another service command complained of the use elsewhere of personnel which it supplied to care for patients being transported from its own debarkation hospital. Other objections arose from the difficulty service commands encountered in property and mess management on hospital cars attached to them but diverted elsewhere for use. In reply to such complaints, The Surgeon General repeatedly explained that centralized control of the movement of hospital cars and hospital trains was necessary to insure the maximum use of all available rail equipment, both Army- and carrier-owned, in the orderly transportation of large numbers of patients.[21]

Measures other than centralization of control were adopted to achieve better use of hospital cars, conserve medical personnel, and relieve railroads of furnishing more sleeping cars. In June 1944 the Transportation Corps requested carriers to return hospital cars in passenger rather than in freight service. In this way hospital cars that had to be moved without patients spent less time idle than they might have otherwise.[22] By the early part of 1945 the Transportation Corps itself began to arrange hospital-car routes and schedules, without reference to railroad representatives. Though this procedure was a departure from the Army's agreement with the railroads, the latter apparently inter-

[20] (1) Memo, CofT for ACofS G-4 WDGS, 16 May 45, sub: Routing Control and Carriers' Equip for Mvmt of Pnts and/or Med Attendants in Groups of 15 or More. . . . TC: 511 (AR 55-130). (2) WD Cir 177, 15 Jun 45.

[21] (1) Ltr, Surg 2d SvC to Brig Gen Raymond W. Bliss, SGO, 3 Feb 44. SG: 531.2 (2d SvC)AA. (2) Diary, Evac Br MRU Oprs Serv SGO, 20 Jun 44. HD: 024.7-3. (3) Ltr, CG Letterman Gen Hosp to Lt Col John C. Fitzpatrick, MRO, 14 Nov 44. HD: 705 (MRO, Maloney Stayback, 127). (4) Memo cited n. 19(4). (5) Ltr, MRO to CG Letterman Gen Hosp, 21 Nov 44. SG: 705.1 (Letterman GH). (6) Ltr, Dep Chief for Hosp and Domestic Oprs, Oprs Serv SGO to Surg 2d SvC, ca. 28 Dec 44. SG: 531.2 (2d SvC)AA. (7) Memo, Maj Frederick H. Gibbs, MAC, for Surg 4th SvC, 29 Jan 45, sub: Hosp Tn Serv, Stark Gen Hosp, with 2 inds. SG: 453 (Stark GH)K.

[22] Ltr, Lt Col I. Sewell Morris, TC, to A. H. Gass, Mil Trans Sec AAR, 6 Jun 44, with reply dated 8 Jun 44. TC: 531.4.

posed no objection. Its chief advantage was that hospital cars could be sent along unauthorized routes (those not normally used by railroad companies) to reduce mileage and to deliver groups of patients at different hospitals. The higher cost which railroads charged for such movements was considered by the Surgeon General's Office to be fully justified by the ends achieved.[23]

In addition to the larger problem of using hospital cars to the best advantage, others were encountered in the operation of hospital trains. One of them, feeding patients on hospital trains, was partially solved by the procurement of Army hospital kitchen cars and the installation of buffet-kitchens in other hospital cars.[24] To govern the procurement of food for these cars, along with the bookkeeping procedures involved, the ASF Control Division, the Surgeon General's Office, and the Office of The Quartermaster General collaborated in the preparation of a standard subsistence procedure for hospital trains in the last part of 1944.[25] Other problems arose in accounting for hospital cars and their equipment, and in their maintenance. In September 1944 a circular governing accounting procedures was published by ASF headquarters, while some months earlier the Transportation Corps prepared technical bulletins on the maintenance of hospital cars.[26] Another problem involved the position of hospital cars in trains. In the winter of 1943–44 the Transportation Corps requested carriers to place hospital cars on regular passenger trains in such a position that the public would not have to use them as passageways. Carriers agreed to place them either directly ahead of or directly behind other passenger cars in the same train. Furthermore the carriers agreed, upon the request of the Chief of Transportation and the recommendation of The Surgeon General, to place "buffer" cars (cars in which no patients were carried) between hospital cars and locomotives when special hospital trains were made up.[27] The carriers also co-operated in observing a request of The Surgeon General that patients be transported only in air-conditioned cars. By Army regulations and an agreement with railroads, patients were authorized "sleeping car accommodations in tourist sleeping cars if available, otherwise standard sleeping cars." Of the entire fleet of Pullman tourist cars, only four hundred were air-conditioned, and it was therefore impossible for carriers always to supply air-conditioned tourist cars when they were requested. For a time during 1944 they supplied higher-priced air-conditioned standard sleeping cars without any increase in cost, but in December of that year they revised an earlier agreement

[23] (1) Memo, CofT for SG (MRO), 14 Feb 45, sub: Routing of Hosp Tn Travel, with inds. SG: 531.4. (2) Ltr, Lt Col E. B. White, TC, to Interterritorial Mil Cmtee, 9 Mar 45. TC: 531.4. After the war ended, in November and December 1945, the Army and Navy agreed upon a procedure for the joint use of Army hospital cars in the United States. This agreement contributed to the conservation of carrier-owned equipment and still greater use of Army-owned hospital cars. ASF Cir 441, 11 Dec 45.

[24] See below, pp. 381–86.

[25] WD Cir 480, 22 Dec 44. Also see WD Cir 184, 21 Jun 45.

[26] (1) ASF Cirs 286, 1 Sep 44; 401, 9 Dec 44. (2) TB 55-285-1, 24 Jul 44; TB 55-285-2, 24 Aug 44, on Echelon Maintenance for Hosp and Kitchen Cars. A complete manual for operation of the new unit cars (TM 55-1254, 15 Dec 45, Car, Railway, Hospital Unit) was issued after the end of the war.

[27] (1) Ltr, Hosp Tn Comdr to CG 2d SvC, 21 Oct 43, sub: Trans Rpt of Hosp Tn Mvmt HT-69, Main 57616, 14-19 Oct 43, with inds. SG: 453.-1. (2) Ltr, CofT (Tfc Control Div) to AAR, 24 Jan 44. TC: 531.4 (Placement of Hosp Cars on Regular Tn). (3) Ltr, SG to SvCs, 2 Dec 44, sub: Use of Buffer Cars in Connection with Mvmt of Pnts by Rail. SG: 453 (SvCs).

with the Army to provide special rates for standard sleeping car equipment.[28]

The problems just reviewed are representative only, in no way intended to be an exhaustive listing, of those encountered by authorities on a higher level than hospital train commanders. These commanders were faced with other problems which were perhaps even more varied and complex. Solutions for most of them had to be found locally, for there was no War Department manual on hospital train operations. During 1945 a series of conferences of hospital train commanders, attended by representatives of The Surgeon General and the Chief of Transportation, were held to discuss such common questions as linen exchange procedures, feeding difficulties, the handling of baggage, entraining and detraining plans, personnel and equipment requirements, means of providing recreation aboard trains, and problems of hospital car maintenance and operation.[29]

Some idea of the scope of hospital train operations may be gained from the following figures. During 1944, 172 hospital trains carrying 37,371 patients were dispatched from the Second Service Command to general and convalescent hospitals scattered throughout the United States. During the period from 26 June 1944 to 15 October 1945, 205 hospital trains evacuated 35,697 ambulatory patients and 17,320 litter patients from Stark General Hospital. From January to August 1945, inclusive, the hospital train detachment of the First Service Command made 232 trips to 1,334 destinations, covering 48,888 miles and moving 67,608 patients. Between July 1944 and December 1945, the Ninth Service Command moved 56,061 patients in hospital cars and 29,439 in Pullmans.[30]

Despite the widespread use of centrally controlled hospital trains, service commands retained throughout the war the authority to arrange with common carriers for the movement of patients as individuals or in small groups. The main difficulty they encountered was in securing accommodations for them in sleeping or parlor cars occupied also by civilians. In November 1943 the ASF Control Division investigated complaints of hospitals about delays in getting reservations for patients and found that they were justified. The average period that elapsed between the time transportation was requested and was made available for 27,265 patients was 3.8 days. In some instances it ranged as high as 15.3 days. Continuation of this situation would mean not only that the treatment of patients would be delayed but also that some hospitals in time would become hopelessly overcrowded. In February 1944, therefore, ASF headquarters directed The Surgeon General, with the assistance of the Chief of Transportation and service commands, to arrange with railroads for securing promptly rail accommodations for Army patients.[31]

---

[28] (1) AR 55-125, 9 Jan 43; C 1, 4 Jun 43; C 2, 4 Aug 43. (2) Memo, CofT for SG, 22 Aug 44, sub: Accommodations in Air-Conditioned Sleeping Cars, with inds. SG: 531.2. (3) WD Cir 240, 7 Aug 45. (4) Ltr, CofT (Tfc Control Div) to GAO (Claims Div), 1 Oct 45. TC: 531.4.

[29] (1) Mins, Hosp Tn Conf, 15-16 Feb 45, Miller Fld, NY; Hosp Tn Unit Comdrs Conf, 10-13 Jul 45, Presidio of San Francisco. HD: 531.4 (Conf). (2) An Rpts, 1st, 2d, 4th, and 9th SvCs, 1944 and 45. HD. (3) Ltr, 9956 TSU Letterman Gen Hosp to SG, 22 Mar 50, sub: Ref Mat for Util of Hosp Tns. HD: 453.1.

[30] An Rpts, 1st, 2d, 4th, and 9th SvCs, 1944 and 45. HD.

[31] (1) AR 55-130, 28 Dec 42, with C 2, 4 Jun 43. (2) WD Cirs 229, 24 Sep 43; 316, 6 Dec 43. (3) History of Control Division, ASF, 1942-45, App, Project 95-2. HD.

In conferences held in Chicago and Washington during April and May 1944, representatives of The Surgeon General, the Chief of Transportation, and the Railroad Interterritorial Military Committee agreed upon procedures for obtaining reservations for individuals and for groups of fewer than fifteen persons. For this purpose, patients were divided into five classes. Class I patients were those who were acutely sick or injured and whose immediate movement to hospitals staffed and equipped to care for them was "a matter of extreme urgency." Class II patients were similar cases whose movement might be delayed safely for forty-eight hours. Class III patients were those who needed to be moved for medical reasons but whose transfer could be delayed approximately seventy-two hours; this group included patients received from theaters of operations at debarkation hospitals. Class IV patients were those being moved, not for medical reasons, but for their own convenience; their transfer might be delayed for approximately six days. Class V patients were those being discharged from the service, being returned to duty, or being sent on sick leave; their movement could be delayed about ninety-six hours. The carriers agreed to appoint special representatives for each individual railroad to assist hospital commanders in obtaining accommodations for patients of all classes within the time limits established for each. Hospital commanders were enjoined to co-operate with such representatives and, when requesting transportation for patients in either of the first two classes, were required to submit certificates attesting that transportation for Class I patients was necessary immediately and for Class II patients within forty-eight hours.[32]

The question of priorities for patients over civilians came up when this agreement was reached. Army authorities agreed with railroad representatives that establishment of such priorities would carry the unintentional implication that railroads were not "doing the job." Therefore they decided against it. In the following June, representatives of The Surgeon General, the Chief of Transportation, and railroad companies maintained a like position when the Office of Defense Transportation proposed a system of priorities. Soon afterward, however, the Interstate Commerce Commission, on the recommendation of the Office of Defense Transportation, issued an order which provided for the dispossession of passengers to obtain accommodations for patients. While this action protected railroads against unwarranted lawsuits by civilians who were displaced, the Surgeon General's Office feared that it might create unjustified hysteria on the part of the public instead of dissuading it from unnecessary travel and, at the same time, might endanger the Army's good relations with the railroads. To avoid the latter contingency, and particularly the unwarranted use of priorities by general hospitals, the Army in October 1944 revised the circular describing the voluntary agreement worked out in May. Restating that agreement, the revised version of the circular required hospital commanders to submit to railroads, along with each request for reservations, certificates attesting the classifica-

[32] (1) Memo, SG for CG ASF thru CofT, 20 Mar 44, sub: Delays in Trans of Pnts to Hosps, with inds. SG: 531.2. (2) Memo, CofT (Mvmt Br) for SG, 16 May 44, sub: Delays in Trans of Pnts to Hosps. Same file. (3) Ltr, CofT to SG, 29 Apr 44, sub: Apmt of RR Rep at US Army Gen Hosps in Arranging Accommodations for Litter and Ambulatory Cases. SG: 705. (4) Ltr, Western Mil Bu to Member RR Assn, 9 May 44, sub: Accommodations for Litter and Ambulatory Cases. SG: 531.2. (5) WD Cir 234, 12 Jun 44.

tion of each patient, those in Classes III, IV, and V as well as in Classes I and II, and indicating the period of time within which accommodations should be provided. In addition it provided that the Interstate Commerce Commission order should be invoked only in accordance with the provisions of this circular. It also forbade the use of priorities to dispossess passengers to secure accommodations for medical attendants returning to home stations.[33] Presumably, so long as railroads lived up to terms of the May agreement, the Army would not dispossess passengers to secure accommodations for patients.

Procedures for Air Evacuation

Air evacuation in the United States in the early part of the war was limited to the movement of individuals or groups of three to four patients from scenes of crashes to hospitals or from one hospital to another. In 1942, for instance, Maxwell Field transported a few patients by plane to Lawson General Hospital, and MacDill Field sent others to both Lawson and Walter Reed General Hospitals. At the time of the North African invasion, the Hampton Roads Port arranged for the flight of a patient suffering from a brain injury to Walter Reed General Hospital.[34] Such flights were exceptional and the first sizable air evacuation of patients in the United States did not occur until the beginning of 1944. For sporadic flights prior to that time, the Air Forces normally set aside no single group of planes, and it was therefore imperative that air evacuation be carried out normally in administrative, training, or transport planes.[35] Moreover, until the latter part of 1942, no personnel was trained especially for air evacuation operations. Air station surgeons either arranged with local operations officers for the transportation of patients by planes belonging to their stations or called upon the surgeons of training centers to supply the necessary accommodations. They either accompanied patients themselves or sent nurses or doctors from air station hospitals as attendants. AAF headquarters authorized SOS installations to submit requests for the air transportation of patients to near-by Air Forces installations, the Air Transport Command, troop carrier commands, and the Air Surgeon's Office.[36]

During the winter of 1943–44 there were widespread demands, for a variety of reasons, for air transportation of patients in the United States. On 16 November 1943, for example, the commander of Ashford General Hospital requested air evacuation to relieve congestion on railroads in that area. A few weeks later the commandant of the School of Air Evacuation suggested it to provide training for air evacuation personnel and to increase the comfort of patients.[37] Early the next Janu-

[33] (1) ICC, Order 213, Title 49, Transportation and Railroads, 27 Jun 44. HD: 531.4. (2) Memo, Col A[lbert] H. Schwichtenberg for SG, 26 Jun 44, sub: Rail Trans of Pnts. SG: 531.2. (3) WD Cir 405, 14 Oct 44. See also WD Cirs 61, 26 Feb 45, and 471, 15 Dec 44.

[34] (1) Ltr, Base Surg AAB MacDill Fld to CG AAF (Air Surg), 17 Nov 42. AAF: 370.05 (Evac Book No 1). (2) Ltr, Surg HRPE to CO Langley Fld, 16 Dec 42, sub: Air Trans for Overseas Sick and Wounded Arriving at HRPE. AAF: 452.1 (Amb Plane).

[35] See below, pp. 429–33.

[36] (1) 3d ind, Hq AAF to Port Surg HRPE, 5 Jan 43, on Ltr, HRPE to CO Langley Fld, 16 Dec 42, sub: Air Trans for Overseas Sick and Wounded Arriving at HRPE. AAF: 452.1 (Amb Planes). (2) Ltr, 6th SvC to AAF (Air Surg), 16 Apr 43, sub: SOP, with incl. AAF: 370.05 (Evac).

[37] Ltrs, CO Ashford Gen Hosp to CO AAB, Richmond, Va., 16 Nov 43; AAF School of Air Evac, Bowman Fld, Ky., 6 Dec 43, sub: Trans of Pnts by Air. AAF: 370.05 (Evac, Book 1).

ary the director of the Surgeon General's Hospital Administration Division conferred with the Deputy Chief of Air Staff on the "feasibility of moving patients by air from port hospitals." [38] The following month, at a conference of service commanders, the commanding general of the Second Service Command stated that air transportation for patients was "most desirable," and suggested its use particularly for small groups who needed to be moved without delay.[39] In April the flight surgeon assigned to Brooke General Hospital propounded still another reason: the evacuation of patients by air would be economical, saving the Government, according to his estimate, at least fifty dollars per patient.[40] A combination of such reasons, along with increases in aircraft production, a shortage of Pullman cars, and the absolute necessity of moving large numbers of patients who arrived in the United States from theaters of operations, were responsible for the extensive use of air evacuation in this country during the latter half of the war.

The first large-scale movement of patients by air in the United States was made in January 1944. At that time three troop carrier command planes, with personnel from the School of Air Evacuation, were sent to Stark General Hospital to move patients being debarked from two hospital ships. In a period of ten flying days, between 7 and 19 January, these planes flew 661 patients in 29 loads to 5 general hospitals. No cases of air sickness occurred and only twelve patients required medication, such as the administration of aspirin or morphine, during flight. The success of this mission prompted the commanding general of the Service Forces to congratulate the Air Forces and to express the hope that patients might be evacuated by air from ports of debarkation "repeatedly in the future." [41]

During the spring of 1944 plans were made to convert that hope into a reality. In April the Air Transport Command was made responsible for the movement of patients by air in the United States (as it had been made responsible earlier for air evacuation from theaters of operations). Soon afterward it assigned to its Ferrying Division as a special mission the movement of about 700 patients from coastal medical installations to various hospitals throughout the United States. The next month the Transport Command delegated its responsibility for domestic air evacuation to the Ferrying Division, and began to earmark transport planes for evacuation only.[42] In June representatives of AAF and ATC headquarters, the Ferrying Division, the Air Surgeon, and The Surgeon General agreed upon procedures for domestic air evacuation operations. When the ASF Medical Regulating Officer desired to move patients by air, he informed the AAF Medical Regulating Officer, requesting necessary arrangements. The latter telephoned the Ferrying Division in Cincinnati, Ohio, to determine availability

[38] Diary, Hosp Admin Div (SGO), 8 Jan 44. SG: 314.8.

[39] Rpt, Conf CGs of SvCs. Dallas, Tex., 17–19 Feb 44. HD: 337.

[40] Ltr, Off Flt Surg Brooke Gen Hosp to CG AAF thru Central Flying Tng Comd, 28 Apr 44, sub: Trf by Air of AAF Pnts from Brooke Gen Hosp to AAF Conv Ctr. AAF: 370.05 (Evac, Book 2).

[41] (1) Ltr, CG ASF to CG AAF, 4 Feb 44. AAF: 370.05 (Evac). (2) Ltr, AAF Sch of Air Evac to CG AAF, 16 Feb 44, sub: Air Evac, with incl. Same file. (3) *The Air Surgeon's Bulletin*, Vol. I, No. 4 (1944), pp. 12–13.

[42] (1) Initial Medical History (11 February 1943 to 30 June 1944), Headquarters Ferrying Division, Air Transport Command. HD: TAS. (2) Memo, Lt Col Richard L. Meiling for Air Surg, 27 Apr 44, sub: Air Evac 19–25 Apr 44. AAF: 370.05. (3) See below, pp. 436–37.

and location of planes and then informed the ASF Medical Regulating Officer if the mission could be accomplished within the time limits desired. If so, the ASF Medical Regulating Officer directed hospitals to prepare patients for the movement planned and the AAF Medical Regulating Officer informed the Ferrying Division of the mission to be accomplished.[43]

The Ferrying Division co-ordinated plans for each flight with the hospital from which patients were being transferred at least 24 hours in advance of the plane's departure. Flight attendants supplied by this Division to care for patients en route also arranged to have them properly tagged for identification and to have their records and valuables carried along with them. To permit hospitals receiving patients to prepare for their reception, flight attendants notified them in advance by telephone of the expected time of arrival.[44]

During the period from April 1944 to August 1945 the Ferrying Division transported about 100,000 patients from debarkation hospitals to general and convalescent hospitals throughout the United States. Each patient was flown an average of 1,388 miles.[45] The procedure by which this was accomplished made it possible, after control of hospital train movements was also centralized in Washington, for the ASF Medical Regulating Officer to co-ordinate the use of planes and trains in domestic evacuation, thereby relieving railroads of a tremendous burden. It also enabled the Regulating Officer to observe more closely than might have been otherwise possible the policy of transferring patients promptly and directly from debarkation hospitals to installations where they would receive final treatment.

---

[43] (1) Rpt, Conf on Air Evac, 7 Jun 44. SG: 580. (2) Memo, SG for CG AAF attn Reg Off, 7 Jul 44. SG: 580.-1.

[44] (1) Organizational History of the Ferrying Division, June 20, 1942 to August 1, 1944. ATC: Hist Div. (2) 1st ind, CG Ferrying Div ATC (Surg) to CG ATC attn Surg, 24 Sep 44, on Ltr, CG 2d SvC to CG ASF attn SG, 29 Aug 44, sub: Air Evac. SG: 580.

[45] Andres G. Oliver and Hampton C. Robinson, Jr., "Domestic Air Transportation of Patients," *The Air Surgeon's Bulletin*, Vol. II, No. 11 (1945), p. 400.

CHAPTER XXII

Providing the Means for Evacuation by Land

Supplying enough ambulances and rail cars of suitable types for the transportation of patients in the United States and in overseas areas was a continuing problem. Plans for improved types were being made before the war started, and when it ended new ones were still being developed and ordered. Numerous difficulties were encountered in this process, as well as in manning and equipping hospital trains.

Motor Ambulances

Of all conveyances the motor ambulance was the most widely used and transported the largest number of patients. The type in greatest use was the general-service ambulance. Capable of serving in training camps in the United States as well as in communications and combat zones of theaters of operations, it was called at different times the field ambulance, the station ambulance, and the cross-country ambulance. Others of more specialized—and therefore more limited—use were the metropolitan and multipatient ambulances.

General-Service Ambulances

Because general-service ambulances were basic conveyances for patients in both peace and war, experiments to improve them were made between World Wars I and II. In 1932 a field ambulance on a (4 x 2)[1] chassis of 1½-ton capacity was developed by the Medical Department Equipment Laboratory and by 1939 it had replaced ambulances of World War I type. Although this ambulance was designed for use at Army posts and camps in the United States as well as for field service with tactical units, it was not entirely satisfactory for either. It rode too roughly and was too poorly heated and ventilated for the comfort of patients in the United States, and it got stuck in the mud too easily for satisfactory service in the field or in forward areas of theaters of operation.[2] The Surgeon General's Office concluded that heavier ambulances, perhaps of the metropolitan type normally used by civilian hospitals, should be used not only at Army hospitals in the United States but also in communications zones of theaters, and that a light ambulance, able to oper-

[1] That is, having four wheels, two of which were attached to the engine drive-shaft.

[2] (1) Ltr, SG to TAG, 21 Feb 34, sub: Repl of Wartime Ambs. HRS: G–4/29094. (2) Ltr, QMG to TAG, 15 Apr 35, sub: Mil Characteristics for Ambs, Light Fld Type. QMG: 451.8. For letters on motor vehicular requirements and assignment of ambulances see files HRS: G–4/29714 and QMG: 451.8; for changes in specifications and rear spring improvements see files SG: 451.8–1 and 451.8–1 (Carlisle Bks).

ate over bad terrain, should be developed for use in combat zones.[3]

Beginning in 1937 the Medical Department and the Quartermaster Corps had experimented with development of such an ambulance. Meanwhile the General Staff reaffirmed its policy of limiting the types of chassis used by the Army in order both to assure the mass production of vehicles and to simplify the procurement and distribution of spare parts as well as the maintenance and repair of vehicles. It announced in August 1939 that all tactical vehicles (that is, those used by table-of-organization units) would be all-wheel-drive types, and that only five chassis would be considered standard for the Army: ½-ton, 1½-ton, 2½-ton, 4-ton, and 7½-ton.[4] The Medical Department Equipment Laboratory and Holabird Quartermaster Depot then concentrated on experiments with a ½-ton (4 x 4) chassis, and in June 1940 The Surgeon General announced that the ambulance built on it would be "accepted as the new cross-country motor ambulance for use in all divisional and corps units in the combat zone."[5] This ambulance, like the one it was to replace, could carry four litter patients. When the first of this type was delivered for testing early in January 1941, the Surgeon General's Office and the Laboratory found that the ambulance which had been developed primarily for use in combat zones rode so comfortably and was so well heated and ventilated that it would serve satisfactorily for hospitals in the zone of interior as well.[6] In short, the new cross-country ambulance was a better general-service ambulance than the 1½-ton (4 x 2) field ambulance.

A change in standard chassis required a change in the new ambulance during 1942. In 1941 two new chassis—¼-ton (4 x 4) and ¾-ton (4 x 4)—were introduced, and the ½-ton (4 x 4) was dropped from the Army's standard list. As early as February 1942 the Quartermaster Corps was anticipating issuing ¾-ton ambulances in place of ½-ton vehicles.[7] About four months later plans for the change had been completed, and ¾-ton ambulances were ordered along with other ¾-ton vehicles. Although similar in appearance to the ½-ton ambulance, the new ¾-ton ambulance had a shorter wheelbase, larger tires, and more clearance under the axle.[8] The Medical Department Equipment Laboratory thought that these differences made it more comfortable for patients and less apt to get stuck in mud and sand.

While the cross-country ambulance was designed mainly for use in theaters of operations, it was used widely in the zone of interior as well. The stoppage of passenger-car production early in the war curtailed the procurement and use of metropolitan ambulances built on pas-

[3] 2d ind, SG to TAG, 3 Jan 40, on Ltr, SG to TAG, 25 Nov 39, sub: Fld Ambs, Motor. SG: 451.8-1. Also see the following T/Os: 8-508, Sta Hosp, 25 Jul 40; 8-507, Gen Hosp, 25 Jul 40.

[4] Ltr AG 451 (6-15-39) Misc-D, TAG to SG, 12 Aug 39, sub: Standardization of Motor Vehs. AG: 451 (8-12-39).

[5] (1) For letters on these experiments see files QMG: 451.8 and 400.112 T-M, 1937-40, and SG: 451.8-1 and 451.8-1 (Carlisle Bks), 1937-40. (2) Ltr, SG to Dir MD Equip Lab, 1 Jun 40, sub: Critical Measurement Data on Cross-Country Amb. HD: McKinney files, Jun 40.

[6] Memo, Col G[arfield] L. McKinney (Planning Subdiv) for SG, 14 Jan 41, sub: New Cross-Country Amb; Insp at Carlisle Bks, 13 Jan 41. Off file, Research and Dev Bd SGO, "Cross-Country Amb."

[7] (1) Ltr QM 451 M-ES, QMG to SG, 14 Feb 42, sub: Reclassification of Amb, Fld, with 3 inds. QMG: 451.8. (2) Memo, TAG for CGs AGF and AAF, C of Arms and Servs, 6 Apr 42, sub: Standardization of Wheeled Motor Veh Chassis and Trailers. AG: 451 (4-4-42).

[8] (1) TM 9-2800, 1 Sep 43, Standard Military Motor Vehicles.

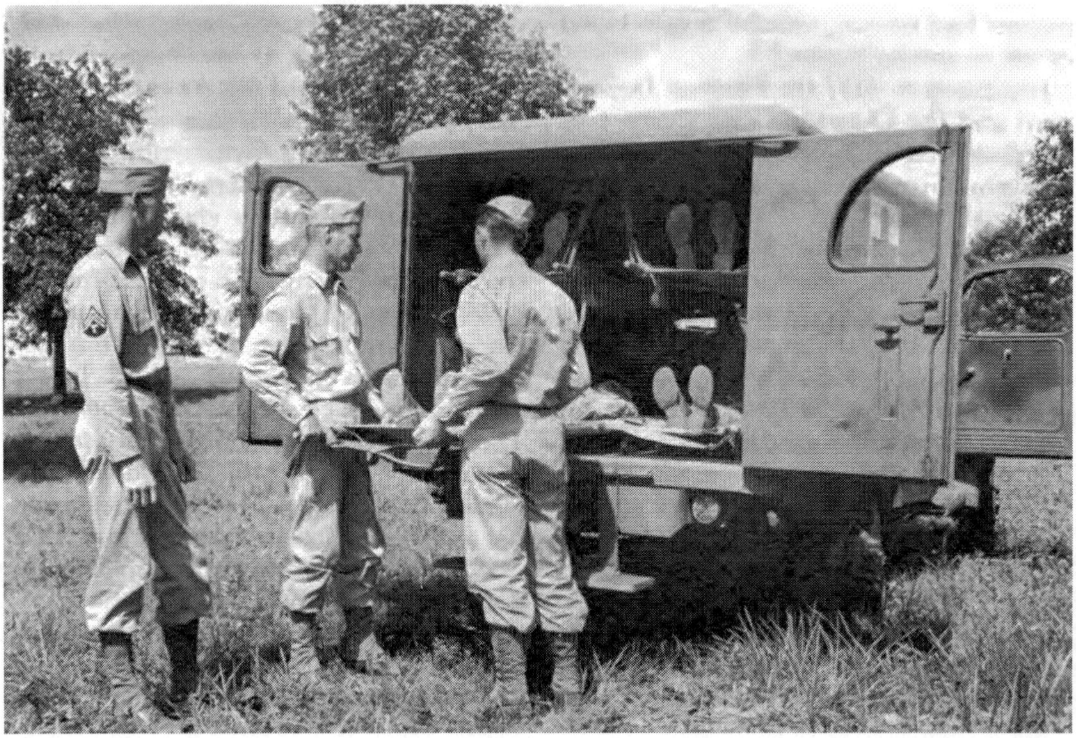

PLACING THE FOURTH LITTER PATIENT IN A FIELD AMBULANCE

senger-car frames.[9] The Medical Department therefore used what was available. As ambulances of the cross-country type were delivered to the Army, they were first distributed to table-of-organization units. Those of the older type (1½-ton field ambulance) that were no longer needed by such units were divided among posts, camps, and stations in the United States.[10] As ambulances of the old type wore out or as requirements exceeded supply, ambulances of the new types were issued to zone of interior installations. In addition, 356 chassis for 1½-ton (4 x 4) trucks were taken from a civilian pool of motor vehicles in 1943 and were used to build modified field ambulances for service in lieu of unavailable metropolitan ambulances.[11] Thus, in addition to the metropolitan ambulances either on hand or procured from available stocks at the beginning of the war, hospitals in the United States used four types of ambulances: the 1½-ton (4 x 2) field ambulance; the 1½-ton (4 x 4) modified field ambulance; the ½-ton (4 x

[9] For letters on efforts to secure additional metropolitan ambulances and their procurement and distribution see file SG: 451.8-1 (1939-43). Also see History of the Automotive Division, War Production Board, 1941-45 (1945). Natl Archives: WPB 020.1.

[10] SG Cir 81, 8 Aug 41, sub: Admin Motor Veh. For letters on distribution and redistribution of field ambulances from tactical units to zone of interior hospitals see files: SG: 451.8-1, AG: 451.8, and HRS: G-4/29714 for 1940-43.

[11] Memo, ACofS for Oprs ASF for CofOrd, 6 May 43, sub: Reqmts for Fld Ambs. AG: 451.8 (5-6-43).

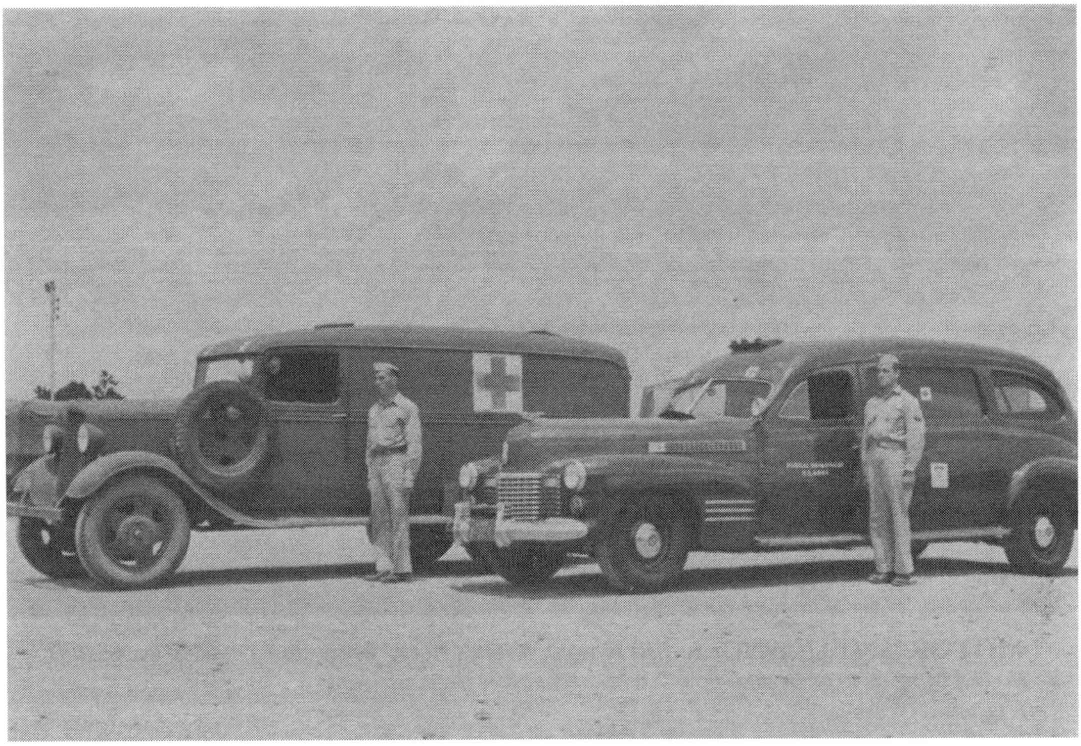

FIELD AND METROPOLITAN AMBULANCES USED IN 1942

4) cross-country ambulance; and the ¾-ton (4 x 4) ambulance.

By the winter of 1942–43 it appeared that the ¾-ton ambulance was not entirely satisfactory for overseas use. SOS headquarters thought it took up too much shipping space, and some theaters expressed dissatisfaction with its performance. The Southwest Pacific, for instance, stated that lighter vehicles with greater traction were needed for the rough muddy trails over which patients had to be transported, while reports from North Africa indicated that the ¾-ton ambulance was difficult to land from lighters, lacked the traction and drive needed in that theater, and had insufficient angles of approach and departure to allow it to operate easily over ditches and hills of rough terrain.[12] The SOS Requirements Division in January 1943 proposed several methods of overcoming these difficulties: shipment of the standard ambulance in a two-unit pack for reassembly in theaters of operations, replacement of its metal body with bows and a tarpaulin top, and provision of "litter kits" for use in adapting stand-

[12] (1) Diary, SOS Hosp and Evac Br, 13, 16, 22, and 28 Jan 43. HD: Wilson files, "Diary." (2) Ltr, CinC SWPA to CG SOS, 21 Nov 42, sub: Improvement of Equip and Orgn, US Army, with 3 inds. SG: 322.15-1. (3) Memo, Col Robert C. McDonald, Hosp and Evac Br Oprs Div ASF for Gen [Le Roy] Lutes, 21 Apr 43, sub: Gen Kenner's Rpts, with incls. HD: Wilson files, "Book IV, 16 Mar 43-17 Jun 43." (4) Ltr, Joseph A. Keeney, Army Med Serv Tec Cmtee to Col Calvin H. Goddard, 7 Jul 52. HD: 314 (Correspondence on MS) XI.

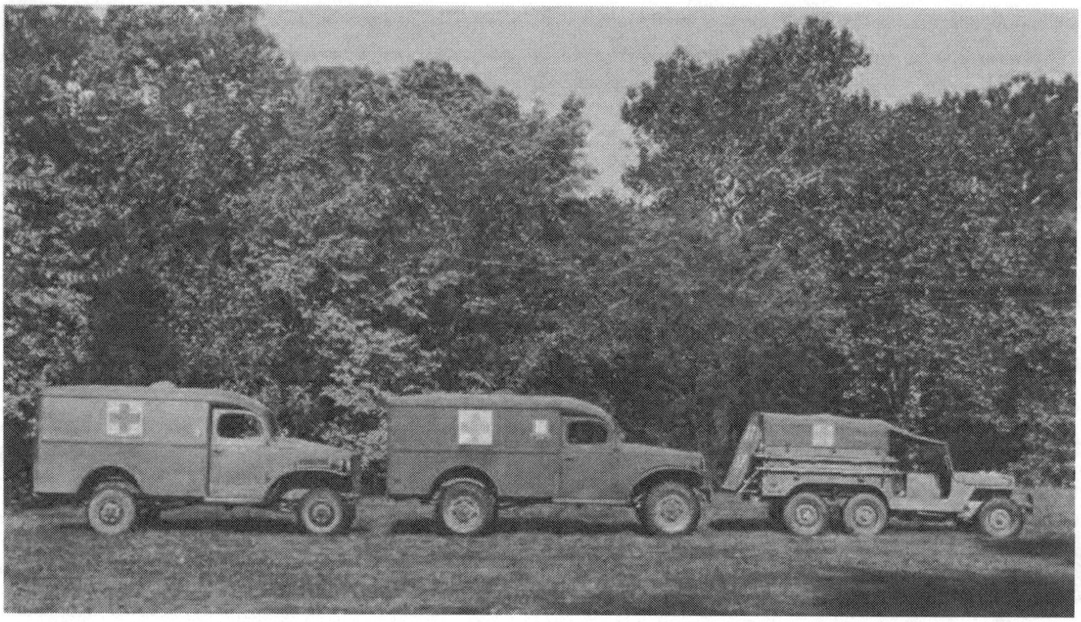

MOTOR AMBULANCES. *Left to right, ½-ton (4x4), ¾-ton (4x4), and ¾-ton (6x6), the last being an experimental vehicle which was never standardized.*

ard vehicles to the transportation of patients.[13]

The Surgeon General's Office countered with a different proposal. The Medical Department Equipment Laboratory had already begun to evaluate experiments of medical units in replacing litter bearers with motor vehicles—particularly ¼-ton (4 x 4) trucks, or jeeps—to transport patients from battalion aid stations to collecting stations. By the middle of 1942 it had decided that none of the standard vehicles of the Army were satisfactory for this purpose. Some were too rough; some had silhouettes that were too high; and others—notably the unprotected and uncovered jeep—were so small that litters protruded over their sides or ends. Consequently the Medical Department Technical Committee and the Surgeon General's Office had proposed in August 1942 the development of a light forward-area ambulance on a nonstandard chassis—a ¼-ton (4 x 4) chassis to which an extra axle and two wheels were added, making it a ¾-ton (6 x 6) chassis. SOS headquarters had disapproved this proposal because it conflicted with the War Department's policy of using only standard chassis.[14] The Surgeon General's Office still believed that this vehicle was a practical solution to the dual problem of saving space on ships and furnishing theaters with ambulances that could be used far forward in rough terrain and in February

[13] Memo, CG SOS for SG, 30 Jan 43, sub: Ambs. SG: 451.8-1.

[14] (1) Mins, MD Tec Cmtee, 17 Aug 42. (2) 1st ind, CG SOS to SG, [29 Aug 42], on unknown basic ltr. (3) Memo, Chief Dev Br Research and Dev Div SGO for Chief Fld Equip Br Research and Dev Div SGO, 3 Sep 42, sub: Forward Area Amb. All in Off file, Research and Dev Bd SGO, "Amb, Forward Area."

1943 recommended again that this type should be developed at once. The SOS Requirements Division referred this recommendation to the Army Ground Forces, principal user of front-line ambulances. Rather than introduce a new type of chassis, AGF headquarters recommended the modification of the ¾-ton (4 x 4) ambulance and the issuance of "litter kits" for use with standard field trucks.[15] The Surgeon General's Office consented, and during the early part of 1943 the Ordnance Department and the Medical Department Equipment Laboratory collaborated in the development of an ambulance on a ¾-ton (4 x 4) chassis that incorporated improvements desired for field use and had a body that could be "knocked down" for shipment. By July 1943 two experimental vehicles had been tested, and in August the Surgeon General's Office recommended that one with plywood and steel paneling be adopted as standard.[16] As the 1944 ambulance procurement program was nearing completion (April 1944), the new "knock down" ambulance was standardized, and the older ¾-ton vehicle, which had been issued widely to units in all areas, was reclassified as a limited standard item.[17]

Metropolitan Ambulances

The possibility of procuring metropolitan ambulances in addition to those on hand or acquired at the beginning of the war was raised in the middle of 1944. Early in June the War Production Board called the attention of ASF headquarters to an opinion of the Ambulance Body Manufacturers Industry Advisory Committee that "The Army may not have considered the need for street ambulances to be used in connection with [Army] hospitals in this country." [18] Referring the matter to the Surgeon General's Office on 21 June 1944, ASF headquarters routinely called for recommendations as to possible Army requirements for "street" ambulances. When The Surgeon General took this opportunity to insist upon the procurement of 200 metropolitan ambulances, ASF headquarters disapproved, stating that no suitable commercial chassis were in production, that the conversion of passenger cars frozen in the civilian pool would be too expensive, and that requirements for metropolitan ambulances could continue to be met by using field (or general-service) ambulances.[19] The Surgeon General's Office then surveyed service command needs and in January 1945 reported its findings. The 149 metropolitan ambulances already in use were so badly worn as to require replacement, and 151 additional vehicles of that type were needed by ASF and AAF hospitals. Accordingly The Surgeon General requested

[15] 1st ind, SG to CG SOS, 5 Feb 43, 2d ind, CG SOS (Reqmts Div) to CG AGF, 18 Feb 43, and 3d ind, CG AGF to CG ASF, 10 Apr 43, on Memo, CG SOS for SG, 30 Jan 43, sub: Amb. AG: 451.8 (1-30-43) and Off file, Research and Dev Bd SGO, "Cross-Country Amb."

[16] (1) Memo, CG ASF for SG, 19 Apr 43, sub: Amb, with ind. SG: 451.8-1. (2) Ord Tec Cmtee, Item 20641, 12 Jun 43. HD: 451.8. (3) Ltrs, MD Equip Lab to SG, 18 Aug, 21 Oct 43, sub: Amb, Cross-Country, Improvements, with inds. SG: 451.8-1.

[17] (1) Memo, CofOrd for CG ASF (Reqmts Div), 10 Mar 44, sub: Truck, ¾-ton, 4 x 4, Amb KD-Standardization and Rev of Mil Characteristics, with 2 inds. AG: 451.2. (2) Ord Tec Cmtee, Item 23100, 9 Mar 44. HD: 451.8. Limited standard vehicles were usable substitutes for standard vehicles and were issued as long as the supply on hand lasted.

[18] Ltr, WPB to ASF, 9 Jun 44. SG: 451.8-1.

[19] (1) Memo, CG ASF for SG, 21 Jun 44, sub: Street Amb for Use in US, with 2 inds. (2) Memo, CG ASF for SG, 20 Jul 44, sub: Amb, Metropolitan, ¾-ton, 4 x 2, with 2 inds. Both in SG: 451.8-1.

ASF headquarters to authorize the development of "substitute standard" metropolitan ambulances by the conversion of light sedans which the War Department had on hand. The Ordnance Department began such a project, but the war ended before it was completed.[20]

Multipatient Ambulances

Toward the end of the war the Medical Department succeeded in getting a multipatient ambulance and thus achieved, in part at least, a goal toward which it had worked in the early war years. From 1939 until the middle of 1943 the Surgeon General's Office and the Medical Department Equipment Laboratory had conducted almost continuous experiments to develop a single large vehicle that could serve not only as a multipatient ambulance both in the zone of interior and in combat areas but also as housing for mobile laboratories, operating rooms, and wards and as a means of transporting surgical, shock, and other specialized teams to areas where they were critically needed.[21] They had experimented with 2½-ton (4 x 2) front-wheel-drive bus-type vehicles, van-type semitrailers pulled by 1½-ton and 2½-ton tractors, and 2½-ton (6 x 6) trucks.[22] These experiments failed mainly because an attempt was being made to use a single vehicle for several purposes, and none possessed all of the characteristics required. For example, the front-wheel-drive bus was a nonstandard vehicle and lacked sufficient traction for cross-country use, while the semitrailer lacked maneuverability in combat areas and was too rough for patients. The 2½-ton (6 x 6) truck, on the Army's standard list, was successfully used in the development of a surgical truck for armored divisions, but the Quartermaster Corps thought that it would be unsatisfactory as an ambulance because full loads of ambulatory patients would overload its front axles and wheels. Thus the Medical Department reached the middle of 1943 without having developed a standard multipatient ambulance. Meanwhile its Equipment Laboratory converted eight experimental, nonstandard, front-wheel-drive bus-type vehicles, which had been procured in 1940 and 1941 and had been found unsatisfactory for field use, into multipatient ambulances for service at ports in the United States. In June four apiece were issued to Letterman and Halloran General Hospitals in place of the passenger buses requested by Letterman, and instead of the additional standard general-service ambulances requested for Halloran by the second Service Command.[23] The next month the Laboratory recommended that the project for the development of a multipatient ambulance be continued, but Surgeon General

[20] (1) Ltr, SG to all SvCs, 26 Sep 44, sub: Amb, Metropolitan, ¾-ton, 4 x 2, Reqmts, with replies. SG: 451.8-1. (2) Ltr, SG to CG 7th SvC, 15 Sep 44, sub: Trans of PW Pnts in Carry-alls, with 7 inds. Ord: 451.8-39. (3) Ord Tec Cmtee, Item 27294, 20 Mar 45, sub: Amb, ¾-ton, 4 x 2, Light Metropolitan. HD: 451.8.

[21] Ltr, MD Equip Lab to SG, 27 Dec 45, sub: Hist of Amb, Bus-Type, Experimental, MD Equip Lab Proj F 2. HD: 451.8.

[22] For documents on these experiments see files for 1940–43 as follows: SG: 451.8–1 (Carlisle Barracks), 451.8–1, 451.2–1, and AG: 451.8.

[23] (1) Ltr, Letterman Gen Hosp to 9th SvC, 22 Mar 43, sub: Req for Passenger Buses, with 2 inds. SG: 451.8–1 (9th SvC). (2) Memo, 2d SvC Ord Br for DepCofOrd Tank-Auto Ctr (Detroit), 24 Apr 43, sub: Motor Vehs, with 6 inds. SG: 451.8 (2d SvC). (3) Ltr, SG to CG ASF, 14 Jun 43, sub: Conversion of Surg Hosp Vehs to Bus-Type Ambs. SG: 451.2–1 (Carlisle Bks).

Kirk directed that it be dropped.[24] During the following year his Office and the Laboratory concentrated on the development of such special purpose vehicles as mobile medical and dental laboratories, optical repair units, and dental and surgical operating trucks.[25]

In the second half of 1944 the question of furnishing multipatient ambulances was reopened. In July Letterman General Hospital asked for the replacement of the four worn-out multipatient ambulances which it had received in mid-1943. To this request Ninth Service Command headquarters added four more for other debarkation hospitals on the west coast (two for Birmingham General Hospital and two for Fort Lewis). By October the number requested for the Ninth Service Command was doubled.[26] Meanwhile, during July and early August, Mitchel Field, which served as a debarkation point for air evacuees, converted four Ordnance maintenance trucks into special multipatient ambulances for the transportation of patients from planes to the Mitchel Field Hospital and from that installation to Halloran General Hospital.

To meet the need thus demonstrated, the Surgeon General's Office proposed on 11 September 1944 the development of a special ambulance to be used only in the United States and to carry twelve to sixteen litter patients. This limitation was expected to eliminate difficulties encountered earlier in attempts to develop multipatient ambulances that could carry either litter or ambulatory patients in both the zone of interior and combat zones. At first ASF headquarters was reluctant to approve a developmental project for a vehicle in small demand. It proposed, instead, that The Surgeon General submit a list of standard military vehicles that would be satisfactory, when modified, for the use intended. Believing that no standard military vehicle was suitable, the Ordnance and Medical Departments decided that front-wheel-drive bus-type vehicles of the kind procured for experimental purposes in 1940 and 1941 should be used. An important factor in this decision was the statement by the company making such vehicles that it had "open production facilities" and could therefore "offer favorable delivery," if standard engines, transmissions, and axles were made available to them.[27] In addition, The Surgeon General pointed out, a pilot model had already been developed in 1940. He requested, therefore, that the Chief of Ordnance be authorized to procure twenty-four such vehicles for Medical Department use. This request was approved by ASF headquarters on 4 November 1944.[28]

---

[24] (1) Ltr, SG to MD Equip Lab, 6 Jul 43, sub: Dropping and/or Suspension of Dev Projects, with ind. SG: 451.8–1. (2) Ltr, SG to CG ASF (Reqmts Div), 22 Jul 43, sub: Bus-Type Amb (Project F–2 and Mobile Hosp Ward (F 15.01)). Same file. (3) Memo, Chief Fld Equip Dev Br SGO for Chief Research Coord Br SGO, 27 Jul 43, sub: Experimental ¾-ton Amb. Off file, Research and Dev Bd SGO, "Bus-Type Amb, F–2."

[25] For full discussions of these projects, see John B. Johnson, Jr, and Graves H. Wilson, A History of Wartime Research and Development of Medical Field Equipment (1946), pp. 295–730. HD.

[26] (1) Memo, CG Letterman Gen Hosp for CG 9th SvC, 20 Jul 44, sub: Repl of Ambs, Bus-type, with 3 inds. SG: 451.8 (9th SvC). (2) Ltr, SG to CG Letterman Gen Hosp, 26 Sep 44, sub: Multi-litter Ambs (Bus-Type), with 2 inds. Same file.

[27] Having "open production facilities" meant that the company's plant could begin production immediately without having to await the completion of other orders.

[28] Ltr, CG ASF (Dir of Sup) to CG 2d SvC, 21 Jun 44, sub: Trucks, 1½-ton, (4 x 4) Ord Maintenance, for Mitchel Fld, with 12 inds. SG: 451.8.

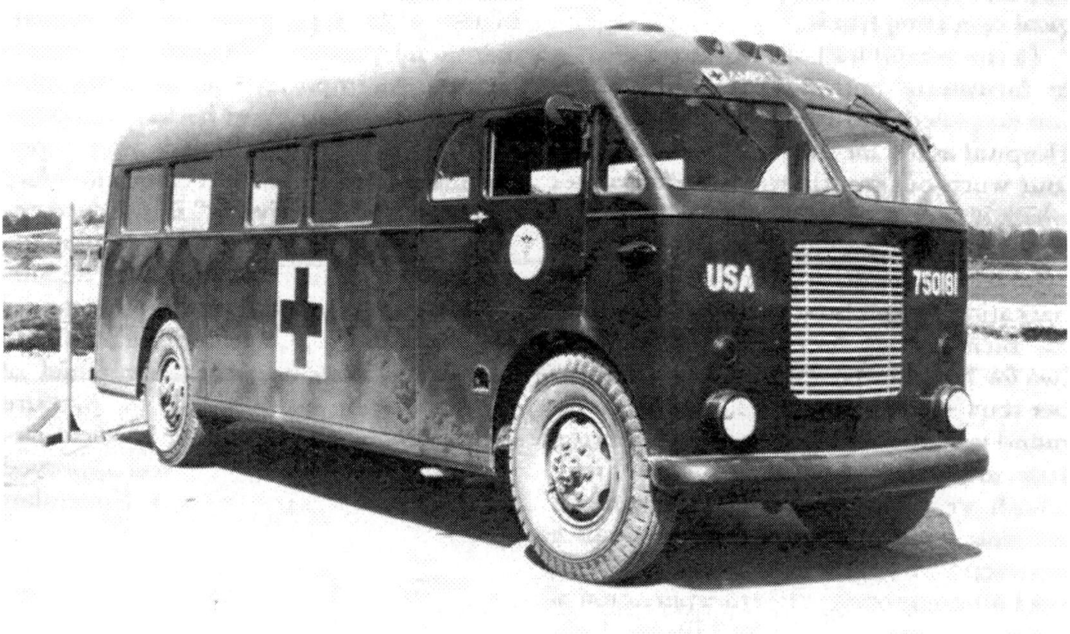

EXTERIOR VIEW OF MULTIPATIENT METROPOLITAN AMBULANCE, 1945

Production of the new 12-litter ambulances began almost immediately after the contract was awarded late in December 1944. Preliminary work on blueprints and specifications had already been completed, and on 8 January 1945 construction of the first model began. At the end of February it was road-tested by Ordnance and Medical Department representatives. By late March the first two were delivered to the Army, and during May—the month when the greatest number of patients arrived from theaters of operations—other multipatient ambulances were ready for delivery to hospitals.[29] Meanwhile, the Surgeon General's Office had surveyed requirements and found that additional ambulances of this type would be needed—forty-seven for service commands and fifty-one for the Air Forces. In June 1945 ASF headquarters approved their procurement. The next month the Ordnance Department began the process of standardizing the new ambulance. Before this was done in Sep-

[29] (1) Ltr, SG to CGs SvCs, 26 Feb 45, sub: Amb, 1-ton, 4 x 2, 12 litter, Metropolitan Front Drive, with replies. SG: 451.8 (SvCs). (2) See letters on development and inspections, modifications in litter supports, and changes in rear springs in Off file, Research and Dev Bd SGO, "Amb, Bus-Type, Experimental, F-2."

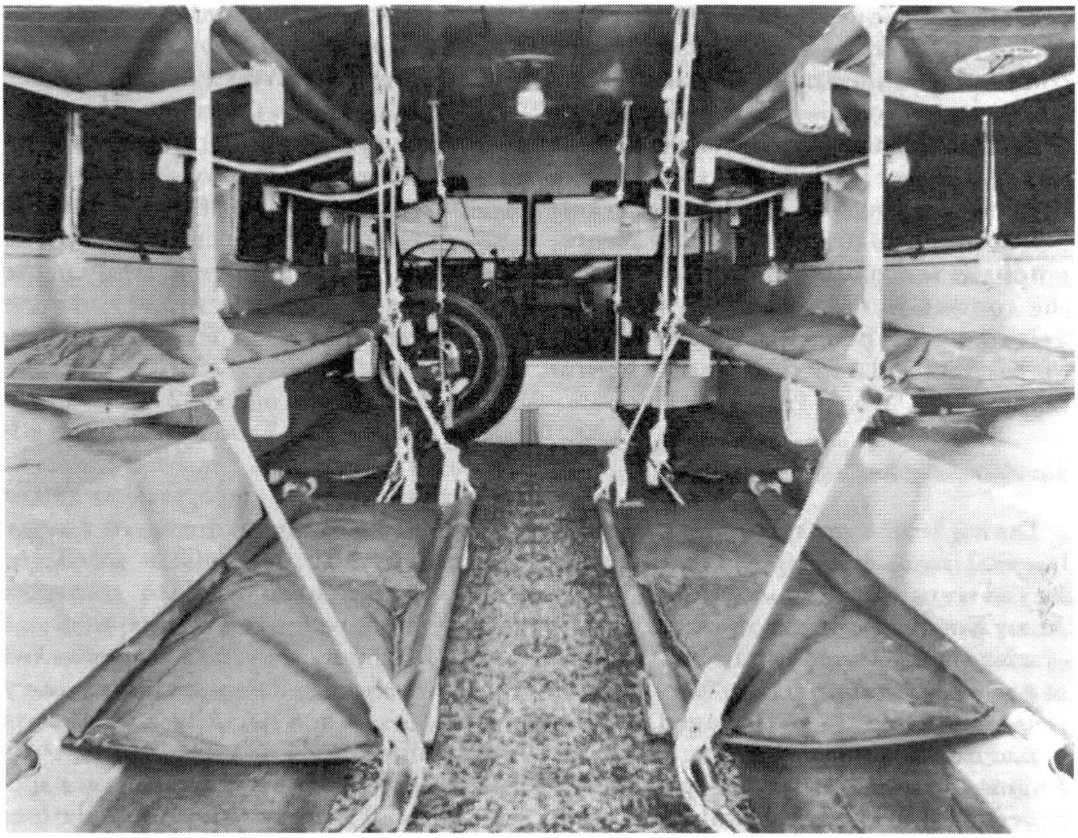

INTERIOR OF THE MULTIPATIENT METROPOLITAN AMBULANCE

tember 1945, V-J Day occurred and the contract for ninety-eight additional multipatient ambulances was canceled.[30]

Hospital Trains

At the beginning of 1939 the Medical Department had no hospital trains on hand and only indefinite plans for procuring them in the event of war. The Army had disposed of its World War I hospital cars because it was cheaper to transport the few patients who required movement in peacetime in Pullman cars and tourist sleepers of regularly scheduled trains. Thereafter the Medical Department had assumed that three types of trains would be used in the event of another war: (1) trains made up entirely of government-owned cars; (2) "semipermanent" trains composed of one government-owned administrative car, called a unit car, and an appropriate number of commercial baggage cars, Pullman cars, tourist sleepers, and chair cars; and (3) improvised trains

[30] (1) Ord Tec Cmtee, Items: 28530, 26 Jul 45; 29055, 13 Sep 45; 29740, 8 Oct 45, sub: Amb, 1½-ton, 4 x 2, 12-litter Metropolitan. HD: 451.8. (2) Memo, SG for CG ASF (Reqmts and Stock Control Div), 6 Sep 45, sub: Ambs. SG: 451.8.

consisting of any available commercial rolling stock. Trains of the last type were considered undesirable because they lacked accommodations for the emergency treatment of patients and for train administration. There were doubts that those of the first type could be constructed in sufficient numbers during wartime. Hence, emphasis was placed upon planning for the conversion of commercial cars into unit cars. Such plans were drawn during the twenties and approved by the General Staff in 1931.[31]

Development of the "Ideal" Unit Car

During 1939 more specific planning for hospital trains was inspired by planning for rail transportation undertaken by the Army Engineers, urged on by the deteriorating international situation. As a part of a more general project to furnish lightweight trains for use on damaged or poorly laid tracks in theaters of operations, the Engineers in January 1939 proposed a government-owned hospital train built from standard military cars (20-ton, 28-foot-long, four-wheeled box cars). It was to consist of a personnel car, a dressing (or operating) car, nineteen ward cars, and a kitchen car, and was to be used, according to the Engineers, to transport patients "from the front line to any point in the Communications Zone or Zone of Interior." The Surgeon General's Office and the Medical Department Board agreed to adopt this train "for planning purposes," believing that they were not thereby eliminating the possibility of using other types of trains in communications zones. On 4 August 1939 the Engineers announced that they were basing plans for all trains in theaters of operations on the use of 20-ton railway cars. Shortly afterward, before committing itself further, the Surgeon General's Office turned to a study of trains used during World War I both in theaters of operations and in the zone of interior.[32]

This study showed that trains made up entirely of government-owned cars had been used effectively in Europe but that the semipermanent, or unit-car, type of train had been more successful in the United States. The unit car had had a kitchen large enough to feed 250 people, space for transporting 28 litter patients, and quarters for 1 officer, 2 noncommissioned officers, and 2 cooks. Among its advantages had been its flexibility, its economy of procurement and operation, and its provisions for feeding patients. As a single car attached to a regularly scheduled train, it had been used to transport twenty-eight or fewer patients; with one or two Pullman cars, it had been attached to regularly scheduled trains to carry more patients; and it had been used, along with Pullman cars, tourist sleepers, chair cars, and baggage cars, to make up a special hospital train with accommodations for over 200 patients. Conversion of a Pullman car into a unit car was thought to have been cheaper than the construction of cars for an entire train. Moreover, since other cars used in connection with it had been owned either by railroads or by the Pullman Company, only the unit car

[31] (1) Ltr, QMG to SG, 29 Dec 21, sub: Disposition of Hosp Cars, with 5 inds. Natl Archives, SG: 531.4-1. (2) Ltr, Bd of Engr Equip to CofEngrs, 9 Mar 31, sub: US Army Specifications, Car, Unit, Hosp, with 2 inds. CE: 531.43, pt 1. (3) US Army Specification 43-13, with drawing 43190, 30 Jul 31. SG: 453.-1. (4) Ltr, SG to *Comite International de la Croix-Rouge, Geneve,* 15 Feb 36. Natl Archives, SG: 322.2-5.

[32] (1) Memo, Engr Bd for CofEngrs, 12 Jan 39, sub: SP 70, Type Plans and Specifications for Motive Power and Rolling Stock on Standard Gauge Rys (Rpt 559, Prelim Rpt on Hosp Tns, Engr Bd, 23 Dec 38), with 9 inds. SG: 453.-1. (2) Rpt, MD Bd MFSS Carlisle Bks, Pa, 30 Mar 39. Same file.

had had to be "deadheaded" (returned empty) to the trains' point of origin. Furthermore, the unit car's kitchen facilities had helped to solve one of the major problems of World War I—the feeding of patients. Because of these advantages, and since the Engineers were already working on plans for cars for completely government-owned trains, the Surgeon General's Office concentrated in the winter of 1939–40 on the development of plans for an "ideal" unit car.[33]

The plans drawn were for a car that differed considerably from the unit car of World War I and to some extent from one that had been planned in 1931. The latter presumably represented an improvement over the World War I car. It was to have side doors for loading patients and, in addition to the kitchen, an operating or dressing room and more space for attendants, but its capacity for patients had been reduced from twenty-eight to ten. In the fall of 1939 the Surgeon General's Plans and Training Division decided to eliminate all spaces for patients, in order to increase the feeding capacity of the kitchen to 500, enlarge the operating room and make an aisle around it, provide roomier quarters for more medical attendants, and furnish storage space for foods and medical supplies. These changes were intended to produce a car which would have most of the facilities planned by the Engineers for the several administrative cars (dressing, kitchen, and personnel) of the proposed overseas train and would be "ideal" for use in mass evacuation in the United States.[34]

After preliminary plans for the unit car had been drawn, the Medical Department Board and the Surgeon General's Office studied "in a new light" the Engineers' proposal to use only lightweight trains in theaters of operations. They found that the General Staff had "not specifically approved" the 20-ton car for a hospital train, but that it had approved (in 1931) the unit car. Moreover, they considered the train proposed by the Engineers to be "unsatisfactory" and "a reversion to that [type] used prior to 1863." Finally, they had an alternative to offer: the unit car "included all the necessary facilities for the care of the sick and wounded" and could be used with commercial cars to make a complete hospital train either in the zone of interior or in theaters of operations. The Surgeon General and the Engineers then reached a compromise on 8 May 1940. The latter agreed with The Surgeon General that, as a first choice, hospital trains in theaters of operations should consist of the unit car and other heavy cars appropriate to it. The Surgeon General agreed that hospital trains of lightweight cars could be used in areas where the construction of roadbeds made the use of heavier equipment impractical.[35] Thereafter, the Surgeon General's Office and the Medical Department Board collaborated with the Quartermaster General's Office and the Pullman Company in completing specifications for the unit car; and with the Engineers in

[33] (1) Memo, Maj H[erbert] E. Tomlinson (SGO) for Col [Robert Du R.] Harden, 25 Aug 39, sub: Hosp Tns in World War. SG: 453.-1. (2) *The Medical Department . . . in the World War* (1923), vol. I, pp. 334–35; (1923), vol. V, pp. 180–86; (1925), vol. VIII, pp. 37–41.

[34] (1) Memo, SG (Capt Joe A. Bain) for QMG, 4 Oct 39, sub: Hosp Unit Car. SG: 453.-1. (2) Memo, SG (Col James E. Baylis, Exec Off) for MD Bd, 6 Feb 40. Same file.

[35] (1) 9th ind, SG to CofEngrs, 15 Apr 40; 10th ind, CofEngrs to SG, 4 Jun 40; 11th ind, SG to MFSS, 8 Jun 40, on Memo, Engr Bd for CofEngrs, 12 Jan 39, sub: SP 70, Type Plans and Specifications for Motive Power and Rolling Stock on Standard Gauge Rys. SG: 453.-1. (2) Notes on Conf on Hosp Tns, TofOpns, by Capt Bain, 8 May 40. Same file.

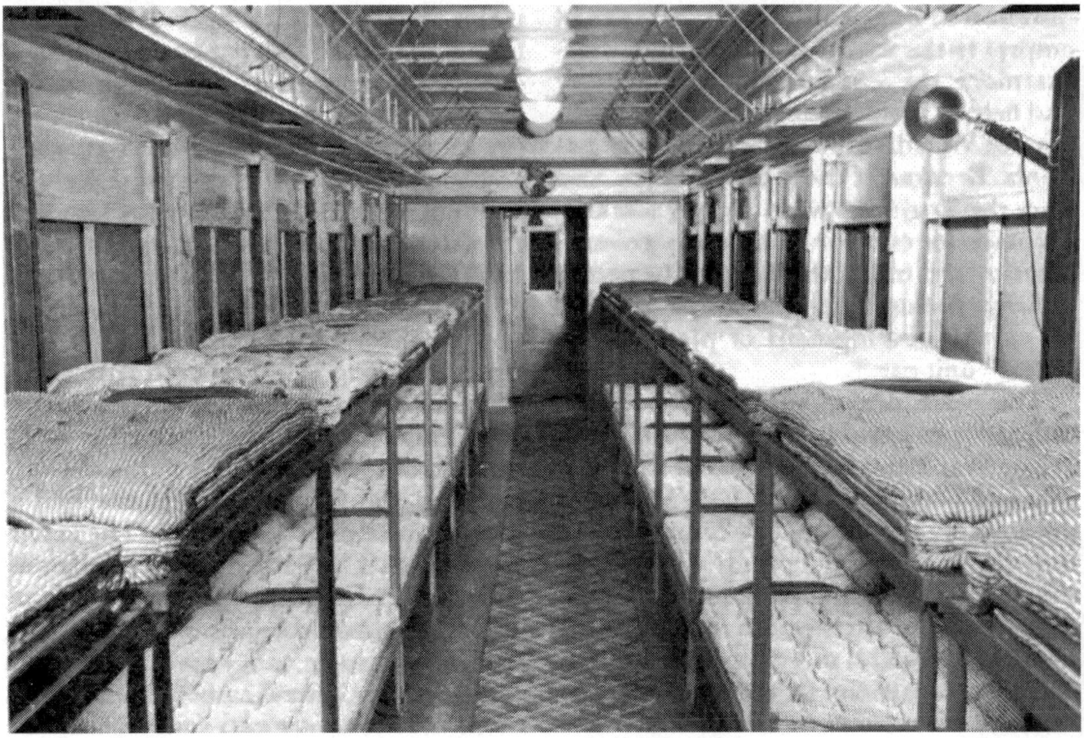

STATIONARY BEDS IN HOSPITAL WARD CAR, 1941

making preliminary designs for cars for the lightweight train.[36]

In the fall of 1940, when the establishment of Army bases in the Atlantic and the prospective passage of selective service legislation created a potential need for hospital trains, the Surgeon General's Office requested that two Pullman cars be converted into unit cars. This request was approved. Furthermore, in December 1940 the Engineers ordered, along with other railway equipment, enough 20-ton cars to test some for use in hospital trains.[37]

Need for Ward Cars and Their Development

About the time the first unit cars were delivered, the Surgeon General's Office found, contrary to its expectations, that government-owned hospital cars of another type would be needed. When the decision was made to eliminate spaces for patients in the unit car, the Planning and Training Division had expected that litter patients would be carried in tourist sleepers. About a year later, in February 1941, it discovered that tourist sleepers, like

[36] (1) Memo, SG for TAG, 6 May 40, sub: Hosp Unit Car. TC: 531.4. (2) Rpts, MD Bd No 190, 27 Aug 40, Hosp Unit Car; No 174, 27 Aug 40, Hosp Tn, Combat Area; No 174, 9 Sep 40, Berth for Hosp Tn. SG: 453.–1.

[37] (1) Memo SG for TAG, 5 Sep 40, sub: Hosp Tns, with 4 inds. SG: 453.–1. (2) Purchase Order 51536, 16 Dec 40, Haffner-Thrall Co, Chicago. CE: 453, pt 6. (3) Extract from History of the Development of Railroad Equipment, prep by Hist Staff, Engr Bd, Ft Belvoir, Va. HD: 531.4.

Pullman cars, had washrooms at either end, instead of straight through-and-through aisles, and that patients on litters could therefore not be carried from sleepers to unit-car operating rooms.[38] For the latter to be of any use, it was necessary to develop a special ward car. During the spring of 1941 the Pullman Company, following recommendations of the Medical Department, prepared plans for converting standard Pullman cars into ward cars. This was to be done by removing existing washrooms and installing other toilet and washing facilities in such a way as to leave a straight aisle; by adding wide side doors to permit easy loading and unloading of litter patients; and by replacing the Pullman berths with sixteen two-tiered stationary beds made by the Simmons Company. Such beds were chosen, instead of Glennan adjustable beds used during World War I, because they were thought to be more comfortable and cheaper to procure. In July 1941 the General Staff approved a request from The Surgeon General for four cars of this type, and contracts were let with the Pullman Company in September. It was then anticipated that a hospital train would consist of one government-owned unit car, two government-owned ward cars, a baggage car, and a variable number of standard Pullman or chair cars. The four ward cars were delivered in November and December 1941.[39] *(Table 17)*

When the Japanese attacked Pearl Harbor, the Army had two unit cars and four ward cars—enough government-owned equipment to serve as the nuclei of two hospital trains. The unit cars had not been used during 1941 because they were not air-conditioned and no ward cars were available for use with them. The ward cars just delivered had not been used either, but they had been favorably received by Medical Department officers who had seen them. Enough rail equipment for six additional hospital trains was needed, according to previous plans, for a full mobilization of the Army.[40]

Ward Dressing Cars Replace Unit Cars

Early in January 1942 the Surgeon General's Office began to plan for additional hospital cars. In the course of a few months the concept of the types of cars needed changed radically. Despite lack of experience with the new unit cars, the Surgeon General's Planning and Training Division decided to abandon them as a type. In view of earlier statements and subsequent experience it is probable that the following factors accounted for this decision. The unit car developed in 1940 had no space for patients. Capable of feeding up to 500 persons, its kitchen could be used to capacity only with trains consisting of about eighteen cars. On such trains, serving food from a unit car to patients in other cars was a real problem. Moreover, since patients transported in the United States did not normally require surgery en route, the operating room of the unit

[38] (1) Ltr, SG (Col Albert G. Love) to Hq 8th CA (Col A[lbert] P. Clark), 19 Mar 40. Off file, Research and Dev Bd SGO. "Unit Car." (2) Memo, Capt Bain for Brig Gen Albert G. Love, 6 Feb 41, sub: Hosp Unit Car. Same file.

[39] (1) Ltrs, SG to Pullman Co, Chicago, 4 Mar, 20 Mar, 2 May, and 9 May 41; Pullman Co to SG, 14 Mar, 22 Apr, 24 Apr, 5 May, and 27 May 41. SG: 453.-1. (2) Ltr, SG to CofEngrs, 31 May 41, sub: Hosp Ward Cars. CE: 453, pt 6. (3) Ltr, SG to TAG, 31 May 41, same sub, with 4 inds. SG: 453. (4) Memo, CofEngrs for QMG, 25 Nov 41, same sub. CE: 453, pt 6.

[40] (1) Rpt, Observer, Second and Third Army Maneuvers, Sabine-Red River-Louisiana-Area, 15–26 Sep 41. SG: 354.2-1 (Maneuvers, Gen). (2) Memo, SG for TAG, 6 May 40, sub: Hosp Unit Car. SG: 453.-1.

TABLE 17—HOSPITAL CAR PROCUREMENT PROGRAM, 1940–45

Ordered		Type of Car	Delivered	Numbers Assigned	Declared Surplus
Date	Number				
Total	380				
November 1940	2	Unit	February 1941	1 and 2 (Changed to 8200–8201, Jul 42 and to 89200–201, Aug 44)	November 1945–February 1946
September 1941	4	Ward	November - December 1941.	1–4 (Changed to 8900–8903, Jul 42).	November 1945–February 1946
March 1942	6	Ward Dressing	July–August 1942.	8917–8922 (Changed to 89000–005, Apr 43).	November 1945–February 1946
March 1942	12	Ward	July–August 1942.	8904–8915	November 1945–February 1946
January 1943	32	Ward Dressing	September - December 1943.	89006–89037	November 1945–February 1946
January 1943	64	Ward	September - December 1943.	8916–8979	November 1945–February 1946
August 1943	40	Kitchen	March - September 1944.	8731–8770	March–June 1946
May 1944	100	New Unit	November 1944–May 1945.	89300–89399	March–June 1946
January 1945	100	New Unit	May–August 1945.	89400–89499	Retained
February 1945	20	Kitchen	March–July 1945.	8711–8730	October - November 1945

Sources: Hosp. Cars in Interchange Service—All Standard Gauge. HD: 453.1 (Hosp. Car Procment). (2) Correspondence filed in AG Technical Records: SG 453.1 and 531.4; TC, same file numbers.

car was larger and more elaborate than was needed.[41]

To replace the unit car the Surgeon General's Office and the Pullman Company developed a ward dressing car in the early months of 1942. It contained a small surgical dressing room and space for thirty litter patients, but it lacked kitchen facilities. It differed from the ward car only in the replacement of a toilet and berths for two patients with an operating or dressing room. This room, which could also be used as a loading room, was equipped with an operating or dressing table, a washstand, a sterilizer, and a locker for surgical instruments. The dressing table could be used in the center of the room, moved down the aisle of the car to a patient's berth, or stored at the side of the car. Food would come from commercial dining cars. Thus the Medical Depart-

[41] (1) Rpt of MD Bd to consider MD Bd Project No 190, Hosp Unit Car, 8 Jul 41. SG: 453.-1. (2) Ltr, SG (Maj Thomas N. Page) to Pullman Co, 13 Jan 42. Off file, Research and Dev Bd SGO, "Hosp Ward Car." (3) Ltr, SG (Lt Col H[oward] T. Wickert) to Pullman Co, 13 Feb 42. SG: 453.-1. (4) Ltr, Lt Col Thomas N. Page to Modern Hosp Pub Co, Chicago, 1 Dec 42. Same file.

ment placed its reliance early in World War II, as it had in World War I before the unit car was developed, upon railroad and Pullman companies for feeding patients. Instead of stationary Simmons beds, two-tiered Glennan adjustable berths were to be used in both ward and ward dressing cars. Chief advantage of the latter was that upper berths could be pulled down to form backs for lower berths and thus make places for patients to sit. To provide enough government-owned equipment for six hospital trains, in addition to that already available for two, the Engineers ordered six ward dressing cars and twelve ward cars in March 1942. They were delivered to the Charleston, New Orleans, San Francisco, and New York Ports in July and August.[42] *(See Table 17.)*

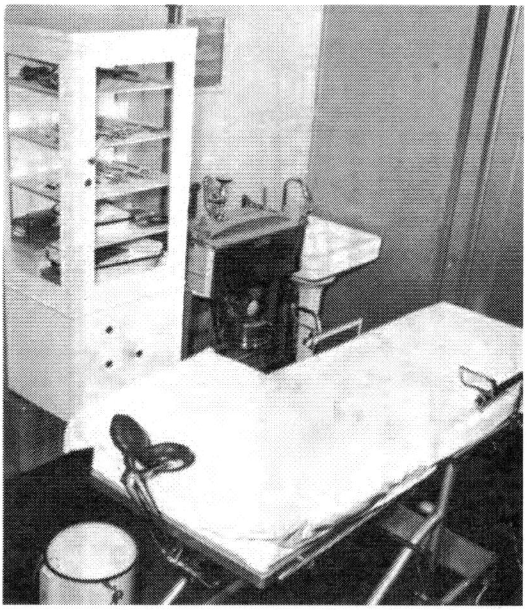

DRESSING ROOM IN HOSPITAL WARD DRESSING CAR, 1942

Air-Conditioning Hospital Cars

About a month before the new cars were delivered, the Surgeon General's Office initiated action to get them air-conditioned. In response to a hospital train commander's request, that Office asked SOS headquarters in June 1942 to have air-conditioning equipment installed in all hospital cars. Action on this request was delayed because of differences of opinion about the more desirable kind of equipment between the Surgeon General's Office on the one hand and the Engineers and the Transportation Corps on the other. Both the Engineers and the Transportation Corps favored the use of ice-activated air-conditioning equipment, apparently because it was simpler to install and because it was commonly used on Pullman cars at the time. The Surgeon General's Office preferred a type of mechanical air-conditioning equipment which was thought to insure more even temperatures and was not dependent upon batteries for operation when hospital cars were standing.[43] A mechanical system of this type, produced by Mountain Aire Products, Incorporated, was installed in one hospital car for testing in the fall of 1942. Subsequently, as a result of these tests, differences of opinion arose

[42] (1) Ltrs, Pullman Co to SG, 13 Jan, 26 Jan, 10 Feb 42, with blueprints, Plan 4103-A, 4103-B. SG: 453.-1. (2) Specifications for Remodeling 18 Pullman Parlor Cars to Hosp Ward Cars for WD, from Pullman Co, 30 Jan 42. Off file, Research and Dev Bd SGO, "Hosp Ward Cars."

[43] (1) Ltr, Med Sec 1927 CASU, Hosp Tn No 1 (San Francisco) to Surg 9th CA, 22 May 42, sub: Air-Conditioning for Hosp Tn No 1, with 5 inds. SG: 453.-1. (2) Memo SPOPM 673, ACofS for Oprs SOS for CofEngrs, 18 Jun 42, sub: Mechanical Air Conditioning for Unit Cars. Same file.

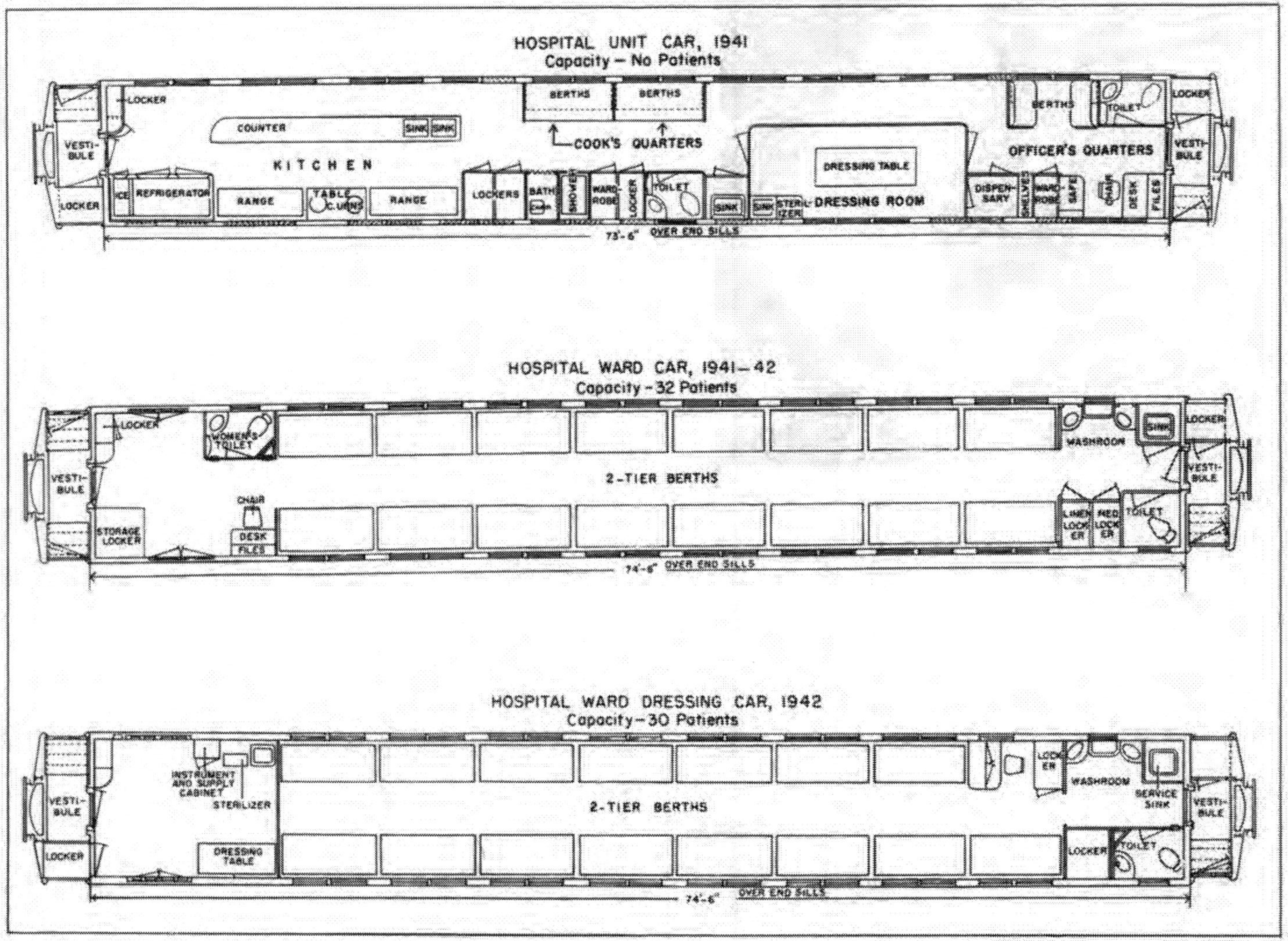

PLANS FOR HOSPITAL CARS, 1941–42

even within the Transportation Corps as to whether this or an ice-activated system was desirable but officially the Transportation Corps in December 1942 recommended installation of ice-activated systems and "declined to accept responsibility" for the performance of Mountain Aire systems. Despite this "veiled threat," the Surgeon General's Office requested that Mountain Aire equipment be installed in all ward and ward dressing.cars. SOS headquarters resolved this deadlock by directing the Chief of Transportation to install air-conditioning equipment in all cars and by allowing him to determine the type of equipment that would meet performance requirements recommended by The Surgeon General.[44] After the Transportation Corps and the Medical Department agreed upon desirable performance standards, the former in the spring of 1943 had ice-activated air-conditioning equipment installed in the ward and ward dressing cars which had been delivered during 1941 and 1942. The installation of such equipment in hospital cars ordered after the fall of 1942 raised no problem, because they were procured with the air-conditioning systems normally used by companies supplying the cars—some mechanical and some ice-activated.[45] Later, during 1945, the Mountain Aire system was removed from the car in which it had been installed and was replaced with an ice-activated system.[46] Toward the end of the war the Transportation Corps as well as the Surgeon General's Office came to prefer mechanical air-conditioning systems, because of the difficulty of icing cars en route and the fear of ice shortages, but they considered a change undesirable at that time lest it delay completion of additional cars being ordered.[47]

Disagreement About the Type and Number of Cars

Soon after the Surgeon General's Office first requested air-conditioning for hospital cars, SOS headquarters raised the question of whether those being procured were of the proper type and number. At that time neither the Surgeon General's Office nor SOS headquarters had had experience in the operation of hospital trains during World War II. Moreover, with the majority of troops still in training in the United States, the ultimate strength of theaters of operations and the number of casualties to be returned to the zone of interior were not yet fully envisioned. Nor was the strain which the war was to put on commercial transportation entirely comprehended. Nevertheless, officers concerned with secret planning for the North African invasion were anticipating the reception of casualties from that operation, and those intimately involved in transportation problems were beginning to be aware of some of the difficulties

[44] (1) Memo, Engr Bd for CofEngrs, 7 Oct 42, sub: Air Conditioning of Pullman Type Hosp Cars, with 2 inds. SG: 453.-1. (2) Memo, CofT (Rail Div) for SGO (Lt Col J. B. Klopp), 12 Dec 42, sub: Mountain Aire Air-Conditioning System, with 4 inds. Same file. (3) Memo, Col H. T. Wickert for Gen [Larry B.] McAfee, 5 Jan 43. Off file, Research and Dev Bd SGO, "Hosp Tns, Air Conditioning."

[45] (1) Memo, CofT (Rail Div) for SG (Col J. B. Klopp), 4 Feb 43, sub: Air Conditioning for Hosp Cars, with incl "Mil Characteristics of Air Conditioning for Hosp Cars." SG: 453.-1. (2) Ltr, CofT for CGs 1st, 2d, 3d, 4th, 8th, and 9th SvCs, 10 Feb 43, sub: Air Conditioning of Hosp Cars. TC: 531.4 (Hosp Cars).

[46] (1) Memo, CofT for SG, 21 Nov 44, sub: Air Conditioning on Ward Dressing Car 89002. SG: 453.1. (2) Memo, CofT (Rail Div) for Procmt Div OCT, Cincinnati, 13 Mar 45, sub: Cooling Syst on Hosp Car 89002. TC: 531.4.

[47] Memo, Sup Div OCT to Rail Div OCT, 19 Jan 45. TC: 531.4.

railroads would encounter in meeting transportation needs of both the civilian population and the armed forces. In this atmosphere the Assistant Chief of Staff for Operations of SOS headquarters, to whose Hospitalization and Evacuation Branch a Medical Corps officer, Lt. Col. William C. Keller, had recently been assigned for the purpose of advising on rail evacuation, issued a directive on 23 July 1942 that provoked a re-examination of the hospital train program. It called upon the Engineers to develop a new type of hospital car, called a rail ambulance car, and suggested that twenty-seven of them—three for each of the nine service commands—should be procured by 1 January 1943. The reason for this directive, apparently, was a belief in SOS headquarters, first, that the hospital cars being procured were of an unsatisfactory type because they had to be supplemented with commercial Pullmans, sleepers, diners, and baggage cars, and second, that available railway facilities would be inadequate when patients began to arrive from theaters in large numbers. The proposed car was to have spaces for twenty to thirty-three patients, depending upon whether berths were two- or three-tiered; quarters for medical attendants, including one officer, one nurse, and four enlisted men; kitchen facilities capable of feeding both patients and attendants; and a dressing room and pharmacy. Because of a developing shortage of Pullman cars and tourist sleepers, lounge cars were to be used for conversion. Each lounge car thus converted would decrease demands of the Medical Department for commercial sleepers and would, at the same time, relieve the railway dining service of some of its load. From seven to eighteen cars of this type could make up complete hospital trains; or single cars, attached to regularly scheduled trains, could move patients in small groups.[48]

The Surgeon General objected both to the proposed type of car and to the suggestion that additional hospital cars were needed. He pointed out that small numbers of patients could still be moved in Pullman cars of regularly scheduled trains. For the mass movement of patients he preferred a complete train made up of government-owned ward and ward dressing cars and commercial baggage, sleeping, and dining cars to one consisting entirely of government-owned rail ambulance cars. A train of the latter type, he contended, was wasteful of both personnel and equipment. One having 10 cars would have 10 dressing rooms and 10 kitchens and would require 10 officers, 10 nurses, and 40 enlisted men. The Surgeon General stated that patients were not put on trains until doctors felt reasonably sure that they would need little treatment in transit. Hence so many dressing rooms were not needed. Moreover, he believed that regular dining car service could be used for feeding patients either in Pullman cars of regularly scheduled trains or in the cars of complete hospital trains. In his opinion the transportation of sick and wounded would rate so high a priority that the Medical Department would always be able to get sufficient commercial cars for its use. Furthermore, the Surgeon General's Office opposed the use of three-tiered berths because it was difficult to get litter patients into the top one.[49]

[48] (1) Memo SPOPM 370.05, ACofS for Oprs SOS for CofEngrs thru SG, 23 Jul 42, sub: Proposed Rail Amb Car. SG: 322.2-5.

[49] 1st ind, SG to CofEngrs, 1 Aug 42, on Memo SPOPM 370.05, ACofS for Oprs SOS for CofEngrs thru SG, 23 Jul 42, sub: Proposed Rail Amb Car; also 2d ind, CofEngrs to CG SOS thru SG, 24 Aug 42; and 3d ind, SG to CG SOS, 29 Aug 42 (init Col H. T. Wickert). SG: 322.2-5.

After first stating that the eight hospital trains which his Office had planned would be sufficient, The Surgeon General reviewed requirements about a month and a half later and concluded in October 1942 that additional trains would be needed. On the basis of four litter patients per 1,000 troops per month from a total overseas strength of 2,500,000, he estimated that 10,000 litter patients would have to be moved from ports to hospitals each month. The eight trains (twenty-four cars) already planned, making three 1,000-mile trips per month, could move 2,160 litter patients per month. For the remainder, The Surgeon General estimated that thirty-two additional hospital trains would be needed. He recommended, therefore, that instead of rail ambulance cars thirty-two ward dressing cars and sixty-four ward cars be procured.[50] This recommendation, as well as types of hospital cars in general, was discussed on 9 October 1942 in a conference of representatives of the Surgeon General's Office, the Engineers, the Transportation Corps, and the SOS Hospitalization and Evacuation Branch.[51] The Surgeon General later expressed the belief that this conference had settled the issue in favor of ward and ward dressing cars.

Before giving The Surgeon General's recommendations formal approval, SOS headquarters asked the Transportation Corps about the prospective availability of commercial diners and sleepers. In this connection it called attention to World War I experience, especially to difficulties in feeding patients.[52] In reply the Transportation Corps emphasized the burden already placed upon commercial dining car service by wartime travel and troop movements and, in addition, raised a new point. Instead of using one ward dressing and two ward cars as the nucleus of a complete hospital train, the Transportation Corps proposed that one rail ambulance car be used for that purpose. If this should be done only 32 hospital cars would be needed, instead of 96, and the remaining 64 cars could be used for regular troop movements.[53] It seems that the Transportation Corps believed that commercial dining cars would not be available in sufficient numbers but that Pullman and tourist sleepers would. SOS headquarters therefore decided not to approve The Surgeon General's recommendation, but directed the Engineers instead to procure thirty-two self-contained rail ambulance cars.[54]

The Surgeon General's Office, which "considered the controversial matter [of the types and numbers of hospital cars required] finally settled" by the 9 October 1942 conference, was displeased with this action and on 18 November asked for another conference "to arrive at a complete and final decision." [55] During that meeting The Surgeon General's representative stated that he preferred ward

[50] 4th ind SPOPH 322.15, ACofS for Oprs SOS to SG, 25 Sep 42; 5th ind SPMCP 322.2-5, SG to CG SOS, 10 Oct 42, on Memo SPOPM 370.05, ACofS for Oprs SOS for CofEngrs thru SG, 23 Jul 42, sub: Proposed Rail Amb Car. SG: 322.2-5.

[51] Rpt, Conf, 9 Oct 42, sub: Adequacy of Hosp Tn Equip. SG: 453.-1.

[52] Memo SPOPH 322.15, CG SOS for CofT, 22 Oct 42, sub: Rail Amb Cars. TC: 531.4.

[53] (1) Memo, Mvmts Div OCT for Maj Gen C[harles] P. Gross, 29 Oct 42, sub: Rail Hosp Tns. TC: 531.4. (2) Memo, CofT (Maj Gen C. P. Gross) for ACofS for Oprs SOS, 30 Oct 42, sub: Rail Amb Cars. Same file.

[54] 6th ind SPOPH 370.05, ACofS for Oprs SOS to CofEngrs thru SG, 6 Nov 42, on Memo SPOPM 370.05, ACofS for Oprs SOS for CofEngrs thru SG, 23 Jul 42, sub: Proposed Rail Amb Car. SG: 453.-1.

[55] (1) Diary, SOS Hosp and Evac Br (Keller), 16 Nov 42. HD: Wilson files, "Diary." (2) Memo, SG for CG SOS, 18 Nov 42. HRS: Hq ASF Control Div file, "Evac."

and ward dressing cars, regardless of the number procured, to rail ambulance cars. In addition the Surgeon General's Office went on record as preferring to feed patients from kitchens improvised in railway baggage cars, if diners should not be available, rather than to agree to the procurement of rail ambulance cars. After this conference SOS headquarters reversed its decision and on 24 November directed the Transportation Corps to procure not less than forty and, if practical, as many as ninety-six ward and ward dressing cars. Contracts for the higher number were let in January 1943.[56] *(See Table 17.)*

Development of a Hospital Train for Overseas Use

In the course of discussions about the numbers and types of hospital cars needed for the zone of interior, the question of trains for theaters of operations came up. Before mid-1942 the Engineers had switched from a 20- to a 40-ton car as the standard for overseas military trains. After studying blueprints and proposals for 40-ton cars, the Surgeon General's Office and the SOS Hospitalization and Evacuation Branch agreed in August 1942 to use them in hospital trains built for theaters of operations.[57] Following Medical Department recommendations, the Engineers completed preliminary drawings and specifications for a combat-zone hospital train of twenty-one 40-ton cars (operating, personnel, kitchen, and ward cars) by the end of November 1942. The Surgeon General's Office then suggested changes in the proposed specifications and in January 1943 recommended to the Chief of Transportation that one train of 40-ton cars should be constructed immediately for service testing and that all trains included in the Army supply program should be procured as soon as possible after completion of such tests.[58]

In February 1943 the Army supply program included forty overseas hospital trains of twenty-one cars each for procurement in 1943 and 1944, but none had been ordered and SOS headquarters doubted that these figures actually represented requirements. The SOS Hospitalization and Evacuation Branch therefore conferred on 18 February 1943 with representatives of the SOS Requirements Division, the Surgeon General's Office, and the Transportation Corps. The Surgeon General's representative informed SOS headquarters that only fifteen overseas trains would be needed in 1943 and five more in 1944. On 23 February 1943 SOS headquarters directed Transportation Corps to procure that number, plus one additional train of ten cars for experimental and training purposes. Soon afterward the War Department learned that the European theater was procuring twenty-three hospital trains in the United Kingdom and on 8 April 1943 the Surgeon General's Office requested the Transportation Corps to have only the experimental train constructed.[59]

---

[56] (1) Memo SPAOG 370.05, ACofS for Oprs SOS for CofT, 24 Nov 42, sub: Ward Cars (Med). TC: 531.4. (2) Memo SPMC 322.2–5, SG for CG SOS, 25 Nov 42. Same file.

[57] (1) Diary, SOS Hosp and Evac Br (Keller), 6–7 Aug 42. HD: Wilson files, "Diary." (2) Memo, ACofS for Oprs SOS for CofT, 10 Aug 42, sub: Conf on Rail Evac. HD: Wilson files, "Book I, 26 Mar 42–26 Sep 42."

[58] 2d ind. SG to CofT (Rail Div), 8 Jan 43, on Memo, Engr Bd for CofT (Rail Div), 30 Nov 42, sub: Lightweight, Combat Zone, Hosp Tn, with 10 drawings and 10 specifications. SG: 453.–1.

[59] (1) Memo, SOS Reqmts Div for SOS Plans Div Hosp and Evac Br, 11 Feb 43, sub: Hosp Cars, with Memo for Record. AG: 531.43 (9–29–42). (2) Memo, SOS Reqmts Div for CofT, 23 Feb 43. AG: 322.38. (3) Memo, CofT for SG, 25 Mar 43, sub: Hosp Tn for Tng Purposes, with 2 inds. SG: 453.–1.

During the latter half of 1943 this train was completed and exhibited to the public on a cross-country trip. It was then used for the evacuation of patients from the California-Arizona Maneuver Area, returned to Hampton Roads for two test runs, sent to Camp Ellis (Illinois) for use in training hospital train units, returned to the manufacturer for the correction of deficiencies, and displayed as a part of the Fifth War Bond Drive in New York City. Complaints about the mechanical aspects of the train were numerous, but the most important from the viewpoint of patient evacuation were that the ward cars were poorly ventilated, crowded even when they carried a normal load of patients (sixteen in each car), and uncomfortably rough even at speeds of less than thirty-five miles per hour.[60] Finding no further need for this train in the United States, the Technical Division of the Surgeon General's Office in July 1944 drafted messages in which the War Department queried the European and North African theaters as to whether or not they could use it. The latter agreed to accept the train and in September 1944 it was taken to Hampton Roads for shipment to southern France.[61]

Improvement of Existing Cars and Procurement of Kitchen Cars

In late 1942 and the first half of 1943, while the types and numbers of hospital cars needed for the zone of interior were being discussed and the program for trains for theaters was being re-examined, experience made it possible to evaluate the hospital unit, ward, and ward dressing cars. The unit cars had proved to be of little use, for reasons already explained. Ward and ward dressing cars appeared to fulfill their purposes and required only minor modification, such as the installation of storage lockers, floor lights, bulletin boards, and bedside holders for patients' food trays. These changes were incorporated in specifications for new cars. They were also made in the ward and ward dressing cars already delivered.[62]

Two major problems in the operation of hospital trains appeared: safeguarding neuropsychiatric patients during transit and feeding patients and medical attendants from commercial diners. Hospital train commanders found that in transporting mentally disturbed patients either restraints and sedation had to be used or additional attendants had to be assigned. As a partial solution to this problem, they recommended the use of wire screens inside car windows.[63] Throughout late 1943 and early 1944, the Medical Department collaborated with the Transportation Corps and the Pullman Company in developing a standard screen to meet this need. It was made of heavy mesh wire and was designed to fit inside the windows of standard tourist and Pullman cars. It was re-

[60] (1) Memo, Col I. Sewell Morris, OCT for Mvmt Div OCT, 4 Nov 43, sub: Hosp Tn for Calif-Ariz Maneuver Area. HD: 453.1 (10-Car Hosp Tn, Overseas). (2) Ltr, CO 3d Hosp Tn to SG, 15 Dec 43. TC: 531.4. (3) Memo, CofT for SG, 20 Apr 44, sub: Ten-Car Hosp Tn. . . . SG: 453.-1. (4) Ltr, CofT to SG, 4 Apr 44, sub: Hosp Tn, Contract W-2789-tc-1201. TC: 531.4.

[61] (1) Draft rad prepared by Tec Div SGO for dispatch to ETO, 1 Jul 44. SG: 322 (Hosp Tn)H. (2) Weekly Diary, Tec Div SGO, 29 Jul-4 Aug 44. HD: 453.1 (10-Car Hosp Tn, Overseas). (3) Routing Forms, AAR, 13 Sep 44. TC: 511 "Main 39595."

[62] (1) Memo, SG for CofT, 4 Mar 43, sub: Hosp Car Changes. SG: 453.-1. (2) Memo SPTSY 453, CofT for SG, 8 Mar 43, sub: Hosp Cars, with Rpt of Insp of Cars being Air-Conditioned. Off file, Research and Dev Bd SGO, "Hosp Tns, Air Conditioning."

[63] (1) Ltr, Hq 2d SvC to Hosp Tn No 2, Ft Monmouth, N.J., and Hosp Tn No 1, Tilton Gen Hosp, Ft Dix, N.J., 3 Apr 43, with 4 inds. SG: 322.2-5. (2) See other train reports, SG: 322.2-5 and TC: 531.4 (Hosp Tn Mvmts).

movable and could be locked in place by means of the standard bunk key carried by all Pullman porters. Issued on the basis of a set of thirty-two (enough for one car) for each hospital train, these guards were helpful in preventing patients from hurting themselves on car windows and from attempting to escape.[64]

The feeding problem was more complicated. Train commanders were almost unanimous in complaints about difficulties of feeding patients from commercial diners. These diners often failed to meet Army standards of sanitation, carried no foods for special diets, served meals that became monotonous, provided midmorning or midafternoon nourishment for patients only at excessive costs, were not open for meals for attendants on night duty, and were often uncoupled at junction points, leaving both patients and attendants without meals for the remainder of their journeys.[65] Moreover, the fear that dining cars would be unavailable for all needs—expressed by SOS headquarters and the Transportation Corps in the fall of 1942—was becoming a reality. The entire problem was discussed in February 1943 in a series of conferences on railway rates between railroad officials and representatives of the Surgeon General's Office, the Transportation Corps, and the SOS Hospitalization and Evacuation Branch. At that time the railroads agreed to supply hospital trains with dining cars or, if diners were not available, with baggage cars that could be used as kitchen cars.[66] Soon afterward the Transportation Corps asked the General Staff for authority to convert twenty-one idle Coast Artillery kitchen cars into hospital kitchen cars. After spending several months modifying and testing one, the Medical Department and the Transportation Corps decided that they were too small and lightweight to operate with fast passenger trains. In July 1943, therefore, they agreed to seek authority to procure forty kitchen cars of the type being built for use with troop trains. Since cars in that number would provide one kitchen car for each group of three ward and ward dressing cars—the same ratio by which kitchen cars were provided for troop cars—ASF headquarters approved the request on 16 August 1943. By December one hospital kitchen car was delivered for service testing, and the remainder, incorporating minor changes made as a result of this test, were delivered during 1944.[67] *(See Table 17.)*

Development of a "New-Type" Unit Car

Within two months after ASF headquarters approved the procurement of hospital kitchen cars and before all ward

[64] (1) Ltr, SG (Tec Cmtee) to CG ASF (Reqmts Div), 22 Jul 43, sub: Window Guards for Hosp Tns. SG: 453.1. (2) Ltr, SG to MD Equip Lab, 15 Sep 43, sub: Window Guards for Tourist and Hosp Ward Cars. Same file. (3) Ltr, SG for CGs all SvCs, 26 Apr 44, sub: Window Guards for Hosp Tns. SG: 453.1 (SvCs).

[65] Reports of hospital train movements are replete with descriptions of difficulties involved. See TC: 531.4 (Hosp Tn Rpts) and scattered rpts in SG: 322.2-5 and 453.1.

[66] (1) Ltr, Interterritorial Mil Cmtee Rail Carriers to CofT (Tfc Control Div), 25 Jan 43, with incls. TC: 531.4. (2) Diary, SOS Hosp and Evac Br (Keller), 24-26 Feb 43. HD: Wilson files, "Diary." (3) Ltr, Interterritorial Mil Cmtee Rail Carriers to SG, 6 Apr 43, with incl. SG: 453.1. (4) Memo W55-33-43, sub: Trans of Hosp Cars and Tns, 10 Aug 43. AG: 531.4 (6 Aug 43).

[67] (1) Memo, CofT (Tfc Control Div) for ACofS OPD WDGS, 2 Mar 43, sub: Kitchen Cars. TC: 531.4. (2) Memo, SG for CofT, 7 May 43, same sub. Same file. (3) Memo, SG for CofT, 29 Jul 43, same sub. SG: 453.1. (4) Memo, Dep Dir of Oprs ASF for CofT, 16 Aug 43, same sub. HD: Wilson files, "Day File, Aug 43." (5) Rpt, 1247 SCSU for CG 2d SvC, 23 Dec 43, sub: Rpt of USA Kitchen Car, 8731. Same file.

and ward dressing cars already ordered had been delivered, the Surgeon General's Office in October 1943 requested that additional cars of still another type be provided. The reason was that a change was gradually being made in the distribution of patients among general hospitals. Establishment of a policy of caring for patients from theaters of operations in hospitals near their homes and designation of particular hospitals for the specialized treatment of certain disabilities meant that patients arriving on a single ship would be distributed among many different general hospitals. For a time the practice of sending a complete trainload of patients (from 200 to 300) to one general hospital continued, and it was often necessary to retransfer patients to other hospitals. During the latter half of 1943, however, the Second Service Command began to try to send patients directly from the debarkation hospital in New York to the general hospitals in which they would receive treatment. This was done by making up trains in sections which could be cut off at intermediate points for routing to different general hospitals. Each section consisted of a combination of ward cars, ward dressing cars, and commercial sleeping cars. The chief difficulty encountered in this practice was in feeding patients. Until kitchen cars were delivered, the entire train had to depend upon uncertain commercial dining car service. Even if kitchen cars had been available, each section separated from the main train would have still been dependent upon commercial dining service.[68] On 15 October 1943, therefore, the Surgeon General's Office requested the Transportation Corps to provide fifty "new type unit cars" by May 1944. These cars, for which a sketch had been drawn by the Hospital Construction Branch, were to be similar to the rail ambulance car designed by the Engineers in the fall of 1942.[69] They were to be used as parts of complete hospital trains; for secondary movements from the main, or primary routes of hospital trains; and for the transportation of small groups of patients on nonhospital trains. Although ASF headquarters had formerly advocated the use of such cars, it replied in November 1943 that no new developmental project should be started unless it was essential to winning the war and directed, as a preliminary step to further action on The Surgeon General's request, an evaluation of the passenger traffic problem with particular reference to the transportation of patients. The next month this headquarters modified its position by authorizing the conversion of the two unit cars that had been delivered to the Army in 1941 into pilot models for the new type.[70]

Reappraisal of the Hospital Train Program

Before the pilot models were completed for service testing, the Surgeon General's Office re-examined the entire hospital train program. Early in 1944, it will be recalled, a group in this Office had completed a detailed study of the anticipated patient load.[71] It was estimated that 30,000 patients per month would have to be moved by train by October 1944 and that at least 75 percent of them would have to be moved in government-owned

[68] (1) Ltr, CO 1247 SCSU 2d SvC to SG, 2 Oct 43, sub: Cons of Hosp Unit Cars. TC: 531.4. (2) Memo, CofT for SG, 23 Sep 43, sub: Govt-Owned Hosp Cars, with 1 ind. Same file.

[69] Memo, SG for CofT, 15 Oct 43, sub: Unit Car, New Type, with Drawing (7 Oct 43). TC: 531.4. See above, pp. 377–80.

[70] Memo, SG for CofT, 18 Sep 43 (corrected 18 Oct 43), sub: Unit Car, New Type, with 5 inds. TC: 531.4.

[71] See above, pp. 323–25.

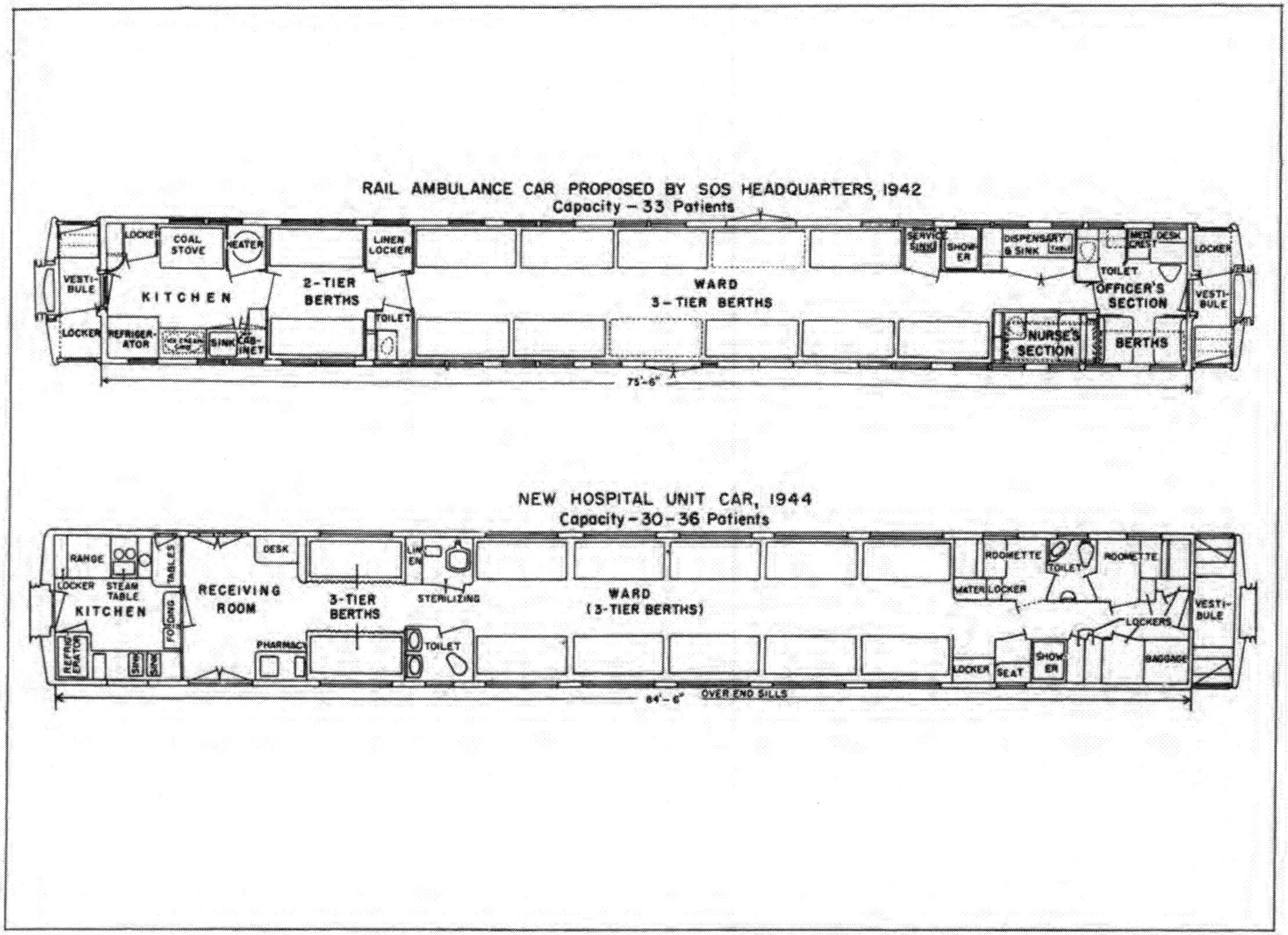

PLANS FOR RAIL AMBULANCE CAR AND NEW HOSPITAL UNIT CAR

cars. Assuming that each car could carry twenty-five patients per trip and could make four trips per month, 225 cars would be needed. Since 120 were already available or authorized, The Surgeon General requested 105 additional hospital cars of the new unit type. At the same time he asked that buffet kitchens be installed in all ward and ward dressing cars. The Transportation Corps agreed with The Surgeon General as to the type of cars desired but believed, on the basis of a study just made, that as many as 200 additional hospital cars would be needed. On 11 April 1944 representatives of ASF headquarters, the Surgeon General's Office, and the Transportation Corps agreed that it would be quicker and more economical to construct new cars than to try to lease commercial cars for conversion. Two weeks later ASF headquarters approved both the alteration of ward and ward dressing cars and the procurement of 100 new cars. Additional ones would not be authorized, it was stated, until military requirements became "firmer."[72] Contracts for altering old cars and building new ones were let with the American Car and Foundry Company in May 1944, and by late fall of that year cars of both types were ready for trial runs.[73]

The new unit car was similar to the unit car of World War I and to the rail ambulance car proposed in 1942 in that it had space for both patients and attendants as well as facilities for caring for patients and for feeding all passengers. It was different in that it was built specifically as a hospital car, instead of being converted from existing rolling stock, and was equipped "with every travel luxury." Ten feet longer than Pullman cars, its body was of steel and was mounted on easy-riding six-wheel trucks. At one end was a stainless steel kitchen, with a refrigerator, an ice cream cabinet, a coal range, sinks, a steam table, and a coffee urn. Both the press and the Army called this the "principal innovation in the new car." Next to the kitchen was a pharmacy and receiving room, with wide doors on each side for loading litter patients. This room could be used also as an emergency operating or dressing room. Adjoining it were two sets of three-tiered berths that could be used for seriously ill patients, for mental patients, or for medical attendants. This section was separated from the main ward by a sterilizer room on one side of the car and a toilet and washroom on the other. The main ward section had a row of five three-tiered Glennan-type berths on each side. They could be adjusted to provide seating space, or the two lower berths could be used for litter patients and the upper berth for ambulatory patients or attendants. Between the main ward and the vestibule were storage lockers and a shower bath on one side of the car, and a roomette each for an officer and a nurse on the other. Each car was carpeted, equipped with special lighting fixtures, and air-conditioned.[74] Although less luxurious and lacking specific accommodations for doctors and nurses, hospital ward and ward dressing cars, after the installation of the kitchenettes in space made available by removal of berths for four patients, could be used in much

[72] Memo, SG for CG ASF, 30 Mar 44, sub: Hosp Cars, ZI, with 4 inds. SG: 322.2-5 and TC: 453.9.

[73] (1) TC-3066, Specifications for Cons of Car, Hosp, 8 May 44. Off file, Research and Dev Bd SGO, "Unit Car, New Type." (2) Memo, CofT (Reqmts Div) for CG ASF (Dir of Mat), 14 Jun 44, sub: Hosp Cars, ZI, with 3 inds. SG: 322.2-5.

[74] (1) *Railway Age*, Vol. 117, No. 26 (1944), pp. 964-66. (2) American Car and Foundry Company, Report to Workers, pp. 76-79. Lib Congress. (3) For details of development see files SG: 453.1, TC: 531.4, and Off file, Research and Dev Bd SGO, "Hosp Unit Car."

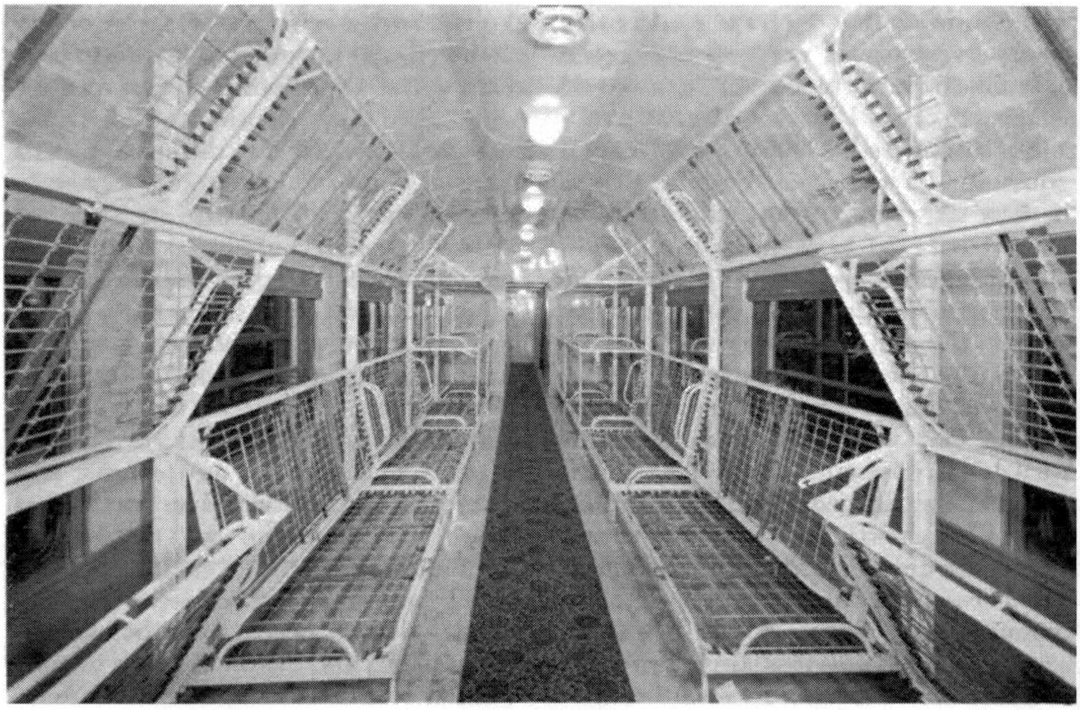

WARD IN NEW HOSPITAL UNIT CAR, 1944 *(note adjustable berths).*

the same way as the new unit cars. Thus by the end of the war, the Medical Department had what were in effect only two types of hospital cars: unit cars and kitchen cars.

With development of the new unit car and modification of ward and ward dressing cars, a change occurred in hospital train movements. Gradually the practice developed of making up hospital trains for a number of destinations and of including in them variable numbers of hospital cars in different combinations. Ordinarily, regardless of the inclusion of hospital cars with kitchen facilities, hospital kitchen cars were used for feeding all patients so long as a number of hospital cars remained attached to the train. This practice was followed because it was more efficient to prepare food in one place than in many different places. All cars of a hospital train did not proceed to the same destination. At "gateways" (railway junctions) separate cars were cut away from the main route and were attached to commercial trains to carry loads of patients to different destinations. After delivering initial loads, cars were often diverted to transport additional groups of patients from one general hospital to another before being used again as parts of a complete hospital train. Whenever cars were separated from hospital trains, their buffet kitchens were used to feed patients.[75] Thus the hospital cars

[75] (1) Rpts, Hosp Tn Conf, 15–16 Feb 45, Miller Fld, SI, N.Y.; 10–13 Jul 45, Presidio of San Francisco. HD: 531.4 (Conf). (2) Records of hospital train movements, filed in OCT, Tfc Control Div, form OCT 145.

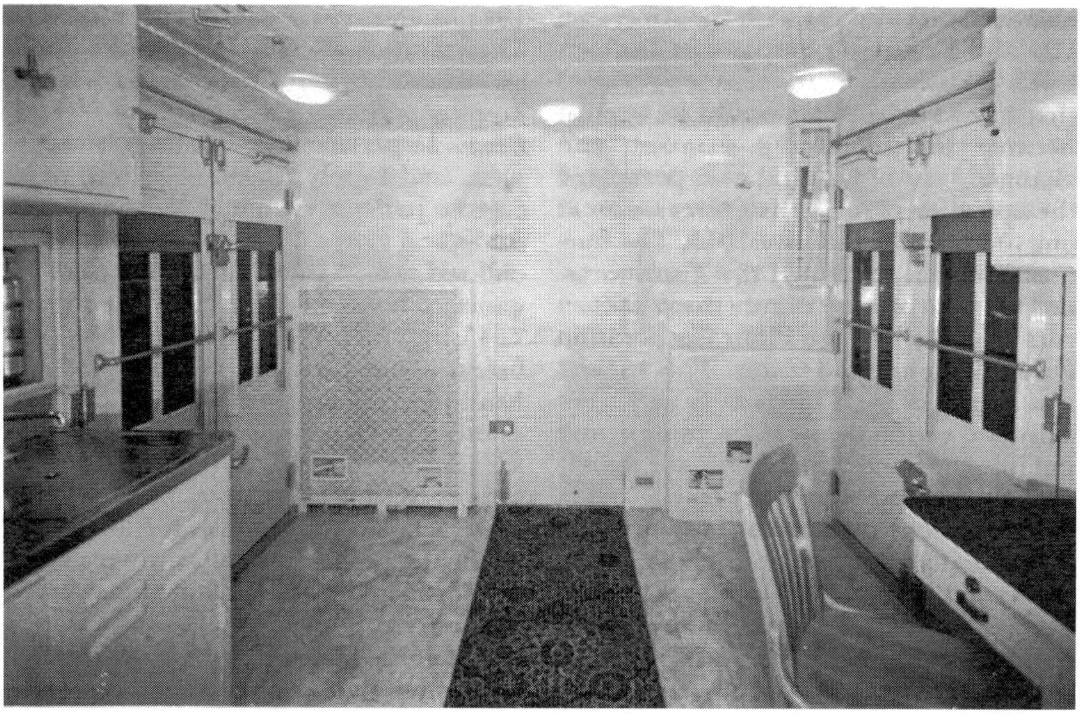

RECEIVING ROOM IN NEW HOSPITAL UNIT CAR, 1944

finally in use in World War II possessed an adaptability which permitted them to be used along with other cars to make up a complete hospital train or singly to transport small groups of patients on commercial trains.

Procurement of Additional Hospital Cars

In the winter of 1944–45 the Surgeon General's Office reviewed the anticipated patient load and re-estimated the hospital and evacuation facilities that would be required. On the assumption that V–E Day would occur in June 1945, it was estimated in December 1944 that the number of patients returned to the United States each month from January through August 1945 would range from 32,000 to 36,000 and would decrease thereafter.[76] A drop in the patient load would result in no less need for hospital cars, for after V–E Day the major portion of patients would arrive at Pacific ports and a car operating from one of them could make fewer round trips and carry fewer patients per month, because of the greater distance to general hospitals, than could one from an Atlantic port. At the same time, railroads were finding it increasingly difficult to supply the Army with enough commercial cars of the desired type. To assure adequate numbers of hospital cars, the Surgeon General's Office on 19 December 1944 asked for 100 additional unit cars as soon as possible. ASF headquarters approved this request,

[76] See above, pp. 327–28.

and contracts were let with the American Car and Foundry Company in January 1945.[77] Meanwhile, it became apparent that more kitchen cars would be needed because the increasing number and changed type of hospital cars permitted the operation of more than forty trains at one time. On 22 January 1945, The Surgeon General requested the Transportation Corps to procure twenty troop kitchen cars from the Defense Plant Corporation for use with hospital trains. This request was approved, and the twenty cars were delivered within the next few months and put into use immediately, without significant alterations.[78] *(See Table 17.)*

The peak of the patient load arriving from theaters of operations came before the second group of 100 unit cars was delivered. In May 1945, when the greatest number of patients in any single month arrived, the Army was using 120 old cars and 100 new unit cars, plus almost 60 kitchen cars. During that month, 47,044 patients were moved by train. This required the use of 1,200 Pullman cars to supplement government-owned cars.[79] Thereafter, the number of patients declined rapidly and by late August 1945, when the last of the cars ordered in January had been delivered, the Medical Department declared surplus thirty-six modified ward and ward dressing cars. After V–J Day the decline in the patient load permitted the disposal of additional cars and by the middle of 1946 the Medical Department retained only 100 unit cars.[80] *(See Table 17.)*

Problems in Manning Hospital Trains

At the beginning of the war the Medical Department had a table of organization for a hospital train unit. Revised early in 1942, it was reissued in April as Table of Organization 8–520. It provided for a self-sustaining unit to operate a complete hospital train with a capacity of 360 patients. To perform its own administrative, mess, and supply functions as well as to care for patients, each unit was authorized 4 Medical Corps officers, 6 nurses, and 33 enlisted men.[81] Eight such units were organized between June 1942 and June 1943, and for a short time there was confusion about their purpose both in SOS headquarters and among service commands. In September 1942, on recommendation of the Surgeon General's Office, SOS headquarters made it clear that such units were intended for service in theaters of operations and were to be employed in the United States on training trips only.[82]

About the same time, there was concern about attendants for patients being transported by train in the United States. After the North African invasion, casualties began to arrive in increasing numbers. Furthermore, hospital cars which the Army had ordered early in 1942 were delivered

[77] (1) History . . . Medical Regulating Service . . . , Tab 5, Hospital Trains. (2) Memo, SG for CG ASF (Planning Div) thru CofT, 19 Dec 44, sub: Hosp Cars, ZI, with incl. SG: 322.2-5. (3) Memo, ASF Planning Div for ASF Reqmts and Stock Control Div, 21 Dec 44, same sub. HRS: ASF Planning Div Program Br file, "Hosp and Evac."

[78] (1) Memo, SG for CofT (Rail Div), 22 Jan 45, sub: MD Kitchen Cars. SG: 453.1. (2) Memo, Maj R. W. Tonning (OCT) for Rail Div OCT, 18 Jun 45, sub: Conv of 20 Trp Kitchen Cars. TC: 531.4.

[79] Information supplied by Troop Movements and Records Section, Traffic Control Branch, Passenger Division, OCT.

[80] (1) Memos, SG for CofT (Mil Ry Serv), 27 Sep 45, 27 Feb 46, and 2 Apr 46, sub: Release of Surplus Hosp Cars. SG: 453.

[81] T/O 8–506, 1 Nov 40; T/O 8–520, 1 Apr 42.

[82] (1) An Rpt, Oprs Serv SGO, 1943. HD. (2) 2d ind, CG SOS to CG 4th SvC, 22 Sep 42, with Memo for Record, on Memo, CG 4th SvC for CG SOS, 29 Aug 42, sub: Hosp Tn. AG: 322.38.

and in August the entire fleet of twenty-four were assigned to service commands.[83] In discharging responsibility for manning them, service commands encountered difficulty in determining how many doctors, nurses, and enlisted men were needed. SOS directives instructed them to use as a guide Table of Organization 8–520, but it applied to an entirely different situation. In the zone of interior hospital trains were to be composed of three hospital cars supplemented with such common-carrier equipment as Pullmans, diners, and baggage cars. They carried varying numbers of patients and depended upon the railroads in the early part of the war for mess service. To supply service command surgeons with a more appropriate guide, SOS headquarters on 24 December 1942 directed The Surgeon General to prepare a manning table for zone of interior hospital trains. Submitted six days later, this table indicated that 2 doctors, 1 nurse, and 14 enlisted men were needed for 100 patients; 2 doctors, 1 nurse, and 16 enlisted men for 200 patients; 3 doctors, 1 nurse, and 19 enlisted men for 300 patients; and 3 doctors, 1 nurse, and 21 enlisted men for 400 patients. Soon afterward SOS headquarters directed the Second Service Command—and presumably others—to use this guide in requisitioning personnel for use aboard hospital trains.[84]

As experience accumulated in transporting increasingly large numbers of patients, ASF headquarters in August 1943 issued a new guide—Table of Distribution 8–1520—which differed from the one prepared by the Surgeon General's Office in December 1942. Whereas the old guide had covered groups of patients ranging by hundreds from 100 to 400, the new one covered groups increasing by twenty-fours from 118 to 358. This change reflected the growing tendency to send small groups of patients to different hospitals instead of making mass movements from a port to one or two hospitals only. The old guide had called for 2 doctors, 1 nurse, and 16 enlisted men for 200 patients; the new one called for 3 doctors, 1 administrative officer, 3 nurses, and 11 to 16 enlisted men for 190.[85] Despite a moderate increase in personnel in the new guide, it proved inadequate, at least in one service command, and was not followed. During the period from 15 March 1944 through 12 May 1944, seventeen hospital trains evacuated patients from Stark General Hospital in the Fourth Service Command. Each carried an average of 190 patients and had assigned as attendants an average of 6 doctors, 3 administrative officers, 5 nurses, and 57 enlisted men.[86] Presumably other service commands also were free to use more attendants than the guide called for.

Another problem which service commands encountered was the manner in which train personnel should be handled administratively. Until the middle of 1943 all commands assigned such personnel to station or general hospitals. Difficulties caused by this procedure were illustrated by the experience of the Second Service

[83] See above, pp. 349, 375.

[84] (1) Ltr SPOPH 322.15, CG SOS to CGs and COs of SvCs and PEs, and to SG, 15 Sep 42, sub: Mil Hosp and Evac Oprs, with incl. AG: 704. (2) 2d ind, CG SOS to SG, 24 Dec 42, with Memo for Record; 3d ind, SG to CG SOS, 30 Dec 42, with incl; and 4th ind, CG SOS to CG 2d SvC, 5 Jan 43, with Memo for Record, on Memo, CG SOS for CG 2d SvC, 21 Nov 42, sub: Auth to Activate Two Hosp Tns. AG: 320.2 (11-21-42).

[85] (1) T/D 8-1520, 12 Aug 43, Hosp Tn, ZI. (2) See pp. 347–48.

[86] Memo, 1st Lt Theodore Kemp, Control Div [4th SvC] for Maj Maxwell, 5 Jun 44, sub: Pers Reqmts for Hosp Tn. HD: 531.4 (Pers Reqmts). There is no indication in the document cited as to the organization to which Major Maxwell was assigned.

Command. For example, officers, nurses, and enlisted men used to operate one of its trains were assigned to Halloran General Hospital. This hospital assigned them to ward duties, maintained their records, paid them, and considered them administratively a part of the hospital staff. In consequence, nurses and enlisted men often worked on wards until the departure time of trains, without opportunities to rest and prepare themselves for trips. To get enlisted men released from ward duties for train trips, the train commander had to request the permission of the commanding officer of the hospital medical detachment who, in turn, had to request permission of the chief of the section for whom these men worked in the hospital. Officers who were assigned to wards lost contact with patients they left behind while away on train trips. Working part of the time in the hospital and part on hospital trains, officers and enlisted men found it difficult to demonstrate to hospital authorities their fitness for promotion and were often passed over when promotions were made. Enlisted men who were absent from the hospital on paydays failed to receive their pay and, unless paid on a supplemental payroll, had to await the next regular payday a month later. The hospital considered this situation just as unsatisfactory as did the train commander because it had officers, nurses, and enlisted men upon whom it could not always depend for hospital service. Nevertheless this system kept all personnel fully occupied in the intervals between train movements, and perhaps some of the problems connected with it could have been solved by minor administrative changes. The Second Service Command however adopted a different solution by requisitioning additional personnel for train operations and assigning it, along with that already available, to a separate unit, the 1247th Service Command Service Unit.[87]

During 1944 other service commands followed this example. The organization of train units that were separate from hospital detachments was discussed at a service commanders' conference in February 1944 and was indorsed by the commanding general of the Service Forces. Afterward, in July 1944, the First, Third, and Ninth Service Commands organized separate train units. At least one of them, the First, placed its train unit under the direct control of the service command surgeon in the spring of 1945. The Fourth Service Command followed a different procedure. In September 1944 a receiving and evacuation detachment, consisting of litter bearers and clerks as well as train personnel, was organized at Stark General Hospital.[88] The organization of separate units, if their members were kept fully occupied, was superior to the use of hospital personnel for train service, since it simplified administration in all respects.

Service command surgeons encountered difficulty in getting adequate personnel allotments for train operations. Having estimates of the potential patient load, the Surgeon General's Office attempted early in 1944 to forestall this difficulty. In April it submitted to ASF headquarters an estimate of medical attendants needed by each service command during 1944 for train operations. ASF headquarters took

[87] (1) Rpt, Hosp Tn 1, Halloran Gen Hosp to CG 2d SvC ASF (Med Br Sup Div), 5 May 43, sub: Rpt of Hosp Tn Mvmt, HT 16-21-1-11, Main 24025, 27-28 Apr 43, with Supp. SG: 531.4. (2) An Rpt, 2d SvC, 1943. HD.

[88] (1) Rpt, Conf CGs of SvCs, Dallas, Tex, 17-19 Feb 44. HD: 337. (2) An Rpts, 1st and 9th SvCs, McGuire and Stark Gen Hosps, 1944, HD. (3) GO 49, 14 Apr 45, Hq ASF, 1st SvC, Boston. HD: 531.4.

the position that service commands should determine their own needs and should submit requisitions accordingly.[89] Under this system, service command surgeons apparently failed to get the strength actually needed for train operations. For example, at the end of 1944 the surgeon of the Second Service Command had an allotment of 589 for assignment to hospital trains, but used 1,175. To make up the difference, he attached to trains 586 persons from other medical installations in the command. The Surgeon General discussed this problem with the Chief of Staff at the end of 1944. As a result service commands got additional personnel. For example, the number assigned to train service in the Second Service Command increased by May 1945 to 1,322—58 physicians, 1 dentist, 75 other officers, 91 nurses, 1,053 enlisted men, and 44 civilians.[90]

Supplies and Equipment for Hospital Trains

Equipment for the care and comfort of patients on hospital trains had to be planned for each hospital car developed, and consideration had to be given to balancing the necessity of items for medical use against the limited amount of space available. Hence, large items of equipment that were fixed parts of hospital cars, such as berths, instrument cabinets, storage lockers, instrument sterilizers, bedpan washers and sterilizers, cooking ranges, refrigerators, coffee urns, and the like, were planned along with cars in which they were to be installed and became a part of the specifications for their construction. Builders of hospital cars normally procured and installed such items, but in some instances the Medical Department procured certain special ones, such as instrument sterilizers and operating tables, for installation by builders.[91]

Supplies and items of equipment that were not fixed parts of hospital cars were listed in tables of allowances and in Medical Department equipment lists. The latter were the more important, because hospital cars carried few items supplied by services other than the Medical Department. By the fall of 1940, when procurement of the first two unit cars was approved, the Surgeon General's Office had developed an equipment list for cars of that type. Like other Medical Department equipment lists, it included such items as drugs and biologicals, gauzes and bandages, surgical instruments, linens, office supplies, and mess equipment.[92] Later, in 1942, when ward and ward dressing cars

[89] (1) Memo, Dep Dir Plans and Oprs ASF for Dir Pers ASF, 26 Apr 44, sub: Reqmts for Med Pers to Cover Rail Mvmts . . . , with incl. HRS: ASF Planning Div Program Br file, "Hosp and Evac, vol. 3." (2) Memo, Dep Dir Plans and Oprs ASF for DepCofS for SvCs ASF, 8 May 44, sub: Est of Numbers of Sick and Wounded Arriving from Overseas, with incl. Same file.

[90] (1) History, Office of the Surgeon, Second Corps Area and Second Service Command From 9 September 1940 to 2 September 1945. HD. (2) Notes for Gen Kirk on Conf with Gen Marshall, Summary: 25 Dec 44. HD: 024 (Resources Anal Div, Jul–Dec 44).

[91] (1) Gen Specifications for Hosp Unit Cars for WD, 4 Jun 40. TC: 453. (2) Rpt of MD Bd, Med Fld Serv Sch, 27 Aug 40. SG: 453.-1. (3) 1st ind, SG to MSO Carlisle Barracks, Pa., 10 Apr 41, on Ltr, MSO Carlisle Barracks, Pa., to SG, 7 Apr 41, sub: Car, Railroad, Hosp Unit, Unit Car No 2. Off file, Research and Dev Bd, SGO, "Hosp Unit Cars." (4) Specifications for Remodeling 18 Pullman Parlor Cars to Hosp Ward Cars for the WD, 30 Jan 42. Off file, Research and Dev Bd, SGO, "Hosp Ward Car." (5) TC US Army Specification No TC-3066, 8 May 44, Construction of Car, Hospital. Off file, Research and Dev Bd, SGO, "Unit Car, New Type." (6) Ltr, SG to CO Hosp Tn SCSU 1247, 27 Jun 45, sub: Sterilizers for Hosp Ward Cars. SG: 453 (2d SvC)AA.

[92] (1) Memo, [Col] A[lbert] G. L[ove] for Lt Col [Francis C.] Tyng, 10 Oct 40, sub: Hosp Unit Car. Off file, Research and Dev Bd, SGO, "Unit Car." (2) Med Equip for Hosp Unit Car, Oct 40. Same file.

were developed, equipment lists were prepared for them also, and when their delivery was expected in the spring of that year the Surgeon General's Office requested SOS headquarters to approve the inclusion of assemblages, packed according to these lists, as authorized items in tables of allowances for hospital cars. Approval was given, and these lists became the official basis for the issuance of equipment and supplies to ward and ward dressing cars when they were first delivered to the Army in the late summer of 1942.[93]

These early equipment lists were necessarily theoretical in nature, because the Medical Department had had no experience, when they were prepared, in operating hospital cars of the types developed during World War II. In 1943 they were revised. Subsequently, as experience accumulated, hospital train commanders proposed further revisions. Their recommendations were at variance with one another, and the Surgeon General's Office had difficulty in deciding which to accept.[94] Hence, at a hospital train commanders' conference in February 1945, a representative of the Surgeon General's Technical Division distributed a tentative equipment list, based upon recommendations already submitted, for consideration by officers who were responsible for the care of patients aboard hospital trains. After discussing the items listed, train commanders and The Surgeon General's representative agreed upon which should be retained, deleted, or added.[95] New equipment lists for ward, ward dressing, unit, and kitchen cars were then published in March 1945.[96] Several months later it appeared that train commanders were dissatisfied with the supplies and equipment agreed upon and at a conference in July 1945 they proposed changes. Some, such as in the substitution of twelve bath towels for twelve hand towels, the Surgeon General's Office approved. Others it refused to authorize because The Surgeon General insisted upon retaining in all hospital cars enough equipment of certain types, such as surgical instruments, to provide for emergencies or accidents that might occur as well as for the routine care of patients en route.[97]

In addition to revising equipment lists, the Surgeon General's Office either developed new items or permitted hospital train commanders to do so. For example, upon a recommendation of the Fourth Service Command, the Surgeon General's Office in 1944 developed a better mattress of a different size for use on hospital trains.[98] Accepting a suggestion from the Second Service Command, it soon afterward developed an adjustable back rest. This item contributed to the comfort of patients by enabling them to change positions while

[93] (1) Memo, Lt Col Thomas N. Page for Lt Col Griffin and Lt Col Hays, 20 Apr 42. Off file, Research and Dev Bd, SGO, "Hosp Ward Cars." (2) Ltr, SG to Reqmts Div SOS, 10 May 42, sub: Med Equip for Hosp Tn, with ind. SG: 453.-1. (3) Memo, CG SOS for CGs 2d, 4th, 6th, 8th, and 9th SvCs and for SG, 26 Aug 42, sub: Control of Hosp Tns. HD: 531.4.

[94] (1) Ltr, CO 2d SvC Hosp Tns 1247th SCSU to SG, 2 Oct 43, sub: Changes to Med Equip, Ward and Unit Cars. SG: 453.-1. (2) Diary, Tec Div SGO, 25 Nov-1 Dec 44. HD. (3) Memo, Post Sup Off [Stark Gen Hosp] to SG, 21 Jan 45, sub: Mess Equip on Hosp Cars, with 2 inds. SG: 453.

[95] (1) Transcript of Proceedings, Hosp Tn Conf, 15-16 Feb 45. (2) Diary, Tec Div SGO, 17-23 Feb 45. HD.

[96] ASF Catalog Med 10-14, Med Equip List, 27 Mar 45.

[97] (1) Transcribed Mins of Hosp Tn Unit Comdrs' Conf, 10-13 Jul 45. HD. (2) Memo, Capt George R. Allen for Dir Tec Div SGO, 30 Jul 45. Off file, Research and Dev Bd SGO, "Unit Car, New Type."

[98] (1) Diary, Tec Div SGO, 3-9 Jun 44, 25 Aug-1 Sep 44. HD. (2) Transcript of Proceedings, Hosp Tn Conf, 15-16 Feb 45. HD.

in train berths.[99] Another example of new equipment was the bath tray. Fitting on the sides of hospital berths, this tray simplified the work of nurses in bathing patients in bed. It was first put in use by the Second Service Command in the latter part of 1944. The Surgeon General's Office adopted the idea and began a development project for such a tray but the war ended before it was standardized.[100]

Items included in the equipment lists of hospital cars were considered to be the minimum in type and quantity that should be kept aboard at all times. Hence, hospital car commanders were authorized to draw equipment and supplies, to replace those used, from any medical supply officer in the United States. Normally, however, home stations made replacements.[101] To avoid bookkeeping, linen was exchanged on an item-for-item basis. Regulations early in the war required hospitals to exchange linen with hospital trains when patients were transferred to their control. It happened frequently that such exchange either delayed train schedules or was not made at all. At the train commanders' conference in February 1945, therefore, it was decided that the exchange of soiled for clean linen would normally be deferred until the end of a trip or until points were reached at which trains stopped for lengthy periods. In cases where soiled linen was not replaced by one of the hospitals to which patients were delivered. that hospital furnished a receipt for the linen it received so that train commanders could draw clean linen from general hospitals at the ends of trips.[102]

---

[99] (1) Ltr, SG to CO 2d SvC Hosp Tns 1247th SCSU, 11 Sep 44, sub: Back Rests. SG: 442.7 (2d SvC)AA. (2) Diary, Tec Div SGO, 28 Apr–4 May 45. HD.

[100] (1) Ltr, Chief Hosp and Evac Br 2d SvC to CG ASF attn SG, 14 Oct 44, sub: Hosp Tns, with incl. SG: 700.7–2. (2) Ltr, SG to CO 2d SvC Hosp Tns 1247th SCSU, 2 Dec 44. SG: 453 (2d SvC)AA. (3) Diary, Tec Div SGO, 21–27 Jul 45. HD.

[101] (1) Diary, Tec Div, SGO, 17–23 Feb 45. HD. (2) ASF Cirs 286 and 401, 1 Sep and 9 Dec 44.

[102] (1) Ltr, CG Lovell Gen Hosp to SG, 8 Feb 45, sub: Linen Exchange for Hosp Cars, with 2 inds and Memo for Record. HRS: Hq ASF Planning Div Program Br file, 370.05 "Hosp and Evac." (2) Transcript of Proceedings, Hosp Tn Conf, 15–16 Feb 45. HD.

CHAPTER XXIII

Providing the Means for Evacuation by Sea

Most of the patients evacuated from theaters of operations to the zone of interior were transported in surface vessels. It is therefore important to consider in the following discussion the types of vessels used, reasons for their employment, and problems encountered in suiting them to the transportation of patients, along with difficulties in furnishing such vessels with the supplies, equipment, and attendants required for the care of patients en route.

Ships' Hospitals and Hospital Ships

At the beginning of 1939 the Army had four transports in which to return patients from overseas bases, such as Hawaii and the Philippines. With the expansion of existing bases and the establishment of new ones in the Atlantic during 1939 and 1940, additional transports were added to the Army's fleet, and efforts were made to enlarge and improve their hospital facilities. These efforts were only partially successful, because funds for such work were limited. Furthermore, the ships themselves were too old to warrant extensive alterations, and the speed with which some were put into transport service left no time for major changes.[1] In view of this situation as well as the probability that large numbers of patients would be evacuated in subsequent months, the New York Port of Embarkation proposed in the fall of 1940 that the U.S. Army Transport *Chateau Thierry* should be converted into a part-time hospital ship, to carry freight and troops on outbound voyages and return with full loads of patients.[2] On recommendation of the chief of his Hospital Construction Subdivision, The Surgeon General disapproved, stating that the proposed transport was not suitable for conversion, that its use would violate the terms of the

[1] The United States Army Transports *U. S. Grant, St. Mihiel, Chateau Thierry*, and *Republic* had been in almost continuous service since World War I. The *Hunter Liggett, Leonard Wood*, and *American Legion* were added in 1939. Others added to meet Army expansion needs were the *Irwin, Kent, Munargo, Orizaba*, and *President Roosevelt (Joseph T. Dickman.)* For their histories, see Roland W. Charles, *Troopships of World War II* (Washington, 1947), pp. 1–68. Information on problems of providing hospital facilities on these ships may be found in SG files: 560–69 (BB), 632.–1 (BB), 632.–2 (BB), 721.5–1 (BB) under name of transport; AG: 571, 573.27; TC: 571.4; and in surgeons' reports attached to voyage reports filed in TC: 721.1. Also see Chester Wardlow, *The Transportation Corps: Responsibilities, Organization, and Operations* (Washington, 1951), pp. 136–44, in UNITED STATES ARMY IN WORLD WAR II.

[2] (1) Ltr, Supt ATS NYPE to QMG thru CO NYPE, 27 Sep 40, with 1st ind. TC: 632 *(Chateau Thierry)*. (2) Ltr, CG NYPE to QMG, 26 Nov 40, sub: Inadequate Hosp Fac on Trans. AG: 573.27 (11–26–40). (3) Ltr, Port Surg NYPE to SG, 29 Nov 40, sub: Inadequate Hosp Fac on Trans. SG: 632.–1 *(Chateau Thierry)*BB.

Geneva and Hague Conventions,[3] and that its employment in the evacuation of small numbers of patients from scattered areas would be uneconomical. He recommended instead that "the idea of developing a hospital ship be given further study," and that the Army continue to use transports for the evacuation of its sick and wounded from overseas areas.[4]

During 1941 the question of whether or not hospital ships would be provided remained unanswered. The question also arose of whether the Army or the Navy would be responsible for the evacuation of Army patients. Existing plans called for the control of all water transportation by the Navy beginning on M-Day (Mobilization Day), and during the early part of 1941, under policies announced by the President, the Navy began to take over Army transports on which hospital areas had been enlarged and improved. Disturbed by this loss to the Navy of evacuation space and fearing a repetition of World War I experiences, when the Navy failed to evacuate patients to the satisfaction of the Army, the surgeon of the New York Port in October 1941 proposed that a hospital ship should be provided for the Army.[5] Reaction in Washington was mixed. Some officers in the G–4 Division of the General Staff, in the Office of The Quartermaster General, and in the Surgeon General's Office were favorably impressed; but the chief of the Surgeon General's Hospital Construction Subdivision doubted "the wisdom and productivity of this proposal."[6] In transmitting it to the General Staff, The Surgeon General asked for decisions as to the policy on evacuation and as to whether the Army or the Navy would be responsible for transporting the Army's patients.[7] The Japanese attack on Pearl Harbor occurred before further action was taken on the New York Port's proposal.

Basic Decisions on Water Evacuation in 1942

Entry of the United States into the war made necessary both immediate and long-range plans for facilities for the evacuation of patients from theaters of operations. An agreement between the Army and Navy soon after Pearl Harbor for the Army to continue to operate transports despite prewar plans to the contrary partially solved this problem,[8] for the Army could continue to evacuate patients aboard them. Other questions remained to be answered: (1) whether or not hospital ships would be

[3] The Geneva Conventions of 1864, 1906, and 1929 established principles for belligerents to follow in the care, treatment, and transportation of the sick and wounded of land warfare; the Hague Conventions of 1899, 1904, and 1907 adapted to maritime warfare the provisions of the Geneva Conventions. The Hague Convention of 1907 was signed by the representatives of forty-three countries, among them the United States, China, France, Great Britain, Germany, Italy, and Japan. In 1942 the Medical Department published an article on the Conventions, along with copies of their texts. Albert G. Love, "The Geneva Red Cross Movement: European and American Influence on its Development," *Army Medical Bulletin*, No. 62 (1942).

[4] (1) Memo, Lt Col John R. Hall, SGO, for Planning and Tng Div SGO, 10 Dec 40, sub: Conv of USAT *Chateau Thierry* into a Hosp Trans Ship. (2) 2d ind, SG to QMG, 28 Dec 40, on Ltr, CG NYPE to QMG, 26 Nov 40, sub: Inadequate Hosp Fac on Trans. Both in SG: 632.-1 (*Chateau Thierry*)BB.

[5] (1) Ltr, Surg NYPE to SG thru CG NYPE, 29 Oct 41, sub: Hosp Ships, with 4 incls. HRS: G-4/29717-100. (2) Memo, ACofS G-4 WDGS for ACofS WPD WDGS, 19 Nov 41, sub: Trf of ATS to Navy. HRS: G-4/29717-51.

[6] Memos, Col A[rthur] B. Welsh for Col [Howard T.] Wickert, undated; Col Wickert for Cols [Harry D.] Offutt and [John R.] Hall, 7 Nov 41, sub: Hosp Ships. HD: 560.2.

[7] 2d ind SGO 541.-2 (BB), SG to AG, 24 Nov 41, on Ltr, Surg NYPE to SG thru CG NYPE, 29 Oct 41, sub: Hosp Ships. HRS: G-4/29717-100.

[8] Wardlow, *op. cit.*, pp. 200–201.

used, and (2) if so, the extent to which they would be used and whether or not the Army or Navy would control them.

Opinions on these points differed during the first half of 1942. General Headquarters approved the use of both transports and hospital ships for evacuation, but believing that the enemy would not respect the terms of the Hague Convention granting hospital ships immunity from attack, GHQ recommended that all plans for evacuation should be prepared with that probability in mind. GHQ also recommended that a decision be sought on whether the Army or Navy would operate hospital ships.[9] Taking the position that transports could be used for evacuation from areas with ample shipping, as demonstrated in World War I, The Surgeon General recommended a continuation of that method for all large theaters; but because of disruption by the war of peacetime transport schedules, he now proposed that two hospital ships (one for the Atlantic and one for the Pacific) should be provided for the evacuation of patients from small scattered bases. He made the latter recommendation contingent upon respect by the Axis Powers for the terms of the Hague Convention—the primary consideration, in his opinion, in any decision to use hospital ships. The Surgeon General also announced that he preferred to evacuate Army patients in ships operated solely under Army control. In any case, he wanted no division of responsibility. The agency responsible for operating ships for evacuation should be responsible also, in his opinion, for the medical care and administrative control of patients aboard them.[10] The Quartermaster General recommended the conversion of two Army transports into vessels that could be used either as hospital ships or as ambulance transports. If employed in the latter capacity they could be operated by the Army Transport Service and would sail under convoy, carrying troops on outbound voyages and returning full loads of patients to the United States.[11] A group of officers in G-4, most of whom were later transferred to SOS headquarters and among whom was a Medical Corps officer (Maj. William L. Wilson), maintained that Convention-protected hospital ships—at least six—should be used in addition to transports to evacuate Army patients from major theaters despite uncertainty about the attitude of the Axis Powers toward the Convention. Furthermore, having ascertained that the Navy had no plans for providing hospital ships for the Army and being convinced by World War I history of the futility of depending upon the Navy for evacuation, this group wanted the Army both to own and to operate the vessels procured for use as hospital ships.[12]

In the first half of 1942 the G-4 group pressed for approval of its plans. After the Bureau of the Budget disapproved supplemental estimates for funds for six hospital ships submitted in January 1942, because the Maritime Commission stated

[9] (1) Memo, Chief Surg GHQ for CofS GHQ, 9 Jan 42, sub: Return of Sick and Wounded from Foreign Theaters. HD: 541 (Trans). (2) Memo, GHQ for ACofS G-4 WDGS, 14 Jan 42, sub: Hosp Ships. . . . HRS: G-4/29717-100.

[10] (1) Memo, SG for ACofS G-4 WDGS, 5 Jan 42, sub: Plan for Water Trans for Sick and Wounded. SG: 541.2. (2) Memo, SG for JCS (Col [Russell I.] Vittrup), 6 Jun 42, with inclosed notes. SG: 560.-2.

[11] Ltr, QMG to TAG, 14 Feb 42, sub: Hosp Space on Army Trans. TC: 632 (Army Trans).

[12] (1) Memo, ACofS G-4 WDGS for TAG, 24 Jan 42, sub: Hosp Space on Army Trans. HRS: G-4/29717-100. (2) Memo, CG SOS for CofSA, 28 Apr 42, sub: Hosp Ships, with 9 incls. HD: Wilson files, "Book IV, 16 Mar 43-17 Jun 43." (3) *The Medical Department . . . in the World War* (1923), vol. I, pp. 357-71.

that it would procure ships required by the Army, G–4 requested the Commission on 12 February 1942 to procure six hospital ships, along with several vessels of other types, for the Army's use. When the Commission replied that hospital ships fell "properly under the cognizance of the Navy Department," G–4's Transportation Branch disagreed and asked the Commission to reconsider its opinion. Receiving no reply to this request by late April 1942, SOS headquarters (recently established and containing many officers formerly in G–4) pursued the matter further. In letters prepared for the signature of the Secretary of War, it urged the Maritime Commission to procure six hospital ships for the Army, whether to be operated by the Army or Navy, and called upon the Secretary of the Navy to settle with the Army this question of jurisdiction. The administrator of the recently established War Shipping Administration, who was also chairman of the Maritime Commission, replied that he could not allocate vessels for use as hospital ships until the Army and Navy had agreed upon "strategic requirements." Because of its close relation to other shipping problems, the Secretary of the Navy proposed that the whole question be referred to the Joint Staff Planners, a group working under the Joint Chiefs of Staff.[13]

The investigation conducted by the Joint Staff Planners and the Joint Chiefs of Staff covered not only the strategic shipping situation but also other matters: the probability of enemy respect for the Geneva and Hague Conventions, the British practice of evacuating patients by sea, and the estimated evacuation requirements for operations in the Pacific and for BOLERO (the build-up of American troops in the United Kingdom for an invasion of the European continent). The views of the Chief of the Bureau of Medicine and Surgery of the Navy and of The Surgeon General of the Army were also sought. The latter restated the position which he had taken earlier. The former believed that both Army and Navy patients should be evacuated by transports that were manned and operated by the Navy but were supplied with enough Army officers and enlisted men to care for Army medical records. If hospital ships should be used, he disapproved painting and marking them as international conventions stipulated. Rather he proposed that they be painted like transports for travel in convoy and reveal their identity as hospital ships only under "desirable" circumstances. In view of agreement between the two medical services on the use of transports for evacuation and in the interest of economy in shipping, the Joint Chiefs of Staff announced on 25 May 1942 that the normal means of evacuating patients from areas with "more or less continuous transportation service" would be by returning troop transports. Since the Army and Navy disagreed on the question of hospital ships, the Joint Chiefs announced a compromise decision in June 1942. Three vessels would be procured and operated as hospital ships under the Hague Convention. They would be built according to plans supplied by the Army, would be operated under the "general direction" of the Army, and would be provided with Army medical complements, but would be converted under supervision of the

[13] (1) Memo, ACofS G–4 WDGS for CofSA, 8 Feb 42, sub: Supp Ests "D," FY 1942. AG: 111 (1–31–42). (2) Ltrs, CofSA for US Mar Comm, 12 Feb, 7 Mar, 1 May 42; US Mar Comm to CofSA, 24 Feb, 4 May 42. SG: 560.–2. (3) Ltr, SecNav to SecWar, 6 May 42, sub: Basis of Responsibility for Procurement and Opr of Hosp Ships. AG: 573.27 (5–6–42).

Navy and would be operated by Navy crews.[14] Although authorized in the middle of 1942, the first of these ships was not placed in service until June 1944.

In the course of these protracted negotiations, the Army—believing that the general problem of evacuating patients from ground operations in overseas theaters was one for solution within the War Department—partially took matters into its own hands.[15] In March 1942 the earlier proposal of The Quartermaster General to convert transports into vessels that could be used either as hospital ships or as ambulance transports was revived by the Transportation Corps. The Surgeon General reversed his prewar position in opposition to the use of ambulance transports and in April supported this proposal as a means of caring for immediate needs. Even if hospital ships should be authorized, he pointed out, their construction would require at least eighteen months.[16] SOS headquarters approved, and late in May 1942 the *Acadia* was withdrawn from regular transport service. From June to October it underwent conversion at the Boston Port of Embarkation, emerging with a capacity of approximately 1,100 troops outbound and 530 patients inbound. Making its first trip as an ambulance transport in December 1942, the *Acadia* continued to sail as such until placed under the protection of the Hague Convention as a hospital ship in May 1943.[17]

Providing Facilities for Evacuation by Transports Early in the War

In view of shipping shortages, uncertainty about the use of hospital ships, and the decision for the Army to continue to operate troop transports, the most obvious method of meeting immediate evacuation needs was the use of transports. Existing regulations required each to have a hospital with beds equal in number to 1 percent of its passenger capacity for cases of sickness en route.[18] Before the war the number of hospital beds on most transports had been increased to provide additional space for patients being evacuated from overseas areas. In March 1942 the Office of the Chief of Transportation proposed that the larger bed capacities be officially authorized for all transports—those to be procured as well as those already in service. Both the Surgeon General's Office and SOS headquarters approved, and in June 1942 the higher ratios were authorized. Changes were made in the fall of that year in the proportion of beds for different types of patients, but not in the total number authorized. The first eight months of the year had shown that 75 percent of the patients evacuated to the United States were mental cases. To provide more accommodations for them SOS headquarters on 8 September 1942 directed the

[14] (1) JMTC 4/M, 9 May 42, Evac of Sick and Wounded from Overseas. SG: 704.-1. (2) JCS 52, 21 May 42; JCS 52/1, 29 Jun 42. Records and Admin Br, Off ACofS G-3 WDGS. (3) Ltr, Bu of Med and Surg USN to JPS, 4 Jun 42, sub: Evac of Sick and Wounded from Overseas. SG: 704.-1. (4) Memo, SG for JCS (Col Vittrup), 6 Jun 42. SG: 560.-2.

[15] Ltr, SecWar to SecNav, 1 May 42, sub: Evac of Army Sick and Wounded from Overseas. AG: 560.

[16] Memo, CofT for CG SOS, 13 Mar 42, sub: Hosp Space on Army Trans, with 2d ind, SG to CG SOS, 8 Apr 42. SG: 632.-1 (BB).

[17] (1) Sailing Orders 82, Vessel: USAT *Acadia*, Outbound Voyage 5, 18 May 42. TC: 565.3 *(Acadia)*. (2) Ltr, Surg NOPE to Col John R. Hall, SGO, 18 May 42, with reply dtd 20 May 42. HD: 560.2 "Hosp Cons Br SGO—Hosp Ships." (3) Memo, Chief Misc Br SOS for Gen [Le Roy] Lutes, 24 Jun 42, sub: Hosp Ships. HD: Wilson files, "Book I, 26 Mar–26 Sep 42." (4) TC: 561–565 *(Acadia)*; and OPD: 370.05.

[18] AR 30–1150, 19 Sep 41.

Chief of Transportation to convert a portion of general ward beds of each ship's hospital into beds for mental patients.[19] Thus during 1942 ratios (expressed in percentages) of hospital beds to troop berths were authorized for various types of transports as follows:

Type of Ship and Patient	*Percent Hospital Beds to Troop Berths*	
	Mar 1942	*Sept 1942*
Owned and permanently converted ships–total	5.0	5.0
Ward	4.0	2.5
Isolation	0.5	0.5
Mental	0.5	2.0
Chartered and fully converted ships–total	4.0	4.0
Ward	3.0	2.0
Isolation	0.5	0.5
Mental	0.5	1.5
Temporarily or hastily converted ships–total	3.0	3.0
Ward	2.0	1.5
Isolation	0.5	0.5
Mental	0.5	1.0

Meeting standards set for ships' hospitals on vessels converted into troop transports depended upon the time available to ports for modifications and improvements. Throughout 1942 transports were hastened into service and sent out heavily loaded, sometimes with numbers of troops that exceeded ships' rated capacities by 10 percent.[20] Changes in hospital areas of such vessels could be made only while they were undergoing initial conversions for the transport service or were in port between voyages for maintenance and repairs. Hence their hospital facilities varied. On some, completely new hospital areas were constructed. On others, existing hospitals were enlarged and improved. As a rule the Transportation Corps submitted to the Surgeon General's Hospital Construction Division for review the plans for hospital areas of vessels being converted. This Division sometimes approved plans that would not have been acceptable under ordinary conditions, but it disapproved others in part or in whole, and thus conversions were sometimes delayed. To prevent such delays and to standardize improvements made at different ports on different types of vessels, the Surgeon General's Office in November 1942 prepared a list of general specifications for ships' hospitals.[21] Early in 1943 the Water Division of the Office of the Chief of Transportation sent it to all ports for use as a guide. Minimum standards thus established were as follows: a "suitable" surgical suite, minimal facilities for pharmacy and laboratory, adequate toilets for the hospital area with separate toilets for isolation wards, safety devices for wards for mental patients, a small X-ray unit with darkroom, berths of not more than two tiers, and beds equal in number to those authorized by SOS headquarters. Preferably, the hospital was to be located slightly aft of midship, not more than one deck below the uppermost "continuous weather deck," adjacent to cabins whose berths could be used for patients, and relatively close to lifeboats. It was to be well ventilated and lighted and was to

[19] (1) Memo, CofT for SG, 28 Mar 42, sub: Basic Plan for Evac of Sick and Wounded. HD: 705. (2) Ltr SPOPM 322.15, CG SOS to CGs and COs of CAs, PEs, and Gen Hosps, and to SG, 18 Jun 42, sub: Opr Plans for Mil Hosp and Evac, with incl. HD: 705.1. (3) Memo, ACofS for Oprs SOS for CofT, 8 Sep 42, sub: Fac for Care of Mental Pnts on Trans. HD: 705 (MRO, Fitzpatrick Daybook).

[20] For example, see Memo, Oprs Off OCT for Water Div OCT, 15 May 42, sub: Increased Trp Capacities. TC: 541.1.

[21] (1) Ltr, SG (Hosp Cons Div) for CofT, 26 Nov 42, sub: Gen Specifications for Hosp Areas on Converted Trans. SG: 632.-1 (BB). (2) Memo, Maj John C. Fitzpatrick for Chief Hosp and Evac Br Plans Div SOS, 17 Sep 42, sub: Rpt of Surv of Ships and Ships' Hosps. HD: 705 (MRO, Fitzpatrick Ref file). (3) Ltr, CofT to Supt ATS NYPE, 3 Oct 42, sub: Hasty Convs. SG: 632.-1 (BB).

have passageways wide enough for the removal of patients on litters.[22]

Construction of new transports offered the possibility of assuring suitable ships' hospitals provided there was effective coordination among the Surgeon General's Office, the Office of the Chief of Transportation, and the Maritime Commission. For a time, plans drawn by the Maritime Commission were not submitted to the Surgeon General's Office and the latter considered hospitals on some of the new vessels unsatisfactory. After a series of conferences early in 1943 the Maritime Commission agreed to submit its plans thereafter to the Transportation Corps and the Surgeon General's Office for review and comment.[23]

Early in 1943 a significant change was made in accommodations for mental patients on transports. Until that time some berths had been enclosed with wire cages, making spaces approximately 6 x 3 x 3 feet each in which seriously disturbed mental patients might be placed to avoid endangering themselves and others. In January 1943 the New York Port surgeon proposed the elimination of such "unnecessary and inhumane" accommodations. The neuropsychiatry section of the Surgeon General's Office supported this proposal. It pointed out that advances in medical practice, such as the use of sedation, hydrotherapy, and diversional activity, with minimum mechanical restraint, made it possible to care for mental patients in specially constructed wards. The Chief of Transportation therefore requested the Maritime Commission to eliminate metal cages from future transports and directed port commanders to remove existing ones and provide suitable security-ward space instead on other transports. Although surgeons of several ports argued that they would then be unable to care for mental patients, especially on long voyages in tropical areas, the Transportation Corps and The Surgeon General remained firm.[24] To guide transport and port surgeons in caring for seriously disturbed patients without metal cages, they issued a memorandum on the care of mental patients on transports in July 1943.[25] Later in the war, as will be seen below, the Army reverted to the use of individual cells for severely disturbed patients.

In the fall of 1942 British vessels, such as the liners *Queen Mary* and *Queen Elizabeth,* which since early 1942 had been carrying American troops overseas,[26] were brought within the program for enlarging the patient-capacity of transports. Since the British did not move helpless patients in transports, the *Queens* had inadequate laboratory and surgical equipment and each had only 175 beds for patients. In October 1942 the Army started arrangements for the installation of a 300-bed hospital on each ship. British officials in Washington were at first unsympathetic to

[22] Ltr, CofT (Water Div) to CGs PEs attn ATS, 26 Jan 43, sub: Gen Specifications for Hosp Areas on Converted Trans, with incl. TC: 632.

[23] Correspondence on ships' hospitals of troop ships and reports of conferences with Maritime Commission representatives are found in SG: 632.-1 (BB) and TC: 632.

[24] (1) Ltr, Surg NYPE to SG (Col Tynes), 19 Jan 43, sub: Psychotic Pnts on Army Trans. TC: 632. (2) Memo, SG for CofT 15 Feb 43, sub: Elimination of Cages for Care of Mental Cases on US Army Trans. SG: 632.1 (BB). (3) Ltr, CofT to US Mar Comm, 27 Feb 43. TC: 632. (4) TC Cir 35, 1 Mar 43, Elimination of Cages for Mental Pnts. (5) Letters from port surgeons at San Francisco and New Orleans containing objections to removal of cages are filed in SG: 632.-1 (BB) and TC: 632.

[25] Ltr, CofT (Mvmt Div) for CGs PEs, 10 Jul 43, sub: Care of Mental Pnts on US Army Trans. TC: 370.05 (Army Vessels).

[26] (1) Wardlow, *op. cit.,* pp. 6, 222–24. (2) Charles, *op. cit.,* p. 309.

the American plan for putting larger hospitals aboard, but changed their attitude after American officials explained that shortages of shipping and lack of hospital ships made it imperative to evacuate patients on transports. Final agreement was that the United States would install a 300-bed hospital on each ship while in an American port. The proportion of beds in general wards, isolation wards, and mental wards would be the same as that already established for hastily converted transports. When completed, each hospital would be operated by American Army personnel. The construction of new hospital areas began early in November when the *Queen Mary* came into port. Several months later work was begun on the *Queen Elizabeth*.[27]

Renewed Efforts to Get Army Hospital Ships, 1942-43

Neither the policy announced by the Joint Chiefs of Staff in the spring of 1942 nor efforts to supply evacuation facilities in compliance with this policy silenced demands for Army hospital ships. As early as April 1942 General Hawley (then Colonel), Chief Surgeon of the U. S. Army Forces in the British Isles (later the European Theater of Operations), announced in a letter to The Surgeon General the policy upon which the European theater was to insist: helpless patients would not be evacuated on ships subject to enemy attack (transports) but only on hospital ships plainly marked and operated under the terms of the Hague Convention. Repeatedly thereafter the European theater requested hospital ships of the War Department, stating in August 1942 that five would be needed by April 1943 and five more by the following September.[28] To these demands were added, in the fall of 1942, requests for hospital ships from ports in the United States that were responsible for evacuating patients from scattered island bases.[29] Some bases were not on the itinerary of regularly scheduled transports and hence needed other means of evacuation. The most logical seemed to be the use of hospital ships on a "pick-up" service. In response to these needs, the Surgeon General's Office in October 1942 recommended the procurement of three hospital ships, in addition to the three already authorized by the Joint Chiefs of Staff. They would be used to collect patients from scattered island bases, to evacuate casualties from large-scale landing operations, or to supplement transports in evacuating patients from the more distant and larger theaters.[30] The Chief of Transportation referred this recommendation to the Joint Staff Planners. Earlier, in August, a request for three Convention-protected ships which General Eisenhower

[27] (1) Memo, ACofS for Oprs SOS for SG, 6 Oct 42, sub: Med Equip and Sups for US Hosp Fac aboard HMT *Queen Mary* and *Queen Elizabeth*. SG: 475.5-1 (BB). (2) Memo, ACofS for Oprs SOS for CofT, 6 Oct 42, sub: Instl of US Hosp Fac on HMT *Queen Mary* and *Queen Elizabeth*. HD: 705 (MRO, Fitzpatrick Daybook). (3) Memo, SOS Hosp and Evac Br for ACofS for Oprs SOS, 2 Nov 42, sub: Add Hosp Fac on Two British Ships. SG: 705.-1 (BB).

[28] (1) Ltr, USAFBI (Chief Surg, Col Paul R. Hawley) to SG, 25 Apr 42. SG: 560.2 (Gr Brit). (2) Rads CM-IN-4037 (11 Aug 42), CM-IN-6044 (17 Aug 42), CM-IN-7813 (21 Aug 42), USASOS (London) to AGWAR; CM-OUT-5084 (16 Aug 42), CM-OUT-7479 (24 Aug 42), AGWAR to USASOS (London). OPD: In and Out Messages.

[29] (1) Diary, Misc Br SOS (Col [William L.] Wilson), 20 Jul 42, HD: 705 (MRO, Extracts from Hosp and Evac Br SOS Diaries). (2) Ltr, CG CPE to CofT, 25 Sep 42, sub: Hosp Ship for the CPE, with 2 inds. SG: 560.-2.

[30] 1st ind, SG to CG SOS, 23 Oct 42, on Memo, CG SOS for SG, 16 Oct 42, sub: Rpt of Progress. SG: 632.-1 (BB).

wanted by the end of September for the North African invasion had also been referred to that group. In both instances, the Joint Staff Planners, weighing the need for vessels to transport troops and cargoes against the need for hospital ships, decided that additional vessels could not be spared for the latter purpose and reaffirmed the existing policy of using transports as the normal means of evacuation. On 12 November 1942 the Joint Chiefs of Staff disapproved requests for additional hospital ships.[31]

Early in 1943 events caused a change in existing policy. To demands of the European theater were added requests of the Southwest Pacific and North Africa for hospital ships not only for evacuation to the zone of interior but more particularly for intratheater use. In February 1943 the Southwest Pacific informed the War Department that it was converting a Dutch ship, the *Tasman,* into a hospital ship, and asked that it be certified under the terms of the Hague Convention.[32] The North African theater, like the European, had adopted a policy of evacuating no helpless patients in transports. Early in March 1943 it refused to load litter patients on the *Acadia,* which was making its second trip as an ambulance transport. Later that month this theater cabled Washington for two hospital ships for use in evacuating patients to the United Kingdom.[33] Concurrently, evidence was accumulating that the enemy would respect the terms of the Hague Convention. Germany and Italy permitted British hospital ships to operate unmolested in the Mediterranean, and they, along with Japan, had announced they were operating their own hospital ships. Furthermore, several Allied Governments, as well as the U. S. Navy, had followed the lead of the British and placed hospital ships under Red Cross (Hague Convention) protection.[34]

Along with insistent demands of theaters for hospital ships and growing evidence of enemy respect for the Hague Convention, it appeared in the first half of 1943 that loss of transport and cargo space through conversion of vessels to hospital use was a less cogent reason than formerly for not authorizing hospital ships. By that time the troop ship fleet had grown through new construction and the conversion of freighters. Moreover, British hospital ships were occasionally being used to transport American patients from the European theater to the United States. A request by that theater in January 1943 that medical personnel and equipment be

[31] (1) Memos, CofT for JPS, 21 Aug and 2 Nov 42, sub: Hosp Ships. TC: 564. (2) JPS 27/5/D, 24 Aug 42; JCS 52/2, 29 Aug 42. HD: 705 (MRO, Fitzpatrick Ref file, Aug 42–May 43). (3) JCS 52/3, 12 Nov 42. Records and Admin Br, Off ACofS G–3 WDGS.

[32] Rad CM-IN-9207, SWPA to AGWAR, 18 Feb 43. HD: 705 (MRO, Fitzpatrick Daybook, Apr 42–Jun 43). For conversion plans for these ships see HD: SWPA 560.2 *(Tasman* and *Maetsuycker);* for letters about certifying the *Tasman* see: TC: 561–565.1 *(Tasman).*

[33] (1) Rpt, 204th Hosp Ship Co, USAT *Acadia,* voyage 2 (8 Feb–11 Mar 43). TC: 721.5 *(Acadia).* (2) Rad CM-IN-14498, NATO to WD, 27 Mar 43. SG: 560.-2 (N. Africa). (3) An Rpt Med Sec NATOUSA, 1943. HD.

[34] (1) Memo, CinC US Fleet, for JCS, 26 May 43, sub: Hosp Ships, incl A to [JPS] 360–9 (JCS 315/2) Memo, JPS for JCS. Records and Admin Br, Off ACofS G–3 WDGS. (2) See list of hospital ships (US Army and Navy, Allied Governments, and Axis Powers) in State Dept file 740.00117 Eur War 1–1648. By May 1943 Japan had 20 hospital ships, while Germany and Italy had 33. The British Commonwealth of Nations had about 30 hospital ships for use in the Atlantic, Mediterranean, and Indian Ocean. The U.S. Navy had converted the *Solace* into a modern hospital ship, and it was at Pearl Harbor on 7 December 1941. It was designated as a Convention-protected ship on 31 October 1942. The Navy ship *Relief* was likewise designated as a hospital ship on 5 February 1943.

transported by these ships on return trips led to a study of the legality of such action by the Army Judge Advocate General. In March 1943 he issued an opinion that hospital ships, whether British or American, might be used for the transportation of medical personnel and equipment without violating the provisions of the Hague Convention.[35] This meant that space on hospital ships could be used for medical transport purposes to compensate, in part at least, for the loss of vessels to ordinary transport service.

Still another factor influencing decisions about hospital ships early in 1943 was the tardiness with which the three ships authorized by the Joint Chiefs of Staff in June 1942 were being made available. The delay was caused largely by division of responsibility for them between the Army and Navy and subsequent misunderstandings over submission of plans and selection of types of hulls. Even the most optimistic estimated in the spring of 1943 that they would not be ready until mid-1944.[36]

In view of these circumstances The Surgeon General raised anew the hospital ship question. He now proposed that hospital ships be provided for the evacuation of all helpless patients. On 30 March 1943 he recommended that the *Acadia* should be registered immediately as a hospital ship under the Hague Convention, "in view of the urgency of the situation in the African theater"; that a second transport should be converted into a hospital ship as soon as possible; that completion of the three ships being built by the Navy should be "expedited"; and that five additional vessels should be procured for use as hospital ships by 1 July 1944.[37] Subsequently, in April 1943, representatives of the Chief of Transportation, the Surgeon General's Office, and the ASF Hospitalization and Evacuation Branch discussed additional details of the proposed program. They agreed that vessels selected for conversion should be suitable for use as hospital ships but should also have some characteristics, such as excessively slow speeds, which made them undesirable for service as transports with convoys. They agreed also that the Army should procure and operate hospital ships and that Army hospital ships should be provided with facilities for emergency diagnosis and treatment only, rather than with elaborate facilities for definitive surgical and medical care as on Navy hospital ships. Finally, they decided that the first step in achievement of this program would be to request the Joint Chiefs of Staff to amend the policy on evacuation facilities established in May 1942. Subsequently, Colonel Fitzpatrick prepared an impressive study for submission on 24 April 1943 to the General Staff. Its crux was the recommendation that the Joint Chiefs of Staff (1) should approve the use of Convention-protected hospital ships as the normal means, when available, of evacuating the helpless fraction of sick and

[35] (1) Ltr, CG SOS ETO to CG SOS, 4 Jan 43, sub: Util of Hosp Ships for Trans Med Units and Sups, with 2 inds. HD: 705 (MRO, Fitzpatrick Daybook). (2) Memo SPJGW 1943/1760, JAG War Plans Div for JAG, 18 Mar 43, sub: Hosp Ships. SG: 560.2.

[36] (1) Memos, CG SOS for VCNO, 14 Jul and 10 Sep 42, sub: Hosp Ships for Evac of Sick and Wounded from Overseas. TC: 564. (2) Memo, Col A[chilles] L. Tynes for SG, 11 Sep 42, sub: Rpt on Conf on Cons of Hosp Ships. SG: 632.-1 (BB). Reports of progress in planning and converting these ships were made currently by OCT to SG and SOS. See files HD: 560.2 (Hosp Cons Br, Hosp Ships, *Hope, Mercy*, and *Comfort*). (4) Ltr, VCNO to CofSA, 18 Dec 42, sub: Procedure for Acquisition and Conv of USS *Comfort* (AH-6), USS *Hope* (AH-7), USS *Mercy* (AH-8). SG: 560.2.

[37] Memo, SG for ACofS OPD WDGS thru CG ASF, 30 Mar 43, sub: Hosp Ships, with 2 inds. SG: 560.-2.

wounded, (2) should authorize steps to implement this revision of policy at the earliest practicable date, and (3) should approve the use of hospital ships on outbound voyages for the transportation of medical supplies and personnel. The War Department General Staff approved this recommendation and forwarded it on 12 May 1943 to the Joint Chiefs of Staff.[38]

The provision of hospital ships for the North African theater did not await this recommendation. In response to North Africa's request for two hospital ships, the Operations Division of the General Staff offered on 7 April 1943, after consultation with both the Chief of Transportation and The Surgeon General, to convert the *Acadia* into a hospital ship if the theater was willing to forego its use in the transportation of troops. After both the Combined and Joint Chiefs of Staff had considered the theater's acceptance of this offer, North Africa was notified on 22 April that the *Acadia* would be converted into a hospital ship. A second ship, the *Seminole,* was selected and approved for use as a hospital ship a week later.[39] Both ships were stripped of armament and other belligerent features; their hulls were painted white with a horizontal green band on each side; and red crosses, which could be illuminated at night, were painted on their sides, decks, and funnels. On 6 May the Secretary of War informed the Secretary of State of the designation of the *Acadia* as a hospital ship; four days later, of the *Seminole.* Structural work required in the conversion of the *Seminole* delayed her departure until September 1943, but the *Acadia,* which had already been fitted out as an ambulance transport, sailed from New York to North Africa on her maiden voyage as a hospital ship on 5 June 1943.[40]

Six days later the Army received full authority to procure and operate its own fleet of hospital ships. On 11 June 1943 the Joint Chiefs of Staff amended the earlier policy, announcing that the helpless fraction of patients would be evacuated in hospital ships if they were available. At the same time they approved the use of hospital ships for the transportation of medical supplies and personnel on outbound voyages. To permit observance of the amended policy, the Joint Chiefs authorized the conversion of slow-speed passenger vessels and of EC–2 cargo ships (Liberty ships) to provide a total of 15 hospital ships by 31 December 1943, 19 by 30 June 1944, and 24 by 31 December 1944. All but three—those already authorized for construction by the Navy—were to be procured, converted, manned, and operated by the Army alone. Since it had already sent the *Acadia* on its maiden voyage as a hospital ship and had begun the conversion of the *Seminole,* the Army thus had authority to place nineteen ad-

[38] (1) Ltr, CG ASF for ACofS OPD WDGS, 24 Apr 43, sub: Hosp Ships, with 9 incls. OPD: 573.27. (2) Memo, CofT for CG ASF, 11 May 43, sub: Hosp Ships. TC: 564. (3) Memo, CofSA for Secretariat JCS, 12 May 43, sub: Hosp Ships, with incl. OPD: 573.27.

[39] (1) Rads CM–IN–14498 (27 Mar 43); CM–IN–6760 (12 Apr 43); CM–IN–12911 (21 Apr 43), NATOUSA to WD. (2) Rads CM–OUT–3358 (8 Apr 43); CM–OUT–5910 (14 Apr 43); CM–OUT–9291 (22 Apr 43); CM–OUT–12622 (30 Apr 43), WD to NATOUSA. OPD: In and Out Messages. Under the CCS plan the British would furnish 10 hospital ships and 6 hospital carriers, and the United States would provide 2 hospital ships as soon as available.

[40] (1) Memo, ACofS OPD WDGS for CofS, 5 May 43, sub: Designation of USAT *Acadia* as Hosp Ship. OPD: 573.27. (2) Ltrs, SecWar to SecState, 6 and 10 May 43. Same file. For plans and problems of conversion see file SG: 632.–1 (BB) and HD: 560.2 (Hosp Ships, Hosp Cons Br).

ditional hospital ships in operation by the end of 1944.[41]

The Hospital Ship Program, 1943–45

Selection of vessels for conversion into hospital ships was important to The Surgeon General because their basic characteristics largely determined the success of conversion. The width of a ship's beam determined whether passageways would be wide enough to permit the handling of litter cases. The size of its superstructure determined whether patients could be located above the water line in areas that had natural ventilation and from which patients might be removed easily if it became necessary to abandon ship. The cruising range of a vessel determined whether it was suitable for transoceanic service, and its speed determined the number of trips per month and thus the number of patients it might evacuate. In June 1943, therefore, The Surgeon General arranged with the Chief of Transportation for joint inspection of vessels before selection for conversion.[42]

The ships chosen represented a compromise. In several instances, vessels were rejected by the Surgeon General's representatives, either because they had speeds of less than ten knots, had fewer than three decks above the water line, or were of too narrow beam. On the other hand, despite its objection to their slow speed and low deck heights, the Surgeon General's Office had to agree to the conversion of six EC–2 cargo ships. The remaining fifteen ships (including the *Acadia* and *Seminole*) were of varying ages and speeds. Seven had been built between 1901 and 1919; seven, between 1920 and 1926. Six had speeds of 10 to 12 knots; four, of 13 to 14 knots; and five, of 15 to 16 knots. Some had been coastwise vessels only and later proved unsuitable for use in the Pacific during stormy seasons.[43] *(Table 18.)*

All of the vessels selected were converted into hospital ships according to plans approved by the Surgeon General's Hospital Construction Branch. Plans for the conversion of the six EC–2's were drawn by Cox and Stevens, naval architects in New York City; those for the remainder, by the Maintenance and Repair Branch of the Water Division, New York Port of Embarkation. A civilian architect from the Surgeon General's Office, assigned temporarily in New York, represented the Medical Department in the initial stages of planning. Subsequently, completed plans were referred to the Surgeon General's Hospital Construction Branch for final approval. In all planning, emphasis was placed on the number of patients' berths that could be provided rather than upon elaborate clinical facilities.[44]

A major problem in planning hospital ships was the location and arrangement of the surgical suite and other professional rooms, wards for different types of patients, and quarters for the ship's crew and

---

[41] (1) JCS 315, 13 May 1943; JCS 315/1, 30 May 43. Records and Admin Br, Off ACofS G–3 WDGS. (2) Memo, JCS for ACofS OPD WDGS, 11 Jun 43, sub: Hosp Ships. OPD: 573.27. (3) Memos, Dir of Oprs ASF for SG and CofT, 18 Jun 43, sub: Hosp Ships. SG: 560.–2.

[42] Memo, Maj Gen Norman T. Kirk (SG) for Lt Col John C. Fitzpatrick, 30 Jun 43, sub: Hosp Ships. SG: 560.–2 (BB).

[43] For correspondence dealing with the hospital ship conversion program, inspection of and acceptance or rejection of certain transports (e.g., *Robin Adair, Manuel Arnos, Utahan, William L. Thompson*), revision and changes in plans for hospital areas, problems of construction, and Medical Department inspections during conversion, see TC: 564, SG: 632.1 (BB), SG: 560.2, and HD: 560.2 (Hosp Ships, Hosp Cons Br).

[44] Tynes, Construction Branch, pp. 94, 113.

TABLE 18—UNITED STATES ARMY HOSPITAL SHIPS IN WORLD WAR II

Name	Vessels Used for Conversion [a]			Patient Capacity [b]	Speed [d] (Knots)	Designation as Hospital Ship			First Voyage [b]			Decommissioning of Hospital Ships	
	Name	Year Built	Place of Conversion			Date	Announcement by WDGO: Number	Announcement by WDGO: Date	Port of Departure	Date	Destination	Announcement by WDGO: Number	Announcement by WDGO: Date
Acadia	Acadia	1932	New York	787	18	3 May 43	27	3 Jun 43	New York	5 Jun 43	N. Africa	17	11 Feb 46
Aleda E. Lutz	Colombie	1931	New York	778	16	13 Feb 45	23	3 Apr 45	New York	18 Apr 45	United Kingdom	33	6 Apr 46
Algonquin	Algonquin	1926	Mobile	454	15	11 Sep 43	65	9 Oct 43	New Orleans	2 Feb 44	N. Africa	6	11 Jan 46
Armin W. Leuschner	Willard A. Holbrook [c]	1921	Mobile										
Blanche F. Sigman	Stanford White	1943	New York	590	11	20 Apr 44	43	29 May 44	New York	7 Jul 44	United Kingdom	47	24 May 46
Charles A. Stafford	Siboney	1918	New York	706	16	16 May 44	61	1 Aug 44	New York	21 Sep 44	United Kingdom		2 Nov 46 [e]
Chateau Thierry	Chateau Thierry	1920	Boston	484	16	29 Nov 43	5	8 Jan 44	Boston	5 Mar 44	N. Africa	17	11 Feb 46
Comfort [d]	C 1–B Hull	1943	San Pedro	705	15	20 May 44			Los Angeles	21 Jun 44	Southwest Pacific		2 Nov 46 [e]
Dogwood	George W. Carver	1943	New York	592	11	3 Feb 44	40	17 May 44	New York	21 Jul 44	United Kingdom	10	25 Jan 46
Emily H. M. Weder	President Buchanan	1920	New York	738	13	2 Mar 44	42	27 May 44	New York	12 Jul 44	Italy	120	18 Dec 45
Ernest Hinds	Kent	1918	San Francisco	288	12	3 Jan 44	19	4 Mar 44	Charleston	14 Jul 44	Italy	88	17 Oct 45
Ernestine Koranda	Dorothy Luckenbach	1919	New York	722	12	11 Dec 44	19	24 Mar 45	New York	13 Apr 45	United Kingdom	117	9 Oct 46
Frances Y. Slanger	Saturnia	1927	New York	1,628	19	13 Feb 45	41	23 May 45	New York	30 Jun 45	United Kingdom	3	7 Jan 46
Hope [d]	C 1–B Hull	1943	San Pedro	705	15	31 May 44			Los Angeles	23 Sep 44	Southwest Pacific		2 Nov 46 [e]
Howard A. McCurdy	President Tyler [c]	1920	Boston										
Jarrett M. Huddleston	Samuel F. B. Morse	1942	New York	582	11	20 Apr 44	46	6 Jun 44	New York	2 Sep 44	United Kingdom	3	7 Jan 46
John J. Meany	Zebulon B. Vance	1942	Boston	582	11	20 Apr 44	47	6 Jun 44	New York	27 Jul 44	Italy	10	25 Jan 46
John L. Clem	Irwin	1918	Mobile	286	12½	24 Feb 44	28	3 Apr 44	Charleston	15 Jun 44	N. Africa	88	17 Oct 45
Larkspur	Bridgeport	1901	Jacksonville	592	10	18 Feb 44	26	30 Mar 44	Charleston	31 Aug 44	United Kingdom	17	11 Feb 46
Louis A. Milne	Lewis Luckenbach	1919	Boston	952	12	19 Sep 44	2	5 Jan 45	Boston	19 Mar 45	United Kingdom	94	22 Aug 46
Marigold	President Fillmore	1920	Tacoma	758	12	24 Feb 44	35	25 Apr 44	Charleston	19 Jul 44	Italy	75	22 Jul 46
Mercy [d]	C 1–B Hull	1943	San Pedro	705	15	31 May 44			Los Angeles	31 Aug 44	Southwest Pacific		2 Nov 46 [e]
Republic	Republic	1907	Mobile	1,242	12	13 Feb 45	62	26 Jul 45	New Orleans	4 Sep 45	Southwest Pacific	17	11 Feb 46
St. Mihiel	St. Mihiel	1920	Boston	504	16	22 Feb 44	25	27 Mar 44	Boston	10 May 44	N. Africa	27	21 Mar 46
St. Olaf	St. Olaf	1942	Boston	586	11	24 Feb 44	51	19 Jun 44	New York	12 Aug 44	United Kingdom	120	18 Dec 45
Seminole	Seminole	1925	New York	454	14	8 May 43	27	3 Jun 43	New York	20 Sep 43	N. Africa	3	7 Jan 46
Shamrock	Agwileon	1907	New York	543	14	3 Aug 43	52	1 Sep 43	New York	4 Sep 43	N. Africa	120	18 Dec 45
Thistle	Munargo	1921	New York	455	14	29 Nov 43	1	4 Jan 44	New York	8 Apr 44	N. Africa	10	25 Jan 46
Wisteria	William Osler	1943	New York	588	11	23 Feb 44	40	17 May 44	New York	16 Jul 44	United Kingdom	75	22 Jul 46

[a] Charles, *op. cit.*, and Bureau of Ships, Navy Department, *Ships' Data U. S. Naval Vessels* (Washington, 1945), vol. III.
[b] Summary charts in History . . . Medical Regulating Service. . . Ships' capacities varied from time to time because of alterations in wards. See lists of capacities, HD: 560.2.
[c] Conversion into hospital ship suspended after V-J Day.
[d] Converted and designated as hospital ship by the Navy for the Army; operated by the Navy for the Army until the spring of 1946; transferred to the Army for operation in April and May 1946.
[e] Decommissioning not announced by General Order. The Secretary of War informed the Secretary of State of this action on 2 November 1946.

medical complement. Experience in planning ships' hospitals for transports and in converting the *Acadia* and *Seminole* served as a guide at first. More satisfactory standards evolved as additional experience accumulated with later conversions. Normally the Surgeon General's Office preferred to have the following located on decks above the water line: quarters for officers, nurses, and medical attendants; the surgical suite; clinical and administrative areas; and wards for litter patients, for patients who had communicable diseases, and for those who were seriously disturbed mentally. Decks at the water line, or just below it, were considered suitable for wards for neuropsychiatric and ambulatory patients, for quarters for the ship's crew, and for galleys and mess rooms. Storerooms, the morgue, and the laundry were placed in lower areas, including the hold. To achieve maximum stability, the surgical suite—consisting of two operating rooms, a sterilizing room, a scrub-up area, rooms for sterile and nonsterile supplies, and an X-ray and darkroom—was preferably placed on the main deck slightly aft of center. To insure freedom from unnecessary traffic, isolation and mental wards were considered best located when they were aft. Clinical and administrative areas, including the dressing room, pharmacy, laboratory, surgeon's office, medical records office, chaplain's office, Red Cross office, transportation agent's office, post exchange, and commissary, were considered best located on the deck above the water line near the forward gangway or side-port entrance, to permit easy access when the ship was in port.[45]

Wards were provided on all ships for patients with communicable diseases, and for mental, medical, and surgical cases. Because of the large number of mental patients requiring evacuation, the Movements Division of the Transportation Corps proposed in the fall of 1943 to devote approximately half the capacity of each hospital ship to accommodations for them. Wards for such patients were equipped for safety with concealed radiators and pipes, shatterproof electric light fixtures, heavy doors with viewing panels, locks which could be operated by a master key, and protective bars over all portholes. For the care of acutely disturbed patients there were steel cells 3 to 4 feet wide and 7 feet long. For patients with mild neuropsychiatric disorders, large wards with minimum security devices were used. Isolation wards for patients with communicable diseases were separated into rooms accommodating no more than eight (and preferably four) patients, and were equipped with separate bathrooms, diet kitchens, linen closets, utility rooms, and scrub-up areas. All wards had two-tiered berths and were provided with adequate administrative areas, such as utility rooms, diet kitchens, and offices.[46] In the summer of 1945 mesh wire enclosures were constructed on the decks of some hospital ships to provide areas where mental patients could get fresh air and exercise.[47]

In addition to the general arrangement of hospital facilities, the Surgeon General's

---

[45] Letters dealing with recommendations made by the Hospital Construction Branch are found in SG: 632.1 (BB), HD: 560.2 (Hosp Cons Br, Hosp Ships, Gen), and HD: 560.2 (Hosp Cons Br, file for each hosp ship). Blueprints and photographs of each hospital ship are located in above files.

[46] (1) Tynes, Construction Branch, pp. 101, 107ff. (2) Memo, CofT for SG, 9 Oct 43, sub: Hosp Ships. SG: 560.2. (3) Memo, SG for CofT, 4 Jan 44, sub: Mental Fac Aboard Hosp Ships. SG: 632.1 (BB).

[47] Memo, CofT for SG, 12 Apr 45, sub: Proposed Location of Mental Pnt Incls on Hosp Ships. SG: 632.1 (BB).

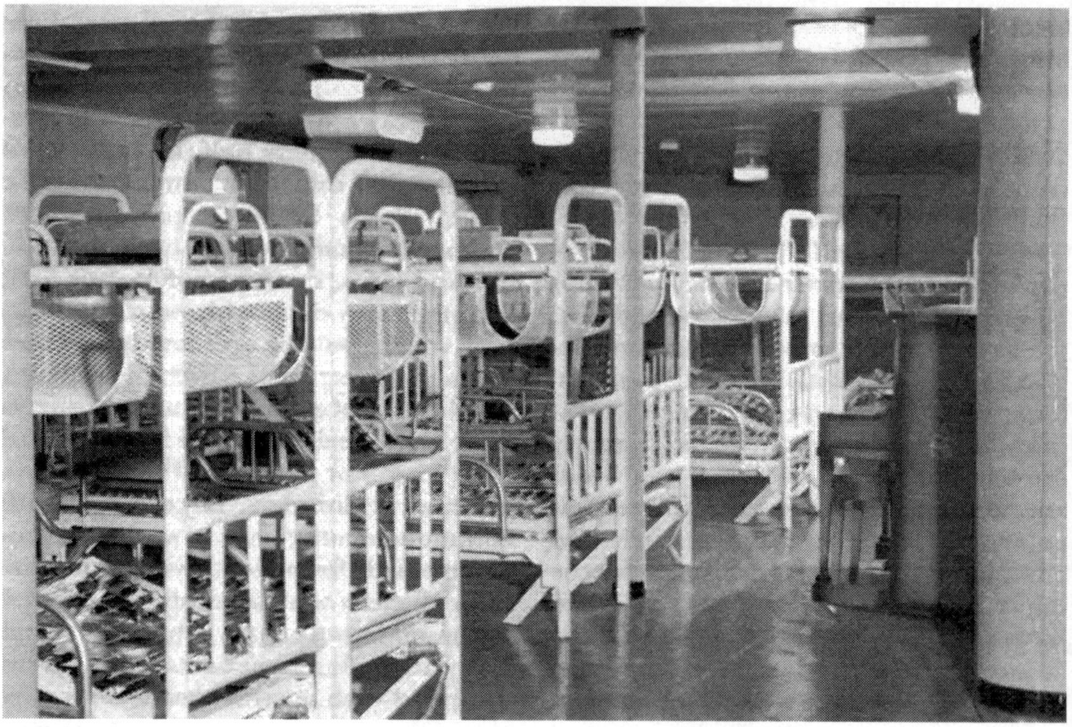

SURGICAL WARD ON USAHS *SHAMROCK*

Office was also interested in features of construction that promoted sanitation and comfort. As a safety precaution and as a buffer against noise, it insisted that bulkheads should be of double-thick fireproof material that was easy to clean. White tile was considered necessary for the decks of washrooms, operating rooms, sterilizing and workrooms, dressing stations, cleaning gear rooms, utility rooms, diet kitchens, prophylactic stations, pharmacies, laboratories and autopsy rooms. For the rest of the hospital area a deck covering of cement composition or of heavy linoleum was considered satisfactory. Deckheads of a material similar to that used for bulkheads were needed as protection against dust in operating rooms, sterilizing rooms, dressing rooms, and smaller wards, and, in addition, as a safety measure—for covering exposed pipes and fixtures—in all mental wards.[48]

Numerous difficulties were encountered in converting the vessels into hospital ships. Lacking a suitable table of organization for hospital ship complements at the beginning of the program, the Medical Department had to estimate the number of officers, nurses, and attendants for whom quarters would be needed on each ship. Late in 1943, when The Surgeon General revised the existing table of organization, some of the conversion plans

[48] (1) Tynes, Construction Branch, pp. 101, 106. (2) Memo, SG for CofT, 26 May 43, sub: Steel Bulkheading in Hosp Ships. SG: 632.1 (BB). (3) Ltr, Water Div NYPE to CofT, 2 Nov 43, sub: Hosp Ships, with 4 inds. Same file.

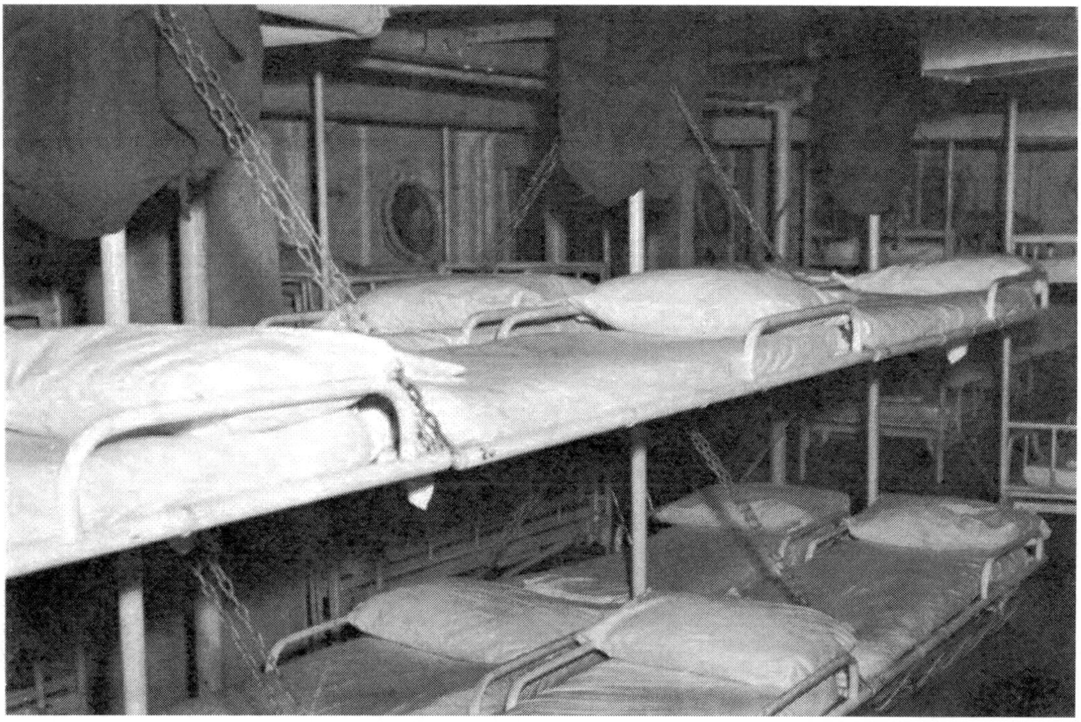

SURGICAL WARD ON USAHS *LOUIS A. MILNE*

already prepared had to be modified to provide different sets of quarters.[49] About the same time, the decision to devote 50 percent of each hospital ship's capacity to accommodations for mental patients caused further revisions in plans already drawn. Changes in the size of the merchant marine crews, along with friction between maritime unions on the one hand and the Transportation Corps and Surgeon General's Office on the other about the size and location of crew quarters, tended to cause revisions in plans. In some instances changes in approved plans were requested by representatives of the Surgeon General's Office (Maj. Howard A. Donald and Lt. Col. Achilles L. Tynes) as they inspected work in progress at various ports.[50] Of perhaps even greater importance were delays in shipyards. Some had difficulty in hiring enough workmen to keep conversion moving along rapidly. Others failed to get materials when they were needed. Still others, heavily committed to the Navy, devoted their workers and materials to naval landing craft with higher priorities.[51]

As a result of these difficulties the entire

[49] For example, see Memo, Lt Col A. L. Tynes for SG, 27 Oct 43, sub: Rpt of Insp of SS *Ernest Hinds*. HD: 560.2 (Hosp Cons Br, Hosp Ship file).

[50] (1) Tynes, Construction Branch, pp. 95–116. (2) Correspondence concerning conversions are filed in SG: 560.2, 632.1 (BB), and in HD: 560.2 (Hosp Cons Br, Gen), 560.2 (Hosp Cons Br, under name of each hosp ship).

[51] (1) Memo, SG for ASF Dir of Mat, 17 Feb 44, with inds. SG: 632.1 (BB). (2) Memo, Col R. M. Hicks (Water Div OCT) for Howard Bruce, 23 Feb 44, sub: Hosp Ship Convs. TC: 564.

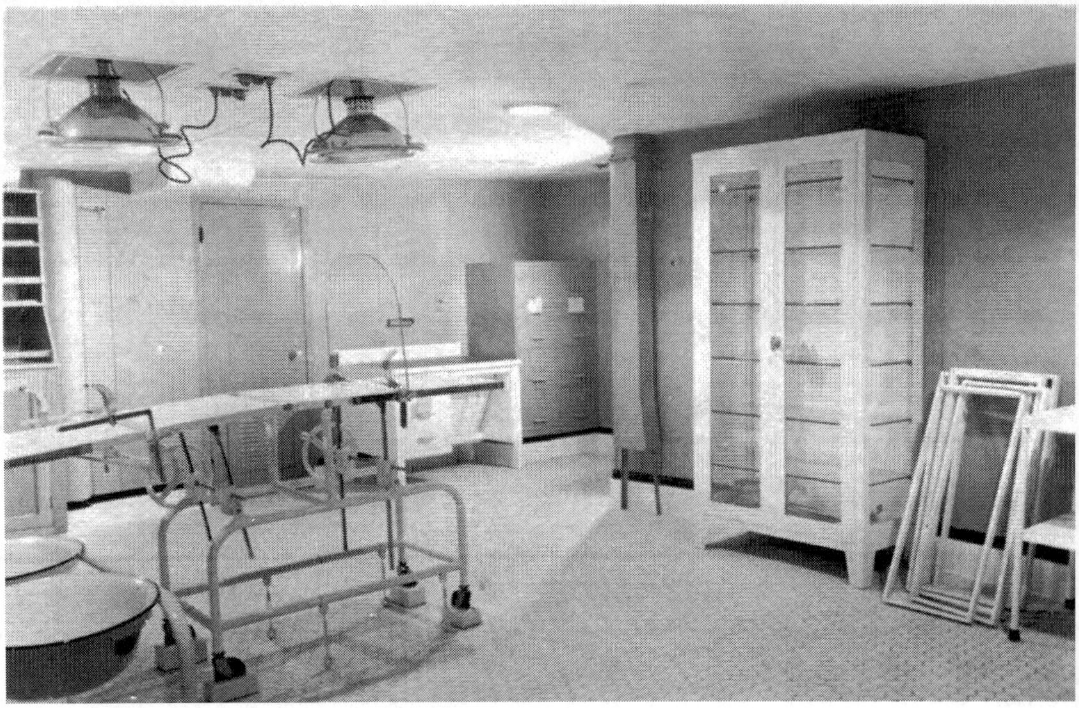

DRESSING STATION ON USAHS *LOUIS A. MILNE*

program was delayed. Only three Army hospital ships were in service by the end of 1943. One per month was placed in service from February through May 1944, and one of the three ships being constructed by the Navy was commissioned the next month. Thus by the end of June 1944 there were nine hospital ships serving the Army, instead of the nineteen anticipated. The next month seven more were completed and in August and September two additional Army hospital ships and the two remaining hospital ships being constructed by the Navy for Army use were ready for their first trips. The final two ships of twenty-four authorized in June 1943 were placed in service in March and April 1945. *(Table 18)* Meanwhile the Southwest Pacific had converted two vessels, the *Tasman* and *Maetsuycker*, for intra-theater use. Although controlled by the American Army, these vessels were Dutch hospital ships, sailing under Dutch registry and certified under the Hague Convention by the Netherlands Government.[52]

As Army hospital ships were readied for service, the problem of naming them arose. The Navy named its hospital ships for abstract qualities and hence designated the three ships it was building for the Army as the *Comfort, Hope,* and *Mercy.*

[52] For further information on these vessels, see TC: 565.1-DB *(Tasman)*; HD: SWPA 560.2 *(Tasman* and *Maetsuycker)*; and State Dept: 740.00117 Eur War 1939/1-1648 (Netherlands Hosp Ships). Also see WD Memo W40-21-43, sub: Use of SS *Tasman* as a Hosp Ship, 20 Oct 43, in AG: 560 (16 Oct 43).

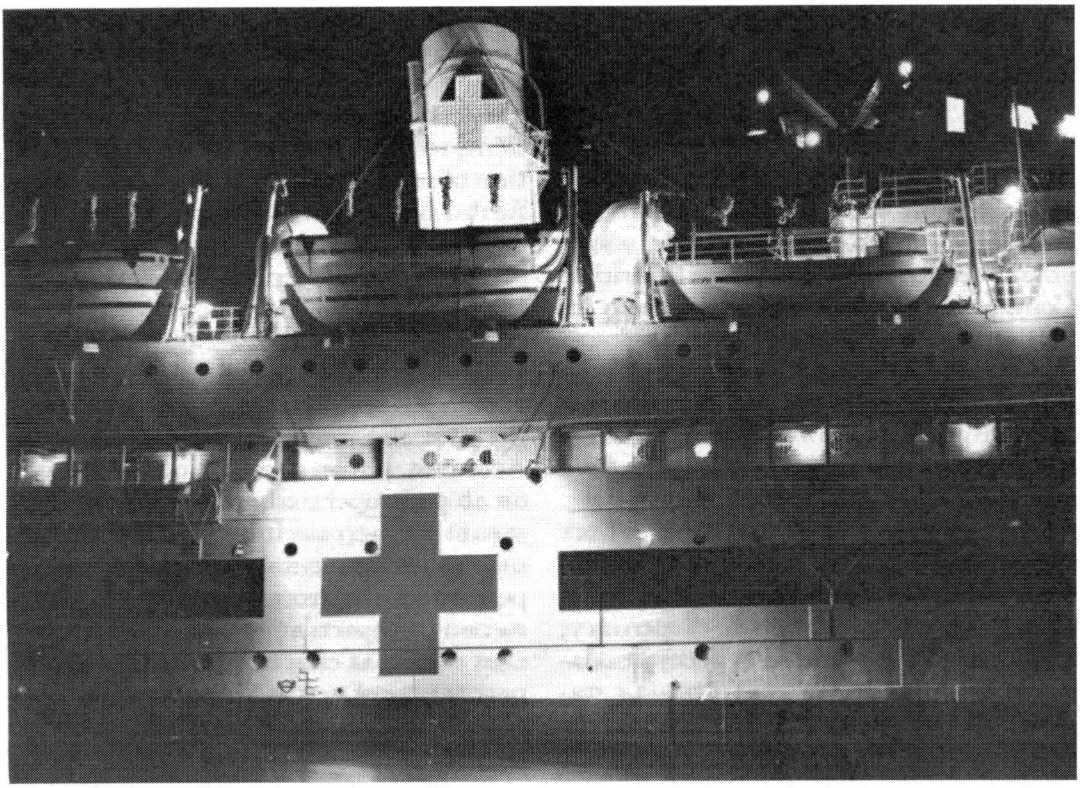

THE USAHS *LARKSPUR*

Trying not to trespass upon this system and at the same time trying to designate Army hospital ships appropriately, the Surgeon General's Office proposed in July 1943 that they be named for flowers. Transportation Corps officials believed that this might complicate rather than simplify their identification as hospital ships. Since all of the vessels being converted were well known in the world's shipping registers, an enemy encountering one could identify it, if designated as a hospital ship under its existing name, by its ascribed physical characteristics and silhouette. It was therefore decided to retain names that were not "entirely inconsistent" with the vessels' new mission and to name others for flowers. In the spring of 1944 the Coast Guard objected to this practice fearing that the Army's naming of hospital ships for flowers would cause confusion with Coast Guard ships carrying the same names. As a result, at the suggestion of the Surgeon General's Office most hospital ships commissioned thereafter were named for deceased Army medical officers and nurses.[53] *(See Table 18.)*

[53] (1) Memos, SG for CofT, 1 Jul 43; CofT for SG, 22 Jul 43, sub: Names for Hosp Ships. (2) Ltrs, USCG to CofT, 3 Mar 44; CofT to USCG, 9 Mar 44. (3) Memos, CofT for SG, 14 Mar 44, 8 Jan 45, sub: Names for Hosp Ships. All in TC: 569.61. (5) TC Cir 80–4, 5 Feb 44, with supp, 25 Mar, 30 May 44, and 10 Feb 45.

Continuation of Efforts To Insure Adequate Hospital Facilities on Transports, 1943-45

Although standards for ships' hospitals had been established by the middle of 1943, meeting these standards continued to involve certain problems. One was to obtain desired modifications of Maritime Commission plans. In reviewing them the Surgeon General's Office sometimes found major faults: failure to comply with directives about the percentage of hospital beds to be provided; unsatisfactory location of hospital areas, as for example in the stern two decks below the lifeboat loading deck, instead of nearer midship and one deck higher; improper arrangement of certain medical facilities, such as the combination of the surgical suite and the dispensary; and failure to provide such accommodations as utility rooms and dressing stations. Unless construction of ships was too far advanced, the Commission generally made the revisions requested by the Surgeon General's Office.[54]

Less success was achieved in negotiations with the British to improve hospitals on their transports. Normally they followed a policy of making few if any structural changes in ex-passenger vessels. In December 1943 this problem was referred to the Combined Military Transportation Committee and, as a result, the Transportation Corps and the Medical Department had to approve specifications for hospital areas aboard British transports that were considerably lower than those for American transports. For example, according to a decision of the Committee, British transports were not required to have wards for mental patients or separate operating and sterilizing rooms. Instead of the latter, they had one room which served as a combination surgeon's office, records room, sterilization room, dressing station, and emergency operating room.[55]

Increases in the number of mental patients to be evacuated and in the proportion of seriously disturbed cases required further changes in transports' hospitals. In the fall of 1943, on the recommendation of the Surgeon General's liaison officer, the Chief of Transportation directed that capacity for mental patients should be increased by 3 percent of the troop capacity of each Army-owned and chartered transport. He also requested the War Shipping Administration to make similar changes on ships it operated for the Army. This meant an increase in authorized accommodations for mental patients from 2 to 5 percent of the troop capacity of Army-owned transports and from 1½ to 4½ percent of that of chartered transports. The percentage of berths for patients of other types remained unchanged. In order to provide additional accommodations for mental patients without diminishing troop capacity, staterooms that were used on outbound voyages for officers and noncommissioned officers were to be altered. "Potential weapons" were to be removed and electrical fixtures supplied with guards; suitable doors were to be installed

[54] (1) Tynes, Construction Branch, p. 117. (2) Ltr, SG to CofT, 16 Sep 43, sub: Gen Arrangement Plans for Hosp Sec on C4-S-B2 Mar Comm Trp Trans. (3) Memo, SG for CofT, 27 Sep 43, sub: Hosp Facs on US Army Trans, C-3 Type. (4) Ltr, Mar Comm to SG, 28 Sep 43, sub: C4-S-B2 Trp Trans, Hosp Spaces. All in SG: 632.-1 (BB).

[55] (1) Ltr. CofT to SG, 18 Dec 43, sub: Proposed Hosp Revision Aboard HMT *Queen Mary*. SG: 632.-1 (*Queen Mary*)BB. (2) Memo, SG for CofT, 17 Feb 44, sub: Comments on Proposed Agreement Conc Minimum Standards Aboard Brit and Amer Trp Ships. SG: 560.-1 (Gr Brit). (3) Ltrs, CofT to CGs PEs, 15 Mar 44; CofT to CGs TofOpns, 19 Apr 44, sub: Minimum Standards on Brit and Amer Trans, with Rpt CMTC, 18 Feb 44, 82d Mtg. TC: 337 (Trp Trans).

and bars placed across portholes; and berths were to be modified so that the lower two could be fixed by bolting or welding and the top one removed before the loading of patients.[56]

About a year later action was taken to provide more suitable accommodations for severely disturbed patients. On 25 October 1944, the Operations Division, War Department General Staff, in a meeting with representatives of the Chief of Transportation, The Surgeon General, and others, decided that transports should have locked cells for some patients and small wards for others. Subsequently, the Transportation Corps announced that individual cells would be provided on transports sailing to the Southwest Pacific equal in number to .75 percent of their troop capacities and on those sailing to other areas equal to .30 percent of their capacities. Approximately half the remaining accommodations for mental patients were to be in small locked wards holding twelve or fewer patients.[57]

A study in the winter of 1944 of the anticipated patient load indicated that, among other measures, fuller use would have to be made of the British *Queens* and "maximum loading" of certain transports would have to be authorized. A series of conferences among Medical Department, Transportation Corps, and British representatives in the European Theater of Operations and in Washington resulted in arrangements in January 1945 to use the *Queen Elizabeth* and the *Queen Mary* on westbound trips primarily for the evacuation of patients. To increase their patient-carrying capacities to 3,500 and 3,000 respectively (the number of patients who could be fed three meals a day from the ships' kitchens), additional pantries had to be installed, accommodations for more medical personnel provided, and facilities for patients modified. These changes were limited mainly to installing rails alongside patients' berths, furnishing additional bedpan washers and sterilizers, and providing food carts for serving hot meals to patients unable to attend mess formations.[58]

To permit the "maximum loading" of seventeen Army and three Navy transports—that is, loading them with the maximum number of patients who could be properly fed and otherwise cared for regardless of lifeboat restrictions—similar changes had to be made aboard these vessels. In March 1945 the Chief of Transportation established the following standards for such changes: additional diet kitchens, food-serving pantries, and food carts should be provided to insure the serving of food in a palatable condition; sufficient bedpan washers and sterilizers should be installed to care for all litter patients; additional mattresses and pillows should be provided; lee rails should be attached alongside the berths of all litter patients and all ambulatory patients who

[56] (1) Ltr, CG USAFFE to TAG, 24 Aug 43, sub: Evac of Psychotic Cases to US, with 2 inds. AG: 704.11. (2) Ltr, CofT to CGs PEs, 18 Nov 43, sub: Increase in Mental Pnt Capacity on Trans. TC: 632 (Army Vessels). (3) Ltr, TAG to CGs AAF, AGF, ASF, Theaters, Def and Base Comds, etc., 8 Jun 44, sub: Procedure for Evac of Pnts by Water or Air from Overseas Comd. AG: 704.11 (3 Jun 44). (4) See pp. 399-400.

[57] (1) Memo OPD 370.05, ACofS OPD WDGS for CG ASF, 27 Oct 44, sub: Evac of Mental Pnts from the SWPA. HRS: ASF Planning Div and Program Br file 370.05, "Hosp and Evac." (2) Memo, Mvmt Div OCT for Water Div OCT, 6 Nov 44, sub: Mental Accommodations on Trp Trans. SG: 705.

[58] (1) Rads CM-OUT-72113 (3 Dec 44); CM-OUT-76241 (12 Dec 44), WD (prepared by Lt Col J[ohn] C. Fitzpatrick) to Hq ComZ ETO. SG: 560.2. (2) Rpt, CMTC 67, 16 Jan 45, sub: Return of Pnts and Other Pers West-Bound on the *Queen Elizabeth* and *Queen Mary*. SG: 705.

could not care for themselves without assistance; and additional dispensaries and surgical dressing rooms should be constructed for the routine dressings and emergency care patients might need en route.[59] These changes increased the capacities of seven transports to an average of more than 1,300 patients each, including mental and litter cases.[60]

Additional Hospital Ships and Modifications for Pacific Service

In authorizing five additional Army hospital ships in December 1944 to help handle the patient load in 1945, the Joint Chiefs of Staff directed that changes in vessels selected should be kept to the minimum necessary to fit them as "ambulance-type hospital ships." Recognizing the necessity of this policy, The Surgeon General agreed that existing deck structures of these ships should be used to the greatest possible extent, but insisted that each ship should have a proper surgery and X-ray department, adequate messing facilities for feeding bed patients, and suitable office space.[61] In this instance the Joint Military Transportation Committee selected the vessels to be used and once again the Surgeon General's Office collaborated with the New York Port of Embarkation in the preparation of plans for conversion. One of these ships was ready for service by April 1945; another, two months later; and the third, in September 1945.[62] Work on the remaining two was suspended after V-J Day and they were again placed in the transport service to return troops from overseas areas.

While plans were being made to put five additional Army hospital ships in service, steps were taken to prepare those already available for Pacific duty. During 1944 the surgeons of some complained that ventilation of these vessels was so poor that patients often found the heat and odors almost unbearable. Early in 1945 representatives of The Surgeon General and the Chief of Transportation agreed that it would be ideal to have hospital ships completely air conditioned, as were those of the Navy, but in view of shortage of time they decided that only portions of them, such as operating rooms, clinics, and certain wards, should be air conditioned and that efforts should be made to increase the exhaust ventilation of other areas. This program was approved for the five newly authorized ships, and during May, June, and July 1945, at least eight others were routed to the New York Port of Embarkation for the installation of air-conditioning equipment.[63]

Medical Attendants for Service on Transports

Determining a Method of Supplying Personnel

The question of how medical attendants were to be supplied to care for patients

[59] (1) Memo, CofT for Dir Nav Trans Serv, 22 Feb 45, sub: Pnt Capacity *Mt. Vernon, Wakefield* and *West Point*. (2) Rads, WD for CGs PEs, UK Base Sec, Hq ComZ ETO, POA, MTO, SWPA, 14 and 22 Mar 45. (3) Ltr, CG NYPE to CofT, 20 Apr 45, sub: Increase of Litter Capacity of Trp Ships. All in TC: 569.

[60] Total patient capacities of the vessels varied from 404 on the *Borinquen* to 2,618 on the *George Washington*. See list of maximum capacities in History . . . Medical Regulating Service . . . , sec 6.

[61] (1) JCS 1199, 16 Dec 44, Hosp Ship Program; JCS 1199/1, 5 Feb 45, same sub. (2) Memo, Col A[chilles] L. Tynes for SG, 21 Dec 44, sub: Plans for Proposed Conv of French Ships, *Athos II* and *Colombie*, into US Army Hosp Ships. Both in SG: 560.2.

[62] See Table 18.

[63] (1) Memo SPTOM 560, Mvmt Div OCT for Water Div OCT, 31 Mar 45, sub: Surv of Ventilation Systs Aboard Hosp Ships. HD: 705 (MRO, Newman Staybacks). (2) Memo, Mvmt Div OCT for Gen R[obert] H. Wylie, 14 Jul 45, sub: Repair Status of US Army Hosp Ships. SG: 705.

being evacuated by Army troop transport arose early in the war. In January 1942, G-4 directed The Surgeon General and The Quartermaster General to include in plans for sea evacuation operations recommendations about the source and use of personnel for ships. In response The Surgeon General proposed the establishment of Medical Department pools at ports in the zone of interior and in theaters of operations. From such pools port commanders in the zone of interior could assign appropriate medical staffs to ships' hospitals on outbound transports and theater commanders could assign additional attendants to care for patients on return trips. After completing voyage assignments, the attendants could return to theater pools by the first available ship. When not on transport duty, they could be used to supplement the staffs of hospitals located near ports either in the zone of interior or in theaters of operations.[64]

SOS headquarters at first partially approved The Surgeon General's plan. On 18 June 1942 it authorized port commanders to establish pools of Medical Department personnel, under control of port surgeons, from which to furnish complements for ships' hospitals. According to a guide supplied by The Surgeon General, the permanent complement aboard each transport was to consist of the ship's surgeon and twelve enlisted men. Before departure of a transport from the United States, a port surgeon was to estimate the number of patients it would return from theaters and, according to a graduated table in the guide, was to assign necessary attendants. In emergencies overseas commanders could supply additional attendants.[65] This system proved inadequate, perhaps for several reasons. Ports in the United States had trouble getting enough medical personnel to operate the system. In the absence of a large backlog of patients in theaters, it was impractical to estimate the number of evacuees to be returned. Finally, port pools were difficult to keep in operation because ships sometimes were diverted and did not return directly to home ports.

The SOS Hospitalization and Evacuation Branch therefore suggested a different plan in August 1942. Calling for the use of table-of-organization units listed in the troop basis, it promised to insure the availability of attendants at all times. Therefore SOS headquarters directed The Surgeon General to prepare an appropriate table. It was to provide not only for units to care for groups of 25, 50, 75, 100, 250, and 500 patients but also for units to serve as permanent medical complements of transports. The latter were to operate ships' hospitals on outbound trips and were to serve as administrative and technical nuclei around which supplementary platoons could function when patients were being returned to the United States. The Surgeon General prepared the table as directed, but protested against its adoption. Because table-of-organization units were inflexible, he contended, they were wasteful of personnel when used in operations characterized by variable factors, such as ships' destinations, length of voy-

[64] (1) Memo AG 573.27 (10-29-41), TAG for SG, 26 Jan 42, sub: Hosp Space on Army Trans. HD: 541 (Equip for Trans). (2) Ltr, SG to TAG, 16 Feb 42, sub: T/O for Hosp Ship and Tabulation of Med Pers Reqmts for ATS to Evac from Overseas, with 5 incls. Same file. (3) Memo, SG to CG SOS (Dir of Oprs), 30 Apr 42. HD: 705 (Hosp and Evac, Col Welsh file).

[65] (1) Ltr SPOPM 322.15, CG SOS to CGs and COs of CAs, PEs, and Gen Hosps, and to SG, 18 Jun 42, sub: Oprs Plans for Mil Hosp and Evac, with incls. (2) Ltr, SG to CGs all PEs, 29 Jun 42, sub: Opr Plans for Mil Hosp and Evac, with 3 incls. Both in HD: 705 (Hosp and Evac).

ages, outbound loads, and the number and type of patients on return trips. Nevertheless, the General Staff supported SOS headquarters and directed the activation of ten platoons in September. The next month, the table of organization for "Medical Hospital Ship Platoons, Separate," was published. It provided for a permanent complement of medical personnel that included one officer and twelve enlisted men for each transport, and for supplementary platoons varying in size from seven to eighty-eight officers, nurses, and enlisted men to care for different numbers of patients.[66]

Publication of this table did not settle the question entirely. In November 1942, when SOS headquarters was about to activate thirty additional platoons, The Surgeon General again objected to their use. Whether because of this objection or for other reasons, SOS headquarters seems to have compromised. Supplementary platoons were organized to serve aboard transports carrying patients, but table-of-organization units to serve as the permanent medical complements were never activated. Instead, SOS headquarters continued to supply personnel for this purpose in allotments to port commanders.[67]

Measures to Conserve Personnel

Steady and large increases in evacuation in the latter half of the war, along with other demands for shares of a limited supply of medical personnel, especially doctors, intensified the problem of providing attendants for patients aboard transports. In the fall of 1943 the use of inflexible table-of-organization units was questioned by the Surgeon General's Personnel Board and by ASF headquarters as being wasteful. The use of theater pools was again considered, but Lt. Col. John C. Fitzpatrick, liaison officer of The Surgeon General with the Chief of Transportation, defended the use of platoons. They constituted the surest way, he insisted, for ASF to discharge its responsibility for the care of patients after they left theater control. In October 1943 representatives of The Surgeon General, the Chief of Transportation, the General Staff, and ASF headquarters reviewed the entire question and decided that "platoons should be modified and retained." They agreed also that maximum use should be made of returning casual medical personnel to supplement the medical service on transports. These measures, they expected, would promote manpower economy.[68]

Modifications were made not so much in platoons themselves as in their use. When the table under which they were organized was revised in October 1943, nurses were eliminated, as the Chief of Transportation recommended. Thereafter they were to be furnished, if needed, by theater commanders.[69] Of more importance, the Office of the Chief of Transportation in November 1943 developed a guide for theaters to use in placing platoons aboard transports. This guide took account of the fact that variations in types

[66] (1) Memo, ACofS for Oprs SOS for SG, 28 Aug 42, sub: T/O for Med Pers on Amb Ships and Trp Trans, with ind. (2) Memo, ACofS for Oprs SOS for Dir Mil Pers SOS, 1 Oct 42, same sub. (3) Memo, SG for CG SOS (Mob Br), 19 Oct 42. All in SG: 320.3. (4) T/O 8-534, 27 Oct 42.

[67] (1) Memo for Record, on Memo, CG SOS for TAG, 14 Nov 42, sub: Constitution and Activation of 30 Hosp Ship Plats, Sep. AG: 320.2 (1 Oct 42) (3). (2) Memo, Hosp and Evac Br Plans Div SOS for Mob Br Plans Div SOS, 8 Dec 42, sub: Med Pers on Army Trans. HD: 705 (MRO, Fitzpatrick Daybook, Aug 42-Jun 43). (3) Memo, CG SOS for CofT, 4 Jan 43, sub: Almts for Ships' Complements. SG: 320.3-1.

[68] (1) Rpt, SG Pers Bd Mtgs, 16 Sep-29 Sep 43. SG: 334.7-1. (2) Rpt, SG Pers Bd to Oprs Serv SGO, 28 Oct 43, sub: Study of MD Pers. HD: 334 (Kenner Bd).

[69] T/O&E 8-534, 21 Oct 43.

of patients required variations in the number of attendants provided. For example, while two 100-bed platoons would be required to care for 100 mental or litter patients, a 25-bed platoon was sufficient for a like number of ambulatory or troop class patients. A 100-bed platoon could care for 150 patients if 75 percent were either ambulatory or troop class. This guide, which geared the size of platoons to the type as well as number of patients, was designed to permit a flexibility in use that would contribute to economy. In November 1943 it was sent to the European theater; the following March, to the North African. In June 1944 it was issued to all theaters in a revised directive on evacuation operations.[70]

Another economy measure was the elimination of small platoons. With actual and anticipated increases in the patient load early in 1944, it was unlikely that those with less than 100-bed capacity would be needed. Small units—of 25-, 50-, and 75-bed capacities—were authorized one Medical Corps officer each, as was the 100-bed unit. Thus the use of small platoons to attend groups of patients numbering 100 or more was wasteful of Medical Corps officers. In April 1944 the Chief of Transportation requested ASF headquarters to convert all platoons of 25-, 50-, and 75-bed capacities, a total of 184, to 100-bed units. This action increased their table-of-organization capacity from 7,275 to 18,400 patients without any increase in the number of Medical Corps officers and with the addition of only 1,964 enlisted men and 184 Dental Corps officers. With the eighty-seven 100-bed platoons already organized, this gave a total table-of-organization capacity of 27,100 patients.[71] When additional platoons were required later, none of less than 100-bed capacity was organized.

Another measure to supply attendants for patients evacuated by transport was the use of medical personnel returning to the United States in a duty status. The number of enlisted men, officers, and nurses in this category increased as the war lengthened and as they accumulated enough overseas service to return home on "rotation." Under an agreement reached in October 1943, the War Department on 8 June 1944 directed theater commanders to form such personnel into provisional medical hospital ship platoons and to return to the United States no Medical Corps officer below the grade of colonel and no nurse whatever without assuring the full use of his or her services en route. Subsequently, in the fall of 1944 and early in 1945, when the Chief of Transportation requested the activation of additional platoons, The Surgeon General disapproved, suggesting instead that theaters be directed to form more provisional platoons.[72]

Other measures were also necessary to

[70] (1) Ltr, CofT to CG ETOUSA 13 Nov 43, sub: Util of Med Hosp Ship Plat, Sep. HD: 705 (MRO, Fitzpatrick Stayback, 498). (2) Rad CM-OUT-7672, WD (Mvmt Div OCT) to CG NATOUSA, 18 Mar 44. SG: 322.8-1. (3) Ltr, TAG to CGs AAF, AGF, ASF, Theaters, Def and Base Comds, etc., 8 Jun 44, sub: Procedure for Evac of Pnts by Water or Air from Overseas Comd, with incl 4. AG: 704.11 (3 Jun 44).

[71] (1) Ltr, CofT to CG ASF thru SG, 1 Apr 44, sub: Reorgn of Med Hosp Ship Plat (Sep). HD: 705 (MRO, Fitzpatrick Stayback, 1077). (2) Memo, CofT for CG ASF, 20 Apr 44, sub: Request for Activation of Add Med Hosp Ship Plats, Sep, with 10 incls. HRS: ASF Planning Div Program Br file, "Hosp and Evac. vol. 3."

[72] (1) Ltr, TAG to CGs AAF, AGF, ASF, Theaters, Def and Base Comds, etc., 8 Jun 44, sub: Procedure for Evac of Pnts by Water or Air from Overseas Comd. AG: 704.11 (3 Jun 44). (2) Ltr, CofT to CG ASF thru SG, 25 Oct 44, sub: Request for Prov Med Hosp Ship Plats, Sep. HRS: ASF Planning Div Program Br file, "Hosp and Evac." (3) Memo, CofT for CG ASF thru SG, 24 Mar 45, sub: Request for Prov Med Hosp Ship Plats, Sep, with 2 incls. SG: 322 (Plat).

provide, within the amount of medical personnel available, sufficient attendants for patients on transports. Attempts were made to increase the use of regularly organized platoons by reducing the time they spent in the United States and in returning to theaters. Although such units were assigned to the Chief of Transportation, for a time the commanders of ports actually controlled them while they were in the United States. In the fall of 1944 their control was centralized in the Movements Division of the Office of the Chief of Transportation. Knowing where platoons were needed as well as schedules of ships leaving from all ports, this Division could arrange for the return of platoons to theaters more quickly than could ports. Later, the War Department suggested that theaters might establish air priorities for them, in order to reduce the time normally required for their return. Another measure taken in the fall of 1944 was the deployment of platoons from "isolated theaters," such as the Middle East, India, and South Pacific, to other more active theaters, such as the European.[73]

Problems in the Use of Platoons

Questions arose about the control of platoons. The first ten were assigned to the New York Port of Embarkation, but all others were assigned to the Chief of Transportation and were attached to ports. In December 1942 The Surgeon General asked where and how they were to be placed aboard transports carrying patients. Representatives of his Office, of the Office of the Chief of Transportation, and of SOS headquarters subsequently decided that platoons should be attached to overseas theaters on a temporary duty basis and that theater commanders should be responsible for placing them on transports as needed.[74] After attachment to theaters platoons came under the administrative control of theater commanders. This step gave rise to complaints that theaters employed them improperly when they were not escorting patients to the United States. One complained of being assigned to work in medical supply; another, of being required to sort mail. Nevertheless the War Department followed a policy of not interfering with theater commanders in the control of platoons attached to their commands and intervened only when the care of patients was affected.[75] When the Southwest Pacific failed to place sufficient attendants on transports evacuating patients during 1944, the Movements Division of the

[73] (1) History . . . Medical Regulating Service . . . , sec 3. (2) Rad CM-OUT-69352, WD to CG USAF POA, 28 Nov 44. TC: 322 (Med Hosp Ship Plats). Similar messages were sent to other theaters. (3) Memo for Record, on draft Rad, WD to SWPA and POA, 26 Nov 44. HD: 705 (MRO, Gay Stayback, 151). (4) Memo, CG ASF for CofT, 8 Dec 44, sub: Request for Prov Med Hosp Ship Plats, Sep. HRS: ASF Planning Div Program Br file, "Hosp and Evac."

[74] (1) Ltr, TAG to CGs NYPE, 1st, 4th, 5th, and 8th SvCs and to SG, 30 Sep 42, sub: Constitution and Activation of 10 Plats. AG: 320.2 (9-30-42) (10). (2) Ltr, TAG to CGs NYPE, 1st, 4th, 5th, 7th, and 8th SvCs and to SG and CofT, 16 Nov 42, sub: Constitution and Activation of 30 Plats (Sep) Ship Hosp. AG: 320.2 (1-10-42) (3) Sec 15. (3) Memo, CG SOS for TAG, 5 Jan 43, same sub. AG: 320.2 (11-21-42). (4) Memo, SG for Hosp and Evac Br Plans Div SOS, 21 Dec 42. SG: 200.3-1 (BB). (5) Diary, SOS Hosp and Evac Br, 22 Dec 42. HD: Wilson files, "Diary." (6) Memo for Record, on Memo, CG SOS for SG, 24 Dec 42, sub: Med Hosp Ship Plat, Sep. HD: Wilson files, "Book 2, 26 Sep-31 Dec 42." (7) Memo, CofT for CGs PEs, 17 Jun 43, sub: Mvmt Orders, Med Hosp Ship Plats, Sep. TC: 322 (Med Hosp Ship Plats).

[75] (1) Ltr, CO 584th MHSP, HRPE to SG, 28 Jan 44, sub: Duties Performed by a Med Hosp Ship Plat Overseas. HD: 705 (Hosp Ship Plats). (2) Memo, MRO (Gay) for Col J[ames] T. McGibony, 15 May 45, sub: Misuse of Med Pers. HD: 705 (MRO, Newman Stayback, 159).

Office of the Chief of Transportation initiated a War Department cablegram to that theater calling attention to "repeated reports" that it both overloaded transports and supplied insufficient medical personnel, even though platoons were available. This message pointed out that the Army would suffer serious criticism unless such practices were corrected.[76] In 1945 reports reached the Surgeon General's Office that nursing care on transports returning from the Pacific was below "desirable standards." Believing the cause of this situation to be an inclusion in provisional platoons of enlisted men not technically qualified to care for patients, the Chief of Transportation had a War Department message sent to the Pacific urging greater selectivity in choosing men for provisional platoons.[77]

The medical hospital ship platoon, a wartime development, seems to have justified its existence. On V-E Day 176 regularly organized platoons were being used to attend patients returning from the European theater, and several months later there were 116 in the Pacific. Altogether there were 332 platoons in service in August 1945.[78] Officers familiar with their work agreed generally that they performed excellently, in view of the difficult mission and adverse conditions—long hours, arduous tasks, and a minimum of leave and recreational opportunities. Moreover, although some felt that dentists, pharmacists, and laboratory technicians were not really needed in such platoons, representatives of the Surgeon General's Office agreed in May 1945, in reviewing experience with such units, that their table of organization needed no change. After the war the Medical Regulating Officer proposed only one change—the second officer in each platoon might be of any branch of the Medical Department instead of specifically of the Dental Corps.[79]

Hospital Ship Complements

Although the Army had no hospital ships in the first part of the war, as already pointed out, efforts were made to get them and the Surgeon General's Office drafted a table of organization for a medical hospital ship company early in 1942. Published in April, it provided for a unit of 14 officers, 35 nurses, 1 warrant officer, and 99 enlisted men to care for 500 patients, and for supplementary units of 2 officers, 4 nurses, and 11 enlisted men for each additional group of 100.[80] The approval in May 1942 of the conversion of the *Acadia* into an ambulance transport and a request in August 1942 by the European theater for three hospital ships made it appear that units organized under this

[76] Draft Rad, WD (Mvmt Div OCT) to CinC SWPA, 9 Oct 44, sub: Evac of Pnts from Milne Bay. HD: 705 (MRO, Fitzpatrick Stayback, 1495).

[77] Draft Rad, WD (Mvmt Div OCT) to CinC AFPAC, CGs SFPE, SPE, LAPE, 20 Jul 45. HD: 705 (MRO, Newman Stayback, 195).

[78] Reports of locations, assignments, and movements of platoons were kept from March 1943 until their inactivation in 1945–46. See monthly reports in TC: 322 (Med Hosp Ship Plats); in HD: 705 (MRO, Stayback files: Fitzpatrick, Jun 43–Apr 44; Zolnaski, Mar–Nov 44), and in SG: 705, Plats, weekly Status Rpts, beginning in Mar 44.

[79] (1) History . . . Medical Regulating Serv . . . , secs 3.7 and 3.8. (2) Memo for Record, Resources Anal Div SGO, 7 May 45, sub: Mtg of T/O Rev Cmtee for Redeployment. HD: 705 (MRO, Newman Stayback, 151). (3) Memo, MRO for Dir Hosp and Dom Oprs SGO, 23 Nov 45, sub: ASF MD T/O&E. HD: 705 (MRO, Hodge Stayback, 514). (4) George F. Jeffcott, A History of the United States Army Dental Service in World War II, Ch. X, pp. 35–42. HD.

[80] (1) Ltr, QMG to TAG, 14 Feb 42, sub: Hosp Space on Army Trans. AG: 573.27. (2) T/O 8–537, 1 Apr 42.

table would be needed. SOS headquarters therefore directed The Surgeon General to plan to supply personnel for them.[81] As a result, four hospital ship companies were activated in October and November 1942. One was placed on the *Acadia* when it became an ambulance transport in December 1942. The other three were not used until the first of the Army's hospital ships went into service in the summer of 1943.[82]

After the Army began to select transports for conversion under the 24-hospital-ship program, the table of organization for hospital ship companies had to be revised. It was designed to supply personnel for ships with 500 or more beds, but those to be converted were to have varying capacities, ranging from about 300 to 700. Moreover, experience aboard the *Acadia* returning patients from North Africa had revealed certain inadequacies in the old table. Furthermore, Army hospital ships were to be manned by both civilians and soldiers—the former to operate vessels and the latter to care for patients. But there were some services which might be performed by either group. Hence a decision had to be made as to which services each was to perform and military personnel had to be provided accordingly.[83]

The division of responsibility for borderline services came up in July 1943 when plans were drawn for the conversion of the transport *Agwileon* into the hospital ship *Shamrock*. The Surgeon General's Hospital Construction Branch discovered that the New York Port of Embarkation had devoted much space considered desirable for litter patients—almost an entire deck located above the water line— to quarters for the merchant marine crew. To increase this vessel's capacity for litter patients, the Water Division of the Office of the Chief of Transportation directed reduction of the area occupied by the civilian crew by cutting down both the size of the crew and the space allowed each of its remaining members. The steward's department was then cut from seventy to thirty-five. Despite some reduction in original space allowance for individual members of the civilian crew, they continued to be provided with more commodious quarters than the Army allowed enlisted men. As a result, The Surgeon General and the Chief of Transportation agreed to use enlisted men as much as possible in order to save space for patients.[84] During the fall of 1943 the respective duties of the civilian and military crews were agreed upon and the table of organization for hospital ship companies was revised. It was published on 7 December 1943 as Table of Organization and Equipment 8–537T, Hospital Ship Complement.[85]

While the new table provided for complements to serve on ships ranging in capacity, by hundreds, from 200 to 1,000

[81] (1) Memo, CG SOS for SG, 22 Aug 42, sub: Add Hosp Ships. SG: 560.–2. (2) Memo, SG for CG SOS, 24 Aug 42, sub: Request for Auth and Activation of Certain Req SOS Med Units. SG: 320.3–1.

[82] (1) Memo, CG SOS for ACofS G–3 WDGS, 10 Oct 42, sub: Deletion of 107th Gen Hosp from Current Trp Basis, with Memo for Record. AG: 320.2 (10–10–42). (2) Diary, SOS Hosp and Evac Br (Fitzpatrick), 31 Dec 42. HD: Wilson files, "Diary." (3) See pp. 398, 403–04.

[83] (1) Ltr, CO 204th Hosp Ship Co to CG NYPE thru Surg NYPE, 8 May 43, sub: Request for Change in T/O. TC: 320.3 *(Acadia)*. (2) Harold P. James, Transportation of Sick and Wounded [1945]. HD.

[84] Memo, Lt Col A[chilles] L. Tynes for SG, 3 Jul 43, sub: Revised Plans for Hosp Ship *Agwileon*. HD: 560.2.

[85] (1) Memo for Record, by Maj Howard A. Donald, SGO, 27 Sep 43, sub: T/O for Hosp Ship Cos. SG: 320.3–1. (2) Rpt of Conf, Med Hosp Ship Complement, 30 Sep 43. SG: 560.–2. (3) Memo, SG for CG ASF, 13 Nov 43, sub: T/O 8–537, Hosp Ship Complement. AG: 320.3 (20 Nov 43) (2).

beds, it differed from the old primarily in the number of enlisted men authorized for nonmedical duties. A comparison of the complement authorized for a 500-bed ship under the new table with that for a vessel of the same capacity under the old one illustrates the changes made. The number of doctors—eight—remained the same. While the number of nurses was reduced from thirty-five to thirty-four, a hospital dietitian was added. The number of dentists was reduced from two to one, but Medical Administrative Corps officers were increased from two to three. One Sanitary Corps officer and one chaplain were added to the commissioned staff. Although the number of technicians was reduced by one, the number of medical supply and administrative men was increased from twelve to seventeen. Greatest changes affected enlisted men in the nonmedical services and were governed by the division of duties between civilian and military crews announced by the Transportation Corps in December 1943.[86] Because the civilian crew was to prepare food for all persons aboard, with the exception of special diets for patients, the seventeen military cooks formerly authorized were reduced to one. Since the military crew was to furnish cooks' helpers, the latter were raised in number from ten to twelve. In addition, the military crew was to supply guards for certain sections of the ship (primarily those occupied by patients), operate the laundry, and supply dining room service for assigned enlisted men, patients, and both civilian and military personnel authorized to eat in the saloon mess. It was also to provide room service for all patients and military personnel. For these purposes forty-seven enlisted men were added. To permit them to serve in wards when not engaged in nonmedical duties, thirty-one were to be trained and classified as ward orderlies.

Division of responsibilities between military and civilian crews in the fall of 1943 did not eliminate all problems involved in using both civilians and enlisted men on hospital ships. In February 1944 the crews of two threatened to strike unless civilians were placed in some of the jobs filled by enlisted men. To avoid an interruption in evacuation operations, The Surgeon General and the Chief of Transportation agreed to a compromise.[87] Responsibility for furnishing dining room service in the saloon mess (for both the civilian and military personnel eating there) and for supplying cooks' helpers was transferred to the civilian crew, and the average number of civilians in the steward's department was increased from about thirty-five to about forty-five. This change removed enlisted men from their point of greatest contact with the civilian crew and was expected to reduce friction between the two groups. While it was not reflected in a reduction of the military crew until early in 1945, the change did affect plans for the conversion of transports into hospital ships, for the drawings already made had to be modified to provide quarters for the additional civilians. Thereafter, the Chief of Transportation supplied the Surgeon General's Office with manning tables for each of the hospital ships being provided, so that accom-

[86] OCT Cir 164, sub: Div of Responsibility Aboard US Army Hosp Ships, 10 Dec 43, (revised 15 Mar 44). HD: 705 (MRO, Fitzpatrick Staybacks, 840, 970).

[87] (1) Memo, Dir Hosp Admin Div SGO for Chief Hosp Cons Br Hosp Div SGO, ca. Feb 44, sub: Qtrs for Civ Crews, Hosp Ships. HD: 560.2 (Hosp Ships, Hosp Cons Br). (2) Memo, SG (Fitzpatrick) for CofT (Water Div), 22 Feb 44, sub: Full Civ Crews Aboard Army-Opr Hosp Ships. HD: 705 (MRO, Fitzpatrick Stayback, 848).

modations for the civilian crew might be planned and, at the same time, as much space as possible be saved for patients.[88]

Early in 1945 the table of organization for hospital ship complements was revised. Two of the five additional hospital ships authorized in December 1944 were to have capacities exceeding 1,000 beds each. The revised table took this situation into account, providing for a complement for a 1,500-bed ship. It also reflected the shift of responsibility for providing cooks' helpers from the military to the civilian crew by reducing the number authorized for a 500-bed ship from ten to two. These two were kept to assist one military cook in the preparation of special diets for patients. The number of "basic" soldiers was also reduced—from twelve to seven. Nevertheless, the total number of enlisted men in the complement for a 500-bed ship was reduced by only five, because two men were added to perform nonmedical functions, the number of technicians was increased from forty-four to forty-eight, and four men were added to conduct educational and physical reconditioning programs. One nurse was eliminated. Otherwise the number of commissioned officers remained the same. The new table also reflected a function not originally anticipated for Army hospital ships—hospitalization of casualties resulting from the initial phases of landing operations. Unlike Navy hospital ships, which were fitted for definitive medical and surgical treatment at sea, Army hospital ships were planned and staffed to transport patients who had already received treatment in shore installations and needed only a minimum of medical and surgical care en route. After some had been used in support of amphibious operations, the suggestion was made that the tables of organization of complements of such ships should be revised to include an appropriate concentration of specialists. The Surgeon General's Office believed that the sporadic use of Army hospital ships for amphibious operations did not justify such action. Therefore the new table authorized the reinforcement of normal complements with special medical professional service teams when hospital ships were used in support of amphibious landings.[89]

Since a hospital ship complement was assigned to each ship, the activation and training of complements was keyed to the program of converting transports to hospital ships. From the time the first four were activated in the latter part of 1942 until the end of January 1945, twenty-five additional complements were organized and trained. Three were used on the *Hope*, *Comfort*, and *Mercy*. Twenty-four were used on hospital ships operated by the Army, while two were never used because completion of the ships for which they had been organized was suspended when the war ended.[90]

Problems in Providing Supplies and Equipment for Hospital Ships and Transports

Furnishing medical equipment and supplies for patients evacuated by sea depended upon many variable factors.

[88] (1) Tynes, Construction Branch, pp. 96–100. (2) Ltr SPTOW 231.81, CofT to SG, 7 Mar 44, sub: Auth Manning Scales Aboard US Army Hosp Ships. SG: 320.4–1. (3) For other manning tables, see HD: 560.2 (Hosp Cons Br, under name of ship).

[89] (1) T/O&E 8–537, 3 Mar 45. (2) Memo, MRO for SG (Orgn and Equip Allowance Br), 16 Jun 45, sub: Recomd Changes in T/O&E. HD: 705 (MRO, Hodge Stayback, 361).

[90] History . . . Medical Regulating Service . . ., sec 4.21, with incl.

Among them were the type of ship (troop transport, ambulance ship, or hospital ship), the size and patient capacity of each, the kinds of patients carried (litter, mental, and ambulatory), and the number of days at sea (determined by the speed of each vessel and the length of its voyage). For this reason the initial issue of medical items, as well as replacement issues after each voyage, required individual consideration by port surgeons and medical supply officers. Before the war they collaborated locally with transport surgeons in determining the needs of each transport and in supplying initial and replacement allowances of medical items.[91] In connection with more general planning for sea evacuation operations early in 1942, The Surgeon General proposed that this system be continued, but that port surgeons be guided by lists of equipment to be supplied by his Office. SOS headquarters announced its approval of this proposal on 18 June 1942.[92] Meanwhile in collaboration with transport surgeons, the medical supply officer of the New York Port had prepared typical requisitions for use in making initial issues of equipment and supplies to transports hurriedly placed in service after the war began.[93]

The Surgeon General's guide, distributed at the end of June 1942, contained lists of equipment and supplies for 60-day voyages for 500-bed hospital ships, 500-bed ambulance ships, and transports carrying outbound troops in multiples of 1,000 and inbound patients in multiples of 100. Among the items included in each list were drugs and biologicals, surgical gauzes, surgical instruments, dental supplies and equipment, laboratory supplies and equipment, X-ray supplies and equipment, operating room equipment, and the like.[94] In the fall of 1942 the Surgeon General's Office revised these lists and in December issued them in a new form.[95]

The problem of equipping and supplying hospital ships assumed new importance after the Army was authorized to provide and operate its own. Vessels selected for conversion under this program were to have patient capacities varying from about 300 to 700. It was therefore necessary for the Surgeon General's Supply Division to prepare individual equipment lists, at least for the first few ships converted.[96] After they were prepared the Transportation Corps was informed of fixed equipment and its dimensions, so that plans could be made for its installation, and medical depots were instructed to make initial issues of supplies and equipment to each hospital ship.[97] In the winter of 1943–44 the Surgeon General's Office developed standard equipment lists for hospital ships with 200-, 500-, and 1,000-bed capacities and for 100-bed expansion

[91] For example, see Ltr, Port MSO NYPE to SG, 30 Mar 42, sub: Med Equip of Trans. HD: 541 (Equip for Trans).

[92] (1) 2d ind, Act SG to CG SOS (Dir Oprs), 8 Apr 42, on Memo, CofT for CG SOS, 13 Mar 42, sub: Hosp Space on Army Trans. SG: 632.-1 (BB). (2) Ltr SPOPM 322.15, CG SOS to CGs and COs of CAs, PEs, and Gen Hosps, and to SG, 18 Jun 42, sub: Oprs Plans for Mil Hosp and Evac, with incl. AG: 704.

[93] Ltr, Surg NYPE to SG thru CG NYPE, 18 Mar 42, sub: Standardized Initial Med Sups for Army Trans, with 2 inds. HD: 541 (Equip for Trans).

[94] Ltr, SG to CGs PEs, 29 Jun 42, sub: Opr Plans for Mil Hosp and Evac, with 3 tables. HD: 705 (Hosp and Evac).

[95] (1) Memo, ACofS for Oprs SOS for SG, 22 Aug 42, sub: Basic Equip Lists for Hosp Ships and Ships' Hosps. AG: 573.27 (8-22-42). (2) Instructions for Transport Surgeons, NYPE, 1943. HD: 560.2 (NYPE).

[96] For example, see (1) Ltr, SG to SPE, 3 Nov 43, sub: Conv of S.S. *President Fillmore* into a Hosp Ship. HD: 560.-2 (Hosp Ships). (2) Ltr SPMC 632.-1 (BB), SG to SFPE, 3 Nov 43, sub: Conv of S.S. *Ernest J. Hinds* into a Hosp Ship. Same file.

[97] Memo, SG for CofT, 26 Nov 43, sub: Med Equip for Ships. SG: 475.5 (BB).

units.[98] These lists were revised, along with those for transports, in March 1944 and again in April 1945.[99]

In addition to medical items ships needed other supplies and equipment. Medical Department units serving on ships needed certain organizational equipment. To meet this need, tables of equipment were issued early in 1943 for medical ambulance ship companies and for medical hospital ship companies.[100] Certain housekeeping items, such as mess equipment, beds, mattresses, and blankets, were required for ships' operating crews as well as for medical staffs and patients. During 1942 the Medical Department and the Transportation Corps worked out a division of responsibility for supplying them. In general the Transportation Corps agreed to furnish all nonmedical items and all mess equipment, beds, mattresses, blankets, and linens not used for "strictly medical" purposes.[101]

In planning to equip the *Hope, Comfort,* and *Mercy,* the Army and the Navy encountered difficulty in dividing items for which each was responsible. The Army understood that the Navy and its contractors were to supply all medical equipment that was fixed, or attached, to these ships and that the Army was to furnish all portable medical equipment. It turned out that the Army had to supply all, including fixed medical equipment, such as dental operating chairs, operating tables, and X-ray machines.[102] Uncertainty existed for a while, also, over whether the Army or the Navy with its contractors was to supply housekeeping items. This matter was clarified in an agreement by which the Navy was to supply all portable messing equipment, linens, and blankets, and its contractors were to furnish all mattresses and pillows except those furnished by the Navy for enlisted crews employed in ships' operations.[103]

During the first half of the war other problems developed in connection with the equipment of ships. The Surgeon General's Office believed that adjustable berths similar to beds used in hospitals were needed for seriously ill patients. As a result, a particular type of adjustable berth, known as a "gatch bed," was developed for use on Army hospital ships.[104] Alternating current (AC) electrical equipment, which the Medical Department had in stock and procured in the early part of the war, was unsuitable for use on ships which had direct current (DC) systems. To solve this problem direct current equipment was procured in a few instances, but generally converters were placed on ships so that equipment in stock could be used. Because of the possibility of creating signals that would reveal ships' positions to enemy naval craft, the use of electrotherapeutic equipment on transports was limited.[105]

[98] Equip Lists Nos 97239–05 (200 bed); 97239–10 (500 bed); 97239–15 (1000 bed); 97239–20 (100 bed expansion units), in ASF Med Sup Catalog MED 3, 1 Mar 44.

[99] (1) ASF, MD Consolidated Equip List No 3, 5 Mar 44. (2) ASF Med Sup Catalog MED 10–4, Apr 45.

[100] T/E 8–538, 20 Jan 43; T/E 8–537, 10 Apr 43.

[101] Memo, SG (Tng) for CofT (Water Div), 14 Sep 42, sub: Med Equip for Hosp Ships, Amb Ships and Trans Ships. SG: 475.5–1 (BB).

[102] Tynes, Construction Branch, p. 92.

[103] See SGO (Hosp Cons Br) correspondence with Cox and Stevens, New York City and with the Navy (BuShips) in HD: 560.2 (Hosp Cons Br, Hosp Ships *Hope, Mercy,* and *Comfort*).

[104] Ltr, SG (Tynes) to CofT (Water Div), 17 Nov 42, sub: Plans for Double Deck Hosp Berth With Gatch Bottom Berth. SG: 427.–4 (BB).

[105] (1) Ltr AH6/S63(665–517), AH7/S63, AH8/-S63, BuShips to SupShip NY, and San Pedro, Calif, 28 Jun 43, sub: Hosp Ships, AH6 to 8, A.C. Power Sups for I.C. Sys. TC: 632 (Hosp Ships). (2) Memo, CG SOS (Lutes) for CofT, 8 Oct 42, sub: Electrotherapeutic and X-ray Equip Aboard US Army Vessels. HD: 705 (MRO, Fitzpatrick Daybook).

A significant development occurred in the latter half of the war in connection with the laundries of hospital ships. Laundries aboard ships were necessary if the quantities of linens carried were not to be inordinate. Yet laundry operations consumed a tremendous volume of fresh water, and while hospital ships could not afford to curtail laundry operations it was imperative that fresh water for other uses receive higher priority. To solve this problem the Surgeon General's Office developed a salt-water washing process. In the summer of 1944 successful tests at the Naval Receiving Station and the Army Medical Center (both in Washington, D. C.) demonstrated that salt-water washing was both safe and efficient. The process that was developed involved the use of salt water and certain detergents for suds and first rinses and of fresh water for the final rinse and sour. This process, ultimately used on all Army hospital ships, reduced by about 80 percent the amount of fresh water ordinarily needed for laundry operations.[106]

[106] (1) Historical Record, Laundry Section, Hospital Division, [SGO], 1 July 1944, pp. 22–25, and exhibit 27. HD: 024. (2) Diary, Hosp and Dom Oprs SGO, 18 Aug 44, par 6, Laundry Sec. HD: 024.7–3.

CHAPTER XXIV

Providing the Means for Evacuation by Air

Experiences of World War II firmly established air transportation as an acceptable if not preferable method of evacuation, not only within theaters but also from overseas areas to the zone of interior and from one point to another within the latter. Because of insatiable demands from all quarters for aircraft, the movement of patients by plane, even more than by surface vessels, had to be fitted in with the transportation of troops and cargo. In theaters this problem was often solved by informal arrangements between local surgeons and air force commanders. In the zone of interior agreement was reached only after a debate over whether special planes would be provided for evacuation alone or whether all transport planes would have a dual purpose—the transportation of troops and cargo in one direction and of patients in the other. The Medical Department wanted special ambulance planes for use in all areas—combat zones, communications zones, and the zone of interior. AAF headquarters, on the other hand, insisted upon maximum use of all planes and therefore adopted a policy of using aircraft with other primary missions for evacuation also. Thereafter, the Medical Department and the Army Air Forces collaborated in arrangements for the adaptation of transport planes to the evacuation mission.

Aircraft

Prewar Plans for Airplane Ambulances

Before the war, plans for the procurement and use of airplane ambulances were nebulous. Perhaps one reason was that there was no tradition of using special planes in wartime for evacuation only. With the development of air transportation during World War I and the years that followed, surgeons of various airfields had experimented with the development and use of small airplane ambulances.[1] Repeatedly in the 1930's The Surgeon General had requested the procurement of at least seven airplane ambulances for the movement of patients in the United States during peacetime and for experiments upon which plans for their use in wartime could be based. In each instance, because of difficulty encountered in securing sufficient funds for the procurement of requisite planes for training and for defense of the United States, the General

[1] David N. W. Grant, "Airplane Ambulance Evacuation," *The Military Surgeon*, vol. 88, No. 3 (1941), pp. 238–43.

Staff, on the advice of the Chief of the Air Corps, had disapproved The Surgeon General's requests.[2] Instead, a policy established as early as 1931 continued in effect. Special airplane ambulances were not normally provided, but regular transport planes were fitted with litter-holding brackets to enable them to move patients from one hospital to another. In exceptional cases only, training centers were permitted to convert small planes into airplane ambulances for crash-rescue work (that is, the rapid removal of persons from airplane accidents to hospitals of their home stations).[3]

During 1940 opinion among medical officials as to the need for airplane ambulances in wartime crystallized. Experience of the Germans in air evacuation during the Polish campaign, an account of which appeared in the *Army Medical Bulletin,*[4] perhaps contributed to this development. The chief of the Medical Division of the Office of the Chief of the Air Corps, the surgeon of GHQ Air Force, and The Surgeon General agreed that two types of planes would be needed—small planes for the transportation of one or two casualties from medical stations in divisional areas to hospitals farther in the rear, and large planes for the removal of greater numbers of patients from evacuation hospitals to general hospitals in communications zones or the zone of interior. They agreed also that such planes should be set aside exclusively for air evacuation and should be under the control of theater headquarters.[5] The Chief of the Air Corps and the General Staff implied approval of these propositions, and the latter on 5 September 1940 directed the Chief of the Air Corps to maintain plans for converting standard transport airplanes and suitable single-engine airplanes to ambulance use.[6]

This directive uncovered an important problem. While the procurement of large ambulance planes was expected to be relatively simple, since either civilian or military transports could be readily converted by the installation of litter racks, the procurement of small airplane ambulances promised to be considerably more difficult. In September 1940 the Chief of the Air Corps stated that no small planes suitable for conversion were either available or anticipated for procurement. The General Staff then verbally modified its directive, relieving the Air Corps of responsibility for maintaining plans for the wartime conversion of single-engine airplanes.[7] Soon afterward, when the Gulf

[2] (1) Memo, ACofS G–4 WDGS for CofSA, 8 Jun 32, sub: Aircraft for Amb Serv. HRS: G–4/29413. (2) Ltr, SG to TAG, 7 Nov 33, same sub, with 3 inds. AAF: 452.1 (Amb Planes). (3) Memo, ACofS G–4 WDGS for CofSA, 22 Nov 33, same sub. HRS: G–4/29413. (4) Ltr, SG to TAG, 5 Sep 34, same sub, with 3 inds. AAF: 452.1 (Amb Planes). (5) Memo, ACofS G–4 WDGS for CofSA, 17 Sep 34, same sub. HRS: G–4/29413.

[3] (1) 2d ind, CofAC to Chief Mat Div AC Wright Fld, 5 Dec 31, on Ltr, Maj Robert [E. M.] Goolrick, AC to CofAC thru Chief Mat Div Wright Fld, 23 Oct 31, sub: Amb Airplanes. AAF: 452.1 (Amb Planes). (2) Memo, Chief Med Sec OCofAC for SG, 25 Jan 38. SG: 451.8–1.

[4] (1) Ltr, SG to CofAC, 5 Apr 40, sub: Airplane Casualty Evac in the German-Polish War. SG: 580.1. (2) *Army Medical Bulletin,* No. 53 (July 1940), pp. 1–10.

[5] (1) Ltr, Surg GHQ AF to Chief Med Div OCofAC, 20 Jun 40. SG: 320.3–1. (2) Memo, Chief Med Div OCofAC for SG, 21 Jun 40. Same file. (3) Ltr, SG to TAG, 11 Jul 40, sub: Air Corps Med Trans Group. AG: 320.2 Med (7–11–40).

[6] (1) 2d ind, CofAC to TAG, 24 Jul 40, on Ltr, SG to TAG, 11 Jul 40, sub: Air Corps Med Trans Group. (2) Memo, ACofS G–3 WDGS for CofSA, 7 Aug 40, sub: Air Amb Serv. (3) Memo, TAG to CofAC, 5 Sep 40, same sub. All in AG: 320.2 Med (7–11–40).

[7] (1) R&R Sheet Comment 1, Exec OCofAC to Tng and Oprs, Plans and Mat Divs OCofAC, in turn, 9 Sep 40, sub: Air Amb Serv. AAF: 452.1–B (Amb Planes). (2) R&R Sheet Comment 3, Plans Div OCofAC to Mat Div OCofAC thru Exec, 17 Sep 40, same sub. Same file.

Coast Air Corps Training Center requested procurement of single-engine airplane ambulances for peacetime crash-rescue work, the Chief of the Air Corps disapproved the purchase of airplanes exclusively for ambulance service, but stated, strangely enough, that small planes already in service might be converted into ambulances.[8] A subsequent investigation confirmed his earlier opinion that light planes in service were not suitable for conversion. Some were too old; others were too small; and still others had openings that were too small to admit litters and were incapable of enlargement without weakening the fuselages of planes.[9] Early in 1941, therefore, the Chief of the Air Corps permitted the conversion into ambulances of three small planes of a new type just being procured—0-49s—provided this action did not seriously delay the assignment of planes to observation squadrons.[10] By July 1941 it was reported that each of these had been converted to carry one litter patient and a medical attendant, in addition to the pilot, and had been assigned to training centers.[11]

Meanwhile the Surgeon General's Office and the Medical Division of the Office of the Chief of the Air Corps had been making plans for the use of airplane ambulances in both forward and rear areas of combat zones. During 1940 and 1941, as will be seen later, they developed a table of organization for units that would evacuate patients in airplane ambulances and requested the publication of information about such units in a Medical Department field manual. They also devoted attention to the problem of developing a small plane suitable for use in front-line areas. From the time when the National Research Council suggested in October 1940 that an Autogiro might solve this problem, the Surgeon General's Office maintained a steady correspondence with the company producing such planes. In September 1941 representatives of that Office and of the Medical Division of the Office of the Chief of the Air Corps witnessed a demonstration of an Autogiro and discussed with company officials the characteristics desired in a front-line airplane ambulance.[12] By the latter part of November the company producing Autogiros submitted drawings for an ambulance. The Air Corps Materiel Division agreed that this type of plane, if successfully developed, would be useful in forward areas, but believed that the one proposed would be unsuccessful because of its weight. It recommended, therefore, that further action on the question of an ambulance Autogiro be suspended until after completion and testing of others being developed for Air Corps tactical missions.[13]

---

[8] (1) R&R Sheet Comment 6, Mat Div OCofAC to Med Div OCofAC, 3 Dec 40, sub: Air Amb Serv. (2) R&R Sheet Comment 7, Med Div to Mat Div, 16 Dec 40, same sub. (3) R&R Sheet Comment 10, Plans Div OCofAC to Exec, OCofAC, 31 Dec 40, same sub, with approval by CofAC. All in AAF: 452.1-B (Amb Planes).

[9] Memo, Fld Serv Sec Mat Div Wright Fld for Tec Exec Mat Div Wright Fld, 17 Jan 41, sub: Info . . . Regarding Amb Airplanes. AAF: 452.1-B (Amb Planes).

[10] (1) R&R Sheet Comment 1, Mat Div OCofAC to Exec OCofAC, 23 Feb 41, Comment 3, Tng and Oprs Div OCofAC to Exec OCofAC, 1 Mar 41; and Comment 4, Exec OCofAC to Mat Div OCofAC, 4 Mar 41, sub: Amb Airplanes. All in AAF: 452.1-B (Amb Planes).

[11] Memo, Mat Div Wright Fld for Mat Div OCofAC, 29 Jul 41, sub: 0-49 Amb Airplanes. AAF: 452.1-B (Amb Planes).

[12] See SG: 452.-1, and Off file, Research and Dev Bd SGO, "Amb Airplane."

[13] (1) Memo, Mat Div OCofAC for Mat Div Wright Fld, 28 Nov 41, sub: Amb Autogiro. AAF: 452.1-B (Amb Planes). (2) Memo, Mat Div Wright Fld for Mat Div OCofAC, 3 Jan 42, same sub. Same file.

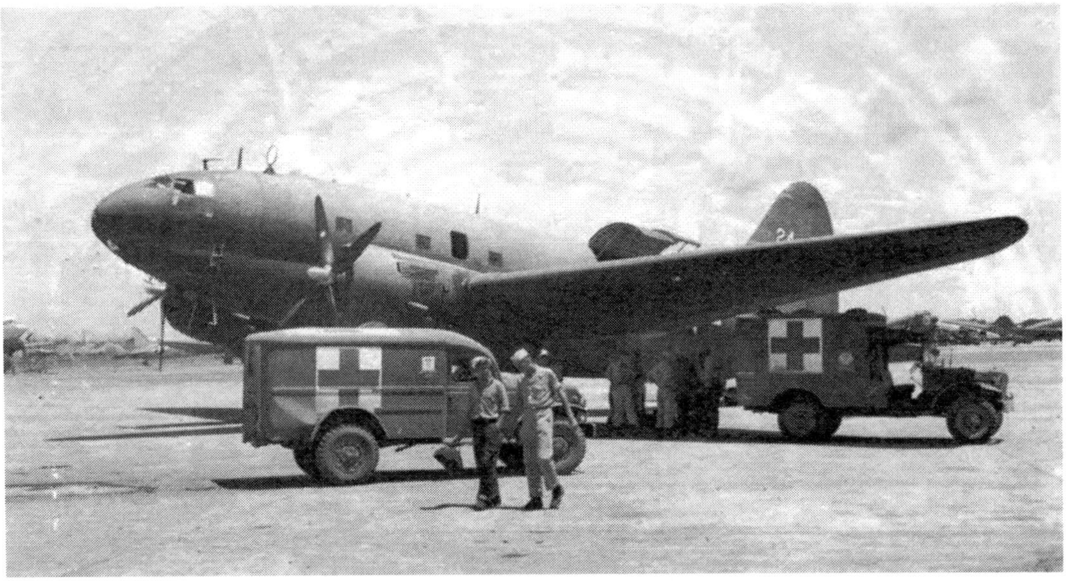

C-46 TRANSPORT PLANE READY TO UNLOAD PATIENTS. *The ambulance on the right is a ¾ ton (4x4) knock-down type.*

Decision Not To Provide Separate Transport Planes for Evacuation

Soon after war began, the need for air evacuation was met by the peacetime practice of using regular transports. The first occasion requiring the movement by air of large numbers of patients occurred in January 1942 during construction of the Alcan Highway to Alaska. The second occurred in Burma in April 1942. In both instances regular transport planes (C-47s) already equipped with litter brackets were pressed into ambulance service.[14]

Successful evacuation by transports did not remove the desire of some military agencies for separate airplane ambulances. In July 1942 the Alaska Defense Command asked for a large airplane ambulance, and was supported in its request by the Western Defense Command. The next month The Surgeon General requested an airplane ambulance for use in transporting patients from the Newfoundland Base Command to the United States. These requests produced a confirmation—in view of the wartime demand for planes for other purposes—of the existing policy of not providing special planes for ambulance service only, but of equipping all transports with litter brackets so they might be used for evacuation as well as for normal missions.[15]

AAF headquarters encountered some difficulty in the observance of this policy.

[14] Frederick R. Guilford and Burton J. Soboroff, "Air Evacuation: An Historical Review," *Journal of Aviation Medicine,* Vol. 18 (December, 1947), pp. 601-16.

[15] (1) Ltr, CG Alaska Def Comd to CG Western Def Comd, 14 Jul 42, sub: Aircraft Amb for Alaska, with 2 inds. AG: 452 (7-14-42). (2) Ltr, CG Eastern Def Comd to CG AAF, 31 Jul 42, sub: Air Amb Evac of Pnts from Newfoundland Base Comd, with 4 inds. SG: 705.-1 (Newfoundland)F.

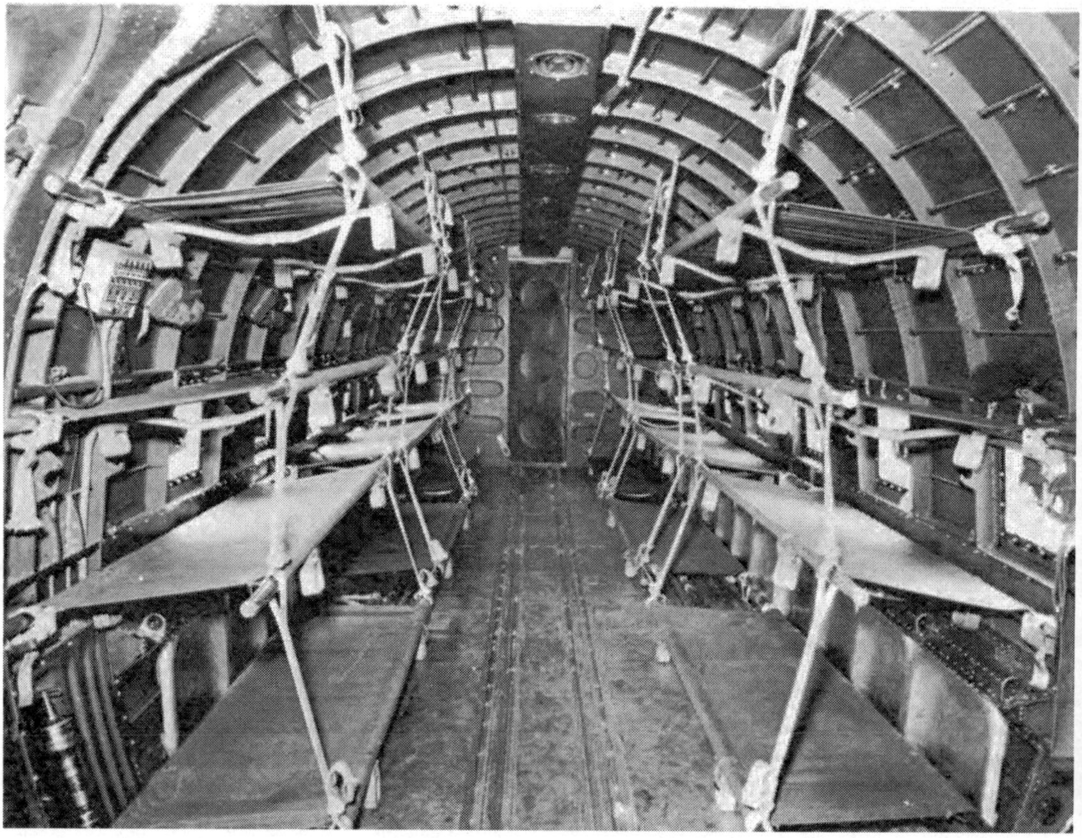

INTERIOR OF C–46 TRANSPORT PLANE, *equipped with webbing strap litter supports.*

Litter brackets were not always installed in transport airplanes, particularly in new types developed to meet wartime needs. In August 1942 the Air Service Command stated that C–53 transport planes were being procured without litter supports and that the makers of these planes considered it impossible, because of difficulty in obtaining parts for litter racks for C–47s, to install them in C–53s before January 1943. The commanding general, Army Air Forces, then directed the Materiel Command to review its transport procurement program to assure the installation of litter supports in planes during their manufacture and to provide for their installation in all C–53s purchased without them.[16] Several months later the Air Transport Command requested that litter supports be provided by manufacturers for all C–46s. Expressing irritation with failure to equip transport planes with litter supports, the AAF Directorate of Military

[16] 1st ind, Chief Fld Serv Air Serv Comd AAF to CG Air Serv Comd AAF, 4 Aug 42, and 3d ind, CG AAF to CG Mat Comd AAF, 21 Aug 42, on Ltr, Chief Overseas Div Air Serv Comd AAF to Chief Fld Serv Air Serv Comd AAF, 20 Jul 42, sub: Litter Racks for C–53 Airplanes. AAF: 370.05 (Evac).

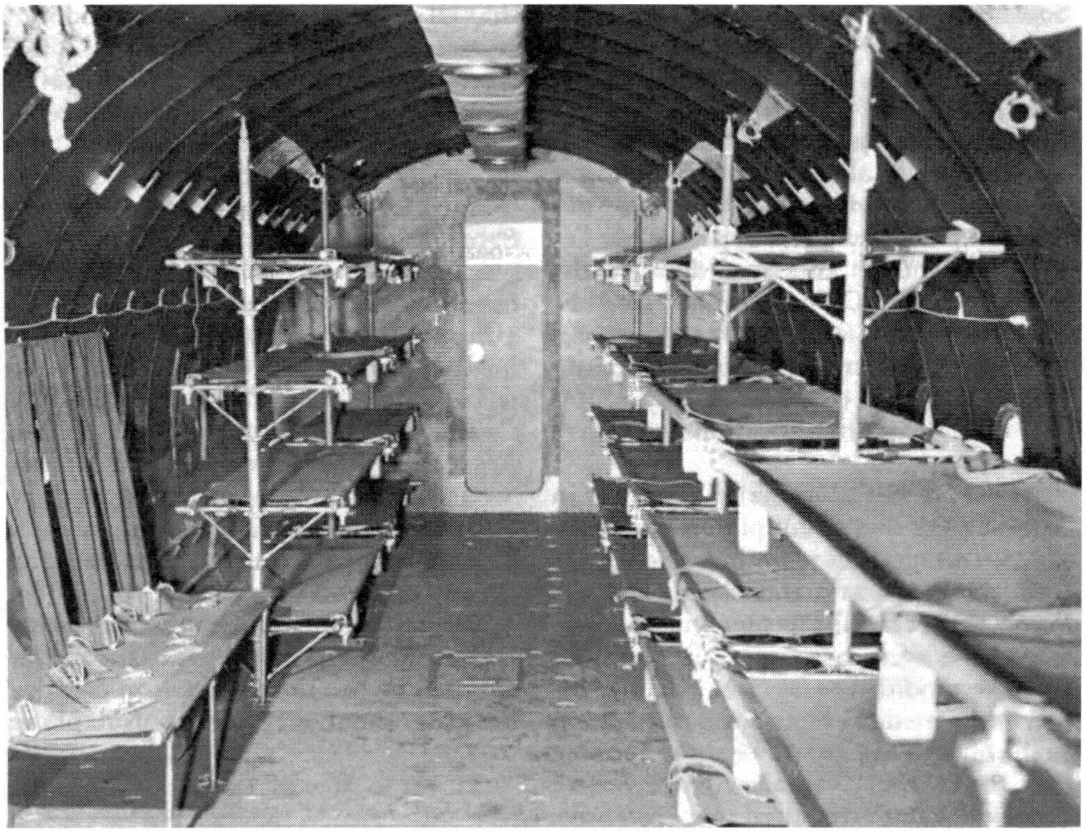

INTERIOR OF C–54 TRANSPORT PLANE *equipped with metal litter supports.*

Requirements called upon the Materiel Command for a report. In reply that Command summarized the situation. All C–47s were completely equipped with litter supports during production. While a shortage of critical materials had prevented installation in the first twenty-four C–46s delivered, all others would come equipped. Beginning in December 1942, all C–53s would be provided with litter brackets by manufacturers. Meanwhile, the Air Forces would install them in 200 planes of that type already delivered. Beginning in January 1943, supports for ten litters would be placed in each C–60. Finally, all new types of transports would be equipped with litter supports when deliveries began.[17]

Small Planes for Ambulance Service at Training Centers

The question of the assignment to training centers of small ambulance planes for rescue work was raised again when the

[17] R&R Sheet Comment 1, CG ATC to Mil Reqmts Dir AAF, 26 Oct 42; Comment 2, Mil Reqmts Dir AAF to Mat Comd AAF, 2 Nov 42; and Comment 3, Mat Comd AAF to Mil Reqmts Dir AAF, 5 Nov 42, sub: Removable Insulation and Litter Supports for C–46 Airplanes. AAF: 370.05 (Evac).

Southeast Air Corps Training Center requested in May 1942 the assignment of one each to its flying training schools. While the AAF Directorate of Military Requirements observed a policy of neither developing nor altering an airplane so as to provide an additional type, it was willing that planes of other types be used to carry patients. It therefore directed the AAF Materiel Command on 18 June 1942 to examine all small transport and liaison planes being procured in order to determine which could be readily adapted, with least modification, to carry litters.[18]

The Materiel Command reported in August 1942 that small planes most suitable for adaptation to ambulance service were the AT–7 and the C–64. The Air Forces had 127 of the former on hand, and 300 C–64s were being procured. Either could be modified to carry at least two litters and a medical attendant, in addition to the pilot. They would be more suitable than the O–49s (L–1s) already converted, because the latter required more extensive modification and carried only one litter and a medical attendant, in addition to the pilot. The Materiel Command therefore requested authority to have a local subdepot modify one AT–7 and to have a manufacturer modify one C–64 in production, in order to determine which would be preferable as an ambulance.[19]

This recommendation was considered by AAF headquarters, along with a request of the Flying Training Command for assignment to the Gulf Coast, West Coast, and Southeast Air Force Training Centers of sixty-two small ambulance planes and of thirteen larger planes of greater cruising range, such as C–60s.[20] On 20 August 1942 the Assistant Chief of Air Staff for Training, A–3, announced that all small planes being procured were earmarked for other missions.[21] AT–7s were in such demand for the navigation training program that C–60s were being modified to supplement them. All C–64s being procured were to be used in communications work, pilot dispersal, and light cargo movement. Consequently it was decided not to modify AT–7s, but to have manufacturers equip all C–64s, beginning in January 1943, with brackets for three litters. Since none of the latter were assigned to the Flying Training Command, the commanding general, Army Air Forces announced on 8 November 1942 that it would have to meet its requirement for airplane ambulances by having litter supports installed in planes already on hand.[22]

The issue of airplane ambulances in the United States came up again on 12 January 1943 when the Air Surgeon proposed the assignment of L–1Bs—liaison planes

[18] Ltr, CG Southeast AC Tng Ctr to CG Flying Tng Comd AAF, 7 May 42, sub: Amb Airplanes, with 5th ind, Dir Mil Reqmts AAF to CG Mat Comd AAF, 18 Jun 42. AAF: 452.–1 (Amb Planes).

[19] (1) Rpt, AAF Mat Ctr Wright Fld, 10 Aug 42, sub: Selection and Modification of Small Aircraft for Amb Serv. (2) R&R Sheet Comment 1, Mat Comd AAF to War Orgn and Mvmt Dir AAF, 16 Aug 42, sub: Amb Airplanes. Both in AAF: 452.–1 (Amb Planes).

[20] Ltr, CG Flying Tng Comd AAF to CG AAF, 5 Aug 42, sub: Amb Airplanes. AAF: 452.–1 (Amb Planes).

[21] R&R Sheet Comment 5, AC of Air Staff for Tng A–3 to War Orgn and Mvmt Dir AAF and Indiv Tng Dir AAF, 20 Aug 42, sub: Amb Planes. AAF: 452.–1–B (Amb Planes).

[22] (1) Interoffice Memo, Capt John P. Marshall Mat Comd AAF to Col Seesums, 19 Aug 42, sub: Amb Airplanes. (2) R&R Sheet Comment 3, Indiv Tng Dir AAF to War Orgn and Mvmt Dir AAF, 5 Oct 42; Comment 7, Indiv Tng Dir AAF to Mat Comd AAF, 22 Oct 42; Comment 10, War Orgn and Mvmt Dir AAF to Indiv Tng Dir AAF, 2 Nov 42, same sub. (3) Memo, CG AAF for CG Flying Tng Comd AAF, 8 Nov 42, same sub. All in AAF: 452.1 (Amb Planes).

modified by manufacturers to carry one litter and one medical attendant, in addition to the pilot—to meet a need expressed by the Second Air Force. Soon afterward the Flying Training Command renewed its attempt to get airplane ambulances. By this time—the spring of 1943—training programs, such as the glider towing program, were being curtailed and small liaison planes (L–1s) formerly used were no longer needed. As a result, some of them were assigned for ambulance service to the Second Air Force, and the Flying Training Command was permitted to modify about 100 liaison-type planes to meet its needs.[23] Soon afterward the AAF Requirements Division announced officially a policy which it had formerly observed without publicity. When a training station needed a special airplane to be held always in readiness purely as an ambulance airplane, its requirement would be treated as a special one and would be met by the conversion of a suitable available plane. Such conversions were to be held to a minimum and were to be made only when specifically approved by AAF headquarters.[24]

The Question of Airplane Ambulances for Use in Combat Zones

After the war began, the Air Surgeon and The Surgeon General continued to plan for the use of small airplane ambulances in combat zones. Their problem in this instance was twofold: (1) to find a suitable plane and (2) to get it delivered in appropriate numbers for use by evacuation units.

Various types of planes were considered. It was agreed that a successful one would have to accommodate at least two litters and a medical attendant, in addition to its pilot, and would have to be able to go in and out of small fields over tops of trees and other obstructions. Before the war, as mentioned above, The Surgeon General had thought that an Autogiro might be developed with these characteristics. In May 1942 an aircraft corporation submitted photographs of a small airplane ambulance which it had developed.[25] Both The Surgeon General and the Air Surgeon proposed that it be studied and demonstrated, even though it could accommodate only a pilot and one patient,[26] but after consultation with the AAF Directorate of Military Requirements the Materiel Command informed the company that the Army had no use for such a plane. It stated that litter bearers were the most effective means for removing casualties from battlefields with rough terrain; that even if the terrain were suitable for landing, a plane was too vulnerable a target to risk in advanced areas; and, finally, that any plane that lacked room for a medical attendant was unsatisfactory.[27] Somewhat later, in June, another manufacturer demonstrated to representatives

[23] (1) R&R Sheet Comment 1, Air Surg to Mil Reqmts Dir AAF, 12 Jan 43, and Comment 3, War Orgn and Mvmt Dir AAF to Air Surg, 16 Mar 43, sub: Airplane Amb (L–1A). AAF: 452.1 (Amb Planes). (2) Routing Slip, [Lt Col] C. W. G[lanz], Mil Reqmts Dir AAF to Col M[ervin] E. Gross, 15 May 43. AAF: 370.05–A (Evac).

[24] AAF Mil Reqmts Policy No. 41, 25 May 43, sub: Amb Airplanes—Provisions for Evac Wounded by Cargo Airplanes. AAF: 370.05–A (Evac).

[25] Ltr, Aeronca Aircraft Corp to Hon John J. McCloy, Asst SecWar, 20 Apr 42, with incl. SG: 452.1. A similar letter to the Commanding General, Army Air Forces is on file in AAF: 452.1–B (Amb Planes).

[26] (1) Ltr, SG to Hon John J. McCloy, Asst SecWar, 5 May 42. (2) Memo, Col David N. W. Grant, Air Surg for Col H[oward] T. Wickert, SGO, 11 May 42. Both in SG: 452.1.

[27] Ltr, Lt Col F. I. Ordway, Jr, AC, Asst Exec Mat Comd to Aeronca Aircraft Corp, 5 May 42. AAF: 452.1–B (Amb Planes).

of the Air Surgeon and The Surgeon General a small plane which he had converted into an ambulance. It was likewise considered unsatisfactory because it also had room for only one patient and a pilot.[28] Meanwhile, the Air Forces had begun the investigation, already mentioned, of small transport and liaison planes which training centers might adapt to ambulance use. Apparently the Air Surgeon believed that this might result in discovery of an existing plane that could be used in combat zones as well as in the zone of interior.[29]

Despite uncertainty about the availability of a suitable plane for use in forward areas, the Air Surgeon continued to plan in those terms. One method of getting approval for his plans was to have airplane ambulances considered as organic equipment of evacuation units. One could assume that upon activation of such units, planes authorized for them would be made available. When the Air Surgeon revised the table of organization for air evacuation units during 1942, he included twenty small planes along with an equal number of flight officers in the table for the air evacuation squadron, light.[30] This table was approved by certain sections of the Air Staff and by the Chief of Air Staff, and one air evacuation squadron, light, was activated on 11 November 1942.[31] When the matter of providing planes for it came up, the Directorate of Military Requirements objected. Not having been consulted in advance, it had made no plans for supplying evacuation units with either planes or pilots. It insisted that litter bearers and automobile ambulances could best move patients from divisional medical stations to rear areas, for pick-up by transport planes. It maintained, therefore, that squadrons equipped with small planes, or "puddle jumpers," were not required and should not be provided.[32] The commanding general, Army Air Forces, supported Military Requirements, and its position was subsequently announced as policy in May 1943.[33]

Consideration of Helicopters for Air Evacuation

Announcement of this policy did not quash the hopes of many, including the Air Surgeon, The Surgeon General, and Army Ground Forces headquarters,[34] that a suitable plane for evacuating patients from front-line areas might be found and its use approved. Late in 1942 a civilian doctor in Virginia had pressed upon the War Department the possibility of using

[28] (1) Ltr, SG to Piper Aircraft Corp, 5 Jun 42. SG: 452.-1. (2) Memo by Lt Col Thomas N. Page, MC, SGO, 7 Nov 42, sub: Air Evac of Pnts. HD: 370.05.

[29] Memo by Lt Col Thomas N. Page, MC, SGO, 7 Nov 42, sub: Air Evac and Air Trans of Med Sups and Pers. HD: 580.1 Air Evac.

[30] (1) R&R Sheet Comment 1, Air Surg to War Orgn and Mvmt Dir AAF, 15 Sep 42, sub: Air Evac, with incl. AAF: 370.03. (2) Rpt of Mtg, ATC, 13 Oct 42, sub: Air Evac of Wounded. AAF: 370.05 (Evac).

[31] (1) R&R Sheet Comment 3, Ground-Air Support Mil Reqmts Dir AAF to Mil Reqmts Dir AAF, 24 Nov 42, sub: Conversion of Airplanes to Evac Wounded. AAF: 370.05 (Evac). (2) Hubert A. Coleman, Organization and Administration, AAF Medical Services in the Zone of the Interior (1948), p. 689.

[32] (1) R&R Sheet Comment 4, Dir Mil Reqmts AAF to AC of Air Staff for Tng, A-3, 31 Oct 42, sub: Conv of Liaison Type Airplanes. AAF: 370.05 (Evac). (2) R&R Sheet Comment 3, Ground-Air Support Mil Reqmts Dir AAF to Mil Reqmts Dir AAF, 24 Nov 42, sub: Conv of Airplanes to Evac Wounded. Same file.

[33] (1) R&R Sheet Comment 1, C of Air Staff to Dir Mil Reqmts AAF, 12 Nov 42, sub: Conv of Airplanes to Evac Wounded. AAF: 370.05 (Evac). (2) Mil Reqmts Policy No. 41, 25 May 43, sub: Amb Airplanes—Provisions for Evac Wounded by Cargo Airplanes. AAF: 370.05-A (Evac).

[34] For the Army Ground Forces' viewpoint, see: 10th ind, CG AGF to CG ASF, 20 Nov 43, on Ltr, Dept of Air Tng Fld Artillery Sch to CG ASF thru Repl and Sch Comd AGF, 7 Sep 43, sub: Air Evac by Light Airplane. AAF: 452.-1 (Amb Planes).

helicopters in front-line medical service.[35] Both the Air Surgeon and The Surgeon General quickly adopted the idea as a solution to the problem of evacuating patients by air from inaccessible areas in combat zones and called upon the AAF Materiel Command for information in this connection.[36] The Command reported early in 1943 that it had been testing helicopters for a period of eight months. Although it had begun the procurement of several types, none of them were expected to be delivered before the middle of 1943. The Command had already given preliminary consideration to the use of helicopters for evacuation and was requiring that they be fitted for the external attachment of "capsules" suitable for carrying litter patients. It was anticipated that this would enable each XR–5 and R–5 helicopter to carry four litter patients and each XR–6 to carry two. In collaboration with the Aero Medical Research Laboratory, the Materiel Command was studying the possibility of modifying XR–5 and XR–6 helicopters so they might carry four and two litters respectively within their fuselages, rather than in externally attached capsules. Meanwhile, it expected that an XR–5 helicopter, with capsules attached, would be ready for testing by September 1943 and that additional ones could be procured, after their use as ambulances had been approved, in from ten to eighteen months.[37]

Progress in the general helicopter program was apparently not as rapid as had been expected. In the winter of 1943–44 the Air Forces had on hand only eight or nine serviceable helicopters and expected that few more would be delivered before the latter half of 1944.[38] The development of an ambulance helicopter had also lagged. Believing that patients should not be transported in capsules beyond the reach of medical attendants except in emergencies, the Air Surgeon succeeded in having a "requirement" established early in March 1944 for a helicopter that could accommodate at least four litter patients and an attendant within its fuselage. In conformity with established policy, the AAF Requirements Division directed that any helicopter developed to meet this requirement should be suitable for basic use as a cargo plane and should be equipped for carrying litters only if this did not interfere with such use.[39] The Air Surgeon also apparently requested the procurement of 150 helicopters for use by his proposed air evacuation squadrons but he reconsidered the matter after discussion with the AAF Requirements Division. In view of the shortage of helicopters of all types and the lack of one that could transport patients within its fuselage, he agreed in March 1944 not to organize helicopter evacuation squadrons but instead to use

[35] (1) Ltr, Dr Huston St. Clair to Maj Gen W[ilhelm] D. Styer, CofS SOS, 23 Nov 42. Off file, Research and Dev Bd SGO, "Amb Airplanes." (2) Ltr, same to Col G[ustave] E. Ledfors, Air Surg Off, 7 Dec 42. AAF: 452.1 (Helicopters). (3) Ltr, Mr. G. H. Dorr, Spec Asst to SecWar to Col W[ood] S. Woolford, Air Surg Off, 31 Dec 42. Same file.

[36] (1) Ltr, SG to Chief Engr Div Wright Fld, 21 Dec 42, sub: Helicopter Dev. AAF: 452.1 (Helicopters). (2) Memo, Air Surg for Mat Comd Wright Fld, [22 Dec 42], same sub. AAF: 452.1 (Amb Planes).

[37] (1) Memo, Mat Comd AAF for SG, 16 Jan 43, sub: Helicopter Dev—Util as Air Amb. (2) Memo, Mat Comd AAF for Air Surg, 3 Mar 43, sub: Helicopter Dev for Air Amb Serv. Both in AAF: 452.1 (Helicopters).

[38] (1) Memo, CG AAF for ACofS G–3 WDGS, [12 Dec 43], sub: Status of AAF Helicopter Program. (2) Ltr, CG AAF to CG Tng Comd AAF, 20 Jan 44, sub: Availability of Helicopter Aircraft. Both in AAF: 452.1 (Helicopters).

[39] (1) Ltr, Mat Div AAF to Mat Comd Wright Fld, 3 Mar 44, sub: Dev of Large Type Helicopters. (2) R&R Sheet Comment 2, Oprs, Commitments, and Reqmts Div AAF to Air Surg, 23 Mar 44, sub: Status of Helicopters. Both in AAF: 452.1 (Helicopters).

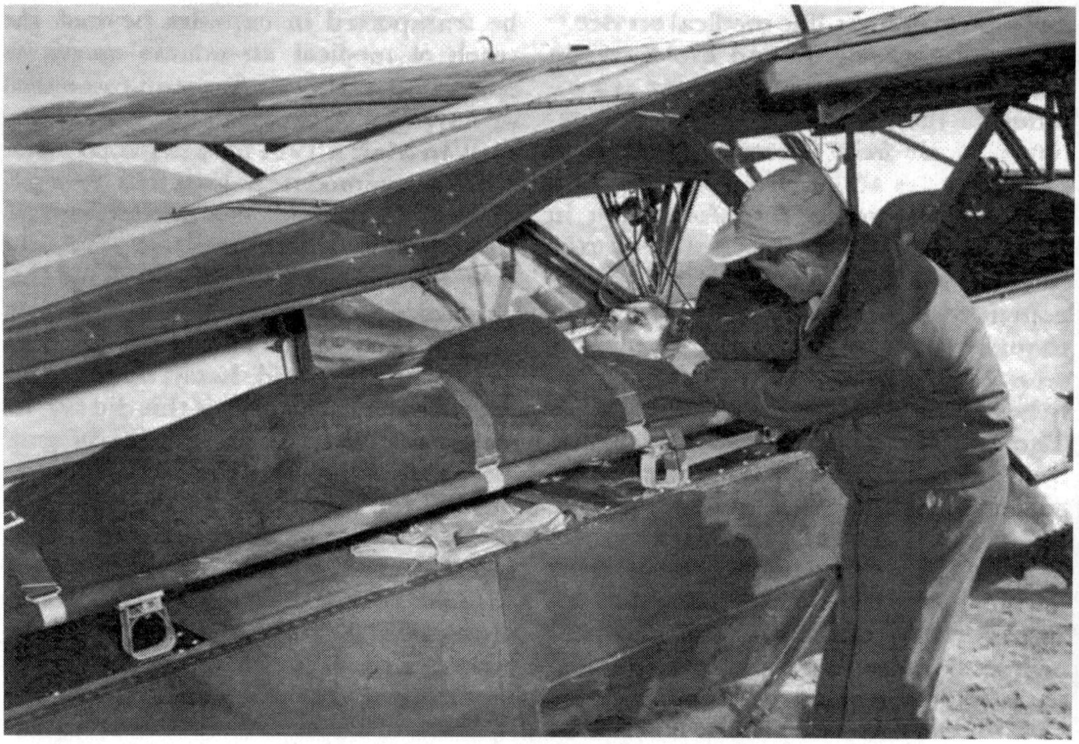

LOADING A PATIENT ON AN L–5 PLANE

for emergency evacuation helicopters ordinarily employed otherwise.[40] Soon afterward he stated that it was AAF policy to use C–64 and L–5 airplanes equipped to carry litters for the evacuation of patients singly or in small numbers.[41] Meanwhile, the general helicopter program continued, and toward the end of the war there were indications that some might soon be modified to carry patients within their fuselages and that they would be available in sufficient numbers for assignment to overseas commands.[42]

Relaxation of the Policy Limiting the Use of Special Planes for Evacuation

Despite AAF policy against the use of airplanes exclusively for evacuation, assignment of additional transport planes to supply enough "lift" for evacuation in addition to normal operations became an accepted practice in the zone of interior

[40] R&R Sheet Comment 1, Air Surg to Oprs, Commitments, and Reqmts Div AAF, 4 Mar 44, and Comment 2, Oprs, Commitments, and Reqmts Div AAF to Air Surg, 7 Mar 44, sub: Use of Helicopters for Air Evac. AAF: 452.1 (Helicopters).

[41] 5th ind, CG AAF (Air Surg) to CG Air Serv Comd, 24 May 44, on Memo, 2d Lt William R. Kee, AC for Air Surg, thru Channels, 17 Apr 44, sub: Evac of Wounded by Air. AAF: 370.05 (Evac). Also see *The Air Surgeon's Bulletin*, vol. I, No. 8 (1944), p. 19 and vol. I, No. 9 (1944), p. 16.

[42] (1) R&R Sheet Comment 1, Reqmts Div AAF to Mat Div AAF, 31 May 45, sub: Litter Capsules for Helicopters. (2) Ltr AG 320.3 (11 Apr 45) OB–I–AFRTH, TAG to CG ETO, 5 May 45, sub: AAF Helicopter Program. Both in AAF: 452.1 (Helicopters).

during the later war years. This practice began in January 1944, when three C–47s were temporarily used to move 661 patients from Stark General Hospital to other hospitals in the zone of interior. Several months later the Air Transport Command temporarily assigned twelve C–47s to its Ferrying Division for a similar "special operation." These operations were so successful that, after the Ferrying Division was made responsible for air evacuation in the zone of interior in May 1944, twelve planes were permanently assigned to that mission. They could, of course, be used for the transportation of other persons and of cargo when not carrying patients. The next month twelve additional C–47s were assigned to provide planes for evacuation. As the number of patients arriving from theaters increased and the calls for air evacuation became more frequent, the number of transport planes assigned to the Ferrying Division for evacuation operations grew until it reached forty-nine by September 1944.[43]

As patients continued to be evacuated from theaters to the zone of interior in regular transport planes, efforts were made during 1944 and 1945 to increase the number of patients they carried. The increase was accomplished in two ways. One was the installation of newly developed webbing-strap litter supports. More patients could be accommodated in planes using these supports than in those equipped with metal-type supports. In the summer of 1944 the Air Forces installed webbing-strap litter supports in C–54s already in use and provided for their installation in others during production.[44] Another method of increasing the use of airplanes for evacuation was to modify the system of determining the number of patients theaters would evacuate by air. In the spring of 1944, it will be recalled, the Air Transport Command authorized theaters to ignore the old system of priorities for air transportation and determine locally the proportion of space on returning transport planes that would be reserved for patients.[45]

Medical Flight Attendants

Early Plans for Medical Personnel for Air Evacuation

Since plans for air evacuation during the period before the war and well into its first year were tentative only, plans for units to be employed in such operations were of necessity also uncertain. In the prewar years The Surgeon General and the Medical Division of the Air Corps collaborated in the development of an organization—sometimes called a task force—that would be used exclusively for the evacuation of patients from forward to rear areas of theaters of operations and perhaps to the zone of interior. While there were differences of opinion on some points—such as the name of the organization, the number of subordinate units it should have, and the amount of personnel

---

[43] (1) Organizational History of the Ferrying Division, June 20, 1942 to August 1, 1944, pp. 271–78. ATC: Hist Div. (2) Initial Medical History (11 February 1943 to 30 June 1944), Headquarters Ferrying Division, Air Transport Command. HD: TAS. (3) Quarterly Medical History, Headquarters Ferrying Division, Air Transport Command, 1 July–30 September 1944. HD: TAS. (4) Memo, Air Surg for SG, 27 Jul 44. SG: 580. (5) Memo, Comdt Sch of Air Evac for CG AAF, 16 Feb 44, sub: Air Evac. AAF: 370.05 (Evac). (6) *The Air Surgeon's Bulletin,* vol. I, No. 4 (1944), pp. 10–11.

[44] (1) 1st ind, CG ATC to ACofS OPD WDGS thru CG AAF, 15 May 44, on unknown basic Ltr. OPD: 580.81. (2) *The Air Surgeon's Bulletin,* vol. I, No. 7 (1944), p. 17.

[45] See above, p. 340.

required for each unit—there was general agreement on major issues. An air ambulance organization should be composed of both Air Corps and medical personnel, the former to maintain and operate ambulance airplanes and the latter to care for patients. This organization should operate under the control of theater headquarters, augmenting surface evacuation, and should perhaps be assigned on the basis of one unit per field army. Medical officers and enlisted men of the organization would not only serve as attendants to patients during flights but would also operate medical stations at large airfields, fifteen to fifty miles from the front, and at small emergency landing fields, two to ten miles from the front. They would collect and transport patients by motor ambulances to such stations, care for them as they awaited air evacuation, and load them on planes for transportation to the rear.[46]

Several tables of organization for an air evacuation unit were developed through the collaboration of the Surgeon, GHQ Air Force; the Medical Division of the Air Corps; and the Surgeon General's Office. One submitted in July 1940 was disapproved by the General Staff because airplane ambulances were included as organic elements of medical rather than Air Corps units of the evacuation organization.[47] Another, submitted by The Surgeon General in October 1940, apparently remained in the G–3 Division of the General Staff without action until the late summer of 1941. It was then revised and resubmitted for approval in November.[48] It was published shortly afterward as the table of organization for a medical air ambulance squadron. This squadron was to be a companion unit for an Air Corps transport group composed of a headquarters squadron, a flight squadron, light, equipped with eighteen single-engine liaison planes for front-line evacuation, and two flight squadrons, heavy, each equipped with twelve two-engine transport planes for intra-theater evacuation. The medical squadron was to consist of a headquarters section, a single-engine transport ambulance section, and two two-engine transport ambulance sections. It was to have 45 Medical Department officers, no nurses, and 218 enlisted men. One unit of this type, the 38th Medical Air Ambulance Squadron, was activated at reduced strength as a test unit in May 1942.[49]

After AAF was charged with responsibility for air evacuation in the summer of 1942, the Air Surgeon's Office developed a new plan for an air evacuation unit, called an air evacuation group. This group was to be composed of a headquarters

[46] (1) Ltr, SG to TAG, 11 Jul 40, sub: AC Med Trans Group. AG: 320.2 Med (7–11–40). (2) Memo, Chief Med Div OCofAC for SG, 3 Oct 40. SG: 320.3–1. (3) 2d ind, SG to TAG, 18 Mar 41, on Ltr, Dir Dept Extension Courses MFSS to SG thru Comdt MFSS, 31 Jan 41, sub: FM 8–5, Mobile Units of MD. AG: 300.7 (1–31–41) FM 8–5. (4) David N. W. Grant, "Airplane Ambulance Evacuation," *The Military Surgeon*, vol. 88, No. 3 (1941), pp. 238–43. (5) FM 8–5, Mobile Units of MD, 12 Jan 42, pp. 157–69.

[47] (1) Ltr, Surg GHQ AF to Chief Med Div OCofAC, 20 Jun 40. SG: 320.3–1. (2) Memo, Chief Med Div OCofAC for SG, 21 Jun 40. Same file. (3) Ltr, SG to TAG, 11 Jul 40, sub: AC Med Trans Group. AG: 320.3 Med (7–11–40). (4) Memo, ACofS G–3 WDGS for CofSA, 7 Aug 40, sub: Air Amb Serv. Same file. (5) Memo, TAG to SG, 5 Sep 40, same sub. Same file.

[48] (1) Ltr, SG to TAG, 29 Oct 40, sub: New T/O Med Bn, Airplane Amb, with 3 inds. (2) DF G–3/42108, ACofS G–3 WDGS to CofAAF, 15 Aug and 27 Oct 41, same sub. (3) R&R Sheet Comment 1, C of Air Staff AAF to CofAC (Med Div), 7 Nov 41, same sub. All in AAF: 320.3 L–1. (4) DF, C of Air Staff to TAG, 19 Nov 41, sub: T/O for Med Airplane Amb Sq. AG: 320.2 (11–19–41).

[49] (1) T/O 8–455, 19 Nov 41, Med Air Amb Sq. (2) Guilford and Soboroff, *op. cit.*

squadron; an air evacuation squadron, light; and three air evacuation squadrons, heavy. While it was anticipated that the heavy squadrons would consist of medical personnel only and would use planes of either troop carrier or air transport commands, the light squadron was to have twenty small planes and twenty pilots assigned as organic elements. The light squadron was to consist of only enlisted men and officers, but the heavy squadron was to have nurses also. The entire group was to have 49 Medical Department officers, 20 Air Corps officers, 78 nurses, and 458 enlisted men. It was anticipated that air evacuation groups would be assigned as the situation required to air forces, theaters, defense commands, task forces, or field armies.[50] The Air Staff having approved the plan for this organization, the I Troop Carrier Command activated such a unit in October 1942, using initially officers and men transferred from the 38th Medical Air Ambulance Squadron. This unit—the 349th Air Evacuation Group—at first consisted of a headquarters squadron and one heavy squadron. In November, when a light squadron and two additional heavy squadrons were activated and assigned to it, the 349th Air Evacuation Group was given the mission of training personnel for air evacuation operations.[51] Meanwhile, as already explained, the Air Staff had decided that transport planes would not be earmarked for evacuation only and that small ambulance airplanes would not be provided for use in forward areas. This decision cut short the life of the squadrons just activated because it destroyed the basic concept underlying their formation.

With the decision to consider air evacuation as a secondary mission of planes engaged in general transport service, a different kind of organization was needed. The Air Surgeon therefore developed a smaller unit, the Medical Air Evacuation Transport Squadron (MAETS), whose table of organization was issued in advance form at the end of November 1942 and was published in regular format in February 1943. This unit had no personnel for the movement of patients in motor ambulances or the operation of medical stations at loading points. It consisted of a headquarters and four evacuation flights, each made up of six flight teams. A commanding officer, a chief nurse, an administrative officer, and 29 enlisted men comprised the headquarters. Each flight, headed by a flight surgeon, consisted of 6 flight nurses and 8 enlisted men, of whom 6 were surgical technicians. Flight teams, made up of one nurse and one technician, could be placed on transport planes as needed.[52] In December 1942 members of the three heavy air evacuation squadrons already activated were used to form six medical air evacuation transport squadrons. The next month the light air evacuation squadron was disbanded and its personnel was absorbed by the 349th Air Evacuation Group. Subsequently, during 1943 and 1944, additional MAETS were organized, trained, and sent overseas.[53]

[50] (1) Coleman, *op. cit.*, pp. 685–87, 703. (2) R&R Sheet Comment 1, Air Surg to Dir War Orgn and Mvmt AAF, 15 Sep 42, with incl. AAF: 370.03. (3) Rpt, Mins of Mtg, ATC, 13 Oct 42, Air Evac of Wounded. AAF: 370.05.

[51] (1) Medical History, I Troop Carrier Command From 30 April 1942 to 31 December 1944. HD: TAS (2) Coleman, *op. cit.*, p. 689. (3) Guilford and Soboroff, *op. cit.*

[52] (1) An Rpt, FY 1943, Oprs Div Air Surg Off. DAF: SGO Hist Br. (2) T/O 8–447, Med Air Evac Trans Sq, 15 Feb 43.

[53] (1) Guilford and Soboroff, *op. cit.* (2) Unit Cards, 801st thru 831st Med Air Evac Trans Sqs, filed in Orgn and Directory Sec Oprs Br Admin Servs Div AGO.

School of Air Evacuation

Charging the 349th Air Evacuation Group with the mission of training personnel for air evacuation operations indicated recognition by the Air Surgeon of the need for specialized training for such work. Despite the fact that it was not to be used in the theaters of operations as originally anticipated, the 349th continued in existence as a training school until June 1943. At that time the Air Forces established a School of Air Evacuation at Bowman Field, Kentucky. This school operated under the Troop Carrier Command until August 1944. Then, after a short period of operation directly under AAF headquarters, it was merged in October 1944 with the School of Aviation Medicine at Randolph Field, Texas. During the period from June 1943 through September 1945 it trained in air evacuation duties 109 medical officers, 1,331 nurses, and 837 enlisted men.[54]

Method of Controlling and Supplying Flight Attendants

Teams of one nurse and one Medical Department technician per plane continued in use throughout the war. As air evacuation operations within the United States began to assume significant proportions early in 1944, ATC headquarters announced in April that additional nurses trained in air evacuation would be assigned to ATC hospitals and would be used, along with enlisted technicians qualified to assist them, to form flight teams for planes transporting patients between hospitals in the United States.[55] When the Ferrying Division took over domestic air evacuation soon afterward, it acquired flight surgeons, flight nurses, and enlisted technicians as part of its bulk allotment of Medical Department personnel for use in air evacuation only.[56] For evacuation within theaters of operations and for flights between theaters and the zone of interior, flight teams were supplied by medical air evacuation transport squadrons. The table of organization for these squadrons was revised in July 1944, reducing the number of enlisted men in squadron headquarters from twenty-nine to twenty-four. Personnel in the squadron's four flights, each of which contained six flight teams, remained unchanged, but the rank of nurses was raised.[57] Squadrons used for intra-theater evacuation were attached to troop carrier commands or to Air Transport Command divisions in theaters. Those for evacuation from theaters to the zone of interior were assigned to ATC wings until the end of 1944. Gradually thereafter the squadrons assigned to ATC wings were disbanded and flight teams used to accompany patients from theaters to the United States were grouped under the 830th Medical Air Evacuation Squadron Headquarters, organized in the office of the ATC surgeon in Washington in November 1944. By the end of the year this squadron consisted of 44 flights; by April 1945 the number had been increased to 56; and by July, to 78. This centralization of administrative and

[54] (1) Coleman, *op. cit.*, pp. 691ff. (2) Guilford and Soboroff, *op. cit.* (3) An Rpt, FY 1943, Oprs Div Air Surg Off. DAF: SGO Hist Br. (4) AAF Reg 20-22, 22 Jul 43.

[55] ATC Memo 25-6, 29 Apr 44, sub: Med Air Evac. AAF: 370.05.

[56] (1) Organizational History of the Ferrying Division, June 20, 1942 to August 1, 1944. ATC: Hist Div. (2) Quarterly Medical History, Headquarters Ferrying Division, Air Transport Command, 1 July-30 September 1944. HD: TAS.

[57] (1) T/O&E 8-447, 19 Jul 44. (2) DF, CG AAF to ACofS G-3 WDGS, 8 Jul 44, sub: T/O&E 8-447, Med Air Evac Sq. AG: 320.3 (2 Jun 44) (1).

operational control resulted in a saving of overhead personnel and permitted the rapid reassignment of flight teams to areas where they were needed most. It also permitted the establishment of a procedure in the spring of 1945 which enabled each flight team to accompany patients to the United States. Formerly, flight teams located along ATC routes had flown from their home stations to stations en route and then had returned to home stations.[58]

The economy of men made possible by air evacuation was a major factor in enabling the War Department to meet the demands for large-scale transportation of patients in 1944 and 1945 with the limited number of attendants at its disposal. Early in 1944, when there was concern in Washington lest there be not only insufficient shipping but also insufficient personnel to move the patient load anticipated for the latter half of the year, the Surgeon General's Office and ASF headquarters asked for an increase in air evacuation from theaters as a means of saving manpower.[59] The saving was possible, for one reason, because air evacuation was so much faster than surface evacuation that patients required the care of only nurses and enlisted technicians. Moreover, for such short periods, fewer attendants per patient were needed. The saving of personnel can be illustrated by comparing the number of attendants required for a trip by hospital ship with the number required for the same trip by planes that did not stop to change medical attendants or to give patients treatment at hospitals en route. In such a case, the transportation of 500 patients by hospital ship required eight doctors, eight other officers, thirty-four nurses, and 135 enlisted men. To transport a similar number of patients by air in one continuous flight required seventeen planes (assuming that each carried thirty patients) with seventeen teams consisting of one nurse and one technician each, or a total of thirty-four persons, together with the personnel rounding out the flights to which these teams were attached—three doctors and six enlisted men. The economy is more strikingly realized if man-days are compared. For example, the transportation of 500 patients across the Atlantic by hospital ship normally required approximately seven days and therefore used about 1,295 man-days of medical attendance, while the same evacuation could be accomplished by airplane within from one to two days, depending upon whether or not an overnight stop was made in Newfoundland, and required from forty-three to eighty-six man-days only.[60]

Efforts To Supply Appropriate Equipment for Air Evacuation

Confirmation as policy during 1942 of the peacetime practice of using operational planes instead of special airplane ambulances for the evacuation of patients required the development of special equipment that could be used easily and quickly to adapt cargo and transport planes to their secondary mission—the

[58] (1) Guilford and Soboroff, *op. cit.* (2) History of the Medical Department, Air Transport Command, 1 January 1945–31 March 1946. HD: TAS. (3) AAF Manual 25–0–1, Flight Surgs Ref File, 1 Nov 45. HD: 321 (AAF).

[59] Memo, CG ASF for ACofS OPD WDGS, 26 Apr 44, sub: Air Evac from ETO and NATO. HRS: ASF Planning Div Program Br file, "Hosp and Evac, vol. 3."

[60] This paragraph is based upon a comparison of the tables of organization of hospital ship complements and medical air evacuation transport squadrons and upon comments by Brig Gen. Albert H. Schwichtenberg on a first draft of this chapter. Also see *Journal of the American Medical Association,* Vol. 141, No. 8 (1949), pp. 540–41.

evacuation of patients. Early in 1942 the Air Forces began to use Douglas removable metal-type litter racks, which had already been designed for this purpose, to enable large cargo planes such as the C–47s to carry eighteen litter patients.[61] These racks had important disadvantages. Their detachable parts frequently were lost or damaged in stowage, and replacements had to be stocked at various fields. Furthermore, it was discovered in the fall of 1942 that standard racks did not accommodate all types of American litters currently in use in combat theaters. The Materiel Center at Wright Field (Ohio) therefore undertook a series of experiments, and by the early part of 1944 it developed litter supports made of webbing straps.[62] They were superior to Douglas metal-type racks in many ways. The racks had to be disassembled after each evacuation mission and stowed in floor compartments while two sets of webbing straps could be spaced and anchored permanently along the roof and side walls of the interiors of planes. Douglas racks weighed nearly 200 pounds in comparison with 110 pounds for webbing-strap supports. Metal supports would accommodate only eighteen litter patients in certain aircraft, but webbing straps would hold twenty-four. Preparation of planes for evacuation with webbing-strap supports could be accomplished in six to eight minutes, a fraction of the time needed to assemble and install metal-type racks. In March 1944, therefore, the use of metal-type racks was curtailed and airplane production was modified to require the installation of the new supports.[63] The Air Forces later issued technical orders to guide those engaged in air evacuation operations in the use of webbing-strap supports in C–47, C–47A, C–46, C–64, and C–54 airplanes.[64]

Litters were important items because they served as patients' beds during flights. Before the war the Air Corps had used a metal litter, based upon the best features of the Navy's Stokes litter. It was noninflammable, easy to disinfect, and could be carried, with a patient strapped in, in either a horizontal or a vertical position, but it was costly, bulky, heavy, and difficult to carry.[65] At the beginning of the war, therefore, the Air Corps substituted for it aluminum-pole litters which had been developed in 1937 especially for Air Corps use. In 1942 growing shortages of aluminum stimulated development of a straight carbon-steel-pole litter. A potential steel shortage in turn brought about the development early in 1943 of both straight and double-folding laminated-wood-pole litters. The latter could be collapsed into a smaller space than others, and it soon came to be generally regarded as the best of Medical Department folding litters and ideal for Air Forces use.[66]

When aluminum and steel again became available in the summer of 1943, the

[61] David N. W. Grant, "A Review of Air Evacuation Operations in 1943," *The Air Surgeon's Bulletin,* vol. I, No. 4 (1944), p. 1.

[62] Tec Instruction 1255, Hq Mat Comd AAF Hq to Tec Exec Mat Ctr, Wright Fld, Ohio, 9 Sep 42, sub: Correction of Standard Type Litter Support Now Being Installed in Army Trans Aircraft. AAF: 452.1–B (Amb Planes).

[63] D. M. Clark, "Litter Support Installations for the C–47 Airplane," *The Air Surgeon's Bulletin,* vol. I, No. 4 (1944), p. 10.

[64] AAF Tec Orders 00–75–1 (1 Jul 44); 00–75–2 (30 Nov 44); 00–75–3 (5 Jan 44); 00–75–4 (15 Jan 44); Air Evac Technique of Loading Pnts in C–47 and C–47A, C–46, C–64, and C–54 Airplanes respectively. AAF: AF Admin Ref Br, Air AG.

[65] John B. Johnson, Jr., and Graves H. Wilson, A History of Wartime Research and Development of Medical Field Equipment (1946), pp. 1–245.

[66] Sup Plan 16, Procurement Div SGO, 20 Oct 43, sub: Litters. Off file, Sup Div SGO, 400.114/3815 (Litter, Steel, Folding).

Air Forces shifted procurement back to straight steel-pole and folding aluminum-pole litters. Those issued were unpopular—the former because of its weight and the latter because it did not fold up well in field use.[67] The folding laminated-wood-pole litter continued to be preferred until February 1944. At that time the Air Forces recommended that straight aluminum-pole litters be procured for the remainder of the war. This change was due not so much to dissatisfaction with the special folding litter as to basic changes in aircraft construction. By the early part of 1944 doors and internal capacities of cargo and transport planes had been so enlarged that difficulties formerly encountered in loading, unloading, and stowing litters were no longer problems in air evacuation. Thus the litter which had been designed originally for Air Force use was supplanted, in Air Force procurement, by the standard Ground Force litter. In the summer of 1945, general preference for straight aluminum-pole and folding laminated-wood-pole litters was sanctioned by keeping only these two types classified as standard.[68]

Supplies and equipment for the care of patients during flight similarly had to be specially designed and selected because weight and space were important factors in air movements. At the beginning of the war, two medical chests had been developed for the Air Corps as Medical Department items. A flight service chest, standardized before and improved during the war, was furnished each air evacuation transport squadron. An airplane ambulance chest, developed by the Air Corps and a plastics corporation in St. Louis, Mo., for issue to each flight team, was lighter and contained a minimum of supplies and equipment to care for the immediate needs of patients.[69] The latter type of chest appears to have been satisfactory only for trips requiring six to nine hours. For shorter trips, like those in the North African campaign, the chest was too large and frequently was not used at all if a nurse had to provide medical care unassisted. For longer ones, medical evacuation personnel considered the chest too small for efficient use.[70] Variation in distances between theaters and the zone of interior and in the types of patients evacuated was so great that standardization of a chest for universal use was impractical. Therefore, improvisations of cabinet-type containers for long trips and the development of experimental kits for short trips continued to the end of the war.[71]

The provision of adequate oxygen equipment and improvement of facilities to control and restrain psychotic patients were other problems the Air Forces faced. The availability of oxygen was essential to minimize physiological changes due to the altitude at which flight was maintained. The Air Forces developed and issued a portable continuous-flow therapeutic-oxygen kit to be used for both air evacuation and air and sea rescue. Beginning in the summer of 1944, each air evacuation team received four of these kits to augment the

[67] See n. 66.

[68] Johnson and Wilson, *op. cit.*, p. 45.

[69] (1) See documents in Off files, Sup Div SGO, 400.112/2642 (Chest, Flt Serv, Empty), and 400.114/3023 (Chest, Amb, Airplane, Empty). (2) T/E 8-447, 30 Nov 42. (3) Ltr, SG to CG SOS, 14 Jan 43, sub: Airplane Amb Chest, with 5 inds. SG: 428.

[70] (1) Weekly Staff Rpts, Staff Mtgs ASO, 13 Sep 43. HD: TAS. (2) Daily Rpt, Sup Div ASO, 3 Oct 44. HD: TAS.

[71] (1) An Rpt, Sup Div ASO, FY 1944. HD: TAS. (2) Daily Rpt, Sup Div ASO, 3 May 45. Same file. (3) Andres G. Oliver and Hampton C. Robinson, Jr., "Domestic Air Transportation of Patients," *The Air Surgeon's Bulletin*, vol. II, No. 11 (1945), p. 401.

standard oxygen system available for the crew and able-bodied passengers.[72] A rather knotty problem developed from the transportation of psychotic patients. Since planes had no facilities for isolation, such patients constituted a potential danger to others during flight. Although the Air Transport Command returned several hundred of them from the Southwest Pacific to the zone of interior during 1944 and 1945, it was not until the end of the war that the Command produced a really suitable flexible restraint.[73]

Although feeding was a normal part of pre- and post-flight care, a serious problem in feeding patients developed when flights extended over long periods of time. Cargo and transport planes had no facilities for cleaning or washing dishes, trays, or silverware; and their crews lacked experience in preparing suitable meals for patients from a limited variety of available foods. By January 1944 this problem became serious and the Air Forces started a survey to find a solution. Nevertheless, provisions for feeding patients being evacuated from theaters continued to be little more elaborate than sandwiches, hot coffee, and cold drinks carried in thermos jugs. Patients transported in the domestic air evacuation system, operated by the Ferrying Division of the Air Transport Command, were more fortunate. In November 1944 Wright Field began testing and later approved for installation in planes of the Ferrying Division a galley unit containing four large cups to heat food, a container for coffee, and two "hot cups" for preparing chocolate, soup, and bouillon, as well as drawers for the storage of food.[74]

Both patients and medical attendants complained of fatigue on long flights, patients because of lying on litters for several hours and medical attendants because of lifting and changing the position of patients frequently. An air mattress was therefore developed by the Air Forces to fit on Army litters. It took little space in stowage, weighed little, inflated easily, and could be washed with soap and water. Authority was granted in January 1945 to issue twenty-four air mattresses to each flight team.[75]

Patients transported by air along both tropical and arctic routes suffered from uncomfortable temperatures in planes when they landed for servicing. Early in 1944 the Air Forces collaborated with the Quartermaster Corps and other agencies in the development of portable air conditioners to cool planes' interiors at stopover points. By August 1944 the Supply Division of the Air Surgeon's Office had issued forty-two air conditioners to the Air Transport Command for use both in the zone of interior and in overseas theaters.[76] In arctic areas, large heaters that could be moved up to planes on the ground were used to warm cargo areas until planes were ready for flight.[77]

---

[72] (1) *The Air Surgeon's Bulletin,* vol. II, No. 3 (1945), pp. 78–79, and vol. II, No. 4 (1945), pp. 106–07. (2) T/O&E 8–447, C 1, 11 Dec 44.

[73] History of the Medical Department, Air Transport Command, 1 January 1945–31 March 1946, pp. 91–97. HD: TAS.

[74] (1) A mimeographed copy of a broad plan to study certain equipment problems in connection with air evacuation of patients, developed around January 1944, may be found in AAF: 370.05 (Evac Book 2). (2) Oliver and Robinson, *op. cit.*, pp. 400–01.

[75] (1) Ltr, CG AAF (Air QM) to CG ASF, 2 Jun 44, sub: Air Mattresses and Pillows. AAF: 427. (2) Rpt, Off of Air Insp (I. B. March) to Air Insp Hq AAF, 21 Aug 44, sub: Summary of Med Insp of ATC and Stas In CBI Wing. HD: TAS (ATC and Misc). (3) T/O&E 8–447, C 2, 25 Jan 45.

[76] (1) An Rpt, Sup Div ASO, FY 1944. HD: TAS. (2) Daily Rpt, Sup Div ASO, 29 Aug 44. Same file.

[77] *The Air Surgeon's Bulletin,* vol. II, No. 10 (1945), pp. 330–31.

Until the fall of 1943 loading and unloading litters in high-door planes were accomplished manually. When air evacuation increased in the latter part of 1943, this method was discarded generally in favor of a fork-lift truck with a "litter adaptor" made from a simple wooden pallet platform used to move and store cargo. The mechanical loading and unloading of patients proved to be rapid, safe, and comfortable and was adopted at most Air Transport Command installations throughout the world by the end of the year.[78]

The exchange of property used in air evacuation constituted a difficult problem. A patient was seldom separated from his litter and blankets until he reached a hospital. When the Air Forces released patients to Ground or Service Forces installations, comparable equipment seldom was returned in exchange and the Air Forces sustained a gradual loss.[79] This was particularly important in the case of litters in the first part of the war because the Ground and Service Forces were using straight-pole litters while the Air Forces preferred and used folding-pole litters. The Air Surgeon and The Surgeon General were acquainted with the problem and by the middle of 1943 began to study means of solving it.[80] A new procedure was established by directives issued by the Air Transport Command in April and the War Department in June 1944. According to it, the Air Transport Command was to furnish necessary medical supplies for use in flight, while commanding officers of medical installations, through medical supply officers, were to be responsible for providing such equipment as litters and blankets. When a hospital requested air transportation for a group of patients, a shipping ticket was to be prepared by its medical supply officer listing necessary litters, blankets, splints, etc. The flight nurse was to turn in the shipping list to the medical supply officer of the receiving hospital where it would be signed and mailed to the originating hospital. Later, the equipment was to be turned in to a depot for return to the theater by boat. If the originating hospital was in the zone of interior, the equipment would be shipped directly to that hospital.[81] This system did not work as well as anticipated. Shipping by water was slow and did not always return property as fast as it was used. As a result, successive efforts were made during 1944 to increase the number of blankets and litters supplied to air evacuation squadrons so that a pool of this equipment could be established overseas.[82]

Changes in the table of organization and equipment for air evacuation squadrons reflected both the development of special equipment for air evacuation operations and attempts to eliminate shortages of equipment in theaters of operations. The table, first published on 30 November 1942, authorized the Air Forces to issue such items as flight clothes and equipment to nurses and enlisted technicians and the Medical Department to issue blankets, litters, and flight service medical chests. As revised in June 1943, this table doubled the allowance of blankets, undoubtedly to

[78] John M. Collins, "Litter Loading Device," *The Air Surgeon's Bulletin*, vol. I, No. 9 (1944), p. 22.

[79] Diary, SOS Hosp and Evac Br (Fitzpatrick), 27 Nov 42. HD: Wilson files, "Diary."

[80] Johnson and Wilson, *op. cit.*, p. 152.

[81] (1) ATC Memo 25-6, Air Evac, 29 Apr 44. AAF: 370.05 (Evac Book 2). (2) Ltr, TAG to CGs AAF, AGF, ASF, Theaters, Def and Base Comds, etc., 8 Jun 44, sub: Procedure for Evac of Pnts by Water or Air from Overseas Comd. AG: 704.11 (3 Jun 44).

[82] Memo SPMOO 400.34 (15 Nov 44), CG ASF (Lutes) for CG AAF, 20 Nov 44, sub: Change 1 to T/O&E 8-447. AG: 320.3 (2 Jun 44).

cover shortages growing out of unsatisfactory operation of the property-exchange system.[83] Medical supplies were to be requisitioned from medical depots operated by the Air Service Command according to requirements determined by the Supply Division of the Air Surgeon's Office.[84] A revision of the table in July 1944 authorized the Air Forces to issue four portable oxygen assemblies per air team, and it increased the number of litters per squadron from 432 to 576. Five months later, a further change reflected the substitution of the Air Forces' newly developed therapeutic-oxygen kit for the portable assembly. It also authorized an increase in straight aluminum-pole litters from 576 to 1,500, and the addition of 3,732 olive drab blankets for each squadron. The increase in litters and blankets was made to cover part of the shortages of these items in the theaters. Another change in the table, published 25 January 1945, added as Air Forces organizational equipment 576 pneumatic mattresses per squadron.[85]

[83] T/E 8-447, 30 Nov 42, with C 1, 14 Jun 43.

[84] Coleman, *op. cit.*, pp. 635-36.

[85] T/O&E 8-447, 19 Jul 44; C 1, 11 Dec 44; C 2, 25 Jan 45.

CHAPTER XXV

Evacuation Units for Theaters of Operations

The evacuation units discussed in preceding chapters were those used primarily in the movement of patients in and to the zone of interior, though some were used also within theaters of operations. Mention has been made earlier, in chapters showing how the zone of interior provided hospital units for overseas service,[1] of other evacuation units that cared for and transported patients from front-line areas rearward through combat zones to mobile hospitals. Certain aspects of these units—such as changes in their organization, personnel, and equipment, and the manner in which they were activated, trained, and used in the United States—need to be considered at this point.

Organization, Personnel, and Equipment

Units designed for the care and transportation of patients in combat zones, as already pointed out,[2] either were organic elements of larger nonmedical organizations such as infantry regiments and divisions, or were separate units intended for assignment to corps and armies. Every regiment and every separate battalion of each arm or service, except medical, had a medical detachment as one of its organic parts. While the size and organization of medical detachments varied according to the size of the units to which they belonged, their functions remained the same. Aid men of the medical detachment accompanied troops into combat, giving casualties emergency medical care at the front lines. Its litter bearers then carried casualties, except those still able to walk, back to aid stations where medical technicians and medical officers treated them for return to duty or prepared them for further transportation. Units that were organic elements of divisions—medical regiments, battalions, or squadrons, depending upon the type of division concerned—collected casualties from aid stations and transported them first to collecting stations and then to clearing stations farther to the rear, sorting them at each station for additional treatment and return to duty or for preparation for further evacuation. Units that were assigned directly to corps and armies, such as medical battalions and medical regiments, collected and treated for return to duty or prepared for evacuation the casualties of their respective areas. In addition, army evacuation units transported casualties from divisional clearing stations to mobile hospitals in army areas and supplied reinforcements for divisional medical services.

[1] See above, pp. 38–49, 144–66, 214–37.
[2] See above, pp. 4, 38–39.

While the system of evacuating casualties through the combat zone was not altered in any significant respect during the war, certain changes occurred both before and during the war in the units operating this system. These changes were designed primarily to achieve mobility, flexibility, and economy.

The medical battalion of the infantry division was developed in the prewar years, it will be recalled,[3] as a result of the emergence of the triangular division to replace the square division. The latter's organic medical unit was a medical regiment which consisted of a regimental headquarters and band, a headquarters and service company, a collecting battalion of three companies, an ambulance battalion of three companies, and a clearing battalion of three companies. It was authorized 66 officers and 980 enlisted men to serve a division of 946 officers, 12 warrant officers, and 21,314 enlisted men.[4] The medical battalion, which served the triangular division of 624 officers, 6 warrant officers, and 14,615 enlisted men, contained 34 officers and 476 enlisted men. It consisted of a headquarters and headquarters detachment, a clearing company, and three collecting companies.[5] Containing litter bearers, collecting-station personnel, and ambulances, each collecting company was capable of supporting a regimental combat team, whether it operated separately or in close conjunction with the division of which it was a part.[6] Although not designed specifically for the purpose, this battalion was used also as the evacuation unit for corps troops. The medical regiment continued in existence, serving National Guard divisions until they were reorganized as triangular divisions in 1942. Like the medical battalion, it also had a function for which it was not specifically designed; that is, it served as an evacuation unit with army troops.[7] Thus medical battalions and medical regiments could be either divisional or nondivisional units, depending upon their assignment and use.

A nondivisional medical unit developed in the prewar years for use in the evacuation system, though not in the actual transportation of patients, was the medical gas treatment battalion. While other medical units had some means of treating at least small numbers of gas casualties, none was adequately equipped to treat the influx of casualties which might result from the use of gas on a large scale. The Surgeon General's Office therefore prepared a table of organization for a medical gas treatment battalion, and the General Staff approved it despite misgivings that such a unit might duplicate the functions of other medical units or of the quartermaster sterilization and bath battalion. The medical gas treatment battalion was made up of a headquarters and three clearing companies. Each of the latter, having two bath and four treatment sections, was expected to bathe and treat gas casualties and to provide them with noncontaminated clothing in preparation for return to duty or for further evacuation to the rear.[8]

[3] See above, pp. 39–40.

[4] T/O 8–21, Med Regt, 1 Nov 40, and T/O 7, Inf Div (Square), 1 Nov 40.

[5] T/O 8–65, Med Bn, 1 Oct 40, and T/O 70, Inf Div (Triangular), 1 Nov 40.

[6] T/O 8–67, Med Co, Collecting, Bn, 1 Oct 40.

[7] FM 8–5, Med Fld Manual, Mobile Units of the Med Dept, 12 Jan 42.

[8] (1) Ltr, SG to TAG, 11 Jun 41, sub: T/Os, with 2 inds. AG: 320.2 (6–11–41). (2) Memo, ACofS G–3 WDGS for TAG, 23 Aug 41, sub: T/O for Med Bn, Gas Treatment, with Memo for Record. Same file. (3) T/O 8–125, Med Gas Treatment Bn, 2 Oct 41, and T/O 8–127, Med Clearing Co, Gas Treatment Bn, 2 Oct 41.

In the first few months after the United States entered the war, the tables of organization of existing combat zone evacuation units were revised and new units were developed for use with new combat organizations. During 1942 the Army Ground Forces experimented with new types of divisions—mountain, jungle, airborne, and motorized.[9] Although organizations of these types were used overseas little, or not at all, the fact that some of them were anticipated for use made it necessary for medical units to be prepared for them. Therefore, during 1942 tables of organization were developed for appropriate medical units for service with new types of forces.[10] Concurrently, changes were made in existing units. To indicate the nature of these changes, it will suffice to consider revisions in the tables of organization of three of the more common types: the medical detachment of the infantry regiment, the medical battalion of the infantry division, and the medical regiment serving the field army.

Unlike the infantry regiment which it supported, the medical detachment's enlisted strength increased appreciably—from 96 to 126—when its table of organization was revised in April 1942. The inclusion of additional surgical technicians accounted primarily for this increase. The number of officers—eight physicians and two dentists — remained unchanged. Changes were made at the same time in the transportation authorized for the detachment. Seven ¼-ton trucks (jeeps), seven ¼-ton trailers, and one 2½-ton truck replaced one motorcycle, fourteen ½-ton trucks, and two 1½-ton trucks.[11]

The infantry division's medical battalion, according to early plans, was to receive an increase in enlisted men and in vehicles as well. Its table of organization issued in April 1942 called for 8 additional enlisted men, an increase in Medical Administrative Corps officers from 5 to 8, a reduction in Medical Corps officers from 27 to 25, and no change in Dental Corps officers (2). The battalion's vehicles, exclusive of trailers, rose from 87 to 93. The addition of trucks accounted for this increase, the number of ambulances—36—remaining the same.[12] About the time this table was published, the War Department ordered a reduction in motor vehicles.[13] The Surgeon General then decided to use the revised version of the table of organization of the medical battalion for motorized divisions being organized, and to develop a new table for the medical battalions of infantry divisions.[14] The new table, submitted for publication in July[15] but issued with an earlier date, reduced the number of motor vehicles by thirteen. None of the vehicles eliminated were ambulances, and trailers were added to replace some of the cargo space lost. Fewer motor vehicles required fewer drivers and mechanics, and hence the new table provided for fourteen fewer enlisted men than formerly. In addition, one Medical Corps officer was eliminated, reducing the total for the battalion from twenty-five to twenty-four. The number of Medical Administrative Corps

[9] Kent R. Greenfield, Robert R. Palmer and Bell I. Wiley, *The Organization of Ground Combat Troops* (Washington, 1947), pp. 336-50, in UNITED STATES ARMY IN WORLD WAR II.

[10] An Rpt, Plans Div Opr Serv SGO, 1942. HD.

[11] T/O 7-11, Inf Regt, Rifle, 1 Oct 40 and 1 Apr 42.

[12] T/O 8-65, Med Bn, 1 Oct 40 and 1 Apr 42.

[13] Ltr SPXPC 320.2 (3-13-42), TAG to CGs AGF, AAF, and SOS, 31 Mar 42, sub: Policies Governing T/Os and T/BAs. AG: 320.2 (3-13-42)(5).

[14] Memo, SG for CG SOS, 6 Jun 42, sub: Changes in T/Os. AG: 320.3 (10-30-41)(2) Sec 8.

[15] Memo, CG SOS for TAG thru ACofS G-3 WDGS, 16 Jul 42, sub: T/Os, Med Bn. AG: 320.3 (10-30-41)(2) Sec 8.

officers (eight) and of Dental Corps officers (two) remained unchanged.[16]

The revision of the table of organization of medical regiments early in 1942 provided for an entirely new type of organization. Instead of having three battalions (collecting, ambulance, and clearing), the new regiment had two battalions that were similar to the medical battalions of infantry divisions, each having three collecting companies and one clearing company. The collecting companies of battalions of medical regiments were almost identical with those of divisional medical battalions, but clearing companies of the former differed from those of the latter in having three instead of two clearing platoons in order to provide increased treatment facilities in army areas. This revision of the medical regiment was based on two of its functions as an army unit: the evacuation of divisional clearing stations and the reinforcement of divisional medical services. Having battalions and companies similar to those of divisional medical battalions, the new medical regiment would simplify the problem of supplying reinforcing units to divisions in combat and, it was anticipated, would permit better ambulance evacuation of divisional clearing stations. This change in the organization of the medical regiment resulted in an increase of Medical Department officers from 66 to 76 and of enlisted men from 980 to 1,078. It also resulted in an increase in vehicles, the number of ambulances rising from sixty to seventy-two.[17] To provide even more ambulances for field armies, if they should be needed, and for communications zones as well, The Surgeon General developed about the same time a table of organization for separate motor ambulance battalions. It was approved and published in April 1942.[18]

In the fall of 1942 the need for economy in personnel and vehicles—which, it will be recalled, affected the organization of hospital units [19]—also resulted in changes in the tables of evacuation units. In response to a War Department directive to reduce personnel and equipment, especially vehicles, in all Army organizations,[20] AGF headquarters established a Reduction Board in November 1942 to review all AGF-type units and to squeeze out the "fat." [21] In the process of shrinking the infantry division as a whole, the Board in March 1943 cut the personnel and vehicles of both the regimental medical detachment and the divisional medical battalion. In the detachment 1 medical officer and 23 enlisted men were eliminated, leaving 7 physicians, 2 dentists, and 103 enlisted men. This cut apparently proved too great, for about four months later twenty-three enlisted men were restored to the regimental medical detachment, bringing the total to 126 for the rest of the war. The only change made in the vehicles of the detachment was the replacement of its 2½-ton truck with a 1½-ton truck. As in the case of the cut in enlisted

[16] T/O 8–15, Med Bn, 1 Apr 42. T/O 8–65, Med Bn, 1 Apr 42, was amended at the end of July to become T/O 8–65, Med Bn, Motorized (C 1, 31 Jul 42).

[17] (1) T/O 8–21, Med Regt, 1 Apr 42. (2) DF G–3/42108, ACofS G–3 WDGS to TAG, 5 Mar 42, sub: Med Regt, with Memo for Record and memos of explanation prepared by SGO. AG: 320.3 (10–30–41) (2) Sec 8.

[18] (1) T/O 8–315, Med Amb Bn, Motor, 1 Apr 42. (2) DF G–3/42108, ACofS G–3 WDGS to TAG, 6 Mar 42, sub: T/Os, with Memo for Record and memos of explanation prepared by SGO. AG: 320.3 (10–30–41)(2) Sec 8.

[19] See above, pp. 131–37, 146–49.

[20] Ltr, TAG to CGs AGF, AAF, and SOS, 2 Oct 42, sub: Review of Orgn and Equip Reqmts. AG: 400 (8–10–42)(1) Sec 22.

[21] Greenfield *et al.*, *op. cit.*, pp. 351–63, discusses the Reduction Board and its work.

men, this change was reversed in July 1943.[22]

Reductions made in both the personnel and vehicles of the divisional medical battalion were more lasting. In March 1943 its Medical Corps officers were decreased from 24 to 22 and its enlisted men from 470 to 430, but its Medical Administrative Corps officers were increased from 8 to 11 and its dentists from 2 to 3. The clearing company of the medical battalion suffered the greatest decrease in enlisted men, twenty being eliminated, of whom twelve were orderlies who normally served in the clearing station. In each collecting company the number of litter bearers was reduced from thirty-six to thirty-one. The Reduction Board believed that the use of jeeps to evacuate casualties from the battlefield warranted this action, but supported the Ground Surgeon in opposing a reduction in the number of ambulances because it believed that twelve would be needed to evacuate casualties from each regiment and would not be available unless included in the table of organization. Nevertheless, the commanding general, Army Ground Forces, directed a cut of two in each collecting company, thereby reducing the number in the entire medical battalion from thirty-six to thirty. Four other motor vehicles, three of which were command cars, were also eliminated.[23] Cuts were made also in the personnel and vehicles of other organic medical units, but being similar in nature to those already described, they need not be discussed here.

Although experience in maneuvers and in theaters of operations indicated that medical battalions and regiments, organized under existing tables, were not entirely suitable for use with corps and army troops respectively, it remained for the Reduction Board of AGF headquarters to initiate a change in corps and army evacuation units. The chief cause of dissatisfaction with existing units was their inflexibility. To provide greater flexibility, permitting the assignment of collecting, clearing, and ambulance companies in any combination required to fit a particular situation, and thereby to promote economy of both personnel and equipment, the Reduction Board in February 1943 proposed the elimination of such large table-of-organization units as the medical regiment and the separate ambulance battalion, and the substitution of small administratively self-sufficient units, such as companies, which could be grouped for training and tactical use under separate battalion and group headquarters detachments.[24] This proposal reflected a general trend in the Army Ground Forces "away from the organic assignment of resources to large commands according to ready-made patterns, and toward variable or *ad hoc* assignment to commands tailor-made for specific missions"[25]—a trend that was to end during 1943 in the disappearance of type armies and corps. In accordance with the Reduction Board's proposal, the Ground Surgeon's Office

[22] T/O 7-11, Inf Regt, 1 Mar 43 and T/O&E 7-11, Inf Regt, 15 Jul 43, 26 Feb 44, and 1 Jun 45.

[23] (1) T/O 8-15, Med Bn, 1 Mar 43; T/O 8-16, Hq and Hq Det, Med Bn, 1 Mar 43; T/O 8-17, Collecting Co, Med Bn, 1 Mar 43; and T/O 8-18, Clearing Co, Med Bn, 1 Mar 43. (2) M/S GNRQT/24549, sub: T/O 8-16, 8-17, and 8-18, with following comments: CG AGF to Reqmts AGF, 5 Dec 42; Reduction Bd to CG AGF, 8 Dec 42; and CG AGF to Reqmts AGF, 9 Dec 42. AGF: 320.3.

[24] (1) M/S GNRQT/31566, Reduction Bd to Reqmts AGF, 10 Feb 43, sub: Med T/Os. AGF: 320.3. (2) An Rpt, Surg First Army, 1941. HD. (3) Memo, Ground Surg for CG AGF, 17 Jun 43, sub: [Anal of Rpts from North Africa]. Ground Med files: Chronological file, Folder 1.

[25] Greenfield *et al., op. cit.*, p. 280. See also pp. 279-99, 351-54.

prepared tables of organization for headquarters and headquarters detachments of medical battalions and groups, and for administratively self-sufficient collecting, clearing, and ambulance companies. The Reduction Board, staff officers in AGF headquarters, and the Surgeon General's Office approved these tables and they were published in May 1943.[26] Thereafter, instead of being rigid table-of-organization battalions and regiments, evacuation units of corps and armies were flexible battalions and groups made up of combinations of collecting, clearing, and ambulance companies that varied as the situation demanded.[27]

A further step in the trend toward the formation of small units that could be used in variable combinations was the development of tables of organization for teams or sections that could be grouped together to form platoons that could be further grouped to form companies. Like other technical services, the Medical Department prepared a table of organization for such units. The Medical Department table, issued in July 1943, provided for administrative, depot, motor ambulance, veterinary, and miscellaneous teams or sections. The three ambulance sections provided for by this table had 3, 6, and 10 ambulances respectively and could be assigned wherever required. One of the miscellaneous sections, the "attached medical section," was designed to provide medical service for nonmedical battalions that were organic parts of larger units but were assigned alone to special missions.[28]

Early in 1944 the general movement already under way to replace Medical Corps officers with Medical Administrative Corps officers wherever possible affected the make-up of evacuation units also.[29] In battalion and group headquarters, for example, administrative officers replaced physicians as operations officers (S–3s). Of perhaps more significance was the substitution in the medical detachments of combat battalions and regiments of Medical Administrative Corps officers for Medical Corps officers as battalion surgeons' assistants. The Ground Surgeon concurred in The Surgeon General's proposal to make this substitution in the medical detachments of coast artillery, antiaircraft artillery, engineer, signal, and ordnance battalions, but he disapproved at first the recommendation that it be extended to the medical detachments of infantry regiments and tank battalions. The latter organizations had such a high percentage of casualties, he stated, that a reduction of Medical Corps officers in their medical detachments would seriously impair the efficiency of their medical services.[30] In February 1944, on the advice of the Fifth Army Surgeon in Italy, the Ground Surgeon reversed himself on this point. Thereafter, in the medical detach-

---

[26] (1) M/S GNRQT/31566, sub: Med T/Os, Comment 5, Ground Med Sec to Reqmts AGF thru Reduction Bd, 11 Mar 43; Comment 6, Reduction Bd to CG AGF, 3 [sic] Mar 43; Comment 7, Sec Gen Staff AGF to Ground Med Sec, 12 Mar 43; Comment 8, Ground Med Sec to Sec Gen Staff AGF, 16 Mar 43; Comment 10, Sec Gen Staff AGF to Reduction Bd, 18 Mar 43. AGF: 320.3. (2) Memo for Record, 29 Mar 43, by Ground Med Sec. Ground Med files: Transfer Binder Journal, 1943.

[27] T/O&E 8–22, Hq and Hq Det, Med Group, 20 May 43; T/O&E 8–26, Hq and Hq Det, Med Bn, Sep, 20 May 43; T/O&E 8–27, Med Collecting Co, Sep, 20 May 43; T/O&E 8–28, Med Clearing Co, Sep, 20 May 43; and T/O&E 8–317, Med Amb Co, Motor, Sep, 20 May 43.

[28] T/O&E 8–500, Med Dept Serv Orgn, 26 Jul 43.

[29] See above, pp. 250–51, 280.

[30] (1) Memo, SG for CG ASF, 25 Nov 43, sub: Conservation of MC Offs. (2) Memo, CG AGF (Ground Med Sec) for CofSA, 22 Feb 44, same sub. (3) DF, ACofS G–3 WDGS to TAG, 1 Mar 44, same sub. All in AG: 320.3 (10–30–41)(2). (4) WD Cir 99, 9 Mar 44.

ment of the infantry regiment, for example, there were five Medical Corps, two Dental Corps, and three Medical Administrative Corps officers instead of seven Medical Corps and two Dental Corps officers. One Medical Corps and one Medical Administrative Corps officer, instead of two Medical Corps officers, served with each of the three battalion medical sections. In the detachment's headquarters there were two Medical Corps officers, instead of one as formerly, to insure a replacement if needed for one of the battalion surgeons.[31]

Further changes were made in existing evacuation units, and new units were proposed and developed in the latter half of 1944 and the early part of 1945. Late in May 1944 a War Department circular directed a reduction in the number of basic privates in all but a few of the Army's table-of-organization units.[32] Basic privates were soldiers in excess of the complement of personnel needed to perform the functions for which units were designed and were provided to serve as replacements for losses occurring in the first phases of combat or, when in garrison, for men who would normally be absent because of furloughs, sickness, and the like. Until May 1944 basic privates represented an addition of about 10 percent to the normal operating strength of a unit. In May the War Department directed that they be reduced by approximately one-half. This led to a reduction in the number of basic privates in the medical battalion of an infantry division from thirty-nine to twenty-two.[33] Separate medical units such as collecting, clearing, and ambulance companies were similarly reduced, but medical detachments serving with cavalry and infantry divisions were exempted.[34]

In the latter part of 1944 the Ground Surgeon proposed changes in the evacuation units of both divisions and armies. It had been recognized for some time, he stated, that the clearing companies of divisional medical battalions needed three—instead of two—clearing platoons, in order to provide one clearing platoon to work with each of three collecting companies in support of the three regimental combat teams of each infantry division. Moreover, reports from theaters of operations, according to the Ground Surgeon, emphasized that the collecting-station platoons of separate collecting companies were not needed in army areas of combat zones. There the need was for more litter bearers. Likewise, the ambulance platoons of separate collecting companies were not required in army areas because separate ambulance companies were authorized as army units. The Ground Surgeon therefore proposed to eliminate collecting companies as army evacuation units, and to substitute for them additional separate ambulance companies and separate litter bearer companies. For the latter he prepared a tentative table of organization. He further proposed that the men and officers formerly assigned to collecting-station platoons of army collecting companies should be used to form third platoons for the clearing companies of divisional medical battalions. Despite the fact that the changes recommended were expected not only to improve the organization of the

[31] (1) M/S, Ground Med Sec to ACofS G-2 AGF, 8 Mar 44, sub: Proposed Changes in T/O. Ground Med files: Chronological file (Col W. E. Shambora). (2) DF, ACofS G-3 WDGS to TAG, 25 Mar 44, sub: T/O&E 8-500 and 8-550, with Memo for Record on change in WD Cir 99 (1944). AG: 320.3 (10-30-41) (2). (2) WD Cir 122, 28 Mar 44.

[32] WD Cir 201, 22 May 44.

[33] T/O&E 8-15, Med Bn, 15 Jul 43, with C 2, 3 Jul 44.

[34] WD Cir 201, 22 May 44.

medical service in division and army areas of combat zones but also to save both commissioned and enlisted personnel, the Deputy Chief of Staff of the Army Ground Forces disapproved the Ground Surgeon's proposal in December 1944 because he considered it undesirable to make such changes "at this late date in the war." [35]

The question of whether or not the medical gas treatment battalion should continue to exist arose in the latter part of 1944. Earlier its table of organization had been superseded by a table providing for a gas treatment team that was smaller and more restricted in its functions,[36] but units already in theaters of operations continued in existence. The Technical Division of the Surgeon General's Office contended in June 1944 that they were not needed because oxygen and drugs could be administered to gas casualties by gas treatment teams and other medical units, the decontamination of equipment and clothing was not a proper function of the Medical Department, and the ability of gas treatment battalions to locate and decontaminate personnel as soon after exposure as necessary was doubtful.[37] The Ground Surgeon also questioned the utility of such battalions and considered them wasteful of personnel.[38] Moreover, since gas warfare had not been used, medical gas treatment battalions in theaters of operations had not performed the functions for which they were intended. Nevertheless, because they had constituted a "convenient reserve," theaters wished to retain them. So also did the Chief of the Chemical Warfare Service. In October 1944, therefore, The Surgeon General requested and received permission to revise and reinstate the table of organization of the gas treatment battalion as an authorized unit.[39]

One of the uses which theaters had made of gas treatment battalions was to hold and care for patients awaiting evacuation at railheads and airports. No unit designed specifically for this purpose had been provided, despite information from North Africa as early as the fall of 1943 that they were needed,[40] and theaters had had to use whatever means were available to meet their needs. This practice had been wasteful of both personnel and equipment. Early in 1945, therefore, after an inspection of the medical service of the European theater by one of his representatives, the Assistant Chief of Staff, G–4, directed The Surgeon General to prepare a table of organization for a medical holding unit.[41] The resulting unit, a medical holding battalion authorized in May 1945, consisted of a headquarters and three holding companies, each capable of han-

[35] (1) Memo for Record, on M/S, Comment 4, Ground Med Sec to ACofS G–1 AGF, 15 Dec 44, no sub. (2) M/S, Comment 1, Ground Med Sec to Gen Staff AGF, 18 Sep 44, sub: T/O&E 8–29 (Proposed) Med Litter Bearer Co, Sep. Both in Ground Med files: Chronological file, Folder 2. (3) M/S, Comment 1, Ground Med Sec for ACofS G–3 AGF, 17 Jun 44, no sub. Ground Med files: Chronological file, Folder 1. (4) Memo, SG for CG ASF, 1 Oct 43, sub: Recomd for Changes in Med Dept Orgn, (SG: 320.3–1) proposed a third platoon for the clearing companies of the medical battalions of infantry divisions. After the war, the third platoon was added (T/O&E 8–18N, Clearing Co, Med Bn, 27 Feb 48).

[36] T/O&E 8–500, Med Dept Serv Orgn, 23 Apr 44.

[37] Diary, Tec Div SGO, 17 Jun 44. HD: 024.7 Oprs Serv.

[38] Ltr, Brig Gen F[rederick] A. Blesse to Col Calvin H. Goddard, 11 Feb 53. HD: 314 (Correspondence on MS) XI.

[39] (1) Diary, Tec Div SGO, 7 and 14 Oct 44. HD: 024.7 Oprs Serv. (2) T/O&E 8–125, Med Gas Treatment Bn, 11 Nov 44.

[40] (1) Memo, CG AAF for SG, 17 Sep 43, sub: Aerial Evac of Casualties. (2) Memo, Dir Hosp Admin Div SGO for Dir Plans Div SGO, 22 Sep 43, no sub. Both in HD: 705 "Hosp and Evac (Holding Unit) MTO."

[41] (1) 2d ind, SG to CG ASF, 3 Mar 45, on unlocated basic ltr. HD: 320.3–1 (T/O&E). (2) An Rpt, Tec Div SGO, FY 1945. HD.

dling 300 patients. Had this battalion not been developed so late in the war, its use would have saved manpower, for it was authorized 26 officers and 404 enlisted men as compared with 45 officers and 411 enlisted men of the medical gas treatment battalions which some theaters used as holding units.[42]

Changes occurred during the war in the equipment as well as the personnel and vehicles of evacuation units. Changes in medical supplies and equipment reflected improvements in items already authorized or additions of items shown by experience to be needed. For example, early in 1944 an improved portable field autoclave replaced an older item of that type in the clearing companies of medical battalions of infantry divisions. At the same time the number of chests of surgical supplies was increased, and portable electric suction apparatus was added to enable clearing stations to aspirate blood from pleural and abdominal cavities.[43] Toward the end of that year and the early part of 1945 a combined otoscope and ophthalmoscope was added to the list of items furnished clearing companies, to permit clearing stations to make better examinations of patients with diseased or injured ears.[44] Other changes were made at intervals in the lists of medical supplies and equipment of evacuation units in order to improve the standard of emergency medical service under combat conditions.[45]

Changes were also made in the equipment of evacuation units to increase their mobility. For example, early in the war the Medical Department developed a pack carrier for battalion medical equipment. This carrier—a canvas container mounted on a wooden frame—permitted the supplies and equipment used in battalion aid stations to be packed in loads (averaging about forty pounds each) that could be carried by individuals of battalion medical sections.[46] Later in the war, after aluminum became available for the purpose, aluminum-pole litters were substituted, it will be recalled, for heavier ones made of steel.[47] Another change contributing to greater mobility in evacuation was the development of litter racks for jeeps, permitting in many instances the substitution of motor for pedestrian evacuation in front-line areas. Although such racks were produced locally for use by evacuation units much earlier, they were not included in tables of equipment as standard items until 1945.[48]

---

[42] (1) T/O&E 8-55, Med Holding Bn, 30 May 45. (2) Ltr, TAG to CinC USAF Pacific and CG USAF POA, 5 Jul 45, sub: T/O&E Med Holding Bn. SG: 320.3.

[43] (1) Ltr, CG AGF to CG ASF thru SG, 10 Nov 43, sub: Proposed Changes in T/O&Es. AGF: 320.3. (2) T/O&E 8-18, Clearing Co, Med Bn, 15 Jul 43, with C 1, 17 Jan 44.

[44] (1) M/S, Comment 1, Ground Med Sec to ACofS G-4 AGF and Reqmts AGF, 23 Aug 44, sub: Addition to T/Es of Certain Med Units. Ground Med files: Chronological file, Folder 2. (2) T/O&E 8-138, Clearing Co, Mountain Med Bn, 4 Nov 44, and T/O&E 8-18, Clearing Co, Med Bn, 14 Feb 45, for example.

[45] Examples of these changes may be found by comparing the T/O&Es of various evacuation units.

[46] (1) An Rpt, Equip Br Tng Div SGO, 1942. HD. (2) Memo, SG for Chief Surg SWPA, 1 Dec 42. SG: 705 (Australia)F. (3) Memo, [Maj] A[lfred] P. T[hom] for Col Shambora, 2 Mar 43, sub: Comments on Lessons Derived from Oprs at Casablanca and Oran. Ground Med files: Chronological file, Training, 1943. (4) T/O&E 7-11, Inf Regt, 15 Jul 43.

[47] (1) John B. Johnson, Jr., and Graves H. Wilson, A History of Wartime Research and Development of Medical Field Equipment (1946), pp. 75-80. (2) For example, T/O&E 8-16, C 1; T/O&E 8-17, C 3; T/O&E 8-18, C 2, all dated 3 Jul 44.

[48] (1) Diary, Tec Div SGO, 3 Jun and 26 Aug 44. HD: 024.7 Oprs Serv. (2) The General Board, U. S. Forces, European Theater, Evacuation of Human Casualties in the European Theater of Operations. Study No. 92. HD. (3) T/O&E 8-16, Hq and Hq Det, Med Bn, 14 Feb 45, and T/O&E 7-11, Inf Regt, 1 Jun 45.

Efforts to increase mobility by reducing the size and weight of equipment were made in the case of evacuation units, as in that of hospital units already discussed.[49] During the winter of 1942–43 the cubage of the equipment (including vehicles) of the infantry division's medical battalion was reduced from about 1,900 to about 1,475 ship tons, a ship ton being 40 cubic feet.[50] Information about the cubage of the equipment of other evacuation units in the fall of 1942 is not readily available, but it is perhaps safe to assume that similar reductions were made in the equipment of those units. After the reductions made in the winter of 1942–43, the cubage of equipment of evacuation units underwent little change until the early part of 1945. At that time there seems to have been a tendency for it to increase slightly. For example, the equipment of the infantry division's medical battalion increased in cubage from about 1,475 to about 1,600 ship tons in February 1945. Similar increases occurred early in 1945 in the equipment of other evacuation units.[51]

Another measure to increase the mobility and improve the standard of combat zone medical service was the development by the Medical Department of certain vehicles for special purposes. The organization and growth of the Armored Force made it apparent during 1941 that new types of medical equipment would be needed. During the fall of that year the Armored Force itself began to experiment with the development of a surgical truck for use as a mobile clearing station. Soon afterward, the Surgeon General's Office secured authority to initiate a research project in that field. During its course, the Medical Department Equipment Laboratory co-ordinated its developmental work with the Armored Force, the Surgeon General's Office, and the Quartermaster Corps. The pilot model of such a truck was delivered to the Laboratory in July 1942. Called a "truck, surgical," this vehicle consisted of a van body mounted on a standard 2½-ton (6 x 6) chassis. Within the body of the truck were a 50-gallon water tank; a sink with hot and cold water outlets; cabinets for supplies, equipment, and accessories; and three dome lights. Medical items such as those used in clearing stations were supplied and installed by the Medical Department. A tent, large enough to shelter twenty litter patients, was supplied to provide space outside the truck for patients awaiting evacuation farther to the rear. These trucks were delivered on a basis of six per division to all armored divisions in the United States during late 1942 and early 1943.[52]

A surgical operating truck for use by auxiliary surgical groups was developed during the latter half of 1943. It differed from the surgical truck of the armored division largely in that it was supplied with greater quantities of more elaborate equipment. While the surgical truck of the armored division had only equipment and supplies for emergency medical treatment to be given inside the truck, the surgical operating truck carried enough surgical instruments and equipment to perform approximately 100 major surgical operations. Surgery was not performed in the truck, but in a tent attached to its rear. The truck served only as a supply and

[49] See above, pp. 146–48.

[50] (1) Memo, CG AGF for ACofS G–3 WDGS, 16 Feb 43, sub: T/O&E, Med Bn. AG: 320.3 (10–30–41)(2) Sec 8. (2) FM 101–10, Staff Offs' Fld Manual—Orgn, Tec, and Logistical Data, 10 Oct 43 and 21 Dec 44.

[51] FM 101–10, Staff Offs' Fld Manual—Orgn, Tec, and Logistical Data, 21 Dec 44 and 1 Aug 45.

[52] Johnson and Wilson, *op. cit.*, pp. 295–339.

sterilizing room. Such trucks, along with auxiliary surgical groups, often served as far forward as divisional clearing stations, supplementing them when the evacuation load was heavy. By the end of October 1945, 207 surgical operating trucks had been delivered for use by the Medical Department. In addition to surgical trucks, the Medical Department developed other special vehicles for use in theaters of operations. They were a mobile dental laboratory truck, mobile optical repair truck, a mobile dental operating truck, and an army medical laboratory truck. Development of these vehicles contributed to the mobility and flexibility of medical service in a fast-moving war.[53]

Activation, Training, and Use in the United States

The responsibility for activating, training, and using in the United States the evacuation units that would operate in combat zones of theaters of operations belonged almost exclusively to the Ground Forces. Before the reorganization of the War Department in March 1942,[54] all field medical units were trained under the supervision of General Headquarters. In the division of responsibility for medical units between the Ground and Service Forces that followed the reorganization,[55] the Ground Forces (successor to General Headquarters) inherited the responsibility for training all medical units used in combat zones and gained in addition the responsibility for preparing their tables of organization and equipment, recommending their inclusion in the troop basis, and activating such units.

Planning for the troop basis during most of 1942 was conducted in terms of standard or fixed organizations. Medical units that were organic elements of combat forces whose structure was fixed by tables of organization, such as infantry divisions, were automatically included in the troop basis along with their parent units. While the structure of combat forces larger than divisions was not governed by tables of organization, corps and armies normally had standard numbers of units of various sorts early in the war. For example, for emergency medical care and evacuation each corps generally had a medical battalion; each army, three medical regiments.[56] In the latter part of 1942 the Ground Surgeon proposed that each Army should have, in addition, a separate ambulance battalion to assist in the evacuation of casualties from divisional clearing stations.[57] Soon afterward, the standard army and corps were abandoned as yardsticks for determining the number of service units needed.[58] In addition, early in 1943, as mentioned above, nondivisional medical units organized under inflexible tables of organization, such as medical regiments, were replaced by flexible battalions and groups made up of variable combinations of separate ambulance, collecting, and clearing companies. While these changes did not affect the automatic inclusion in the troop basis of medical units that were organic elements of com-

[53] Johnson and Wilson, *op. cit.*, pp. 354–96, 407–35, 444–75, 534–66.

[54] See pp. 54–55.

[55] See above, pp. 58–59.

[56] (1) Greenfield *et al.*, *op. cit.*, pp. 276–80, 352–54. (2) Orgn of Major Units, incl to Ltr, TAG to CGs AGF, AAF, and SOS, 31 Mar 42, sub: Policies Governing T/Os and T/BAs. AG: 320.2 (3-13-42)(5).

[57] M/S, Ground Med Sec to [ACofS] G-4 [AGF], 10 Aug 42, sub: Revision of Type Army and Type Army Corps Trps—Med. HD: 322 AGF (Units, Med) 1942.

[58] Greenfield *et al.*, *op. cit.*, pp. 354–71.

bat forces still organized under tables of organization, they did require the establishment of a new basis for estimating the evacuation units that would be needed for service with corps and armies. Thereafter, this basis was a ratio of medical companies to divisions or to a certain number of troops. For example, it was considered that an army or task force needed a collecting company and a clearing company for each of its infantry divisions; and an ambulance company for every group of 12,000 soldiers.[59] On this basis the Ground Surgeon proposed in November 1943 that a troop basis having 105 combat divisions should include 105 collecting, 105 clearing, and 105 ambulance companies.[60] The troop bases subsequently approved did not follow this recommendation. For example, in April 1944, when planning was in terms of 89 divisions, the troop basis included 162 collecting, 104 clearing, and 75 ambulance companies.[61] The discrepancy between the ratio recommended by the Ground Surgeon and that in which separate medical companies were authorized can perhaps be explained by the fact that the troop basis was determined in the latter part of the war more by requests of theaters for units of specific types than by recommendations of staff officers in Washington.[62] In May 1945, just before the war in Europe ended, there were in the troop basis for the support of 89 divisions the following corps and army evacuation units: 137 collecting companies, 75 clearing companies, 96 ambulance companies, and headquarters detachments for 80 medical battalions and 16 medical groups. All but one of these units, an ambulance company, had already been deployed to theaters of operations.[63]

The activation and training of medical evacuation units were so closely intertwined with the activation and training of other Ground Forces units that any account of them would reflect generally a larger picture already described in considerable detail elsewhere.[64] Medical units that were organic elements of any of the combat arms or of any service other than medical were activated and trained along with their parent organizations. Corps and army medical units were activated according to a schedule based upon recommendations of the Ground Surgeon. During most of 1942 they were trained under the supervision of division commanders. In the latter part of that year and the early part of 1943, however, AGF headquarters established special local headquarters (Headquarters and Headquarters Detachments, Special Troops) to supervise the training of all nondivisional AGF-type service units, including those of the Medical Department. At least one of these headquarters had a Medical Corps officer on its staff. The Ground Surgeon exercised general supervision over the technical training of all Ground Forces medical units and, on the basis of inspections and reports, kept AGF headquarters

[59] (1) Ltr, CG AGF to CofSA, 11 Jul 43, sub: Change to T/O 8-27 and 8-28, with incls. AGF: 320.3. (2) T/O&E 8-27, C 1, and T/O&E 8-28, C 1, both dated 5 Aug 43. (3) FM 101-10, 12 Oct 44.

[60] M/S, Comment 2, Ground Med Sec to Plans [Div] AGF. 2 Nov 43, with 2 incls, Anal of 1944 Trp Basis and Summary of Trp Basis Study. Ground Med files: Chronological file, Folder 1.

[61] Troop Basis, Calendar Year 1944, 1 Apr 44 Revision. AG: Ref Collection.

[62] See above, pp. 219–22.

[63] The War Department Troop Basis, 1 May 45. AG: Ref Collection.

[64] Robert R. Palmer, Bell I. Wiley and William R. Keast, *The Procurement and Training of Ground Combat Troops* (Washington, 1948), pp. 426–560 in UNITED STATES ARMY IN WORLD WAR II.

informed as to the state of their readiness for shipment to theaters of operations.[65]

Details of the training of Medical Department units will be included in a volume on that subject planned for this series, but one aspect of their training needs to be considered here. Unlike station and general hospital units that were trained by the Army Service Forces, evacuation units trained by the Ground Forces were charged with actually providing medical service concurrently with their training in the zone of interior. To carry out this dual mission, they needed both personnel and equipment, but they suffered from a shortage of both. Lack of a sufficient number of Medical Corps officers in the Army Ground Forces prevented the assignment of full complements to units in training. Although the ratio of assigned to authorized Medical Corps officers varied from time to time and from unit to unit, it was often less than 50 percent.[66] Early in 1943 the shortage was so great that the Deputy Chief of Staff of the Army directed the Army Ground Forces to amend the tables of organization of medical units for which it was responsible by including in each a remark that medical and dental officers would be furnished "only as required and available within the continental limits of the U. S."[67] Early the next year the Ground Surgeon reported that with one exception—the 92d Division—it was possible to assign only one Medical Corps officer, instead of the seven authorized, to each infantry regiment participating in maneuvers in Louisiana.[68]

The shortage of equipment did not last as long as the shortage of personnel. It was most severe during 1942 and the early part of 1943.[69] At that time the Ground Surgeon reported that repeated requests of the Surgeon General's Office to issue fuller allowances of supplies and equipment always met with the same answer—that production was great enough to meet only the needs of units scheduled for early shipment to theaters of operations.[70] By the middle or latter part of 1943 the supply situation had improved and by the end of the year some units reported that they had on hand approximately all of their equipment.[71] Early in 1944 the Ground Surgeon reported that all medical units engaged in maneuvers in Louisiana had about 95 to 100 percent of their equipment with them.[72]

Despite shortages of equipment and personnel, evacuation units discharged their mission of furnishing medical service

[65] (1) Memo, Asst Ground Surg for [ACofS] G–4 [AGF], 15 Nov 42, sub: Activation Plan for Non-Div Med Units. (2) M/S, Ground Med Sec to [ACofS] G–3 [AGF], 30 Jan 43, sub: Rpt on Readiness of Type Med Units. Both in Ground Med files: Chronological file, Folder 1. (3) An Rpt, Surg Third Army, 1942. HD.

[66] For example, see An Rpts, Surgs Second and Third Armies, 1942, 67th Med Group, 1943, and 66th Med Group, 1944. HD.

[67] Memo, Dep CofSA for CG AGF, 10 Mar 43, sub: Availability of Physicians. Ground Med files: Chronological file, Folder 1. For an example of this remark see T/O&E 7–11, Inf Regt, 15 Jul 43.

[68] Memo, Ground Surg for ACofS G–4 AGF, 26 Feb 44, sub: Rpt of Insp, Louisiana Maneuver Area, 22–24 Feb 44. Ground Med files: Chronological file (Col W. E. Shambora).

[69] An Rpts, Surgs Second and Third Armies, 1942; Surg 4th Motorized Div, 1942; Surg 5th Inf Div, 1942; and 30th, 31st, and 65th Med Rgts, 1942. HD.

[70] M/S, Comment 7, Ground Med Sec to Ordnance [Sec, AGF], 23 Dec 42, sub: Equip for Certain Units, Third Army. Ground Med files: Chronological file, Folder 1.

[71] An Rpts, Surg Second Army, 1943; Surg 4th Inf Div, 1943; 31st, 67th, 69th, 341st, and 343d Med Groups, 1943. HD.

[72] Memo, Ground Surg for ACofS G–4 AGF, 26 Feb 44, sub: Rpt of Insp, Louisiana Maneuver Area, 22–24 Feb 44. Ground Med files: Chronological file (Col W. E. Shambora).

while still in training. While in garrison, Ground Forces medical units were not dependent upon the issuance of their own organizational equipment for use in medical service, because The Surgeon General had established a policy before the war—and it was continued—of supplying dispensary buildings erected in training areas of Army camps with medical supplies and equipment from station stocks.[73] Medical units of infantry divisions normally supplied personnel for the operation of six to seven of such dispensaries in their own divisional areas. Each dispensary generally served a particular segment of a division. For example, each regimental medical detachment operated a dispensary for all persons in the infantry regiment to which it belonged. The medical service rendered by dispensaries consisted of routine immunizations, blood-typing, monthly physical inspections, and daily sick calls. Soldiers found by medical examination at sick call to need hospital care were usually transported to station or regional hospitals in ambulances of divisional medical battalions. Ambulances and aid men also accompanied troops on long marches and on all training exercises of a dangerous nature, such as firing on ranges. In order to interfere with training formations as little as possible and to give as many men as possible experience in providing actual medical service, the personnel of divisional medical units often served in dispensaries on a rotational basis.[74] Nondivisional medical units, such as army medical regiments and groups, also operated dispensaries in garrison—sometimes for their own personnel only and sometimes for persons belonging to other units as well. In addition, units of these types were at times split up to supply medical service for troops in widely separate areas. For example, during 1943 a detail of twenty-five enlisted men and twelve ambulances of the 1st Medical Regiment gave ambulance service to various infantry units stationed in northern California, while various collecting and clearing units of the Regiment handled the medical service of troops in southern California, and a platoon of one of its clearing companies served an artillery training center at Yakima, Wash.[75]

On maneuvers Ground Forces medical units used organizational equipment which had been issued to them for training purposes or for later use in theaters of operations. It was the Ground Surgeon's opinion that such experience was invaluable and that no medical unit should be shipped to theaters of operations without having first become acquainted with its own equipment through use.[76] Divisional medical units operated in support of the divisions to which they belonged, setting up aid, collecting, and clearing stations, and evacuating and caring for both actual and simulated casualties.[77] Nondivisional units performed a variety of functions, in addition to caring for corps and army troops and evacuating casualties from divisional clearing stations. For example, during maneuvers in 1942 the 68th Med-

[73] The Annual Report, Surgeon First Army, 1941, spoke of the establishment of this policy. Its continuance was mentioned in the Annual Reports, Surgeons, Camp Hood (Texas) and Indiantown Gap Military Reservation (Pennsylvania), 1942.

[74] An Rpts, Surgs, 4th Motorized Div, and 65th, 69th, 79th, 86th, 98th, and 99th Inf Divs, 1943. HD.

[75] An Rpts, 1st and 31st Med Groups, 1943; 264th Med Bn, 1943; and 66th Med Group, 1944. HD.

[76] Interv, MD Historian with Col Shambora, 22 Apr 49. HD: 000.71.

[77] An Rpts, Surgs, 4th Motorized Div, and 65th, 69th, 79th, 86th, 98th, and 99th Inf Divs, 1943. HD.

ical Regiment operated the following installations: a convalescent hospital, a medical supply depot, clearing stations for depot and army troops, and an infirmary for corps troops. During maneuvers in 1943 the 134th Medical Regiment established aid and prophylactic stations in towns within the area of operations, maintained clearing stations for army troops, evacuated casualties from division and army clearing stations to evacuation hospitals and from the latter to named station hospitals, and provided personnel for the operation of a provisional medical supply depot.[78] Regardless of the missions assigned, Ground Forces medical units on maneuvers gained valuable practical experience and at the same time supplied medical service for the troops with which they operated.

[78] An Rpts, Surg Second Army, 1942; 1st, 31st, 67th, 69th, 134th, and 341st Med Groups, 1943. HD.

Summary and Conclusions

In concluding this volume with a brief review of the general subject it is pertinent to give first of all certain summary figures which indicate the Medical Department's total accomplishment in the field of hospitalization and evacuation during the war. In the period from January 1942 through August 1945, there were approximately 5,100,000 admissions to Army hospitals in theaters of operations and 8,900,000 to hospitals in the zone of interior.[1] In the same period, more than 518,500 patients were debarked by the Army at ports plus 121,400 by aircraft in the United States for transportation to zone of interior hospitals. *(Table 16)* Meanwhile, evacuation units that were organized and trained in the United States transported many thousands of patients from front-line areas to medical stations and hospitals in theaters of operations. The number of patients on the registers of hospitals in theaters reached a peak of almost 266,500 at the end of January 1945.[2] In a single month—May 1945—more than 57,000 patients were evacuated from theaters to the zone of interior. And by the end of June 1945 the number of patients on the rolls of Army hospitals in the United States rose to more than 318,000. *(Table 13)* The manner in which the Medical Department prepared for and discharged this unprecedented task of hospitalization and evacuation has been the subject of this volume. From the details already presented, certain generalizations can be made and certain conclusions drawn to emphasize some of the problems involved in the accomplishment of this mission.

Like the rest of the Army and the War Department, the Surgeon General's Office and the Medical Department were in the midst of preparations and therefore not ready for a global war when it overtook them in December 1941. The partial mobilization that began with the passage of the Selective Training and Service Act in the fall of 1940 had caused only a partial adjustment from peacetime to what might be expected in wartime. Tables of organization, tables of equipment, and equipment lists of medical units had been revised, but more with considerations of desirability than possibility in mind. Data on hospitalization and evacuation in World War I had been analyzed and were available as a basis for estimating requirements. They had already been used in the establishment of an authorized ratio of beds to troops for hospitals in the United States, but whether or not World War I experience would be applicable to World War II remained to be seen. Hospitalization and evacuation units had been organized and were being trained, but they were few in number. Also, there was uncertainty as to the role of these particular units—whether they would remain in the

[1] These figures are "preliminary pending publication of final tabulations based on the individual medical records." Memo, Eugene L. Hamilton, Chief Med Statistics Div SGO for Clarence Smith, Historical Unit AMS, 3 Mar 53, sub: Hosp Admissions during World War II. HD: 705.

[2] *Statistical Review, World War II*, App R, p. 237.

United States as training units or be sent overseas as functional units. Plans had been made to call others into active service in the event of war, that is, reserve hospital units affiliated with civilian schools and hospitals. With regard to hospital service in the United States and its territories, experience in expanding hospital facilities had shown the undesirability of depending upon existing buildings and had revealed many unsatisfactory features in plans for cantonment-type hospitals. Blueprints were drawn, therefore, for hospitals of a new type, to be of two-story semipermanent construction. An improved general-service ambulance had been developed and put into use; but plans for motor vehicles of other types, such as multipatient ambulances, were still in the experimental stage. Two unit and four ward cars for hospital trains had been delivered, but they had not yet been used in the actual transportation of patients. Although the ships' hospitals of some transports had been enlarged and improved, it was uncertain whether the Army or Navy would operate transports, and therefore evacuate patients from overseas areas during wartime. Moreover, basic decisions as to whether hospital ships would be authorized or not, and as to whether the Army or the Navy would operate them, remained to be made. Evacuation from theaters and transportation of patients from ports to general hospitals in the United States proceeded according to peacetime procedures, with little indication of changes that would be required for a wartime load. Plans for air evacuation were in the hopeful more than the practical stage. And plans for the internal administration of hospitals and the global operation of a system of hospitalization and evacuation were in terms of expanding peacetime procedures rather than of substituting new procedures designed for the task that lay ahead. Finally, a shortage of medical supplies and equipment plagued medical officers from the highest to the lowest levels of command.

Reasons for the unpreparedness of the Medical Department for war—or at least some of them—are reasonably clear. Planning of the Army for many years had been in terms of defending the United States against sudden attack, and even during the period of peacetime mobilization there was uncertainty as to whether United States troops would be employed overseas. Furthermore, appropriations for preparedness were meager, and there was hesitancy even on the part of the President to appear aggressive in planning for a possible war. Finally, the Surgeon General's Office—and perhaps the entire Medical Department—found it difficult, apparently, to break peacetime habits of thought and action and to plan imaginatively for the accomplishment of its mission during a possible future war.

For the Medical Department, as for the rest of the Army, the first year and a half of the war was a time of meeting emergency needs and completing mobilization, while at the same time preparing for full scale war. Needs of the moment received first consideration. As they were met, emphasis gradually shifted to evaluating experience as it accumulated and to planning more effectively for the future. Despite many difficulties, sufficient hospitals were constructed and placed in operation to meet the Army's requirements during its rapid growth and training in the United States. The necessity of speed and economy, however, dictated abandonment of new plans for hospitals of semipermanent construction and the erection of cantonment-type hospitals on unsatisfactory existing plans, with attendant alterations, additions, and repairs. Eventually, availability of materials and general dissatisfaction with the hospitals under construction resulted in the erection of buildings of a third type—one-story buildings of brick or tile—considered by the Surgeon General's Office to be the best for emergency construction. Toward the completion of the construction program, efforts were made to co-ordinate plans of the Army for hospital construction with those of other agencies and with postwar needs. Concurrently with the establishment of additional hospitals in the United States, hospitalization and evacuation units were sent overseas, and others were organized and placed in training for later service. Contrary to earlier plans, standard Army hospital units rather than affiliated reserve units constituted the primary means of meeting the first needs for hospitals overseas. Some of the latter—as well as nonaffiliated hospital units—remained in training in this country for long periods after their activation, and the question arose of whether or not they might be used—as evacuation units were—to provide medical service concurrently with and as a part of their training in the United States. The Surgeon General withstood the demands of higher headquarters to plan toward that end, and the problem of making effective use of numbered hospital units in the United States remained unsolved. By the spring of 1943, after the most urgent needs of theaters had been met, measures were taken to evaluate their existing facilities for hospitalization and evacuation and to plan more effectively to meet their future needs.

The early part of the war was also a time of establishing basic policies and procedures that were to endure throughout the conflict. An early decision of importance was that the Army would operate transports and evacuate patients aboard them. A corollary decision toward the middle of 1943 was that the Army would also operate hospital ships to supplement the space available for evacuation on transports. Procedures that required only minor adjustments later in the war were established to co-ordinate the activities of theaters, ships' surgeons, ports of embarkation, and corps areas (later called service commands) in the evacuation of patients from theaters to hospitals in the zone of interior. In addition, a procedure for evacuating patients from theaters in regularly scheduled transport airplanes was also established, but it was policy during this period to keep air evacuation to a minimum. Despite the wishes of The Surgeon General and the Air Surgeon, AAF headquarters ruled that airplanes would not normally be set aside or built for evacuation only. Hopeful plans for forward-area air evacuation were thereby shelved. Procedures were also developed—albeit directives announcing them were unclear and in some instances contradictory—for the movement of patients by hospital train in the United States. While hospitals and the hospital system in the zone of interior continued for the most part to operate under peacetime procedures, the designation of general hospitals as centers for specialized treatment and the establishment of a policy of hospitalizing patients near their homes occurred early in 1943. These actions came too late to influence the location of general hospitals, and had not had time by the middle of 1943 to affect appreciably procedures for evacuation in the zone of interior. The desirability of shortening the length of time patients stayed in hospitals was recognized and efforts toward that end were begun. They pertained primarily to procedures in administrative channels outside Army hospitals. Finally, attempts of the Air Surgeon to set up separate convalescent facilities for Air Forces patients, along with an awareness by the Surgeon General's Office and other Medical Department officers of the desirability of convalescent-reconditioning programs, caused the establishment early in 1943 of convalescent centers and annexes—the forerunners of convalescent hospitals of later years.

The early period of the war also afforded an opportunity to review plans already made and to adjust them to the new situation. The mobility of war on land masses and the character of operations in island areas highlighted the necessity of modifying existing hospitalization and evacuation units. In some instances, new units were developed. In others, theaters were left to adapt existing units to new uses. Several conditions—shortages of personnel and shipping space, and the nature of combat operations—combined to initiate a trend that was to be carried to greater lengths later—the reduction of personnel and equipment authorized for units and installations of all types and sizes. In this connection, certain other practices began: the substitution of Medical Administrative for Medical Corps officers in administrative positions in theater of operations units and in zone of interior installations, and the replacement of general service men with limited service men, civilians, and enlisted women in hospitals in the United States. Experience with unit cars for hospital trains revealed their impracticability, and the Surgeon General's Office substituted for them a new type of car, called a ward dressing car. The Office successfully opposed a proposal to develop at this time a fourth type of car—one that would include not only a dressing room and berths for patients but also a small kitchen. The Surgeon General's recommendation for the development of a forward-area ambulance was disapproved by higher authority, but the general-service ambulance was modified to facilitate its shipment to and use in theaters of operations. Experiments with multipatient ambulances were unsuccessful, but other vehicles—such as surgical trucks—were developed for use in the evacuation system in theaters.

The task of providing hospitalization and evacuation in the first year of the war was complicated by the fact that it had to be accomplished while a major reorganization in the War Department was taking place. The creation of three major commands — Ground, Air, and Service Forces—required delineations of responsibility for hospitalization and evacuation, and raised questions concerning the extent of The Surgeon General's authority. Responsibility for units to be used in theaters of operations was readily divided between The Surgeon General and the Ground Surgeon, but the Air Surgeon's responsibility and authority, and his relationship with The Surgeon General, were not sufficiently delineated to prevent recurring instances of friction between them; particularly when the Air Surgeon attempted to set up a completely separate hospital system for the Air Forces. The establishment within ASF headquarters of a group concerned with hospitalization and evacuation and headed by a Medical Corps officer had a variety of effects. This group assumed the lead in planning and in coordinating the activities of the many agencies involved in evacuation operations, with the full concurrence, apparently, of the Surgeon General's Office. When it entered the field of hospital operations it encountered opposition. Whether the good it accomplished in this field counterbalanced the ill-feeling and friction which it engendered is difficult to determine accurately even now. Progress had been made by the middle of 1943 in composing differences and solving problems arising from the reorganization, but further adjustments in relations and authority remained to be made in the latter part of the war.

The last two years of the war were characterized by the necessity of providing hospitalization and evacuation for an all-out war with more limited resources than had been anticipated. The problem of estimating requirements therefore demanded continual and increasing attention. By the latter half of 1943 it began to be evident that estimates based on World War I statistical data were too high for World War II. In the fall of 1943, when evacuation policies were established and bed ratios were authorized for theaters for the first time, there occurred the first attempt to use World War II experience as a source of data for estimating requirements. Soon afterward the Surgeon General's Office completed an estimate of the patient load for 1944 for use in planning evacuation from theaters and in determining hospitalization for both theaters and the zone of interior. Facilities provided on the basis of this estimate seemed excessive during 1944 and, as the personnel situation became more restrictive, various agencies of the War Department urged retrenchment. Reductions followed in the ratio of beds (to troops) authorized for station hospitals in the United States and for fixed hospitals in most theaters of operations. Early in 1945, when requirements increased, general and convalescent hospitals in the United States had to be expanded rapidly, more hospital train cars had to be procured, and additional hospital ships had to be rushed to completion. Experience in estimating requirements during 1944 and 1945 pointed up the importance of collecting casualty and disease data early in the war for planning purposes. It also highlighted the necessity and difficulty of correlating far in advance estimates of requirements with estimates of the time when they would occur. Furthermore, it emphasized the importance of co-ordinating plans for hospitalization in theaters with plans for evacuation and for hospitalization in the zone of interior in order to avoid duplication and the uneconomical use of limited resources.

Limited resources affected hospitalization and evacuation in more ways than in demanding repeated estimates of requirements. Shortages of personnel led to widespread application in the latter half of the war of practices already begun on a small scale. Further reductions occurred in the relative amounts of personnel authorized for hospitalization and evacuation units as well as for named hospitals in the United States. Medical Administrative Corps officers were used more extensively to replace Medical Corps officers in administrative and semiprofessional positions; and limited service enlisted men, civilians, and enlisted women replaced the major portion of able-bodied enlisted men in zone of interior installations. The extent to which reductions and substitutions of personnel were made supports the belief that hospitalization and evacuation organizations were overgenerous in their use of personnel at the beginning of the war. It also suggests that the Medical Department might have avoided many difficulties in adjusting to changes eventually required by circumstances and higher authorities if it had been more realistic in the first place, reducing amounts of personnel authorized for various units and installations to that actually required and using from the start greater proportions of Medical Administrative Corps officers, limited service enlisted men, civilians, and enlisted women. Personnel shortages also required the adoption of new practices in the latter half of the war, such as the use of provisional platoons to care for patients on transports, the employment of enemy protected-personnel in the medical service of theaters and the zone of interior, and the substitution of small units that could be used in flexible combinations for larger rigid table-of-organization units, such as regiments and battalions, in combat areas.

Restrictions on new construction in the latter part of the war led to the practice of expanding existing hospitals by using medical-detachment barracks for hospital patients, theater-of-operations-type barracks for detachments, and post barracks for convalescent patients. While several station hospital plants were converted into general hospitals, earlier plans and proposals to meet in the same manner a growing need for general hospital beds in the latter part of the war proved impractical because of a shortage of specialists to man additional general hospitals. Toward the end of the war, the removal of restrictions on the use of certain materials formerly in short supply permitted a program of hospital improvement to correct some of the deficiencies in cantonment-type buildings erected earlier. Although hospital construction was curtailed about the middle of 1943, the major portion of the program of constructing hospital cars and ships occurred after that time—primarily because the need for them was either not fully comprehended or not recognized in the form of authorizations earlier. Demands from theaters in the Pacific in the latter part of the war focused attention upon the need for prefabricated hospital buildings for use in overseas areas. The war ended before this need could be satisfactorily met.

Important changes were made in the zone of interior hospital system in the latter part of the war—partly because of limitations upon available resources but also for other reasons, such as competition between the Air Surgeon and The Surgeon General for the control of segments of hospitalization, the desirability of providing a helpful psychological atmosphere for convalescent patients, and the emergence of new needs. The existing program of specialization in general hospitals was extended to promote the effective use of scarce specialists. The development of regional hospitals represented an attempt to eliminate duplication inherent in the operation of dual sets of hospitals (Air and Service Forces) by providing hospitalization on a regional or geographic instead of a command basis. The establishment of convalescent hospitals not only provided a better psychological environment for convalescent patients but also permitted their care in less expensive facilities than general hospitals. The operation of specific general hospitals solely for prisoner-of-war patients reduced administrative and security problems and contributed eventually to personnel economy. Although there were no significant changes in the system of hospitalization and evacuation in overseas areas, efforts were made to provide theaters with additional types of units, such as medical holding battalions, mobile army surgical hospitals, and convalescent camps, in order to meet existing and emerging needs effectively. Changes did occur in the system of evacuation from theaters to the United States. Aside from improvements in procedures already established, the most important modification was the creation of a Medical Regulating Unit in Washington to centralize control over the use of hospital beds and over the flow of patients and to co-ordinate the movement of patients by sea, rail, and air. This step reflected a growing use of hospital ships, airplanes, and government-owned hospital cars in the evacuation process, contributed to stricter observance of the policies of caring for patients in specialized centers and in hospitals near their homes, and revealed the desirability of locating general and convalescent hospitals in relation to population density rather than troop concentrations.

In connection with changes in the hospitalization and evacuation system came changes in the internal organization and procedures of zone of interior hospitals. They occurred near the end of the war and came largely as a result of emphasis by ASF headquarters on the achievement of efficiency and economy through management engineering. Attempts to standardize hospital organization—a prerequisite to the simplification of administrative procedures—amounted to conformance with the standard organization of ASF posts more than improvements and innovations in hospital organization as such. The introduction of management engineering led to work-load studies, work-simplification measures, and the streamlining of certain administrative procedures, especially those affecting the length of time patients remained in hospitals and, consequently, the number of beds required. Another factor affecting bed requirements—the performance of adequate diagnostic procedures to permit the admission to hospitals of only those patients needing hospital care—was not touched, and the work of dispensaries in this respect remained "one of the weakest links in the whole medical program." [3]

Growth of the patient load in the later war years, coupled with changing policies, procedures, and circumstances, led to the development of new transportation facilities for evacuation. Despite its earlier objection to a proposal for a hospital car with a dressing room, berths for patients, and a small kitchen, the Surgeon General's Office adopted the idea when its necessity became obvious. That Office also promoted the procurement of kitchen cars for hospital trains when it became apparent that railroad companies would be unable to supply the Army with sufficient dining cars. To assist in the movement of patients from ports to near-by hospitals, The Surgeon General proposed, and higher authority approved, the development of a multipatient ambulance. A front-line ambulance was developed experimentally, but it was not authorized for procurement because ASF headquarters and the War Department General Staff insisted upon the use of standard Army vehicles only. Toward the end of the war litter racks that could be attached to jeeps to enable them to evacuate patients from forward areas were standardized for issuance to evacuation units. While airplane ambulances were never authorized or developed, improvements in litter supports permitted increases in the capacities of transport planes for evacuation. Eventually, an increase in the availability of planes led to a modification of existing policy and the as-

[3] Comment by Dr. Eli Ginzberg, formerly Dir, Resources Anal Div SGO, incl to Ltr to Col Calvin H. Goddard, 5 Nov 51. HD: 314 (Correspondence on MS) V.

signment to several commands of planes for use primarily in the movement of patients.

Further adjustments to the new organization of the War Department occurred in the latter half of the war. The Surgeon General expanded and strengthened his Office, particularly the divisions concerned most immediately with hospitalization and evacuation. Concurrently, ASF headquarters abolished its Hospitalization and Evacuation Branch and transferred many of its functions and some of its personnel to the enlarged and strengthened Surgeon General's Office. Eventually, The Surgeon General was restored to his former position of having direct contact with the War Department General Staff. Meanwhile, though still under ASF headquarters, his Office developed means of exercising closer supervision over service command hospital activities, and limits of the respective jurisdictions of the Air Surgeon and The Surgeon General gradually evolved. The Surgeon General was never in a position, though, to exercise a controlling influence over the entire hospitalization and evacuation system of the Army. Perhaps an important reason for this was that, as a result of the dual position he held, he seemed at times to be bidding against himself. As The Surgeon General of the entire Army, he was responsible—to some extent, at least—for apportioning medical resources among major commands (Air, Ground, and Service Forces) and between the zone of interior and theaters of operations. On the other hand, as surgeon on the staff of the commanding general, Army Service Forces, he was responsible for providing as good a medical service in the zone of interior as possible. This required him to act in a disinterested manner on matters involving him as an interested party. Nevertheless, despite difficulties caused by its organizational structure, the War Department and its agencies, including the Surgeon General's Office, managed successfully with limited resources to provide adequate hospitalization and evacuation for an Army of over 8,000,000 men engaged in a global war.

List of Abbreviations

AAF	Army Air Forces
AAR	Association of American Railroads
AC	Air Corps
ACofS	Assistant Chief of Staff
Act	Acting
Add	Additional, addition
Admin	Administration, administrative, administrator
AFPAC	U. S. Army Forces, Pacific
AG	The Adjutant General, Files of
AGF	Army Ground Forces; Army Ground Forces, Files of
AGO	Adjutant General's Office
AGWAR	Adjutant General, War Department
Almt	Allotment
Amb	Ambulance
AML	Army Medical Library
An	Annual
Anal	Analysis
AR	Army Regulations
ASF	Army Service Forces
Asgmt	Assignment
ASO	Air Surgeon's Office
ATC	Air Transport Command; Air Transport Command, Files of
ATS	Army Transport Service
Auth	Authority, authorized, authorization
AWC	Army War College, Files of
Bd	Board
Bn	Battalion
BPE	Boston Port of Embarkation
Br	Branch
C	Chief
CA	Corps area
CASU	Corps Area Service Unit
CBI	China-Burma-India
CCS	Combined Chiefs of Staff
CDD	Certificate of disability for discharge
CE	Chief of Engineers, Files of; Corps of Engineers

CG	Commanding General
CinC	Commander in Chief
Cir	Circular
Civ	Civilian
CMTC	Combined Military Transportation Committee
Cmtee	Committee
CO	Commanding Officer
Co	Company
CofAC	Chief of the Air Corps
CofEngrs	Chief of Engineers
CofF	Chief of Finance
CofOrd	Chief of Ordnance
CofSA	Chief of Staff, U. S. Army
CofT	Chief of Transportation
Comd	Command
ComZ	Communications zone
Conf	Conference
Cons	Construction, constructing, consultant
Conv	Convalescent, conversation, conversion
Co-ord	Co-ordination
CPA	Central Pacific Area
CPE	Charleston Port of Embarkation
DAF	Department of the Air Force
Def	Defense
Dep	Deputy
Det	Detachment
Dev	Development
DF	Disposition form
Dir	Directorate, director
Distr	Distribution
Div	Division
Dom	Domestic
D/S	Disposition slip
EM	Enlisted men
Engr	Engineer, engineering
Equip	Equipment
Est	Estimate
Estab	Establish, establishment
ETOUSA	European Theater of Operations, U. S. Army
Evac	Evacuation, evacuating
Fac	Facility, facilities
Fld	Field
FM	Field manual

FY	Fiscal year
Gen	General
GHQ	General Headquarters
GO	General Order
HD	Historical Unit, Army Medical Service, Walter Reed Army Medical Center (formerly Historical Division, Office of The Surgeon General)
Hist	History
Hosp	Hospital, hospitalization
Hq	Headquarters
HRPE	Hampton Roads Port of Embarkation
HRS	Historical Records Section, Departmental Records Branch, Adjutant General's Office
IAS	Informal action sheet
IG	The Inspector General; The Inspector General, Files of
Incl	Inclosure, inclosed
Ind	Indorsement
Indiv	Individual
Info	Information
Init	Initialed
Insp	Inspection
Instl	Installation
Interv	Interview
JAG	The Judge Advocate General
JCS	Joint Chiefs of Staff
JMTC	Joint Military Transportation Committee
JPS	Joint Staff Planners
Lab	Laboratory
LAPE	Los Angeles Port of Embarkation
Ltr	Letter
MAC	Medical Administrative Corps
Mar Comm	Maritime Commission
Mat	Material, Matériel
MC	Medical Corps
MD	Medical Department
MFSS	Medical Field Service School
MHSP	Medical hospital ship platoon
Mil	Military
Min	Minute
Misc	Miscellaneous
Mob	Mobilization
MOOB	Mobilization and Overseas Operations Branch, Office of The Surgeon General

MOOD	Mobilization and Overseas Operations Division, Office of The Surgeon General
MPD	Military Personnel Division
MR	Mobilization Regulations
MRO	Medical Regulating Officer
MRS	Memo routing slip
MRU	Medical Regulating Unit
M/S	Memorandum sheet or slip
MSO	Medical Supply Officer
MTOUSA	Mediterranean Theater of Operations, U. S. Army
Mvmt	Movement
NATOUSA	North African Theater of Operations, U. S. Army
n d	No date
NOPE	New Orleans Port of Embarkation
NP	Neuropsychiatric, neuropsychiatry
NYPE	New York Port of Embarkation
OCE	Office, Chief of Engineers
OCofAC	Office, Chief of the Air Corps
OCS	Office, Chief of Staff, U. S. Army
OCT	Office of the Chief of Transportation
Off	Office, officer
OO	Office Order
OPD	Operations Division, War Department General Staff
OPMG	Office of The Provost Marshal General
Opr	Operation
Ord	Ordnance; Chief of Ordnance, Files of
Orgn	Organization
OSW	Office, Secretary of War, Files of
PE	Port of embarkation
Pers	Personnel, personal
Plat	Platoon
PMG	The Provost Marshal General
PMP	Protective Mobilization Plan
Pnt	Patient
POA	Pacific Ocean Area
Procmt	Procurement
Prov	Provisional, provision
Ptbl	Portable
PW	Prisoner of war
QMG	The Quartermaster General
Rad	Radiogram
Recomd	Recommendation
Reg	Regulation, regulating

Regt	Regiment
Repl	Replacement
Req	Required
Reqmt	Requirement
Res	Reservation, resolution, reserve
Rev	Revision
Rpt	Report
R&R Sheet	Routing and record sheet
RR	Railroad
Ry	Railway
SCSU	Service Command Service Unit
SecWar	Secretary of War
Sep	Separate
Serv	Service
SFPE	San Francisco Port of Embarkation
SG	The Surgeon General; The Surgeon General, Files of
SGO	Surgeon General's Office
SHAEF	Supreme Headquarters, Allied Expeditionary Forces
SOS	Services of Supply
SPA	South Pacific Area
SPE	Seattle Port of Embarkation
S/S	Summary sheet
Sta	Station
Str	Strength
Sup	Supply
Supp	Supplement
Surg	Surgeon, surgical
Surv	Survey
SvC	Service command
SWPA	Southwest Pacific Area
Syst	System
TAG	The Adjutant General
TAS	The Air Surgeon's Historical Division, Files of
T/BA	Table of basic allowances
TC	Transportation Corps; Chief of Transportation, Files of
T/E	Table of equipment
Tec	Technical
Tel	Telephone
Temp	Temporary
Tfc	Traffic
TM	Technical manual
Tn	Train
Tng	Training

T/O	Table of organization; theater of operations
T/O&E	Table of organization and equipment
TofOpns	Theater of Operations
Trans	Transportation; transports
Trf	Transfer
Trp	Troop
T/S	Transmittal sheet
USAF	United States Air Forces
USAFBI	U. S. Army Forces in the British Isles
USASOS	U. S. Army, Services of Supply
USFET	U. S. Forces, European Theater
Util	Utilization, utilities
Veh	Vehicle
WAAC	Women's Army Auxiliary Corps
WAC	Women's Army Corps
WD	War Department
WDCSA	Office, Chief of Staff, U. S. Army, Files of
WDGS	War Department General Staff
WDMB	War Department Manpower Board
WPB	War Production Board
WRGH	Walter Reed General Hospital
ZI	Zone of interior

Bibliographical Note

Primary Sources

The most important collections of source material for this volume were the central files of the Surgeon General's Office and the files of the Historical Unit, Army Medical Service, Walter Reed Army Medical Center. The central files of the Surgeon General's Office for the war period have been retired and are now in the custody of The Adjutant General. They contain official correspondence, memoranda, and reports originating in the Surgeon General's Office, as well as numerous documents received by this Office from other sources, both military and civilian. These files, like those of most Army agencies, are arranged by subject under a numerical or decimal system. For example, documents on the construction of hospitals are filed under 632; of cars for hospital trains, under 531.4; and of hospital ships, under 560. To include here all of the numerical classifications of documents used in the preparation of this volume, or even those used most often, is both undesirable and unnecessary because the list would be too long and would duplicate information readily available in footnotes throughout the volume.

The files of the Historical Unit are extensive, having been built up by the Historical Division, Office of The Surgeon General (predecessor of the Historical Unit) during the war years. Of particular importance in the Historical Unit files are the annual reports submitted during the war by The Surgeon General, divisions of the Surgeon General's Office handling hospitalization and evacuation matters, surgeons of large commands, and commanding officers of hospitalization and evacuation units and installations that ranged from 3,000-bed hospitals to separate ambulance companies. Although these annual reports obviously must be used with caution, because surgeons and commanders in some instances undoubtedly attempted to present the most favorable view possible of their activities, they contain a wealth of information not otherwise available. In addition, many of them contain excellent discussions of Medical Department shortcomings, because they afforded surgeons and commanders an opportunity to complain about matters over which they were disturbed but had no control. The absence of complete sets of annual reports of the Air and Ground Surgeons for the war years is regrettable. The Historical Unit also has custody of wartime working files of several divisions of the Surgeon General's Office. The most important among them for this volume were those of the Mobilization and Overseas Operations Division, the Medical Regulating Unit, and the Resources Analysis Division. To supplement these papers, the Unit periodically borrowed wartime documents from current office files of the Medical Facilities Planning Branch (formerly Hospital Construction Branch), Medical Statistics Division, Resources Analysis Division, Supply Division, and Medical Research and Development Board of the Surgeon General's Office. The Historical

Unit also has a large decimal file; most of the papers in it, however, are carbon copies of those in The Surgeon General's central files. Supplementing these files and sometimes serving as a clue to the location of other important documents are the diaries of divisions of the Surgeon General's Office covering the period from the fall of 1943 to the end of the war. In addition, the Historical Unit has a copy of the testimony and report of the Committee to Study the Medical Department (1942) and a compilation of recommendations of the Committee and actions on them by the Surgeon General's Office. Portions of these documents were extremely useful for information on relations between the Surgeon General's Office and the SOS Hospitalization and Evacuation Branch and on developments in hospitalization and evacuation up to the end of 1942. Also of interest for this volume, the Historical Unit has microfilm of The Adjutant General's unit cards (large cards giving in abbreviated form the chronology and history of individual military units) of Medical Department organizations, including hospitalization and evacuation units. (The original cards are filed in the Organization and Directory Section, Operations Branch, Administrative Services Division, Adjutant General's Office.) Other documents and materials belonging at present to the Historical Unit were used in this study, but it is unnecessary to mention them specifically.

When this volume was written, the Historical Unit had in its custody, on indefinite loan, three blocks of files of considerable significance. The Wilson files—so called because they were built up and used by Col. William L. Wilson, M. C.—were on loan from the Historical Records Section, Departmental Records Branch, Adjutant General's Office. Covering a period from May 1941, when Colonel Wilson was in G–4, until June 1943, shortly after he left ASF headquarters, these files are actually unofficial records of the ASF Hospitalization and Evacuation Branch. They contain a full set of staybacks, a diary, a decimal file, a subject file, and a file of operational plans submitted by medical installations in the United States. The Ground Medical Section files, containing papers from the Ground Surgeon's Office, were on loan from Headquarters, Army Field Forces, Fort Monroe, Va. Important but not as extensive as would be desired, these files contain several sets of staybacks and many annual reports of Army Ground Forces medical units. On loan from the Air Forces, but recently returned to the Historical Division, Office of The Surgeon General, Department of the Air Forces, were files of the Air Surgeon's Historical Division. In addition to annual reports and wartime histories of many AAF medical installations and commands, these files contain several folders of the Air Surgeon's correspondence, including interoffice memos, on hospitalization and evacuation.

Next in importance to the files of the Surgeon General's Office and the Historical Unit for this study were certain files of ASF headquarters and the War Department General Staff, which are in the custody of the Historical Records Section, Departmental Records Branch, Adjutant General's Office. The most useful ASF files were those of the Control and Planning Divisions, and the folders dealing with Medical Department activities that were kept and used during the war by Generals Somervell, Styer, and Lutes. Of the General Staff files, those of G–4 were naturally most rewarding, but those of G–1, G–3, and OPD were also consulted with success in many instances. Conclusive information, particularly about controversies or disputes that reached high levels of authority for decision or solution, could be found often only in the files of the Chief of Staff, U. S. Army, the Assistant Secretary of War for Air, and the Secretary of War. Other files in the custody of The Adjutant General which it was frequently necessary to use were those of the technical services that assisted the Medical Department in its hospitalization and evacuation operations; among them were the Quartermaster Corps, the Corps of Engineers, and the Transportation Corps. While the wartime files of AAF and AGF headquarters were available and useful, it was particularly disturbing to be unable to find among them anything resembling central files of the offices of the Air and Ground Surgeons. Finally, and certainly not of least importance, were the files maintained by The Adjutant General during the war. Because his Office was the War Department's office of record, all official communications to and from the General Staff found their way into the AG files.

Printed primary sources were also used in the preparation of this volume, but because of the wide circulation they enjoyed it is unnecessary to indicate the depositories in which they are located. Obviously Army regulations, War Department circulars, field manuals, technical manuals, tables of organization and equipment, and the like, are basic sources for any military history. Of interest because they helped the writer fit the history of hospitalization and evacuation into a larger picture are the biennial reports of the Chief of Staff of the Army and the annual reports of the Secretary of War. Although no systematic search was made of Congressional committee reports, a few were used when they appeared to have a direct bearing on the subject under consideration.

As noted at greater length in the preface, the writer also derived much information from interviews and correspondence with persons active in Medical Department affairs during the war.

Secondary Sources

While there are no published monographs or special studies on Army hospitalization and evacuation during World War II, there are a number of unpublished preliminary histories and historical monographs on Medical Department activities that have been helpful to the writer of this volume. Among them are a group of studies prepared by the Historical Division, Office of The Surgeon General, immediately after the end of the war. They are the following: [Samuel M. Goodman], A Summary of the Training of Army Service Forces Medical Department Personnel, 1 July 1939–31 December 1944; Harold P. James, Transportation of the Sick and Wounded; John B. Johnson, Jr., and Graves H. Wilson, A History of Wartime Research and Development of Medical Field Equipment; Richard L. Laughlin, [History of] Reconditioning [in the U. S. Army in World War II]; Edward J. Morgan and Donald O. Wagner, The Organization of the Medical Department in the Zone of the Interior; and Richard E. Yates, The Procurement and Distribution of Medical Supplies in the Zone of Interior during World War II. Two unpublished histories prepared by Florence A. Blanchfield and Mary W. Standlee, Organized Nursing in the Army in Three Wars (1950) and The Army Nurse Corps in World War II (1950), supplied background information for the discussion of the "shortage" of nurses in zone of interior hospitals. Hubert A. Coleman, Organization and Administration, AAF Medical Services in the Zone of Interior (1948), was particularly helpful in the preparation of sections on AAF hospitalization and evacuation. Parts of this work are essentially copies of histories or reports submitted by AAF medical installations to the Air Surgeon's Office and like all such documents must be used with care. The chapters actually prepared by Coleman and his assistants are scholarly and reliable. The Historical Unit has copies of all of the works named above. Two of my colleagues, Blanche B. Armfield and John H. McMinn, deserve special mention because they not only made available drafts of chapters of volumes which they are preparing on Medical Department organization and personnel, respectively, but they also gave the author full benefit of their knowledge both through frequent discussions and through criticisms of his manuscript.

A variety of other unpublished histories were consulted, often with unexpectedly good results. Wartime histories of the Planning and Control Divisions of ASF headquarters supplied information that undoubtedly existed in documents which could not be located in ASF files. Histories of Medical Department activities of the Air Transport Command, its Ferrying Division, I Troop Carrier Command, and the Fourth Air Force were used to supplement information found in the files of AAF headquarters. Wartime histories of Medical Department activities in overseas commands, on file in the Historical Unit, supplied information that occasionally threw light upon some aspects of zone of interior hospitalization and evacuation.

Another group of documents which the author used, but with caution, needs to be mentioned. While some purport to be histories, all of them are in fact final reports of the offices concerned. On file in the Historical Unit, they are as follows: Margaret D. Craighill, History of Women's Medical Unit [Office of The Surgeon General]; History of Medical Liaison Office to the OCT and Medical Regulating Service, Office of The Surgeon General; History, Office of the Surgeon, Second Corps Area and Second Service Command, from 9 September 1940 to 2 September 1945; Historical Record, Laundry Section, Hospital Division, [Office of The Surgeon General]; History of the Organization and Equipment Allowance Branch, [Office of The Surgeon General]; Rene M. Juchli, Record of Events in the Treatment of Prisoners of War, World War II; and Achilles L. Tynes, Data for Preparation of Historical Record of Construction Branch of the Surgeon General's Office during the Expansion Period of the Army and World War II.

Published histories, or those well along in the publication process, used in the preparation of this volume need only to be listed. Among them are several volumes (including three in manuscript form) of the UNITED STATES ARMY IN WORLD WAR II: Ray S. Cline, *Washington Command Post: The Operations Division* (Washington, 1951); Stetson Conn and Byron Fairchild, Defense of the Americas, Vol. I (MS.); Kent R. Greenfield, Robert R. Palmer and Bell I. Wiley, *The Organization of Ground Combat Troops* (Washington, 1947); Ulysses Lee, The Employment of Negro Troops (MS.); Maurice Matloff and Edwin M. Snell, *Strategic Planning for Coalition Warfare, 1941–42* (Washington, 1953); John D. Millett, *The Organization and Role of the Army Service Forces* (Washington, 1954); Robert R. Palmer, Bell I. Wiley and William R. Keast, *The Procurement and Training of Ground Combat Troops* (Washington, 1948); Jesse A. Remington and Lenore Fine, The Corps of Engineers: Construction in the United States (MS.); Erna Risch, *The Quartermaster Corps: Organization, Supply and Services,* Vol. I (Washington, 1953); Mattie E. Treadwell, *The Women's Army Corps* (Washington, 1954); Chester Wardlow, *The Transportation Corps: Responsibilities, Organization, and Operations* (Washington, 1951); and Mark S. Watson, *Chief of Staff: Prewar Plans and Preparations* (Washington, 1950). Use was also made of Wesley F. Craven and James L. Cate (eds.), *The Army Air Forces in World War II* (Chicago, 1948 and ff). Other published histories consulted were: Percy M. Ashburn, *A History of the Medical Department of the United States Army* (Boston, 1929); Roland W. Charles, *Troopships of World War II* (Washington, 1947); Engineer, Office of the Chief, General Headquarters Army Forces, Pacific, *Engineers in Theater Operations* in ENGINEERS OF THE SOUTHWEST PACIFIC, 1941–45, Vol. I. (1947); *Logistical History of NATOUSA-MTOUSA* (Naples, Italy, 1945); *The Medical Department of the United States Army in the World War,* Vol. I (Washington, 1923), Vol. V (Washington, 1923), Vol. VIII (Washington, 1925), and Vol. XIII (Washington, 1927); William C. Menninger, *Psychiatry in a Troubled World* (New York, 1948); and Howard A. Rusk, "Convalescence and Rehabilitation," in Morris Fishbein (ed.), *Doctors at War* (New York, 1945). Various useful historical articles were found also in *The Air Surgeon's Bulletin,* the *Army Medical Bulletin,* the *Journal of Aviation Medicine,* and *The Military Surgeon.*

UNITED STATES ARMY IN WORLD WAR II

The following volumes have been published or are in press:

The War Department
Chief of Staff: Prewar Plans and Preparations
Washington Command Post: The Operations Division
Strategic Planning for Coalition Warfare: 1941-1942
Strategic Planning for Coalition Warfare: 1943-1944
Global Logistics and Strategy: 1940-1943
Global Logistics and Strategy: 1943-1945
The Army and Economic Mobilization
The Army and Industrial Manpower
The Army Ground Forces
The Organization of Ground Combat Troops
The Procurement and Training of Ground Combat Troops
The Army Service Forces
The Organization and Role of the Army Service Forces
The Western Hemisphere
The Framework of Hemisphere Defense
Guarding the United States and Its Outposts
The War in the Pacific
The Fall of the Philippines
Guadalcanal: The First Offensive
Victory in Papua
CARTWHEEL: The Reduction of Rabaul
Seizure of the Gilberts and Marshalls
Campaign in the Marianas
The Approach to the Philippines
Leyte: The Return to the Philippines
Triumph in the Philippines
Okinawa: The Last Battle
Strategy and Command: The First Two Years
The Mediterranean Theater of Operations
Northwest Africa: Seizing the Initiative in the West
Sicily and the Surrender of Italy
Salerno to Cassino
Cassino to the Alps
The European Theater of Operations
Cross-Channel Attack
Breakout and Pursuit
The Lorraine Campaign
The Siegfried Line Campaign
The Ardennes: Battle of the Bulge
The Last Offensive

The Supreme Command
Logistical Support of the Armies, Volume I
Logistical Support of the Armies, Volume II

The Middle East Theater
The Persian Corridor and Aid to Russia

The China-Burma-India Theater
Stilwell's Mission to China
Stilwell's Command Problems
Time Runs Out in CBI

The Technical Services
The Chemical Warfare Service: Organizing for War
The Chemical Warfare Service: From Laboratory to Field
The Chemical Warfare Service: Chemicals in Combat
The Corps of Engineers: Troops and Equipment
The Corps of Engineers: The War Against Japan
The Corps of Engineers: The War Against Germany
The Corps of Engineers: Military Construction in the United States
The Medical Department: Hospitalization and Evacuation; Zone of Interior
The Medical Department: Medical Service in the Mediterranean and Minor Theaters
The Ordnance Department: Planning Munitions for War
The Ordnance Department: Procurement and Supply
The Ordnance Department: On Beachhead and Battlefront
The Quartermaster Corps: Organization, Supply, and Services, Volume I
The Quartermaster Corps: Organization, Supply, and Services, Volume II
The Quartermaster Corps: Operations in the War Against Japan
The Quartermaster Corps: Operations in the War Against Germany
The Signal Corps: The Emergency
The Signal Corps: The Test
The Signal Corps: The Outcome
The Transportation Corps: Responsibilities, Organization, and Operations
The Transportation Corps: Movements, Training, and Supply
The Transportation Corps: Operations Overseas

Special Studies
Chronology: 1941–1945
Military Relations Between the United States and Canada: 1939–1945
Rearming the French
Three Battles: Arnaville, Altuzzo, and Schmidt
The Women's Army Corps
Civil Affairs: Soldiers Become Governors
Buying Aircraft: Materiel Procurement for the Army Air Forces
The Employment of Negro Troops
Manhattan: The U.S. Army and the Atomic Bomb

Pictorial Record
The War Against Germany and Italy: Mediterranean and Adjacent Areas
The War Against Germany: Europe and Adjacent Areas
The War Against Japan

Index

☆ U.S. GOVERNMENT PRINTING OFFICE: 1989 242-456/00014

Made in United States
Orlando, FL
04 November 2026

90201205R00291